SECOND EDITION

CONCISE TEXT OF

# NEUROSCIENCE

# Anterior Cerebral Territory in Axial

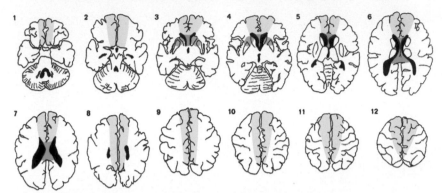

# Cortical Branches     # Cortical Functions

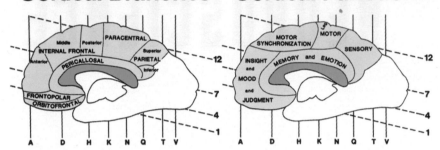

# Anterior Cerebral Territory in Coronal

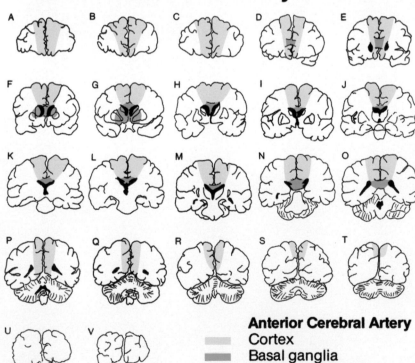

**Anterior Cerebral Artery**
Cortex
Basal ganglia
Corpus callosum

# Middle Cerebral Territory in Axial

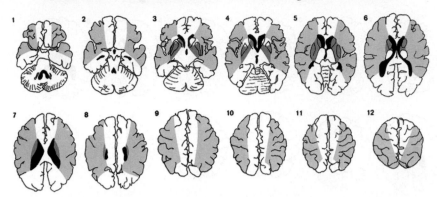

# Cortical Branches

PRECENTRAL
CENTRAL
Anterior
PARIETAL
Posterior
PREFRONTAL
ANGULAR
TEMPORAL
Occipital
ORBITOFRONTAL
Pole
Anterior
Middle
Posterior

12
7
4
1

A D H K N Q T V

# Cortical Functions

MOTOR
SYNCHRONIZATION
MOTOR
SENSORY
Face Arm Trunk Hip
Eyes
Symbolism
INSIGHT
and
MOOD
and
JUDGMENT
UNDERSTANDING
Writing
and
Names
Invol. eye
functions &
vis. compreh.
SPEAKING
HEARING
Speech
NAMING
ORIENTATION

12
7
4
1

A D H K N Q T V

insular cortex – autonomic function and taste

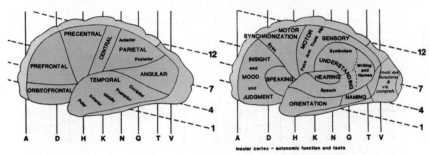

# Middle Cerebral Territory in Coronal

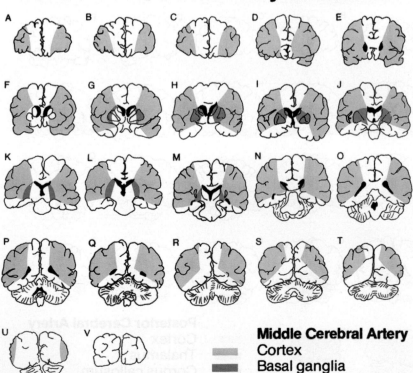

A  B  C  D  E

F  G  H  I  J

K  L  M  N  O

P  Q  R  S  T

U  V

**Middle Cerebral Artery**
Cortex
Basal ganglia

# Posterior Cerebral Territory in Axial

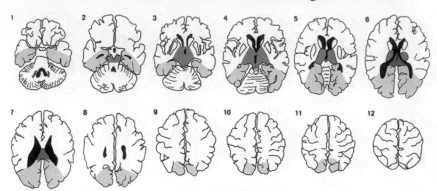

## Cortical Branches

## Cortical Functions

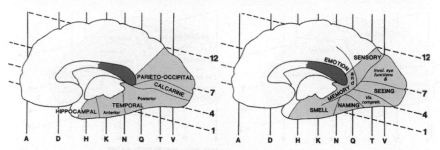

Cortical Branches labels: PARIETO-OCCIPITAL, CALCARINE, Posterior, TEMPORAL, Anterior, HIPPOCAMPAL

Cortical Functions labels: EMOTION and, SENSORY, Invol. eye functions &, MEMORY, SEEING, SMELL, NAMING, Vis. compreh.

# Posterior Cerebral Territory in Coronal

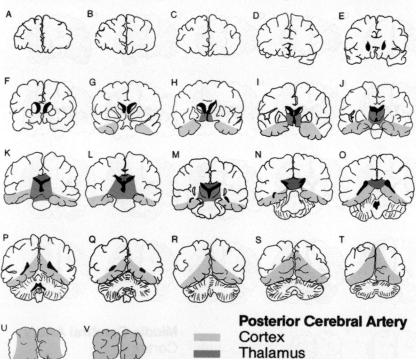

**Posterior Cerebral Artery**
Cortex
Thalamus
Corpus callosum

Preceding pages: Correlation of Cerebral Vascular Territories with Cerebral Function by CT[1,2] or MRI. Reprinted courtesy of Eastman Kodak Company.

## Cerebral Territories in Axial:

In each territory, numbered axial sections correspond to numbered broken lines in the figures directly below. Match *your* CT or MRI lesion to the appropriate territory. Note the number of axial planes in which a lesion is located. Find this numbered plane on the cortical schematic to identify the arterial branch supply and cortical function(s) of that area.

## Cortical Branches/Cortical Functions:

*Medial* surfaces of the brain are shown in anterior and posterior cerebral territories. Lateral surfaces are shown in the middle cerebral territory. Damage to the cortex, fiber tracts (not shown), or both causes loss of indicated function(s).

## Cerebral Territories in Coronal:

Lettered coronal sections correspond to lettered solid lines in the figures directly above. Match *your* CT lesion to the appropriate territory. Note the letter of the coronal plane in which a lesion is located. Find this plane on the cortical schematic to identify the arterial branch supply and cortical function(s) of that area.

L. Anne Hayman, MD
Department of Radiology
Baylor College of Medicine
Houston, Texas

Stephen A. Berman, MD
Department of Neurology
Baylor College of Medicine
Houston, Texas

Vincent C. Hinck, MD
Department of Radiology
Baylor College of Medicine
Houston, Texas

1. Berman SA, Hayman LA, Hinck VC. Correlation of CT cerebral vascular territories with function. I. Anterior cerebral artery. AJR 1980;135:253–257.
2. Hayman LA, Berman SA, Hinck VC. Correlation of CT cerebral vascular territories with function. II. Posterior cerebral artery. AJR 1981;137:13–19.

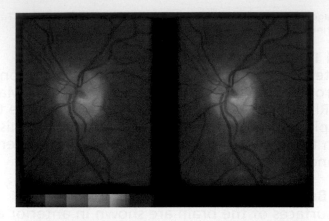

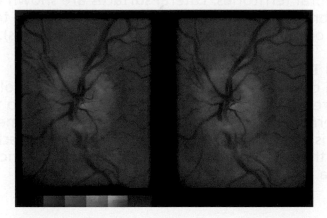

**Papilledema.** These photographs of the papilla demonstrate the progression of papilledema in a single individual. The first image is a normal papilla. Note that the blood vessels radiate outward from the center of the papilla. The blood vessels are full, but not swollen. The margin between the pale papilla and the deeply colored retina is sharp. When viewed in 3-D, the papilla is depressed, forming a pit. The remaining images show successive stages of papilledema caused by increasing intracranial pressure. Note how the margin of the papilla becomes wider and more blurred and the vessels become swollen as the intracranial pressure increases. When viewed in 3-D, the margin of the papilla protrudes further and further into the chamber of the eye with increasing pressure.

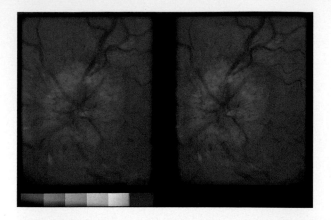

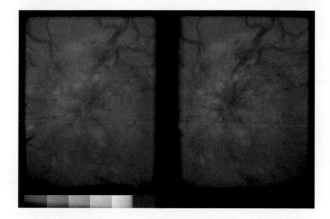

Each frame of this figure consists of a pair of stereoscopic images. These images can be viewed in 3-D with a commercial viewer (available from electron microscope supply companies) or, more simply, by learning how to create the 3-D image without a viewer. To see the figure in 3-D without a viewer, hold the figure at a comfortable distance with the bottom margins of the pair of images parallel to an imaginary axis running between your two eyes. Look through the figure as if you were focusing on a distant object. Three unfocused images will appear. Slowly attempt to focus on the middle image while ignoring the other two. This will not be easy at first, but gets easier with practice. Part of the trick is to allow your brain to bring the image into focus slowly and not to consciously focus on it. When the image comes into focus, it will be seen in three dimensions. (Micrographs courtesy of Dr. Martyn Wills.)

SECOND EDITION

CONCISE TEXT OF
# NEUROSCIENCE

SECOND EDITION

## CONCISE TEXT OF
# NEUROSCIENCE

## ROBERT E. KINGSLEY, PhD

South Bend Center for Medical Education
Indiana University School of Medicine

Illustrated by
Jacqueline Schaffer
Mollie Dunker
and
Caitlin Duckwall

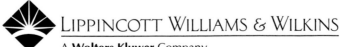
LIPPINCOTT WILLIAMS & WILKINS
A **Wolters Kluwer** Company
Philadelphia • Baltimore • New York • London
Buenos Aires • Hong Kong • Sydney • Tokyo

*Acquisitions Editor:* Paul J. Kelly
*Developmental Editor:* Kathleen H. Scogna
*Marketing Manager:* Christine Kushner
*Project Editor:* Karen M. Ruppert
Cover Illustration "Slice of Life" by Donna Krin Korkes

The publisher is not responsible (as a matter of product liability, negligence or otherwise) for any injury resulting from any material contained herein. This publication contains information relating to general principles of medical care which should not be construed as specific instructions for individual patients. Manufacturers' product information and package inserts should be reviewed for current information, including contraindications, dosages and precautions.

*Printed in the United States of America*

First Edition, 1996

**Library of Congress Cataloging-in-Publication Data**
Kingsley, Robert E.
    Concise text of neuroscience / Robert E. Kingsley; illustrated by
Jacqueline Schaffer, Mollie Dunker, and Caitlin Duckwall.—2nd ed.
        p.   cm.
    Includes bibliographical references and index.
    ISBN 0-683-30460-7
    1. Neurosciences.    I. Title.
    [DNLM: 1. Nervous System. 2. Neurosciences.   WL 100 K55c 1999]
    RC341.K56   1999
    612.8—dc21
    DNLM/DLC
    for Library of Congress                                              99-20294
                                                                              CIP

*The publishers have made every effort to trace the copyright holders for borrowed material. If they have inadvertently overlooked any, they will be pleased to make the necessary arrangements at the first opportunity.*

To purchase additional copies of this book, call our customer service department at **(800) 638-3030** or fax orders to **(301) 824-7390.** International customers should call **(301) 714-2324.**

00 01 02 03 04
1 2 3 4 5 6 7 8 9 10

Dedicated to
*W. vB. and R. D.*
whose deaths from neurological disease
have helped to inspire and motivate me,
*to my parents*
for all they have taught me,
*to my wife and children*
who make it all worthwhile,
*and to the underappreciated medical student*
in whom the future of medicine rests.

# Preface

The goals of *Concise Text of Neuroscience*, second edition, remain the same as those of the first: to provide a practical, concise, and integrated text of neuroscience with major emphasis on clinical neurology for first-year medical students. The basic pattern of the chapters remains unchanged. Anatomical descriptions and a discussion of the physiology are presented first, followed by a section on neurology.

## CHANGES TO THIS EDITION

Every chapter has been revised. My goal was to produce a clearer and more consistent style of presentation that would make the subject matter easily accessible to students. Many of the learning aids in the previous edition have been refined with students' needs in mind. More than 100 of the first edition's illustrations have been revised to improve clarity, and more than 40 new figures have been added. The cases are now presented in a consistent, more detailed format that closely follows standard practice for clinical presentation. The cases therefore serve to familiarize students with the proper format before they begin their clinical rotations. A new summary format makes it easier to review the chapter content. In response to suggestions from students and faculty, answers to the popular "Further Application" questions are included in a new appendix. Also in response to readers' suggestions, the etymologies of many new words have been added to the text, and the glossary has been greatly expanded. Finally, the type of references included at the end of chapters have been changed to emphasize recent review articles rather than chapters from encyclopedic texts.

## NEW FEATURES

Several new features have been added to this edition. Perhaps the most prominent one is the high-resolution multiplanar magnetic resonance imaging (MRI) atlas that replaces the mini-atlas in the first edition. While there are many fine brain atlases available, few MRI atlases are suitable for first-year medical students. I hope this atlas will help to fill that void. And in keeping with the emphasis on neurology, a new appendix briefly discusses the principal imaging methods used in neurological diagnosis.

## REORGANIZATION

In addition to these global changes, the second edition has undergone some minor reorganization. The most obvious change is the division of the chapter on the basal ganglion and cerebellum into two separate chapters. The chapters dealing with neurotransmitters, the basal ganglion, pain, and the cerebral cortex in particular have been extensively revised and updated with new, clinically useful material. In keeping with my general philosophy, however, I have avoided discussing the very latest research findings because I think this kind of information is more of a distraction than a help to the first-year medical student.

All of these changes have increased the size of the book. This expansion is modest, however, and does not constitute an increased learning burden for the student. Most of the added girth comes from the more detailed presentation of the cases and the addition of two new appendices, "Answers to Further Applications Questions" and "Neuroimaging Techniques." Some material has been deleted as partial compensation for these additions.

# Contributors

Steven R. Gable, M.D.

Virginia Hellenga, M.S.

T. R. Kingsley, Ph.D.

Victor F. Jones II, M.D.

Susan L. Stoddard, Ph.D.

# Acknowledgments

A work of this complexity cannot be completed by one person, and I am grateful for the help I have received from many people. I would like to thank Susan Stoddard, who not only literally lent her brain to this project but compiled and labeled all of the MRIs used in the atlas; Virginia Hellenga, who contributed her expertise in Greek and Latin to correct and extend the many etymologies in the text and to expand the glossary; and T. R. Kingsley, who wrote and revised the neuroembryology appendix. Special thanks are due to Steve Gable, Paula Russell, and Devin Zimmerman, who have taught me much neurology, brought many cases to my attention, and generously make their clinic, their patients, and their time available to me for the presentation of patients to my students. Without their generous support, this book would not be possible.

I owe special thanks also to Richard Coggeshall, David Colquhoun, Jaime Dant, Mary Donigan, Steve Flieslor, Lars Johnsson, Kent Morest, Pasko Rakic, Larry Squire, and Gary Wright, who generously searched for and lent me original micrographs and illustrations. I thank Vic Jones and John Harding, who provided me with numerous images of neuropathology and helped me to read and understand the films; Barb Brown and the staff at the Magnetic Resonance Imaging Center, who tracked down cases and reprinted film for me, often on very short notice; Gary Wright, Ed McKee, and Carl Marfurt, who read selected chapters and offered much valuable advice; Connie Gordon, who scanned images, composed figures, edited manuscripts, and nagged me appropriately; and Jeromy Townsley and Kathleen Drajus, who retrieved numerous articles from the Ruth Lilly Medical Library for me.

Finally, I extend my thanks to the staff at Lippincott Williams & Wilkins, who turned a plethora of computer files into a book—a remarkable achievement in my estimation. I especially thank Tim Satterfield and Paul Kelly for their strong support and encouragement and Kathleen Scogna, who edited every chapter and ruthlessly held my feet to the fire of succinctness, clarity, and consistency. To the extent that these three goals have been achieved, she deserves much of the credit. Despite all of this help, errors of commission and omission inevitably seem to find their way into a manuscript, and for these I apologize.

*R.E. Kingsley*
*South Bend, 1998*

# Contents

# 1

# The Gross Structure of the Nervous System

The mammalian nervous system is an information processing system that regulates all of the physiological functions of the organism. In addition, the nervous system performs unique functions that operate independently of the other organ systems of the body. These independent functions provide memory, consciousness, rationality, language, and the ability to project our mental self-image forward and backward in time. The nervous system performs these functions by manipulating information about the external and internal environments. This information consists of *representations of the external world* in which the organism exists. These representations take the form of electrical potentials and protein structures that are incorporated in the structure of the nervous system. The manner in which these representations of the world are *created, transformed, and manipulated* by the nervous system to affect the behavior of the organism is the subject matter of neuroscience.

This book introduces you to the small segment of neuroscience that is important to physicians. The principal topics addressed are the anatomy, physiology, and clinical neurology (nervous system disease) of the human nervous system. The general plan is first to describe the relevant anatomy of a functional system and to follow that with a discussion of its physiology. The neurology associated with that system is presented and in most chapters illustrated with case histories.

This chapter describes the surface features of the nervous system. The deep structures of the nuclei and tracts are discussed in succeeding chapters. This description is not meant to be complete; rather it provides an overview for purposes of orientation and familiarization. It is essential that every physician know the structures described in this chapter, because they form the basis for visualization of the brain and ability to communicate about the brain with others. The purpose of this chapter is to establish a foundation that will enable you to develop a workable association between names and visualized structures, an association that is indispensable to understanding.

## ORGANIZATION OF THE NERVOUS SYSTEM

The nervous system is composed of two types of cells, **neurons** [G. *neuron*, sinew, nerve, string] and **glia** [G. *gloia*, glue], and three layers of connective tissue that form the **meninges** [G. *meninx*, pl. *meninges*, membrane]. The meninges enclose the **central nervous system (CNS)** and separate it from the **peripheral nervous system (PNS)**. The CNS and its meningeal covering are surrounded by bone; the skull and the spinal column.

Neurons are cells with three morphologically distinct components: a **soma** [G. *soma*, body], an **axon**, and **dendrites**. The axon and dendrites are processes that extend from the soma, or cell body. Axons from many neurons may be collected into bundles known as **tracts** in the CNS or **nerves** in the PNS. An aggregation of neuron somas is called a **nucleus** in the CNS or a **ganglion** in the PNS. Glia is cells that are interspersed among the neurons. The details of the cellular components of the nervous system are discussed in Chapter 3.

The CNS consists of the **brain**, the **brainstem**, the **cerebellum** [L. *cerebellum*, brain], and the **spinal cord** (Fig. 1.1). The brain can be further divided into the **cerebral hemispheres**, the **basal ganglia** [G. *ganglion*, pl. *ganglia*, nerve bundle] (telencephalon), and the **thalamus** [G. *thalamus*, chamber] (diencephalon). The brainstem consists of the **midbrain** (mesencephalon), the **pons** [L. *pons*, bridge] (metencephalon without the cerebellum), and the **medulla** [L. *medius*, middle] (myelencephalon). The cerebellum and spinal cord are not grossly subdivided. A general description of these structures follows.

## THE EXTERNAL COVERINGS OF THE CNS

The tissue of the nervous system is soft and fragile. Although it can hold its shape outside the body and does not need skeletal support, it does require skeletal protection from external insults. Therefore, the brain and spinal cord are contained within the rigid framework of the skull and spinal column. While the spine is modified to allow some flexibility, on the whole the central nervous system is encased in a formidable suit of armor. If for any reason the cranial or spinal contents increase in volume—for example, because of the growth of a tumor—this protective covering becomes a liability. Since the skull cannot expand, the intracranial pressure rapidly increases, causing specific and important neurological signs (discussed later).

Within this bony covering, the central nervous system is further enclosed by the meninges, which consist of a series of three membranes (Fig. 1.2). The outermost membrane is the **dura mater** [L. *dura mater*, hard mother], a tough, resilient sheet of connective tissue that encloses the brain and spinal cord. It is perforated in many places to allow for the entrance of cranial nerves and blood vessels. At each of these perforations the dura adheres to the penetrating structure and forms a tight seal. The **pia mater** [L. *pia mater*, tender mother] is the innermost layer that closely adheres to the surface of the CNS. The **arachnoid** [G. *arachne*, spider] lies between them.

### The Cerebral Dura Mater

The cerebral dura mater consists of two layers, an inner **meningeal** and an outer **endosteal** layer. The endosteal layer adheres closely to the inner surface of the skull and serves as its inner periosteum (Fig. 1.3). It is attached tenaciously to the skull by small strands of fibrous connective tissue. The major meningeal arteries lie between the dura and the skull. Also, many small arteries pass from the dura mater into the bones of the skull. If the dura is violently separated from the skull, these arteries may tear and bleed. Forced by the high arterial pressure, the blood dissects a space between the dura and the skull, forming an **epidural hematoma**. This injury occurs most frequently after skull fractures. *If the fracture lacerates one of the meningeal arteries,* death can occur within minutes. The more common **subarachnoid hematoma** occurs when bleeding occurs between the brain and the dura. This injury may follow a severe blow to the head that displaces the brain within the cranium but does not fracture the skull. The displacement may *rupture one or more of the veins* lying on the surface of the brain, causing bleeding. Since bleeding is from veins, the blood is under low pressure. Consequently, the bleeding may last for days or even months and may lead to neurological symptoms so far removed from the initial injury that diagnosis is difficult.

The endosteal and meningeal layers are tightly attached to one another and form one continuous membrane throughout most of the dura. But at certain places the layers separate to form a cavity, or **sinus** (Fig. 1.3). The **superior sagittal sinus** [L. *sagitta*, arrow] is V-shaped. The walls of this sinus are formed from the meningeal layers, while its roof is composed of the endosteal layer. The inferior

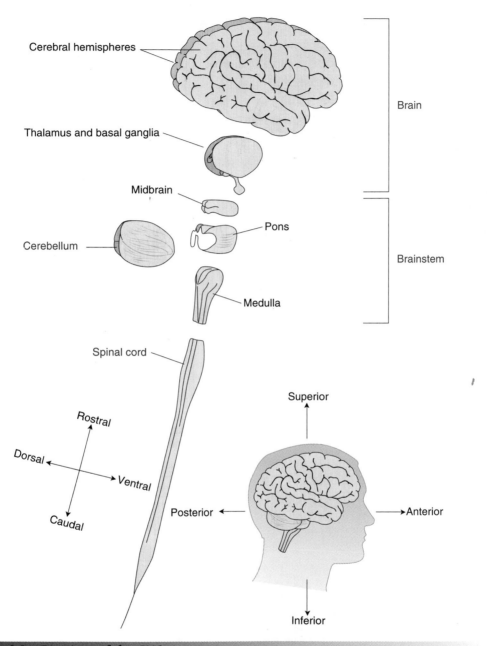

**Figure 1.1    Divisions of the CNS**

The relations of the various major divisions of the CNS are shown. The term *brain* as used here is the embryonic forebrain; the term *brainstem* is the embryonic midbrain and hindbrain. The terms *superior* and *inferior, anterior* and *posterior* are descriptive and are traditionally used to describe direction for the telencephalon, diencephalon, and cerebellum. The terms *dorsal* and *ventral, rostral* and *caudal* are commonly used for the remaining divisions. Rostral and caudal may be used for all parts of the central nervous system, rostral meaning toward the head and caudal, toward the tail. Many authors use posterior and anterior interchangeably with dorsal and ventral. The choice is mostly a matter of style.

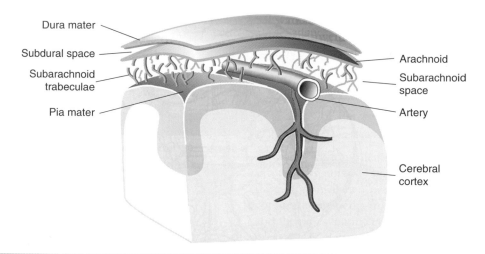

**Figure 1.2    Relations among the three meningeal layers**

The pia mater adheres closely to the brain surface and even follows the blood vessels deep into the tissue of the brain. The arachnoid and the dura mater, normally closely adherent to one another, are shown separated here for clarity.

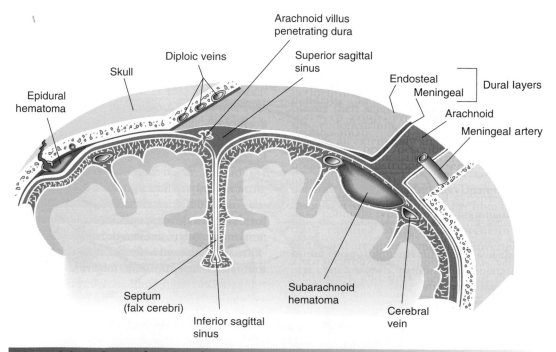

**Figure 1.3    Relations between the dura mater and the vasculature of the brain**

The meningeal and endosteal layers separate to form the sinuses. Two meningeal layers come together to form a septum, here the falx cerebri. Arachnoid villi are sites where CSF is returned to the vascular space. Hematomas can develop between the arachnoid and the pia mater (subarachnoid hematoma) or between the skull and the dura mater (epidural hematoma). Epidural hematomas rapidly expand because they are caused by arterial bleeding. Subarachnoid hematomas, caused by venous bleeding, expand slowly over days to months.

sagittal sinus is formed simply by a separation between the meningeal layers. These sinuses form part of the venous drainage system of the brain, which is described later.

At the inferior margin of a sinus, the two meningeal layers of the dura fuse to form a two-layer dural fold, or **septum**, that separates the cranium into major compartments (Figs 1.3 and 1.4). The most conspicuous of these septa is the **falx cerebri** [L. *falx*, sickle], which lies between the two cerebral hemispheres in the midsagittal plane. At the anterior margin it is attached to the ethmoid bone. It arches posteriorly until it meets another septum, the **tentorium cerebelli** [L. *tentorium*, tent], at the oc-

cipital pole of the skull. The inferior border of the falx remains unattached, leaving a space between it and the floor of the skull. The diencephalon and corpus callosum lie within this space.

The tentorium separates the cerebellum from the cerebral hemispheres. It is attached to the skull at the margin of the petrous bone and along the inferior part of the occipital bone. The medial, or central, edge of this septum is unattached; it joins the free edge of the falx. This free border of the tentorium circumscribes a space, the **tentorial incisure**, through which the brainstem passes. Together the falx and the tentorium separate the interior of the

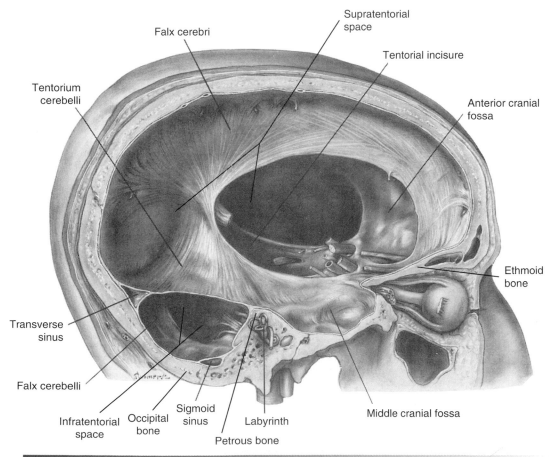

Falx cerebri

Supratentorial space

Tentorial incisure

Tentorium cerebelli

Anterior cranial fossa

Ethmoid bone

Transverse sinus

Falx cerebelli

Infratentorial space

Occipital bone

Sigmoid sinus

Labyrinth

Petrous bone

Middle cranial fossa

**Figure 1.4   The septa of the dura mater**

This sagittal view of the head with part of the skull and all of the brain removed shows the position and relations of the various septa. The tentorial incisure marks the border through which the brainstem must pass from the infratentorial space into the supratentorial space, which are separated by the tentorium cerebelli. (Reprinted with permission from Mettler FA. Neuroanatomy. 2nd ed. St. Louis: Mosby, 1948.)

cranium into three compartments. Inferior to the tentorium is the **infratentorial space**, which contains the cerebellum and brainstem. Superior to the tentorium is the **supratentorial space**, which contains the two cerebral hemispheres divided by the falx. The posterior cranial fossa is congruent with the infratentorial space, and the pairs of anterior and middle cranial fossae are contained within the supratentorial space.

## The Spinal Dura Mater

At the level of the spinal cord, the meningeal layer of the dura separates from the endosteal layer. The endosteal layer blends into the periosteum at the foramen magnum. Because the meningeal layer does not adhere to the vertebra, an **epidural space** is created between it and the bone (Fig. 1.5). The spinal dura, like the intracranial dura, envelops the nerve roots

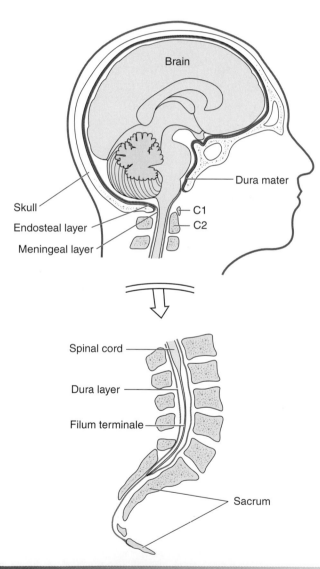

**Figure 1.5   The spinal dura**

At the transition between the intracranial dura and the spinal dura, the endosteal layer of the intracranial dura separates from the meningeal layer and fuses with the periosteum of the bone. The spinal dura is composed only of the meningeal dura layer and does not adhere to the vertebral bones.

as they leave the spinal cord, forming a tight seal at the intervertebral foramina. At the caudal end of the spinal cord, the spinal dura closely adheres to the **filum terminale**. Together they attach to the coccyx and merge with the periosteum (Fig. 1.5).

## The Pia Mater

The surface of the central nervous system is covered with a connective tissue membrane, the pia mater. In contrast to the dura and arachnoid, the pia closely follows all of the surface undulations of the nervous tissue (Fig. 1.2). In the spinal cord, special extensions of the pia form triangular connections between the lateral surface of the spinal cord and the adjacent dura. These **dentate ligaments** anchor the spinal cord to the dura.

## The Arachnoid

The inner surface of the dura is lined with the arachnoid. Because the arachnoid membrane does not adhere to the pia, there is a space between them. Traversing this space is a delicate lacework of connective tissue that resembles a spider's web, the **arachnoid trabecula** (Fig. 1.2). This space, the **subarachnoid space**, is filled with **cerebrospinal fluid (CSF)**. Although narrow over most of the cerebrum, this space is wider over the spinal cord. In some places the subarachnoid space is so large that these areas are called **cisterns** (Fig. 1.6). The cisterns are in communication with one another, allowing the free flow of cerebrospinal fluid over the entire external surface of the brain, brainstem, and spinal cord.

The **lumbar cistern** is noteworthy because it provides a convenient location for sampling CSF. It is easily reached by inserting a needle between the lumbar vertebrae. Because the only neural structures within this cistern are spinal nerves, a needle can be safely inserted without inflicting damage, since it will slide between the nerves. Once the needle is in place, CSF can be sampled and its pressure measured. Contrast material can be injected to replace the withdrawn CSF to make the outlines of the dural sac visible on plain x-ray, creating a **myelogram**. Although the noninvasive

magnetic resonance imaging (MRI) technique is frequently used instead, the myelogram is still useful in emergencies and for patients who cannot undergo MRI (Fig. 1.7).

## THE CEREBRAL HEMISPHERES

The telencephalon is the most prominent feature of the mammalian nervous system. The visible superficial portions of the telencephalon are the two cerebral hemispheres. The hemispheres are separated by the **longitudinal cerebral fissure** and joined by a massive collection of axons, the **corpus callosum** [L. *corpus*, body, and *callosus*, hard] (Figs. 1.8 and 1.9). The cerebral hemispheres are formed by growth of the superficial embryonic telencephalon. This growth is so extensive that the telencephalic surface, the **cerebral cortex** [L. *cortex*, bark], becomes wrinkled during development. This wrinkling greatly increases the cortical surface area within a minimum volume. A convex extension of the cortical surface is a **gyrus** [G. *gyros*, circle], and a concave fold is a **sulcus** [L. *sulcus*, furrow or ditch]. A particularly deep sulcus is commonly called a **fissure**.

*The pattern of gyri on the surface of the hemispheres is not random.* Within any mammalian species, the pattern of gyri and sulci is remarkably similar among individuals. They are useful landmarks that must be memorized. Using these patterns, the human cerebral hemisphere can be divided into five **lobes** (Figs. 1.9 and 1.10). The largest sulcus is the **lateral fissure**, which separates the **temporal lobe** from the remaining cortical mass. Joining the lateral fissure at nearly right angles, the **central sulcus** separates the **frontal lobe** from the **parietal lobe**. The parietal lobe is separated from the **occipital lobe** [L. *occiput*, back of the head] by the **parieto-occipital sulcus**, on the medial wall of the hemisphere. The **insular lobe** is not visible from the surface. It is buried beneath the lateral fissure and covered by the lips of the frontal, parietal, and temporal lobes. These lips, known as the **operculum** [L. *operculum*, cover or lid], arise during development as the expanding frontal, parietal, and temporal

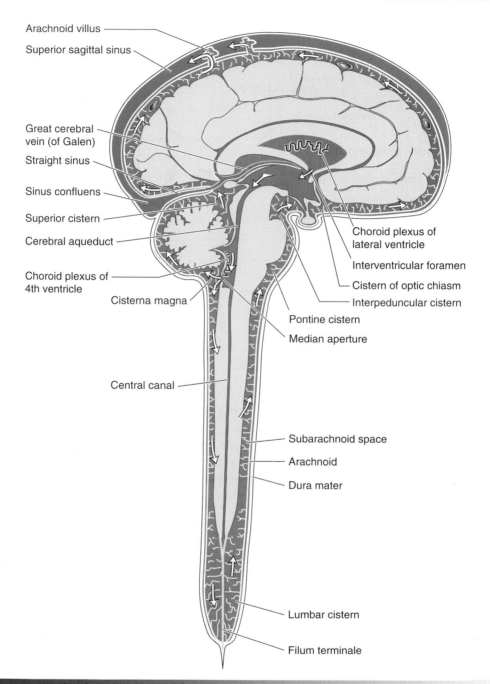

Arachnoid villus

Superior sagittal sinus

Great cerebral
vein (of Galen)

Straight sinus

Sinus confluens

Superior cistern

Cerebral aqueduct

Choroid plexus of
4th ventricle

Cisterna magna

Choroid plexus of
lateral ventricle

Interventricular foramen

Cistern of optic chiasm

Interpeduncular cistern

Pontine cistern

Median aperture

Central canal

Subarachnoid space

Arachnoid

Dura mater

Lumbar cistern

Filum terminale

**Figure 1.6   The distribution and flow of CSF**

This sagittal view of the CNS shows the location of the various cisterns. *Arrows* indicate the direction of CSF flow from points of secretion in the choroid plexus to its final reabsorption in the arachnoid villi. CSF passes from the ventricular compartments into the cisterns through the two lateral apertures and the medial aperture in the fourth ventricle. Within the ventricular compartment the two intraventricular foramen and the cerebral aqueduct are narrow passages that can be easily occluded, causing hydrocephalus.

lobes overrun the insula, much like lava flowing down a mountain. The meeting between the operculum from the temporal lobe and the operculum from the parietal and frontal lobes forms the lateral fissure.

## The Frontal Lobe

Largest of the five lobes, the frontal lobe is greatly expanded in the human relative to the other primates. On its superolateral surface (Figs. 1.8 and 1.11), the **precentral** gyrus spans the hemisphere from the lateral fissure to the longitudinal cerebral fissure that separates the two hemispheres in the sagittal plane. Anterior and perpendicular to the precentral gyrus are three parallel gyri, the **superior, middle**, and **inferior** frontal gyri. On the inferior surface (Fig. 1.11) at the most medial edge of the hemisphere lies the **gyrus rectus**, so named because it is unusually straight. The **olfactory tract** [L. *olfacto,* smell (something)] with its terminal **olfactory bulb**, lies adjacent to the gyrus rectus in a depression known as the **olfactory groove**. Directly over the orbit lie several small gyri known collectively as the **orbital gyri**.

## The Parietal Lobe

The anterior margin of the parietal lobe is denoted by the central sulcus, while the anterior portion of its inferior border is defined by the lateral fissure. Its most posterior regions are ill-defined on the lateral surface. The hemisphere must be viewed from the medial side (Fig. 1.9) to locate the definitive landmark that separates the parietal lobe from the occipital lobe, the parieto-occipital sulcus. This sulcus extends somewhat onto the superior surface of the hemisphere. The posterior boundary of the parietal lobe can be delineated on the lateral surface by projecting an imaginary extension of the parieto-occipital sulcus across the lateral aspect of the hemisphere (Fig. 1.10).

On the superolateral surface of the parietal lobe (Fig. 1.11), the **postcentral gyrus** lies parallel to the central sulcus. The **supramarginal gyrus** lies at the posterior termination of

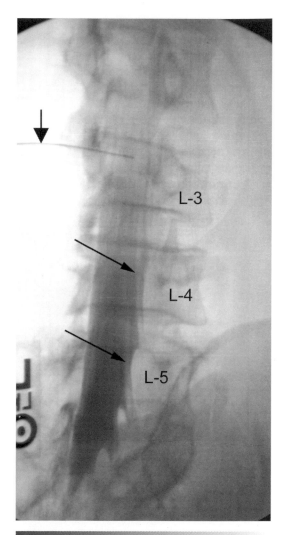

**Figure 1.7 Myelogram of the spinal cord**

Radiopaque contrast fluid was injected into the lumbar cistern to replace some of the CSF. The contrast fluid is dark in this image, allowing the spinal nerves of the cauda equina to appear light (*long arrows*). The injection needle is also visible (*fat arrow*). (Courtesy of St. Joseph Medical Center, South Bend, IN.)

the lateral sulcus. The **angular gyrus** lies posterior to the supramarginal gyrus at the termination of the sulcus that separates the superior and middle temporal gyri, the **superior temporal sulcus.**

The most prominent feature of the medial surface of the parietal and frontal lobes is the corpus callosum, a massive collection of **axons**

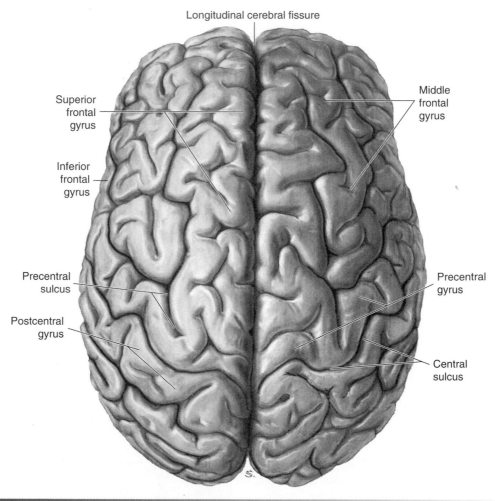

Longitudinal cerebral fissure

Superior
frontal
gyrus

Middle
frontal
gyrus

Inferior
frontal
gyrus

Precentral
sulcus

Precentral
gyrus

Postcentral
gyrus

Central
sulcus

**Figure 1.8   Superior surface of the cerebral hemispheres**

The cerebral hemispheres are separated by the longitudinal cerebral fissure. Note the location of the central sulcus, the precentral and postcentral gyri, and the three frontal gyri. (Reprinted with permission from Mettler FA. Neuroanatomy. 2nd ed. St. Louis: Mosby, 1948.)

[L. *axis,* axis; G. *axon,* axle] connecting the two hemispheres. This structure extends the entire length of the parietal lobe and well into the frontal lobe (Fig. 1.9). The posterior bulge is the **splenium** [G. *splenion,* bandage], and the bend at the anterior pole is the **genu** [L. *genu,* knee]. The **body** of the corpus callosum is between these two landmarks. Along its superior margin lies the **callosal sulcus** and superior to it, the **cingulate gyrus.** The cingulate gyrus is defined on its superior margin by the **cingulate sulcus** [L. *cingulum,* girdle, from *cingo,* surround].

### The Occipital Lobe

Lying posterior to the parieto-occipital sulcus is the occipital lobe, which is relatively small on its lateral aspect (Fig. 1.9). It is divided nearly in two on its medial surface by the **calcarine sulcus** [L. *calcar,* spur shaped]. This sulcus joins the parieto-occipital sulcus and then extends along the medial wall of the temporal lobe. A cross-section cut from fresh material perpendicular to the calcarine sulcus shows a white stripe that follows the sulcus and the gyrus on either side. This stripe is a unique feature, the **line of Gennari,** which confers on this part of the cerebral cortex its special name, the **striate cortex**.

## The Temporal Lobe

Inferior to the lateral sulcus and its imaginary extension and anterior to the parieto-occipital sulcus and its imaginary extension, is the temporal lobe (Fig. 1.10). Running approximately in the anterior posterior plane and parallel with the lateral fissure are three gyri, the **superior, middle,** and **inferior temporal gyri** (Fig. 1.11). The **superior temporal sulcus** separates the superior temporal gyrus from the middle temporal gyrus and extends into the parietal lobe, terminating at the angular gyrus.

The medial surface of the temporal lobe contains several important structures. Most prominent is the **uncus** [L. *uncus,* hook] (Figs. 1.9 and 1.12), a medial protrusion of the temporal lobe. Deep to it lies the **amygdaloid complex** [G. *amygdale,* almond], a group of several related nuclei. The **parahippocampal gyrus** is lateral to the uncus and is bounded on its lateral aspect by the **rhinal sulcus** anteriorly and the **collateral sulcus** posteriorly. The parahippocampal gyrus extends along the medial aspect of the temporal lobe, wraps around the splenium of the corpus callosum, and becomes continuous with the cingulate gyrus (Fig. 1.9). Deep to this gyrus lies the **hip-**

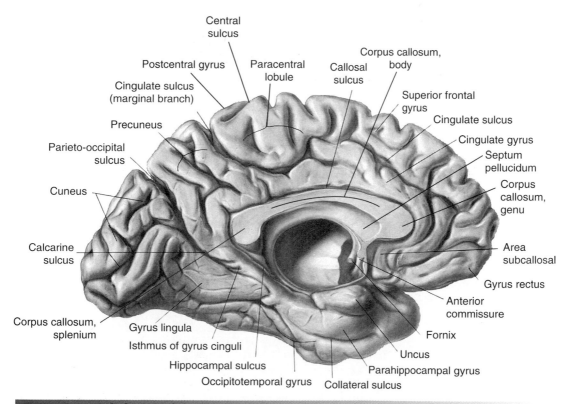

**Figure 1.9. Medial view of the left cerebral hemisphere**

The corpus callosum has been cut in the midsagittal plane. The postcentral gyrus can be reliably identified by following the cingulate sulcus to its marginal branch. Follow the marginal branch to the superior surface of the hemisphere; the postcentral gyrus lies immediately anterior to it. Moving anteriorly one finds the central sulcus. This method is especially useful when interpreting MRIs. The parieto-occipital sulcus is easily identified on the medial surface of the hemisphere. It meets the calcarine sulcus nearly at a right angle in most brains. (Reprinted with permission from Mettler FA. Neuroanatomy. 2nd ed. St. Louis: Mosby, 1948.)

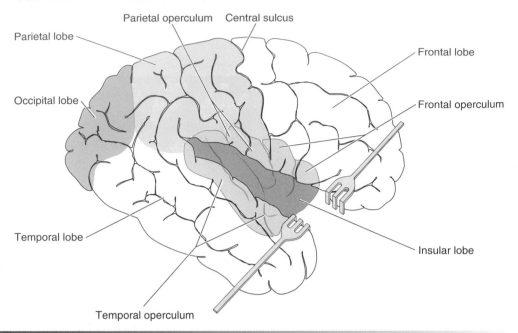

**Figure 1.10 Lateral view of the cerebral hemisphere**

The temporal lobe has been pulled away from the frontal and parietal lobes, revealing the insular lobe deep within the lateral fissure. The cerebral cortex that lies over the insular lobe is generically known as the operculum. Note the landmarks that indicate the remaining lobes. The boundaries of the occipital lobe are not obvious on the lateral view. The demarcation between the temporal lobe and the parietal lobe is not designated by any specific landmark.

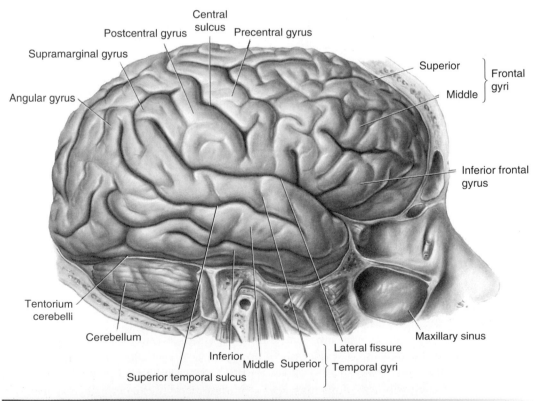

**Figure 1.11 The lateral surface of the cerebral hemisphere**

The superior temporal sulcus terminates in the parietal lobe with the angular gyrus wrapped around it. Similarly, the supramarginal gyrus lies at the posterior termination of the lateral fissure. (Reprinted with permission from Mettler FA. Neuroanatomy. 2nd ed. St. Louis: Mosby, 1948.)

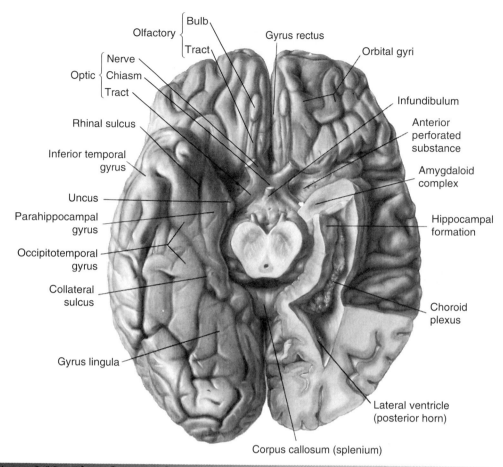

Bulb
Olfactory
Tract
Optic
Nerve
Chiasm
Tract
Gyrus rectus
Orbital gyri
Infundibulum
Rhinal sulcus
Inferior temporal gyrus
Anterior perforated substance
Uncus
Amygdaloid complex
Parahippocampal gyrus
Hippocampal formation
Occipitotemporal gyrus
Collateral sulcus
Choroid plexus
Gyrus lingula
Lateral ventricle (posterior horn)
Corpus callosum (splenium)

**Figure 1.12   The inferior surface of the brain**

The brainstem has been removed at the level of the cerebral peduncles. Note the uncus, which is a useful landmark. On the right side of the figure, part of the temporal and occipital lobes have been removed to reveal the amygdaloid nuclear complex, which lies deep to the uncus. The hippocampal formation lies posterior to the amygdala and within the parahippocampal gyrus. Note also the relationship between the optic nerve, chiasm, and tract. (Reprinted with permission from Mettler FA. Neuroanatomy. 2nd ed. St. Louis: Mosby, 1948.)

pocampal formation, an important structure of the temporal lobe that cannot be seen from the surface.

### The Insular Lobe

Widening the lateral fissure brings the insula into view. This small cortical area is completely covered by the operculum of the overlying frontal, parietal, and temporal lobes (Fig. 1.10). Little is known about the functions of the insula, and little is to be gained from learning the names of its gyri.

### Cortical Maps

About the turn of the century, a number of neuroanatomists proposed systems by which the cerebral cortex could be subdivided into anatomically distinguishable areas. Most of these systems were based on histologic distinctions. Brodmann's map (Fig. 1.13) delineates more than 50 regions. Although originally differentiated by their histologic features, many of the cortical areas have subsequently been found to correlate well with neurophysiological and neurological func-

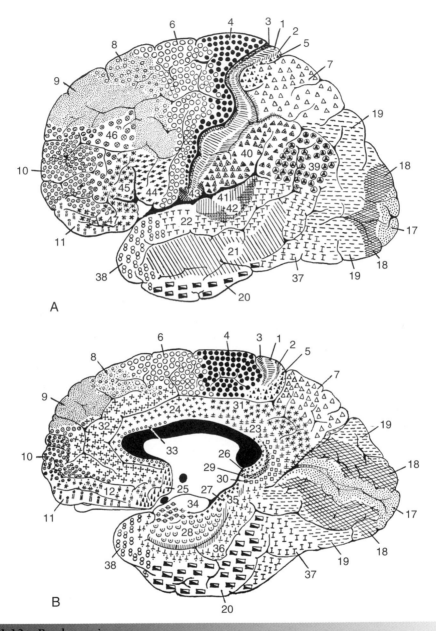

**Figure 1.13   Brodmann's map**

Brodmann divided the human cerebral cortex into more than 50 areas according to their histologic differences. Since some of these areas have distinct neurological functions associated with them, many people refer to them simply by their Brodmann number. Some of these functionally significant regions are pointed out in the text. (Modified from Brodmann K. Vergleichende Lokalisation lehre der Grosshirnrinde in ihren Prinzipien dargenstellt auf Grund des Zellenbaues. Leipzig: Barth, 1909.)

tion. Therefore, Brodmann's map retains a certain popularity, and many areas of the cerebral cortex are simply designated by their Brodmann number. In subsequent chapters the Brodmann number of cortical areas will be mentioned when the numbered area is associated with specific neurological functions. However, most Brodmann areas have no clear correlation with function, so memorizing the entire map is pointless.

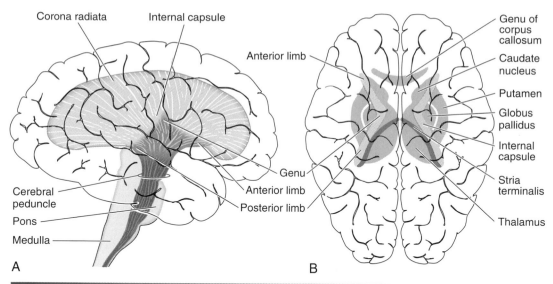

**Figure 1.14 The corona radiata and internal capsule**

**A.** The corona radiata is a narrow band of axons leaving the cerebral hemisphere. The structure resembles a crown; hence its name. These same axons form a more compact bundle; they are called the internal capsule at the level of the basal ganglia and thalamus. Fibers that continue caudally beyond the thalamus become the cerebral peduncles just before they enter the pons. **B.** Viewed from above with the superior half of the cerebral hemispheres removed, the internal capsule is V shaped. Three divisions, the anterior and posterior limbs and the intervening genu, are usually identified. The anterior limb separates the putamen and globus pallidus from the caudate, and the posterior limb separates them from the thalamus.

## THE BASAL GANGLIA AND THALAMUS

Two massive structures lie at the base of the cerebral hemispheres: the basal ganglia and the thalamus. The basal ganglia are a collection of closely associated nuclei that lie deep in the telencephalon and present no surface features. The thalamus is the diencephalon. Both the thalamus and the basal ganglia contain large numbers of cells organized into nuclei. Consequently, the details of these structures cannot be appreciated from gross specimens. This chapter only briefly describes their superficial features; details of their internal structure are discussed in Chapters 5 and 8.

### The Basal Ganglia

The basal ganglia and thalamus, when separated from the cerebral cortex, appear as a large bulbous structure. Dividing this body approximately in two is a massive fiber tract, the **internal capsule**, the principal tract connect-

ing the brain with more caudal structures. The internal capsule is broad and fan-shaped as it leaves the cerebral cortex (Fig. 1.14). In this superior position it resembles a crown of radiating fibers; hence this part of the internal capsule is known as the **corona radiata**, or radiating crown. As the internal capsule descends between the thalamus and basal ganglia, many fibers are given off to these structures and the internal capsule becomes smaller and develops a sharp bend, the **genu of the internal capsule**. The genu separates the **anterior** from the **posterior limb**. As the internal capsule descends further, it becomes even more compact and finally emerges at the rostral end of the midbrain as a round structure known as the **cerebral peduncle** [L. *pes*, foot]. The various divisions of the internal capsule are important landmarks.

The **globus pallidus** [L. *globus*, globe, and *pallidus*, pale] and the **putamen** [L. *puto*, prune], two principal nuclei of the basal ganglia, are nested between the limbs of the internal cap-

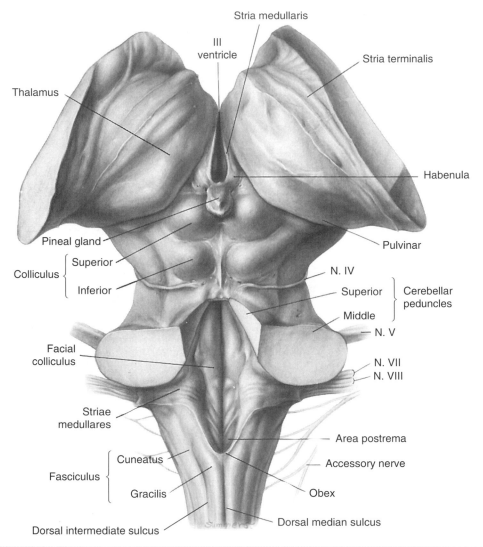

Stria medullaris
III ventricle
Stria terminalis
Thalamus
Habenula
Pineal gland
Pulvinar
Superior
Colliculus {
Inferior
N. IV
Superior } Cerebellar peduncles
Middle
N. V
Facial colliculus
N. VII
N. VIII
Striae medullares
Area postrema
Cuneatus
Accessory nerve
Fasciculus {
Gracilis
Obex
Dorsal median sulcus
Dorsal intermediate sulcus

**Figure 1.15  Dorsal view of the brainstem**

(Reprinted with permission from Mettler FA. Neuroanatomy. 2nd ed. St. Louis: Mosby, 1948.)

sule, on its lateral aspect. The anterior limb separates the head of the **caudate nucleus** [L. *cauda*, tail] from the globus pallidus and putamen (Fig. 1.14). The caudate nucleus, the putamen, and the globus pallidus are the major nuclei of the **basal ganglia**.

### The Thalamus

The **thalamus** is a paired structure that lies medial to the posterior limb of the internal capsule. Based on its embryologic development, it is divided into three regions, the dor-

sal thalamus (usually simply called the thalamus), the **hypothalamus**, and the **epithalamus**. It is a complex structure, and more than 50 nuclei have been described by various authors. The nuclei that are important to the practice of medicine are described in later chapters. The discussion here is limited to the external features that constitute orientation landmarks.

When viewed from the dorsal aspect (Figs. 1.14, 1.15, and 1.16), the principal body of the thalamus can be distinguished from the head of the caudate by a ridge that courses diago-

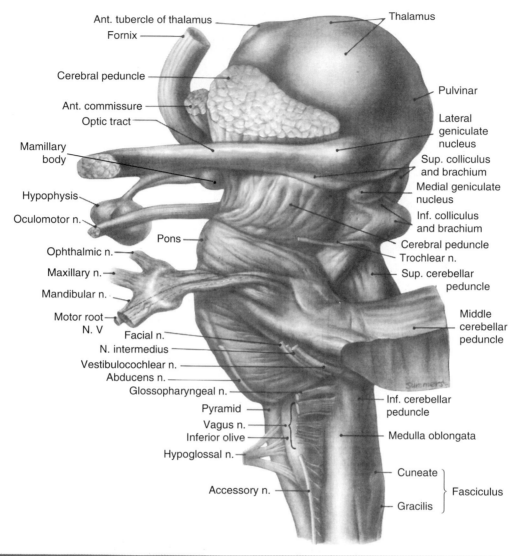

Ant. tubercle of thalamus
Fornix
Cerebral peduncle
Ant. commissure
Optic tract
Mamillary body
Hypophysis
Oculomotor n.
Pons
Ophthalmic n.
Maxillary n.
Mandibular n.
Motor root N. V
Facial n.
N. intermedius
Vestibulocochlear n.
Abducens n.
Glossopharyngeal n.
Pyramid
Vagus n.
Inferior olive
Hypoglossal n.
Accessory n.

Thalamus
Pulvinar
Lateral geniculate nucleus
Sup. colliculus and brachium
Medial geniculate nucleus
Inf. colliculus and brachium
Cerebral peduncle
Trochlear n.
Sup. cerebellar peduncle
Middle cerebellar peduncle
Inf. cerebellar peduncle
Medulla oblongata
Cuneate
Gracilis
Fasciculus

**Figure 1.16   Lateral view of the brainstem**

(Reprinted with permission from Mettler FA. Neuroanatomy. 2nd ed. St. Louis: Mosby, 1948.)

nally across it and medial to the internal capsule. This ridge is a fiber tract, the **stria terminalis** [L. *stria*, furrow, and *terminalis*, terminal]. Medial and ventral to the stria terminalis lies the thalamus; lateral and dorsal is the caudate. Most of the fibers in the stria terminalis originate in the amygdala and terminate in the hypothalamus, septal nuclei, and nucleus accumbens.

The principal structures of the epithalamus are the **habenula** [L. *habenula*, strap], the **stria medullaris**, and the **pineal gland** [L. *pineus*, like a pine cone]. The habenula is a nucleus at the posterior limit of the thalamus that forms a ridge on the lateral wall of the third ventricle. The stria medullaris thalami is a tract that courses along the medial wall of the thalamus, connecting the habenula with the **septal nuclei**, parts of the hypothalamus and the anterior nuclear group of the principal thalamus. Details of these nuclear structures are discussed in Chapter 14. In the midline and merging with the habenula on either side is the pineal gland (Fig. 1.17).

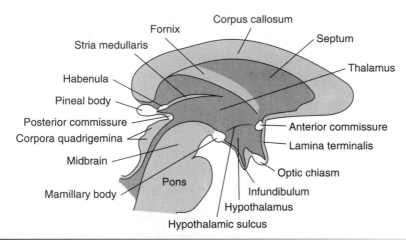

**Figure 1.17    Paraventricular structures of the brain**

This medial view of the brainstem is sectioned in the midsagittal plane, revealing the medial wall of the third ventricle.

Viewed from the lateral aspect of the thalamus, the **optic tract** (cranial nerve [CN] II) wraps around the side of the cerebral peduncle and terminates at the lateral geniculate nucleus (Fig. 1.16). From the ventral aspect (Fig. 1.12) the left and right optic tracts can be followed rostral to the point of their union in the **optic chiasm** [G. *chiasma*, two crossing lines (as in the Greek letter Χ)]. From the optic chiasm, the **optic nerves** extend to the eyes. It is customary in neuroanatomy to describe collections of axons in the central nervous system as tracts, fascicles, peduncles, or striae. In the peripheral nervous system collections of axons are called nerves. However, a confusing exception to this rule applies to the axons coursing between the eye and the brain. Centuries ago, anatomists agreed that the axons coursing between the eye and the optic chiasm would be called the optic nerve and the portion of these same axons that travels from the optic chiasm to the lateral geniculate body would be called the optic tract. In both cases, the axons are true creatures of the CNS. However, since lesions to the optic nerve produce strikingly different visual deficits from lesions to the optic tract, this unconventional nomenclature is extremely useful. Details of the visual pathways are discussed in Chapter 12.

The most inferior portion of the thalamus is the hypothalamus, a diencephalic derivative that is separated from the principal body of the thalamus by the **hypothalamic sulcus** (Fig. 1.17). Its small size belies its importance. The hypothalamus participates in the regulation of the endocrine system, thermoregulation, hemodynamics, and complex behavior. Some of these functions are discussed in Chapter 14. The **infundibulum** [L. *infundibulum*, funnel] is a protuberance that extends out of the ventral surface of the hypothalamus. It connects the hypothalamus with the **pituitary gland** [L. *pituita*, thick nasal secretion] or **hypophysis** [G. *hypo*, below, and *phyo*, grow; i.e., undergrowth] (Fig. 1.16), an endocrine organ of some significance. The paired structures known as the **mammillary bodies** mark the most posterior extent of the hypothalamus (Fig. 1.17). The optic chiasm marks its anterior border.

## THE BRAINSTEM

The embryonic mesencephalon (midbrain), metencephalon (pons without the cerebellum), and myelencephalon (medulla) together make up the brainstem, a long cylindrical structure at the base of the brain. A phylogenetically older part of the nervous system, the brainstem serves diverse functions. Many of these functions are primitive and independent of conscious control, such as vomiting, breathing, and the regulation of blood pressure, blood gas concentration, and body temperature. The brainstem is also the exit point for all of the cranial nerves except the olfactory, optic, and accessory nerves. Sensory information from the spinal cord and cranial nerves and motor commands from the cerebral cortex and cerebellum all pass through the brainstem. Much of this information is modified by brainstem structures. Therefore, this region has great clinical significance.

Only the ventral surface of the brainstem can be seen in the intact brain because the cerebral hemispheres and cerebellum lie over the dorsal surface. Therefore, when studying the external features of the brainstem, it is convenient to remove these structures, as has been done in Figures 1.15 and 1.16.

## The Midbrain

The **midbrain**, or **mesencephalon** [G. *mesos,* middle, and *enkephalos,* brain], is most easily appreciated from its dorsal aspect, where four bumps, the **corpora quadrigemini** [L. *corpus,* pl. *corpora,* body; *quadri,* four; and *geminus,* pl. *gemini,* twin], are readily identified. The rostral pair are known as the **superior colliculi** [L. *collis,* hill] and the caudal pair, the **inferior colliculi** (Fig. 1.15). Immediately caudal to the inferior colliculi and very close to the midline are the **trochlear nerves** [G. *trochilia,* pulley] (CN IV), leaving the brainstem on its dorsal surface and wrapping around the lateral aspect of the cerebral peduncles. From the ventral surface of the brainstem (Figs. 1.16 and 1.18), the most prominent features of the midbrain are the cerebral peduncles. There is a deep space, the **interpeduncular fossa**, between them. Emerging from the interpeduncular fossa are the **oculomotor nerves** (CN III). The mammillary bodies lie just rostral to CN III, forming the rostral border of the interpeduncular fossa.

## The Pons

The pons forms a bridge between the medulla and the midbrain. It is dominated by the hemispheres of the cerebellum, which are attached to the pons posteriorly and must be removed to view the dorsal surface of the pons. The cerebellum is described separately. The most conspicuous external feature of the pons other than the cerebellum is the great bulbous body that forms its ventral surface. Known as the **basis of the pons**, this structure is composed of a large body of gray matter, the **deep pontine nucleus**. Axons originating in the deep pontine nuclei form the rest of the basis of the pons. They collect as a great bundle that enters the cerebellum (Fig. 1.18). These fibers are known as the **middle cerebellar peduncle**.

Several pairs of cranial nerves can be identified from the ventral surface of the pons. The largest and most conspicuous is the **trigeminal nerve** (CN V). This nerve leaves the pons near the lateral edge close to but not at the rostral border. The remaining cranial nerves associated with the pons are at the **pontomedullary** junction, the ridge in the basis of the pons that marks its most caudal extent. The most medial pair of nerves is the **abducens nerve** [L. *abducens,* leading away] (CN VI). More lateral are the **facial** and **vestibulocochlear nerves** [L. *vestibulum,* entrance, vestibule, and *cochlea,* snail shell]. Of these two, the facial nerve, the more medial, leaves the brainstem from the ventral aspect, and the more lateral vestibulocochlear nerve leaves from the dorsolateral surface.

## The Medulla

The medulla is the most caudal division of the brainstem. A deep furrow in the midline, the **ventral medial fissure** runs parallel to the long axis of the medulla on its ventral surface. Another furrow, the **ventral lateral sulcus**, lies parallel to it. Between these two landmarks is a conspicuous protuberance, the **medullary pyramid**. Its protrusion from the base of the medulla is caused by a large fiber tract, the corticospinal tract. The ventral medial fissure extends rostrally to the basis of the pons, where it terminates. At approximately the junction between the medulla and the spinal cord it is less distinct, as its cavity is partly filled with fibers. These fibers are axons of the corticospinal tract that are crossing the midline. This crossing is called the **pyramidal decussation** [L. *decussatio,* in the form of an X]. Although it is more clearly seen in histologic

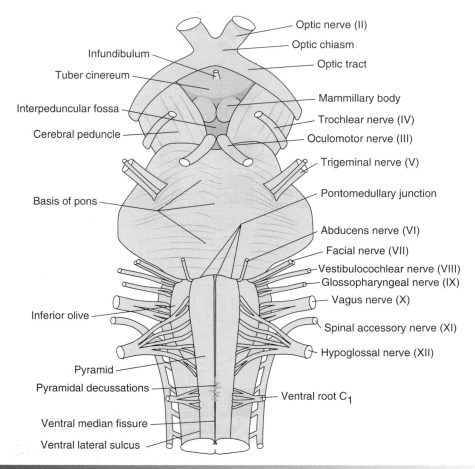

Optic nerve (II)
Optic chiasm
Optic tract
Infundibulum
Tuber cinereum
Interpeduncular fossa
Cerebral peduncle
Mammillary body
Trochlear nerve (IV)
Oculomotor nerve (III)
Trigeminal nerve (V)
Basis of pons
Pontomedullary junction
Abducens nerve (VI)
Facial nerve (VII)
Vestibulocochlear nerve (VIII)
Glossopharyngeal nerve (IX)
Vagus nerve (X)
Inferior olive
Spinal accessory nerve (XI)
Hypoglossal nerve (XII)
Pyramid
Pyramidal decussations
Ventral root C$_1$
Ventral median fissure
Ventral lateral sulcus

**Figure 1.18   Inferior view of the brainstem**

Note the location of the cranial nerves in relation to the major structures of the brainstem.

cross-sections, it is an important gross land-mark, marking the approximate transition be-tween the spinal cord and brainstem.

Lateral to the medullary pyramid is another bump on the side of the medulla, the **inferior olive** (Figs. 1.16 and 1.18). The **hypoglossal nerve** (CN XII) leaves the medulla between the medullary pyramid and the inferior olive. The **vagus** and the **glossopharyngeal nerves** (CN X and IX) leave the medulla at the dorsal margin of the inferior olive. Two pairs of ridges or tubercles can be seen on the dorsal aspect of the medulla. These tubercles run par-allel to the long axis of the medulla and are separated from each other by the **dorsal inter-mediate sulcus** (Fig. 1.15). Deep to these tu-bercles lie important sensory fiber tracts, the **fasciculus gracilis** [L. diminutive of *fascis,* bun-

dle, and *gracilis,* slender] (medial) and the **fasci-culus cuneatus** [L. *cuneatus,* wedge shaped] (lateral). The gracile tubercles are separated at the midline by the **dorsal medial sulcus.** At the rostral extension of the gracile tubercles the **area postrema** forms a slight ridge that looks like a **V** across the surface of the medulla. The midline origin of this eminence is the **obex** [L. *obex,* barrier].

### The Cerebellum

The cerebellum, which lies on the dorsal sur-face of the pons, is its most conspicuous fea-ture (Fig. 1.1). To remove the cerebellum from the main body of the pons, one must sever three pairs of fiber tracts, the **cerebellar pe-duncles** (Figs. 1.15 and 1.19). They are named according to their anatomical location; that is,

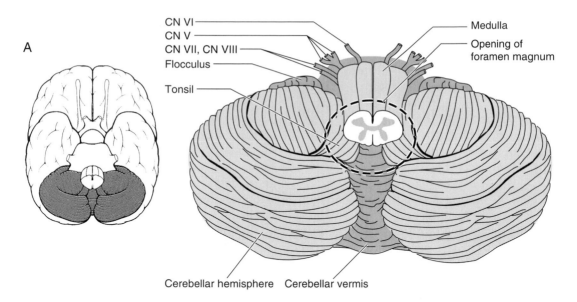

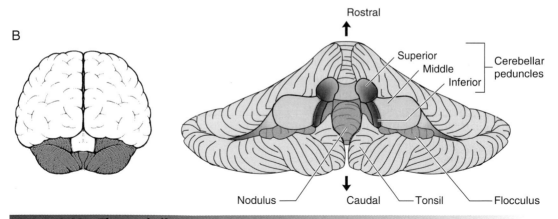

**Figure 1.19   The cerebellum**

**A.** An inferior view of the cerebellum, seen as if looking through the foramen magnum into the cranium. Note the portion of the tonsil, a structure that can herniate into the foramen magnum. Herniation can cause compression of the brainstem, which effectively separates it from the spinal cord. **B.** A view of the ventral surface of the cerebellum detached from the brainstem showing the relation of the cerebellar peduncles to the cerebellar hemispheres. Note the lateral position of the flocculus.

they are **superior, middle,** and **inferior.** The superior peduncles connect the cerebellum to the midbrain; the middle peduncles attach it to the pons; and the inferior peduncles communicate with the medulla and spinal cord. The cerebellar peduncles are best appreciated in histologic sections. All information entering and leaving the cerebellum must pass through these fiber tracts.

The body of the cerebellum is divided into two **hemispheres** and a midline structure, the **vermis** [L. *vermis,* worm] (Fig. 1.19). The surface is elaborated into a series of deep ridges or folds known as **folia** [L. *folium,* pl. *folia,* leaf] because of their resemblance to the leaves of the cedar tree. As with the cerebral cortex, the folia greatly increase the surface area of the organ without increasing its volume. The deepest folia are called fissures, and some authorities divide the cerebellum into lobules according to these fissures. The appropriateness of these divisions is the subject of lively debate among anatomists, physiologists, and physicians. Because the clinically relevant functional organization of the cerebellum does not follow the physical divisions based on the fissures, they are not discussed or elaborated here. Memorizing their names is unnecessary. The **tonsil**, however, is a lobule of the cerebellum that all physicians should know because it can be squeezed into the foramen magnum in conditions that cause the intracranial contents to shift. This situation is discussed later in the chapter.

More clinically interesting is the phylogenetically oldest part of the cerebellum, the **flocculonodular lobe** (Fig. 1.19). The **flocculus** [L. diminutive of *floccus,* tuft of wool] is a small lobe of the cerebellum immediately adjacent to the inferior cerebellar peduncle. The **nodulus** [L. diminutive of *nodus,* knot] is a midline structure between the pair of floccular lobes and is the most caudal segment of the vermis. During embryogenesis the separation of the flocculonodular lobe is the first division of the cerebellum, which attests to its ancient origin. This lobe is noteworthy because injury to it produces unique clinical symptoms (discussed in Chapter 9).

## THE SPINAL CORD

The most characteristic physical feature of the adult spinal cord is that it retains the segmental organization with which it was endowed during embryonic development. Therefore, the spinal cord is composed of 31 segments that, although not identical, are essentially similar in structure (Fig. 1.20).

At the spinal cord, the **dorsal medial sulcus** and the **ventral medial fissure** are continuous with these structures in the medulla. Lateral to the dorsal medial sulcus is the **dorsal root entry zone**, a continuous line along the spinal cord into which small fascicles or bundles of axons enter the spinal cord (Fig.

1.21). A number of these fascicles together form a **dorsal root**. The cells that give rise to the dorsal root axons are **pseudounipolar sensory** neurons (see Chapter 3). With only one exception,[1] the cell bodies of sensory pseudounipolar neurons lie in dense collections of cells called peripheral ganglia. Such a ganglion, a **dorsal root ganglion**, is associated with each dorsal root. In a similar fashion, the **ventral root exit zone** lies lateral to the ventral medial fissure, and the fascicles that originate from it collect to form the **ventral root**. The cells from which the axons of the ventral root originate are **multipolar motor neurons** (see Chapter 3). These cell bodies lie within the spinal cord; no ganglions are associated with the ventral roots.

The ventral root and the dorsal root of each spinal cord segment anastomose to form a single **spinal nerve**. Each pair of spinal nerves leaves the protection of the spinal column through an **intervertebral foramen** [L. *foramen,* opening] (Fig. 1.22). Since each pair of spinal nerves is associated with a vertebra, it is convenient to name spinal nerves according to their associated vertebra (Fig. 1.23). The one exception is in the cervical region, which contains an extra pair of nerves relative to the number of vertebral segments. The first pair of nerves are anomalous, having only ventral roots. Therefore, by convention the first 8 pairs of spinal nerves are called **cervical**; the next 12, **thoracic**; the next 10 are divided equally between **lumbar** and **sacral**; and the last pair are **coccygeal**. Consequently, the first 7 pairs of spinal nerves in the cervical region exit rostral to the vertebrae for which they are named. All other spinal nerves exit caudal to the vertebrae for which they are named.

At the cervical and lumbar enlargements, spinal nerves **anastomose** [G. *anastomosis,* outlet] with adjacent spinal nerves, forming cords that divide and reanastomose. This complicated formation is called a **plexus** [L. *plexus,* pl. *plexus,* braid]. There are two principal plexus, the brachial and the lumbosacral. The **peripheral nerves** emerge after the last

[1]The mesencephalic root of CN V (see Chapter 11).

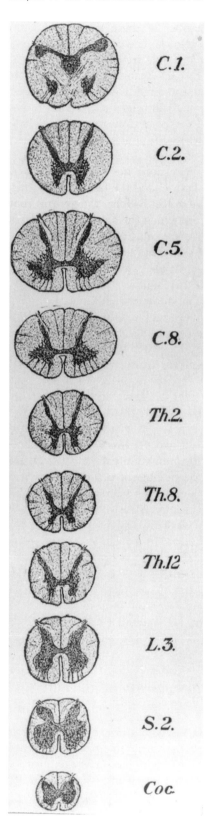

C.1.

C.2.

C.5.

C.8.

Th.2.

Th.8.

Th.12

L.3.

S.2.

Coc.

**Figure 1.20    Cross-sections of the spinal cord**

Note the relative size of the spinal cord at various levels and the differences in the shape of the gray matter. Levels are as indicated: *C,* cervical; *Th,* thoracic; *L,* lumbar; *S,* sacral; *Coc,* coccyx. (Reprinted with permission from Lewis. Gray's Anatomy. Philadelphia: Lea & Febiger, 1924.)

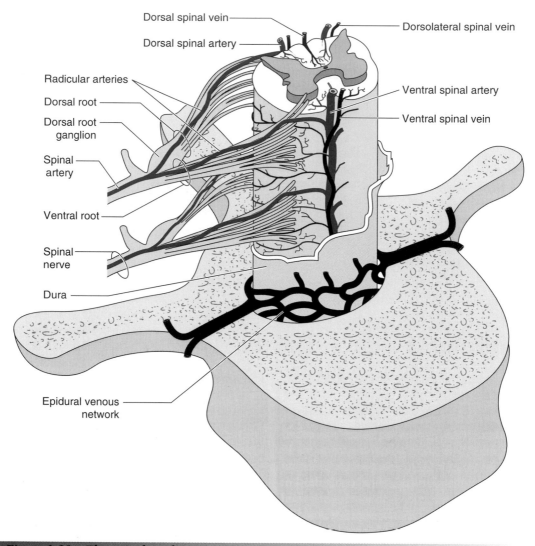

Dorsal spinal vein
Dorsal spinal artery
Dorsolateral spinal vein
Radicular arteries
Dorsal root
Dorsal root ganglion
Ventral spinal artery
Ventral spinal vein
Spinal artery
Ventral root
Spinal nerve
Dura
Epidural venous network

## Figure 1.21   The spinal cord

An oblique view of the spinal cord with the dura removed. The dorsal and ventral roots enter the cord as a continuous series of rootlets. The radicular arteries supply each segment of the spinal cord, but not all segments are equally robust. The dorsal spinal arteries and the ventral spinal artery provide intersegmental anastomoses between the radicular arteries. Venous drainage follows the arteries. A large epidural venous network lies on the ventral surface of the spinal cord.

anastomosis (Fig. 1.24). Axons from several adjacent spinal nerves may be found in a single peripheral nerve; conversely, axons from a single spinal nerve may segregate and be found in several peripheral nerves. This re-arrangement of axons has significant neuro-logical implications that are discussed in Chapter 5.

*The dorsal root is a pure sensory nerve, and the ventral root is a pure motor nerve.*[2] When the dorsal and ventral roots merge to form the spinal nerve, this nerve and all of its deriva-

[2]Ventral root afferent fibers have been described, but their clinical significance has yet to be established.

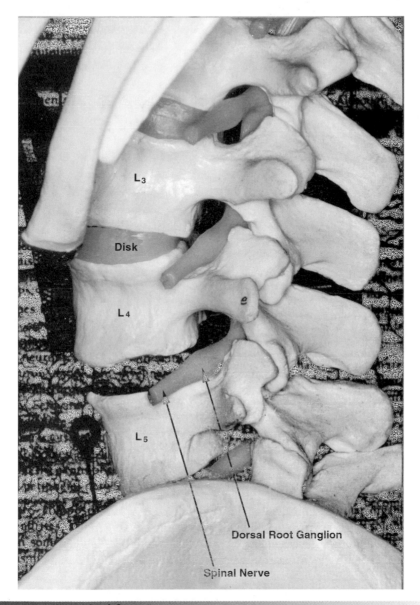

**Figure 1.22    Intervertebral foramina**

This lateral view of a skeletal model shows intervertebral discs and spinal nerves. The spinal nerves leave the protection of the vertebrae by passing through the intervertebral foramen. These foramina can become sites of nerve entrapment.

tives contain both afferent (sensory) and efferent (motor) axons. Thus, any trauma that affects a spinal nerve, the brachial and lumbar plexus, or a peripheral nerve produces complementary sensory and motor findings. Conversely, pure lesions to the dorsal or ventral roots produce pure sensory or motor findings,

respectively. This is a very important diagnostic principle.

The spinal cord itself is shorter than the vertebral column that protects it because the embryological extension of the spinal cord stops sooner than does the extension of the vertebral column. As the vertebral column

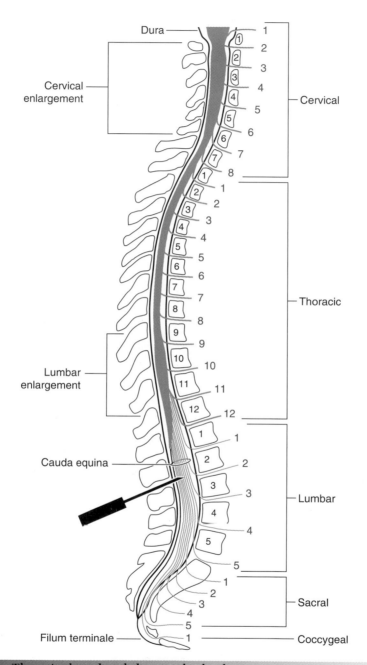

## Figure 1.23   The spinal cord and the vertebral column

The spinal roots and the spinal cord segment from which they emanate are named for the vertebrae. Cervical roots 1 to 7 exit above the vertebrae for which they are named, while the remaining roots exit below. In the region of the cervical enlargement, the spinal cord completely fills the vertebral foramen. The cauda equina, which lies below approximately L2, consists of the elongated spinal roots from the lumbosacral spinal cord. A needle can be safely inserted into the lumbar cistern at L2, as shown. The needle slips harmlessly between the spinal roots, and there is no danger of penetrating the spinal cord.

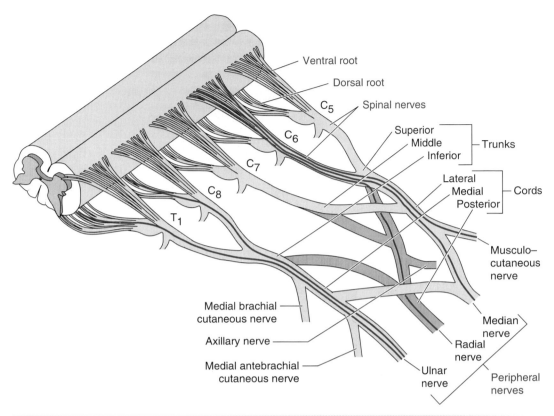

Ventral root
Dorsal root
C₅
Spinal nerves
C₆
Superior
Middle — Trunks
Inferior
C₇
Lateral
Medial — Cords
C₈
Posterior
T₁
Musculo–
cutaneous
nerve
Medial brachial
cutaneous nerve
Median
nerve
Axillary nerve
Radial
nerve
Medial antebrachial
cutaneous nerve
Ulnar
nerve
Peripheral
nerves

**Figure 1.24   The spinal roots, spinal nerves, and peripheral nerves**

Spinal roots are either sensory (dorsal roots) or motor (ventral roots). Spinal nerves are mixed, serving both motor and sensory functions. The axons from individual spinal nerves separate and reanastomose with axons from other spinal nerves as they pass through the plexus of the brachial and lumbosacral regions. Therefore, peripheral nerves can be motor, sensory, or mixed. As illustrated here, spinal segment C6 supplies axons to the median and radial nerves. Segments C8 and T1 both supply axons to the ulnar nerve. Examples of mixed innervation are not shown for simplicity.

continues to develop, it carries the spinal nerves with it, greatly elongating the lumbar and sacral roots within the central vertebral foramen (Fig. 1.23). Because this extension of the lumbar and sacral spinal nerves resembles a horse's tail, it is frequently called the **cauda equina.** In the adult the spinal cord extends only to about the level of the L2 vertebra. The **filum terminalis** [L. *filum,* thread, and *terminus,* end], a fine strand of connective tissue, extends from the last segment of the spinal cord to the coccyx, where it fuses with the periosteum.

The spinal cord is also characterized by two swellings or enlargements. The **cervical** and **lumbar enlargements** correspond to areas of the spinal cord that innervate the extremities (Figs. 1.20 and 1.23). Not surprisingly, more internal neuronal support is required to manage the sensorimotor requirements of the extremities than is required for the trunk. This increased requirement is reflected in the increased size of the spinal cord in these areas. Also, the rostral portion of the spinal cord is larger than the caudal region because all of the axons serving the entire spinal cord must pass through the cervical regions, whereas only those that serve the lumbosacral regions are present at more caudal levels. For these reasons the spinal cord is very closely confined within the central foramen of the cervical vertebrae.

## THE PERIPHERAL NERVOUS SYSTEM

The functional boundary between the central and the peripheral nervous system lies at the junction where oligodendrocytes meet Schwann cells along the axons that form the cranial and spinal nerves. The PNS is composed of three parts: (*a*) somatosensory or **afferent** neurons, (*b*) motor or **efferent** neurons, and (*c*) **autonomic** neurons. Autonomic neurons are discussed in Chapter 13. The PNS is distinguished from the CNS by other less precise but more easily visualized criteria. For example, unlike the CNS, the PNS is not surrounded by bone and is therefore quite susceptible to injury. Also, the CNS is contained within the meninges, while most of the PNS is not. The distinction between the two systems based on the differences in the cells that envelop the axons, however, is the only clinically useful criterion.

In a peripheral nerve, individual axons are enveloped in a loose connective tissue, the **endoneurium** (Fig. 1.25). Small groups of axons are closely associated within a bundle called a **nerve fascicle**. The fascicle is defined by a sheath of connective tissue, the **perineurium**, which imparts mechanical strength to the peripheral nerve. In surgical procedures it can hold sutures without tearing. In addition to its mechanical strength, the perineurium is a diffusion barrier, isolating the endoneural space around the axons from the surrounding tissue. This barrier helps to preserve the ionic milieu of the axon. Several fascicles together form **fascicular bundles** within an extensive multilaminated perineurium. The fascicular bundles in turn collectively form the peripheral nerve that is embedded in loose connective tissue called the **epineurium.**

The fascicular bundles are not continuous throughout the peripheral nerve. They divide and anastomose with one another as frequently as every few millimeters (Fig. 1.26). However, the axons within a small set of adjacent bundles redistribute themselves within the same set of bundles so that the axons re-

main in approximately the same quadrant of the nerve for several centimeters. This arrangement is a practical concern to the surgeon who must stitch a severed nerve. If the cut is clean, it may be possible to suture individual fascicular bundles together. If they are anastomosed in this way, there is a high probability that the distal segment of nerves synapsing with muscles will be sutured to the central stump of motor axons and the same for sensory axons. In such cases good functional recovery is possible. If a short segment of the nerve is missing, the fascicles in the various quadrants of the two stumps may no longer correspond with one another. In this case good functional recovery depends on whether the surgeon can maintain the original axial orientation, since the axons maintain themselves within the same nerve quadrant over long distances. If the nerve is badly mangled, however, good axial alignment may not be possible, and functional recovery is greatly compromised.

## THE NEUROVASCULATURE

It is essential that the physician have a good understanding of the vasculature of the nervous system, because many neurological difficulties are caused by problems with the blood supply. A good knowledge of the brain's vasculature will help you to evaluate various differential diagnoses and find lesions. Furthermore, many neurovascular problems are treatable. Appropriate diagnostic evaluation is essential for optimal treatment in such cases.

### The Carotid Circulation

The brain is supplied by only two pairs of arteries, the **carotid arteries** and the **vertebral arteries**. The internal carotid artery enters the base of the skull and divides into the **middle cerebral artery** and the **anterior cerebral artery** (Fig. 1.27). The middle cerebral artery ascends to the lateral surface of the hemisphere through the lateral sulcus. From the lateral sulcus, branches of the middle cerebral artery spread across the lateral aspect of the frontal, parietal, and temporal lobes (Fig. 1.28A). These branches do not extend to the

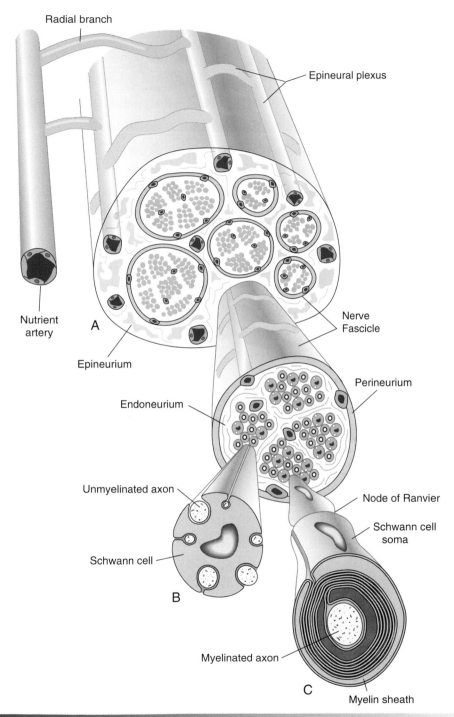

**Figure 1.25    Structure of the peripheral nerves**

**A.** Peripheral nerves are divided into fascicles by the perineurium, a tough connective tissue that isolates the fascicle both physically and chemically. Nutrient blood vessels supply peripheral nerves via a large number of radial branches along its length. These radial branches supply an extensively collateralized network of vessels within the nerve that further collateralize and penetrate the individual fascicles. **B.** Several unmyelinated axons within a fascicle are enveloped in a Schwann cell. **C.** One Schwann cell forms the myelin for a single myelinated axon. Myelin structure is discussed in Chapter 2.

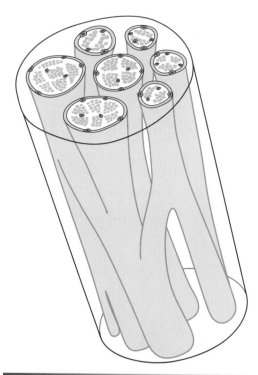

### Figure 1.26 Relation of nerve fascicles within a nerve

Individual fascicles divide and reanastomose along the length of a peripheral nerve. Over a short distance, the fascicles remain in approximately the same quadrant of the nerve. Over larger distances, considerable reorganization usually occurs.

margins of these lobes, and a definite watershed describes an arc around the lateral surface of the hemisphere (Fig. 1.28*C*). It is important to know the watershed boundary because the cerebral cortex served by these arteries has different functions, and by carefully identifying the functional loss one can determine which artery is compromised.

The anterior cerebral artery follows a course on the medial surface of the hemisphere, arcing around the corpus callosum (Fig. 1.28*B*). Branches of the anterior cerebral artery ascend the medial surface of the hemisphere. They extend over the medial ridge onto the most superior aspect of the lateral surface of the frontal and parietal lobes and then descend to meet but not anastomose with the ascending branches of the middle cerebral

artery that arise from below. The lack of anastomoses means that the brain, like the heart, is likely to suffer ischemic damage from thromboses and emboli because there is no well-developed collateral circulation.

### The Vertebrobasilar Circulation

The two **vertebral arteries** enter the skull separately through the foramen magnum and course along the ventral lateral aspect of the medulla (Fig. 1.27). They merge at approximately the pontomedullary junction, forming the **basilar artery.** The basilar artery follows the midline of the pons to its rostral border, where it divides into the two **posterior cerebral arteries.** These arteries send branches to the inferior surface of the temporal lobe and to the occipital lobe.

The basilar artery gives rise to many important branches. The **paramedian** and **circumferential** branches perfuse the basis of the pons (Fig. 1.29). Another branch, the **labyrinthine artery**, supplies the inner ear. In addition, the **superior cerebellar artery** and the **anterior inferior cerebellar artery (AICA)** are branches of the basilar artery that supply most of the superior region of the cerebellum. In most persons the **posterior inferior cerebellar artery (PICA)** is derived from the vertebral artery. It perfuses the rest of the cerebellum and the lateral aspect of the caudal medulla (Fig. 1.27). The superior cerebellar artery and the AICA also supply portions of the pons.

The thalamus and basal ganglia are supplied by branches of several major cranial arteries (Fig. 1.30). The thalamus is supplied principally by **thalamic** branches of the posterior cerebral artery. The adjacent caudate nucleus and globus pallidus are supplied by the **striate branches** [L. *striatus,* striped] from the middle cerebral artery, the **lateral striate arteries.** The head of the caudate is supplied by the **medial striate artery**, a branch of the anterior cerebral artery. The choroid plexus of the third ventricle is supplied by the **posterior choroidal artery** [G. *chorioeides,* skinlike], derived from the posterior cerebral artery, and by the **anterior choroidal artery**, derived from the middle cerebral artery. These branches are

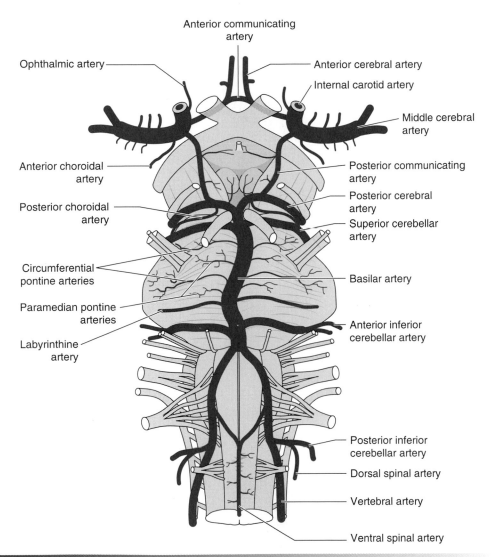

Anterior communicating
artery

Ophthalmic artery

Anterior cerebral artery

Internal carotid artery

Middle cerebral
artery

Anterior choroidal
artery

Posterior communicating
artery

Posterior choroidal
artery

Posterior cerebral
artery

Superior cerebellar
artery

Circumferential
pontine arteries

Basilar artery

Paramedian pontine
arteries

Anterior inferior
cerebellar artery

Labyrinthine
artery

Posterior inferior
cerebellar artery

Dorsal spinal artery

Vertebral artery

Ventral spinal artery

**Figure 1.27    Principal arteries supplying the brainstem**

The carotid arteries supply the anterior and middle cerebral arteries and via the posterior communicating arteries, the basilar artery. The blood supply to the brainstem and cerebellum is derived from the vertebral arteries and the basilar artery. These arteries give rise to a number of penetrating branches, the most important of which are illustrated here.

small relative to the main vessel, which they leave at right angles. They commonly rupture at the junction, producing an intracerebral hemorrhage.

The vertebral arteries also supply the rostral spinal cord. The vertebral arteries give rise to caudally directed branches that fuse with one another at the midline to form the **ventral spinal artery** (Fig. 1.27). Since this fusion

takes place near the level of the inferior olive, the ventral spinal artery courses nearly the full length of the medulla and the entire length of the spinal cord. The most medial structures of the medulla are supplied by the ventral spinal artery, while the more lateral paramedian structures are supplied by branches of the vertebral arteries. The posterior inferior cerebellar artery and the dorsal spinal artery supply

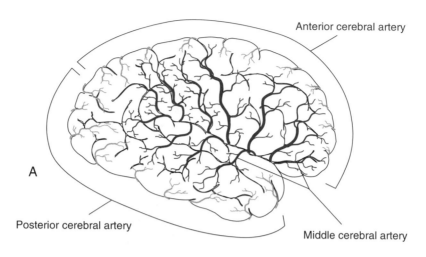

Anterior cerebral artery

A

Posterior cerebral artery

Middle cerebral artery

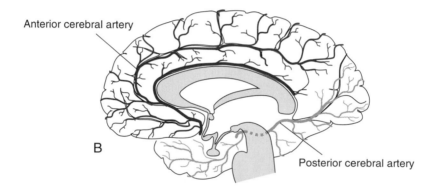

Anterior cerebral artery

B

Posterior cerebral artery

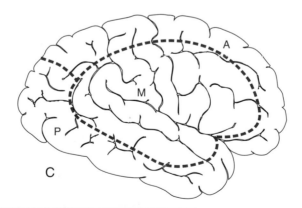

C

## Figure 1.28   Terminal distribution of the cerebral arteries

**A.** The principal blood supply to the lateral portion of the cerebral hemisphere is derived from the middle cerebral artery. The superior, posterior, and inferior boundaries are supplied by the anterior and posterior cerebral arteries. These systems do not anastomose, and there is a definite watershed at their margins (**C**). **B.** The medial portion of the cerebral hemisphere is supplied by the anterior and posterior cerebral arteries; their distributions are illustrated here. The posterior cerebral artery supplies the medial and inferior surface of the temporal lobe. **C.** The watershed boundaries are superimposed on a lateral view of the hemisphere. Distribution of arteries: *A,* anterior cerebral; *P,* posterior cerebral; *M,* middle cerebral.

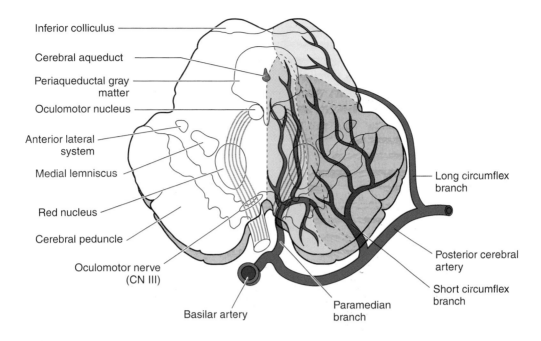

Inferior colliculus

Cerebral aqueduct

Periaqueductal gray matter

Oculomotor nucleus

Anterior lateral system

Medial lemniscus

Red nucleus

Cerebral peduncle

Oculomotor nerve (CN III)

Basilar artery

Paramedian branch

Long circumflex branch

Posterior cerebral artery

Short circumflex branch

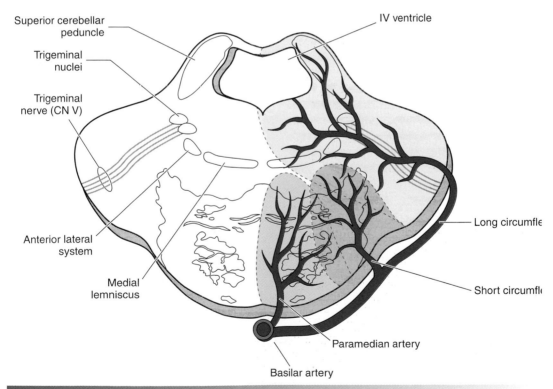

Superior cerebellar peduncle

Trigeminal nuclei

Trigeminal nerve (CN V)

Anterior lateral system

Medial lemniscus

IV ventricle

Long circumfle

Short circumfl

Paramedian artery

Basilar artery

Figure 1.29     Perfusion patterns of the pons

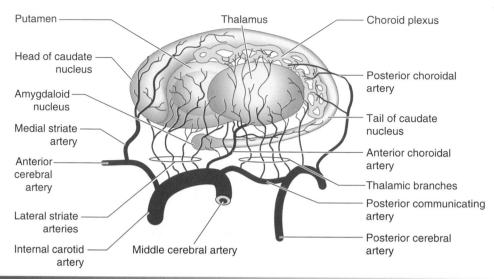

Putamen — Thalamus — Choroid plexus

Head of caudate nucleus

Amygdaloid nucleus

Medial striate artery

Anterior cerebral artery

Lateral striate arteries

Internal carotid artery

Middle cerebral artery

Posterior choroidal artery

Tail of caudate nucleus

Anterior choroidal artery

Thalamic branches

Posterior communicating artery

Posterior cerebral artery

**Figure 1.30    The thalamostriate circulation**

The blood supply to the choroid plexus, thalamus, and basal ganglia is derived from short penetrating branches, which in turn are derived from the posterior and middle cerebral arteries.

the dorsal and lateral portions of the medulla (Fig. 1.31).

Because the **dorsal spinal arteries** are branches of the vertebral arteries that arise near the lateral border of the medulla, each wraps around the medulla to reach the dorsal surface and then travels caudally, in parallel with its mate from the opposite side, along the dorsal surface of the medulla and spinal cord. The dorsal spinal arteries are most conspicuous at medullary and high cervical levels and less conspicuous at low cervical levels, where they merge. After merging, the dorsal spinal artery usually does not descend the entire length of the spinal cord but peters out by midthoracic levels (Fig. 1.32).

### The Circle of Willis

In most persons the posterior circulation derived from the vertebrobasilar system and the anterior circulation derived from the carotid system anastomose through the pair of **posterior communicating arteries**. The two anterior cerebral arteries are joined by the single **anterior communicating artery**. These anastomoses create a circular pathway of arteries, the **circle of Willis** (Fig. 1.27).

### The Spinal Cord Circulation

In addition to the blood supplied by branches of the vertebral arteries to the cervical spinal cord (see page 31), there is a segmental blood supply to the spinal cord. In theory every spinal nerve carries with it a **spinal artery** that divides into a **dorsal** and **ventral radicular artery** [L. *radix,* root]. These radicular arteries follow the dorsal and ventral roots, respectively (Figs. 1.21 and 1.32). This radicular system of arteries is the major source of blood to the spinal cord below the cervical region. These radicular arteries anastomose with the dorsal or ventral spinal arteries, as appropriate, forming a rich collateral network.

As a practical matter, both the number of radicular arteries and their distribution vary widely in the adult. In particular, only about half of the dorsal radicular arteries fully develop and join the dorsal spinal artery, and only about a third of the ventral radicular arteries join the ventral spinal artery (Fig. 1.33). Given the capriciousness of the development of this arterial network, it is not surprising that certain areas of the spinal cord are particularly vulnerable to injury following the loss of a single spinal artery. In general this vulner-

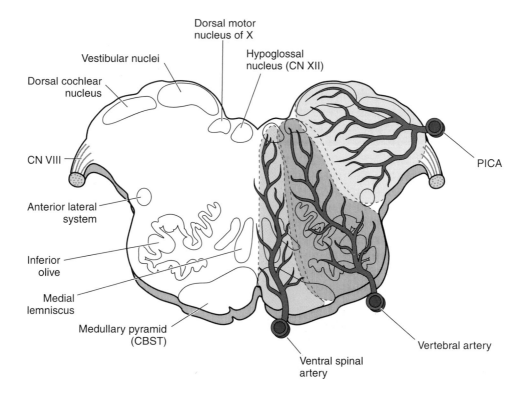

Dorsal motor
nucleus of X

Vestibular nuclei

Hypoglossal
nucleus (CN XII)

Dorsal cochlear
nucleus

PICA

CN VIII

Anterior lateral
system

Inferior
olive

Medial
lemniscus

Medullary pyramid
(CBST)

Vertebral artery

Ventral spinal
artery

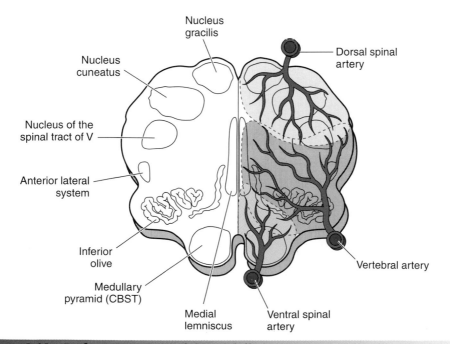

Nucleus
gracilis

Nucleus
cuneatus

Dorsal spinal
artery

Nucleus of the
spinal tract of V

Anterior lateral
system

Inferior
olive

Medullary
pyramid (CBST)

Vertebral artery

Medial
lemniscus

Ventral spinal
artery

**Figure 1.31    Perfusion patterns of the medulla**

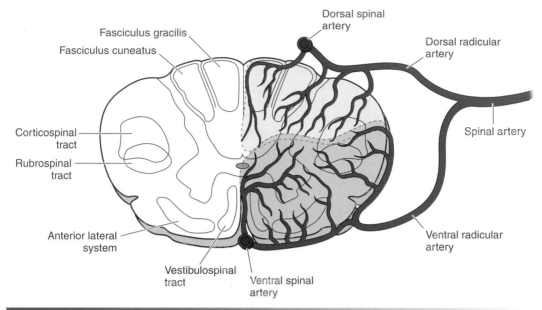

**Figure 1.32    Perfusion patterns of the spinal cord**

ability is greatest at the thoracic levels because the intercostal arteries that give rise to the spinal arteries are themselves poorly anastomosed. **Infarction** [L. *infarcire,* to stuff in] of the thoracic spinal cord is frequently associated with dissecting aortic **aneurysms**[3] [G. *aneurysma,* wide] or surgery that occludes a single intercostal artery.

Vascular compromise of certain areas of the spinal cord can also occur due to the sparse anastomotic connections between the dorsal and ventral circulations. Following *occlusion* of the ventral spinal artery (**ventral [anterior] spinal syndrome**), perfusion from the dorsal spinal arteries is usually not sufficient to prevent infarction of the ventral half of the spinal cord in the region of the occlusion (Fig. 1.33).

## The Blood Supply of Peripheral Nerves

Peripheral nerves are supplied with a rich vasculature (Fig. 1.25). Vessels extrinsic to the nerve run parallel to it and extend branches

that penetrate the epineurium every few millimeters. These epineural vessels branch and anastomose, forming a rich plexus of vessels. These vessels, in turn, send branches into the perineurium of the fascicles. The perineurial plexus then sends penetrating branches into the endoneurium. Within the endoneural space is an extensively anastomosed microvascular network consisting of arterioles, capillaries, and venules. This highly collateralized network affords a wide safety margin against vascular insult.

## The Cerebral Venous Sinuses

In the brain, the penetrating veins of the cerebral cortex closely parallel the penetrating arteries. However, once on the surface of the brain, these veins empty into a series of **sinuses** that are formed by a separation of the endosteal and meningeal dural layers of the dura mater (Fig. 1.3). The sinus drainage system is unique to the CNS. Unlike veins, the sinuses have no valves and being composed of tough connective tissue, are not distensible. They provide a path

---

[3]An aneurysm is any widening, or ballooning, of an artery. In some cases, particularly with the larger arteries, the intima may separate from the arterial wall, a condition described as a dissecting aneurysm.

of exceptionally low resistance by which blood can leave the cranium (Fig. 1.34).

The venous sinus system drains from the **superior sagittal sinus** into a pair of **transverse sinuses** formed where the tentorium cerebelli meets the dura mater. Each transverse sinus follows the margin of the occipital bone to the petrous bone, where it becomes the **sigmoid sinus**. The sigmoid sinus follows

an S-shaped medial course to the point where it exits the skull as the **internal jugular vein** (Fig. 1.34).

Several other sinuses are tributaries to this system. Most notable is the **inferior sagittal sinus**. This sinus is formed at the free inferior edge of the falx cerebri and drains toward the posterior, becoming the **straight sinus** at the tentorial incisure. It passes directly posterior

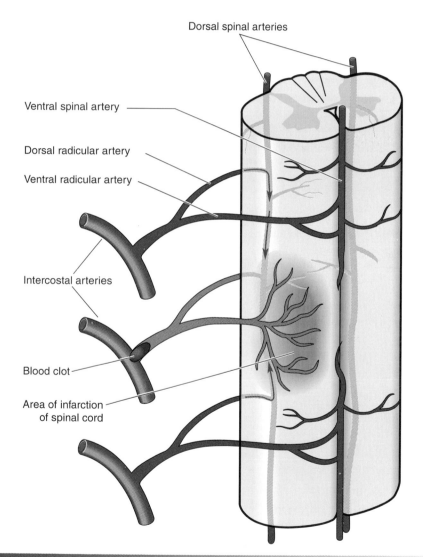

Dorsal spinal arteries

Ventral spinal artery

Dorsal radicular artery

Ventral radicular artery

Intercostal arteries

Blood clot

Area of infarction of spinal cord

## Figure 1.33    Radicular arteries of the spinal cord

Not all of the 31 potential pairs of radicular arteries develop completely. Therefore, some parts of the spinal cord are perfused by only one or two radicular arteries. Loss of a single radicular artery at these sites can result in ischemic infarction of the spinal cord. The upper lumbar and thoracic spinal cord are particularly vulnerable in this way.

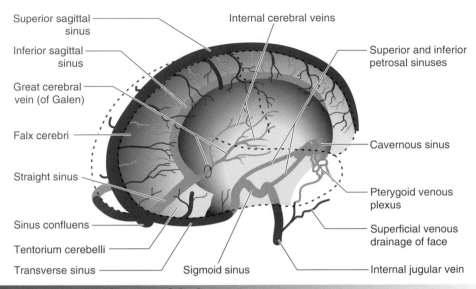

Superior sagittal sinus
Inferior sagittal sinus
Great cerebral vein (of Galen)
Falx cerebri
Straight sinus
Sinus confluens
Tentorium cerebelli
Transverse sinus
Internal cerebral veins
Superior and inferior petrosal sinuses
Cavernous sinus
Pterygoid venous plexus
Superficial venous drainage of face
Internal jugular vein
Sigmoid sinus

**Figure 1.34   Venous drainage of the brain**

The superficial veins of the brain drain into the various interconnected sinuses. The venous blood flows to the transverse sinus at the posterior of the brain. After passing through the sigmoid sinus, the blood finally leaves the cranium through the internal jugular vein. An alternative pathway runs through the cavernous and pterygoid sinus.

to join the superior sagittal sinus and the two transverse sinuses at the **sinus confluens.**

The straight sinus, in addition to receiving blood from the inferior sagittal sinus, receives blood from large internal cerebral veins that drain the basal ganglia, thalamus, and related structures. These internal veins converge to form the **great cerebral vein (of Galen)**, which flows directly into the straight sinus.

The **cavernous sinus** lies at the base of the brain in the sella turcica. It envelops several important structures, including the pituitary gland; the internal carotid artery; and several cranial nerves, including the oculomotor, trochlear, abducens, and the maxillary division of the trigeminal. It receives blood from the anterior inferior portion of the brain, the ophthalmic veins, and the sphenoparietal sinuses. The cavernous sinus drains toward the posterior into the transverse sinus, through the **superior** and **inferior petrosal sinuses.** This sinus can also drain interiorly into the extracranial **pterygoid venus plexus** [G. *pterygoid,* winglike] and from there into facial veins and finally the internal jugular vein.

## The Venous Drainage of the Spinal Cord

The pattern of veins in the spinal cord closely follows the pattern of arteries. They consist of the **ventral** and **dorsal spinal veins** and **radicular** veins (Fig. 1.21). In addition to these veins, which are found in the subarachnoid space, an extensive and delicate **epidural venous network** receives blood from the radicular veins. This **rete** envelops the entire length of the spinal cord and extends to the **clivus** under the pons, where it joins the cavernous sinus. Branches from the rete also drain into the segmental veins associated with the vertebra, and these veins drain into the vena cava.

## Abnormalities of the Neurovasculature

Normal persons exhibit considerable variation in the arrangement of the major arteries at the base of the brain. The point at which the basilar artery forms from the union of the vertebral arteries can lie almost anywhere along the base of the medulla and pons. In those for whom this junction is more rostral than normal, arteries that normally arise from the basilar artery simply arise from one of the vertebral arteries instead. In addition, in some persons the posterior communicating arteries can be as large as the basilar artery or, conversely, be missing altogether. These anomalies usually occur only on one side.

## VASCULAR PLASTICITY

The vascular system has the potential to reorganize itself in response to long-standing atherosclerotic disease. Under normal circumstances blood pressure on either side of a vascular anastomosis is roughly balanced. Therefore, little blood flows from one side to the other. If pressure on one side gradually diminishes, blood naturally flows from the high- to the low-pressure side. Over time the small anastomotic vessels enlarge to accommodate the additional flow. This important adaptive response can help to prevent cerebral ischemia in those with long-standing atherosclerotic disease. With regard to cerebral blood flow, this accommodation occurs primarily in two areas, the circle of Willis and the ophthalmic artery.

Under normal circumstances the blood pressure is equal at all of the arteries supplying the circle of Willis, and little blood flows through the communicating arteries. Consequently, the communicating arteries are normally small and cannot immediately deliver the required amounts of blood if one of the major arteries is suddenly occluded. However, in cases of slowly developing stenosis of one of the four major nutrient arteries, such as the development of an atherosclerotic plaque at the carotid bifurcation, the communicating arteries gradually expand and establish a sufficient collateral circulation to maintain normal brain function.

An alternative path can establish itself in response to slowly developing internal carotid stenosis. This path arises from the external carotid circulation via branches of the facial, maxillary, and frontal arteries. These arteries anastomose with the ophthalmic artery, the first intracranial branch of the internal carotid.

These anastomotic connections are normally small and insignificant. However, in the face of developing stenosis of the internal carotid, they can enlarge. As the internal carotid stenosis develops, pressure in the ophthalmic artery falls. Pressure in the facial, maxillary, and frontal arteries remains normal. This hemodynamic imbalance reverses the blood flow in the ophthalmic artery, converting it to a nutritive artery of the brain (Fig. 1.35).

## ARTERIOVENOUS MALFORMATIONS

During development, for reasons that are not understood, shunts develop between some arteries and veins in nervous tissue. Known as an **arteriovenous malformation**, or **AVM**, this abnormality is composed of a tangle of vessels with abnormally thin walls that shunt blood directly from the arterial to the venous circulation. There is no capillary bed (Fig. 1.36). Because the vessel walls are delicate, they are common sites of intracerebral hemorrhage. They can also be the source of focal seizures (see Chapter 15). AVMs lie undetected in the brain until they cause neurological signs. They can sometimes be isolated by applying vascular clips. Alternatively they may be occluded with injected beads, polymers, or fine wires. Treatment is always complicated and dangerous. Many AVMs cannot be treated by any method.

## BERRY ANEURYSMS

Intracranial bleeding can also be caused by leaking or ruptured aneurysms. One type of aneurysm is an improper local development of the arterial wall that creates a point of weakness. This weakened arterial wall balloons outward under pressure (Fig. 1.37). Named for their berrylike appearance, **berry aneurysms** in the brain are usually (more than 90%) seen in the arteries associated with the anterior circle of Willis. They may lie dormant for years before leaking or rupturing, causing an intracranial hemorrhage that is commonly fatal. If the patient survives the original bleed, the neck of the aneurysm can often be occluded with a small steel clip.

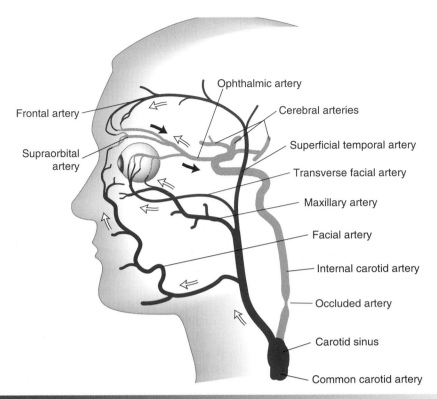

**Figure 1.35  Alternative perfusion pathways**

The ophthalmic artery is the first intracranial branch of the carotid artery. In cases of gradual stenosis of the internal carotid artery, the flow of blood through the ophthalmic artery can be reversed, transforming it into a nutritive artery of the brain. The collateral circulation in this situation is derived from the facial, maxillary, and superficial temporal arteries. *Open arrows,* normal blood flow; *solid arrows,* reversed flow.

## THE VENTRICULAR SYSTEM

The nervous system is a hollow organ. Four cavities within the brain, called ventricles, form a continuous space (Fig. 1.38). The largest of these are the paired **lateral ventricles,** which lie within the cerebral hemispheres. These ventricles reflect the superficial form of the cerebrum; hence, the **anterior horn** is found within the frontal lobe, the **posterior horn** lies within the occipital lobe, and the **inferior horn** penetrates the core of the temporal lobe. The **body of the lateral ventricle** connects the anterior and posterior horns and lies deep to the frontal and parietal lobes.

The **third ventricle** lies in the midline between the two halves of the diencephalon. It is a thin, narrow structure that communicates with the lateral ventricles through a pair of passages, the **intraventricular foramina.** Toward the posterior, the third ventricle narrows at the rostral end of the midbrain to form the very narrow and relatively long **cerebral aqueduct,** which opens into the **fourth ventricle.**

The fourth ventricle is a large space lying dorsal to the pons and medulla and ventral to the cerebellum. A pair of **lateral recesses** in the fourth ventricle course under the cerebellum and communicate with the subarachnoid space through **lateral apertures** into the pontine cistern. In the midline, the fourth ventricle opens into the cisterna magna through a single **medial aperture.** Hence the ventricular system and the subarachnoid space are continuous. These apertures are the only pathways between the ventricular system and the subarachnoid space.

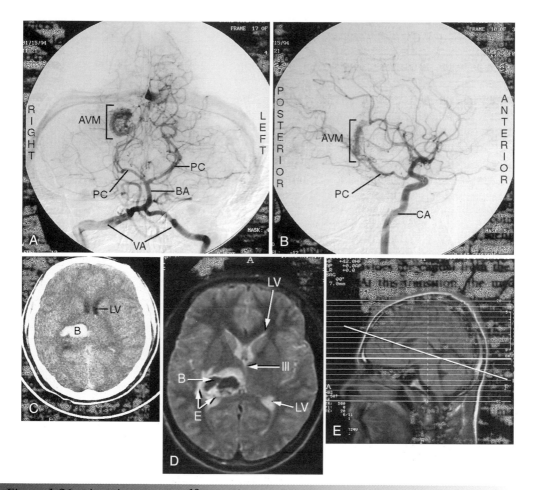

**Figure 1.36    Arteriovenous malformation**

**A.** An anterior-posterior view arteriogram revealing an *AVM* derived from the posterior cerebral (*PC*) artery. The contrast material used to opacify the blood vessels was injected into the left vertebral artery (*VA*) and transported into the basilar artery (*BA*) and the two posterior cerebral arteries. Some contrast material also flowed back into the right VA. **B.** A lateral arteriogram from the patient shown in **A.** The contrast material was injected into the carotid artery (*CA*). The AVM is supplied by both the PC and the CA. **C.** Computed tomography (CT) from the same patient showing fresh blood in the brain (*B*) after a leak from the AVM. The anterior horns of the lateral ventricles (*LV*) are just visible in this section. The CSF appears dark in a CT. **D.** A T2-weighted MRI from the same patient, illustrating the fresh blood (*B*) seen in the CT. This MRI also reveals edema (*E*) surrounding the blood. The lateral ventricles (*LV*) and third ventricle (*III*) are also shown. **E.** A T1-weighted MRI scout view of the brain in the midsagittal plane. The *heavy horizontal line* indicates the plane of the MR image in **D.** The *heavy diagonal line* indicates the plane of the CT section shown in **C.** Ordinary CT sections of the brain are parallel to this plane. (Courtesy of The St. Joseph Medical Center, South Bend, IN.)

## CEREBROSPINAL FLUID

The ventricles and subarachnoid space are filled with a normally clear, colorless fluid, the CSF. An actively secreted product of the choroid plexus, a highly vascularized tissue that partially lines the ventricles, CSF resembles plasma; however, it differs from plasma in several important respects. Table 1.1 summarizes the comparison between plasma and CSF.

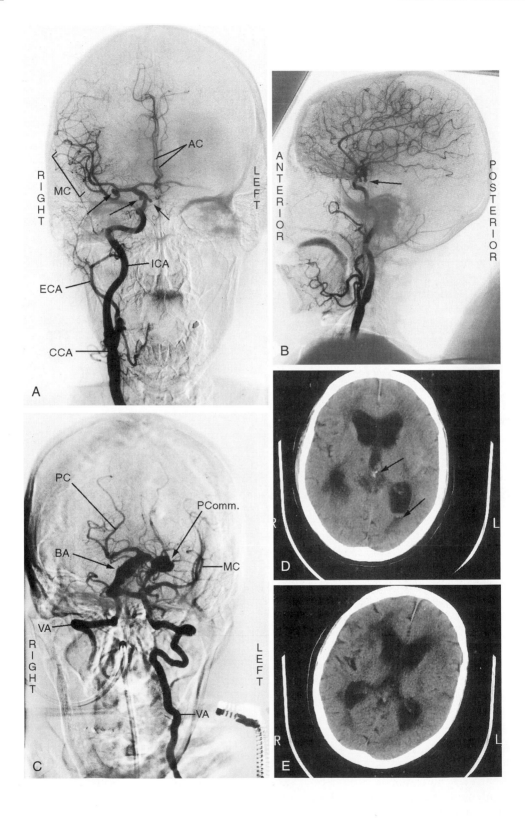

Specifically, physicians should remember that *CSF normally contains less than 50 mg/dL protein* and *no more than 5 cells/mL*. Normal CSF pressure at the lumbar cistern is less than *200 $mm_{H_2O}$* when the patient is recumbent.

## Production and Circulation of CSF

CSF is produced at a relatively constant rate of 400 to 500 mL/day. It stands to reason that it must be reabsorbed at the same rate. Reabsorption is accomplished through **arachnoid villi,** small structures that communicate between the subarachnoid space and the dural sinuses (Figs. 1.3 and 1.6). They are particularly numerous in the sagittal sinus. CSF can freely pass through an arachnoid villus into the venous blood if CSF pressure (normally about 9 mmHg with the person recumbent) is slightly higher than venous pressure (normally about 5 mmHg). Blood is unable to pass into the subarachnoid space when venous pressure exceeds CSF pressure.

## Hydrocephalus

**Hydrocephalus** is a condition in which the balance between CSF in production and reabsorption is disturbed. It can be caused by any one of three events: (*a*) excess production of CSF with normal reabsorption, (*b*) normal CSF production with decreased reabsorption, and (*c*) blockage of the CSF circulation between the sites of production and reabsorption. In the first two conditions, called **communication hydrocephalus**, CSF freely circulates among the ventricles and the subarachnoid space. In the latter condition, called **noncommunicating hydrocephalus**, CSF circulation is interrupted.

In communicating hydrocephalus, CSF production exceeds reabsorption. Initially, to accommodate the increased volume of CSF, extracellular fluid is squeezed out of the neural tissue into the vascular space, where it is removed from the brain. As this squeezing occurs, the ventricles enlarge. As the process continues, neural tissue erodes. Eventually the increased volume of CSF can no longer be accommodated. **Intracranial pressure** increases because the skull, which encases the brain and CSF compartments, is not expandable.

Noncommunicating hydrocephalus occurs when the ventricular circulation is impaired. The excessive CSF is confined to the portion of the ventricular system isolated from the subarachnoid space. CSF circulation is often blocked at the cerebral aqueduct, because it is both very narrow and long. This blockage can be caused by the accumulation of debris caught in the aqueduct. Occlusion can also be directly caused by an expanding mass compressing the quadrigeminal plate. In such cases the lateral and third ventricles enlarge, but the fourth ventricle retains its normal size.

## Figure 1.37  Berry aneurysm

**A.** An anterior-posterior view arteriogram following dye injection into the right common carotid artery (*CCA*). Three berry aneurysms (*arrows*) are visible. *ICA*, internal carotid artery; *ECA*, external carotid artery; *MC* arteries derived from the middle cerebral artery, colloquially known as the candelabra; *AC*, anterior cerebral arteries (note filling of both right and left AC arteries). **B.** A lateral view arteriogram from the same patient following dye injection into the right common carotid artery. The *arrow* points to two berry aneurysms. The MC candelabra is well demonstrated superior to the aneurysms. **C.** An anterior-posterior view of a different patient illustrating a fusiform aneurysm of the basilar artery (*BA*) and another aneurysm of the posterior communicating artery (*Pcomm*). The dye was injected into the left vertebral artery (*VA*) and crossed over into the right VA, partially filling it. The right posterior cerebral (*PC*) and right middle cerebral arteries (*MC*) are also filled. **D.** A CT image of the patient in **C,** showing enlarged ventricles and fresh blood (*arrows*). This patient had been lying on his back for some time before the CT was taken. During that time fresh blood in the lateral ventricle settled under the influence of gravity at the back of the posterior horn (*bottom arrow*). A subsequent CT taken two days later (**E**) still shows enlarged ventricles but no fresh blood. (Courtesy of The St. Joseph Medical Center, South Bend, IN.)

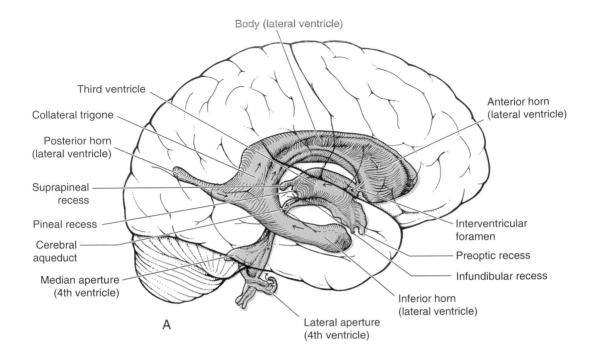

Body (lateral ventricle)

Third ventricle

Collateral trigone

Posterior horn
(lateral ventricle)

Suprapineal
recess

Pineal recess

Cerebral
aqueduct

Median aperture
(4th ventricle)

Anterior horn
(lateral ventricle)

Interventricular
foramen

Preoptic recess

Infundibular recess

Inferior horn
(lateral ventricle)

Lateral aperture
(4th ventricle)

A

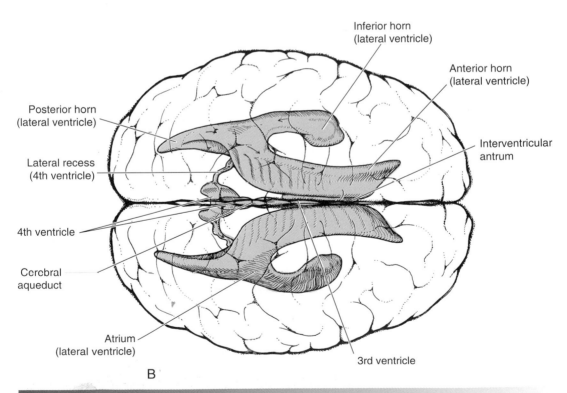

Inferior horn
(lateral ventricle)

Anterior horn
(lateral ventricle)

Posterior horn
(lateral ventricle)

Lateral recess
(4th ventricle)

4th ventricle

Cerebral
aqueduct

Interventricular
antrum

Atrium
(lateral ventricle)

3rd ventricle

B

## Figure 1.38   The ventricular system

The ventricles of the human brain are shown here in lateral (**A**) and superior (**B**) views. Note the location of the lateral and medial apertures of the fourth ventricle and the path that CSF produced in the lateral ventricles must flow (*arrows*) to reach the apertures and exit into the subarachnoid space. The CSF is eventually reabsorbed from the subarachnoid space into the bloodstream. (Modified from Baily P. Intracranial Tumors. 2nd ed. Springfield, IL: Charles C. Thomas, 1948.)

| Table 1.1 | Comparison Between CSF and Plasma | |
|---|---|---|
| **Component** | **CFS** | **Serum** |
| Protein | 35 mg/dl | 7000 mg/dL |
| Glucose | 60 mg/dl | 90 mg/dL |
| Red cells | 0/mL3 | na |
| White cells | <5/mL3 | na |
| $Na^+$ | 138 mEq/l | 138 mEq/L |
| $K^+$ | 2.8 mEq/L | 4.5 mEq/L |
| $Ca^{++}$ | 2.1 mEq/L | 4.8 mEq/L |
| $Mg^{++}$ | 0.3 mEq/L | 1.7 mEq/L |
| $Cl^-$ | 119 mEq/L | 102 mEq/L |
| pH | 7.33 | 7.41 |

The major constituents of CSF and serum are listed here along with their normal values. The values listed in boldface should be memorized.

If one of the intraventricular foramina is blocked, only the corresponding lateral ventricle enlarges (Fig. 1.39).

Not all hydrocephalus is associated with an increase in intracranial pressure. For example, **normal-pressure hydrocephalus** occurs in newborn infants with obstruction of the cerebral aqueduct. They have enlarged ventricles and an enlarged cranium. In infants the cranial sutures have not closed, so the skull expands, allowing an increase in ventricle size without a dramatic increase in CSF pressure (see Appendix 1). Unfortunately, the dilation of the ventricles is so great that it causes neuronal damage by thinning the cerebral cortex. These children become neurologically compromised. To prevent or minimize damage, a tube is placed in the ventricular system and through it CSF is shunted into the jugular vein or the peritoneal cavity, where it can be reabsorbed. These shunts are fitted with a one-way valve that preserves the integrity of the CSF space and regulates pressure.

Normal-pressure hydrocephalus is also seen in the elderly. In these cases the ventricles enlarge but CSF pressure remains relatively normal. The cause of this syndrome is uncertain but is believed to be impaired reabsorption. The patients become demented and develop urinary incontinence and disturbances of gait. Senile normal-pressure hydrocephalus is easily confused with senile dementia. It is important to differentiate senile hydrocephalus from senile dementia because the hydrocephalus responds well to treatment. There is no effective treatment for dementia.

Increased intracranial pressure can also be caused by an intracranial mass, such as subarachnoid hematomas or tumors. As these masses expand, intracranial pressure increases in much the same way as with hydrocephalus. Unlike communicating hydrocephalus, in which the pressure is applied evenly throughout the ventricular system, or noncommunicating hydrocephalus, in which the pressure is applied evenly above the ventricular block, expanding masses apply the pressure asymmetrically, distorting the shape of the brain. Initially some of the pressure can be relieved by increased reabsorption of CSF and a corresponding collapse of the ventricles. This strategy soon fails, and pressure increases rapidly, presenting complications in management of the patient. Perhaps the greatest difficulty is with decreased perfusion of the brain. It is intuitively obvious that cerebral perfusion pressure must equal mean arterial pressure minus intracranial pressure; therefore, cerebral blood flow decreases as intracranial pressure increases. As cerebral perfusion decreases, clouding of consciousness, coma, and eventually death ensue (see Chapter 15).

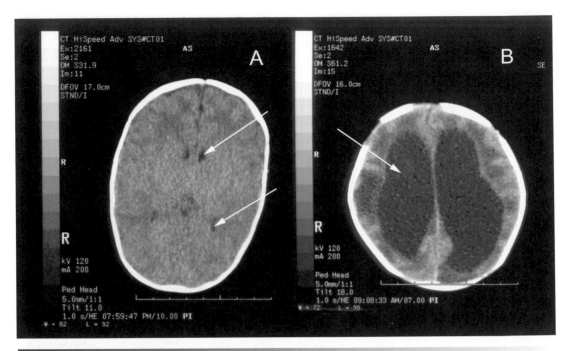

Figure 1.39  Hydrocephalus

The CSF in the ventricles appears dark in CT (*arrows*). The ventricles of a normal infant (**A**) are small. The *arrows* point to portions of the anterior and posterior horns. In an infant with hydrocephalus (**B**) the ventricles are greatly enlarged (*arrow*). (Courtesy of the St. Joseph Medical Center, South Bend, IN.)

Increased CSF pressure can be relieved by inserting a needle into the lumbar cistern. However, a rapid removal of CSF from the lumbar cistern and the associated decrease in CSF pressure may shift the contents of the cerebrum. If this occurs, the cerebellar tonsils may be thrust into the foramen magnum, strangling the medulla and cervical spinal cord, a condition that is frequently fatal. Obviously, before sampling CSF, the physician is obliged to rule out all causes of increased intracranial pressure.

## THE BLOOD-BRAIN-CSF COMPARTMENTS

The nervous system consists of three fluid compartments: (*a*) the **vascular**, (*b*) the **CSF**, and (*c*) the **neuronal** or **extracellular** compartments (Fig. 1.40). These compartments do not freely communicate with one another. The interface between the vascular system and the extracellular compartment of the CNS is called the **blood-brain barrier.** The other two interfaces, the **blood-CSF barrier** and the **CSF-brain barrier**, have until recently received little attention.

## Blood-Brain Barrier

The interface between the vascular system and the CNS occurs in the capillaries. This interface is often called a barrier because it prevents most macromolecules from passing between the two compartments. The endothelial cells that line the capillaries in somatic tissue have 10-nm open spaces between the cells. Macromolecules can pass freely into and out of the vascular space. In contrast, the endothelial cells that line the capillaries of the CNS have tight junctions between them. These tight junctions almost completely prevent macromolecules from entering or leaving the CNS. Even ionic species can be excluded by these specialized endothelial cells. Some molecules can pass from the

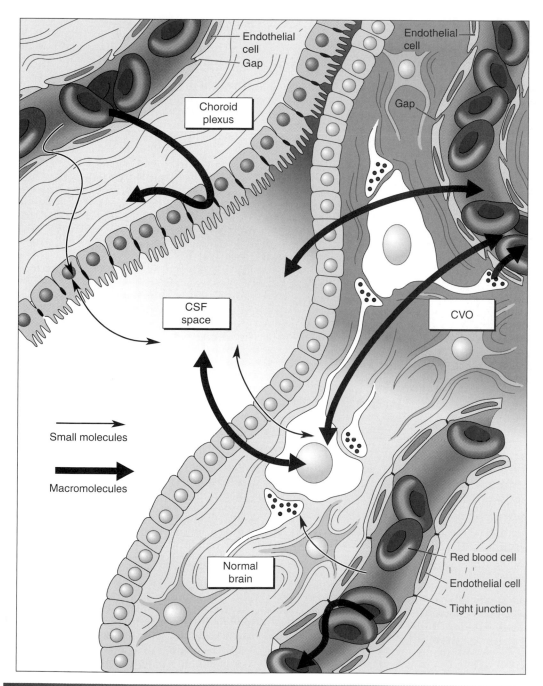

## Figure 1.40    The three fluid spaces of the nervous system

Specialized endothelial cells with tight junction are the principal barrier between the blood compartment and the neural tissue. The tight junctions in epithelial cells form the barrier between the blood compartment and the CSF. Macromolecules pass freely between the CFS and the neural tissue. A circumventricular organ (*CVO*) is shown at the upper right of figure. CVOs provide for a relatively free exchange of macromolecules among the three compartments.

blood into the brain extracellular space. In almost every instance, however, these molecules have a special transport mechanism. For example, amino acids have three specific transport systems designed for acidic, neutral, and basic amino acids. D-Glucose also has a specific transporter. Some other lipid-soluble molecules can cross the blood-brain barrier. Astrocytes (see Chapter 2), which line the external surface of the CNS capillaries, also help to maintain the extracellular milieu. Their most important function in this respect seems to be related to their ability to regulate the extracellular concentration of $K^+$ ions.

The blood-brain interface has considerable clinical significance. As a barrier, it prevents many useful drugs, such as most antibiotics, from reaching the brain. The exclusion of antibiotics from the brain seriously complicates the management of CNS infections. In contrast to antibiotics, opioids readily pass through the blood-brain barrier, which in part explains their effectiveness. The blood-brain barrier breaks down in certain pathological conditions. For example, the vasculature within rapidly growing neoplasms is not an effective barrier. The endothelial cells lack the tight junctions found in normal brain capillaries. The loss of this barrier affects the relative hydration of the neoplasm, which allows it to be differentiated from healthy brain tissue by MRI (see Appendix 4).

### Blood-CSF Barrier

There is also a barrier in the choroid plexus between the vascular compartment and the CSF. In the choroid plexus the endothelial cells of the capillaries do not come in direct contact with the CSF compartment but are a part of the stroma. The standard fenestrated junctions of these endothelial cells allow macromolecules to pass easily from the vascular compartment into the stroma. The barrier between the choroid plexus and the CSF is formed by the epithelial cells, which have tight junctions. Thus isolation of the CSF compartment from the vascular compartment is achieved while still allowing macromolecules access to the stroma of the choroid plexus.

### The CSF-Brain Interface

The interface between the brain and the CSF is formed by the ependymal cells that line the ventricular walls. The outer surface of the brain is lined with the pia mater. Because there are no tight junctions between these cells, there is no significant diffusion barrier between the CSF and the brain. Therefore, macromolecules freely move between the CSF and the intercellular space of the CNS.

## THE CIRCUMVENTRICULAR ORGANS

The barrier between the vascular system and the neurons of the central nervous system is circumvented at specific places in the brain. These sites, known as **circumventricular organs (CVOs)**, exist in close association with the CSF. CVOs are highly specialized. They contain neurons and have unusual capillaries. In some CVOs the neurons have specialized receptors for specific macromolecules, especially the neuroactive proteins. Others have specialized secretory properties. The receptor CVOs are the **area postrema**, the **subfornical organ**, and the **organum vasculosum**. The secretory CVOs are the **medial eminence**, the **neurohypophysis**, the **subcommissural organ**, and the **pineal gland** (Fig. 1.41). Circumventricular organs have a higher capillary density than the surrounding neural tissue (Fig. 1.42). In addition, these capillaries are structurally quite different from the capillaries of the brain. Unlike the capillaries in ordinary neural tissue, CVO capillaries have a pericapillary space, fenestrations between the endothelial cells, and surface pits (Fig. 1.43).

CVOs are the functional interface between the nervous system and the endocrine system. Evidence suggests that specialized receptors line the surface of the endothelial cell pits, where they bind circulating peptides. Once bound, the peptide is transported into the CVO, where it can act on neurons. Thus the brain can be partly regulated by circulating hormones.

The brain is also an endocrine organ. It releases into the blood peptides that affect re-

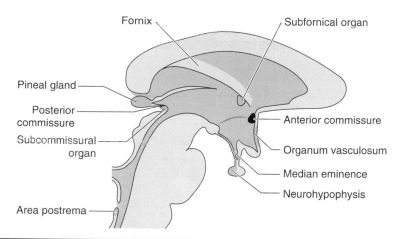

**Figure 1.41    Circumventricular organs**

This sagittal view of the third and fourth ventricles shows the locations of the circumventricular organs (*red*).

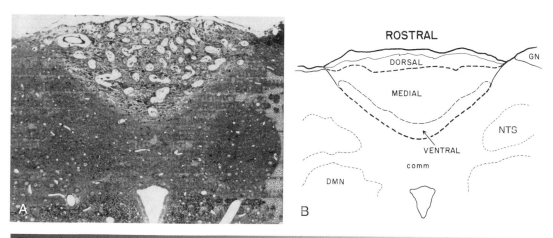

**Figure 1.42    Histology of CVOs**

**A.** The area postrema of the rat is clearly distinguished from the surrounding neural tissue by the density of its capillary bed (45 ×). **B.** The same area identifying major structures: *NTS,* nucleus of the tractus solitarius; *DMN,* dorsal motor nucleus of the vagus; *GN,* gracilis nucleus. (These structures are discussed in subsequent chapters.) (Reprinted with permission from Shaver et al. J Comp Neurol 1991:73–82.)

mote targets. The best-documented role of the brain as an endocrine organ is its release of oxytocin and vasopressin from neurosecretory granules into the perivascular space of the neurohypophysis (a CVO). Within the neurohypophysis these hormones diffuse into the capillaries through fenestrated endothelial cells. Another CVO, the median eminence, is an interface between the nervous system and the pituitary gland. The median eminence not only deposits hormonal signals (releasing factors) into the hypophyseal portal bloodstream, it receives feedback signals in the form of circulating hormones. These systems are discussed in detail in Chapter 14.

Many high-molecular-weight neuroactive peptides that cannot cross the blood-brain interface are nevertheless found in the CSF. They appear to be secreted by some CVOs and perhaps detected by other CVOs. Therefore, it

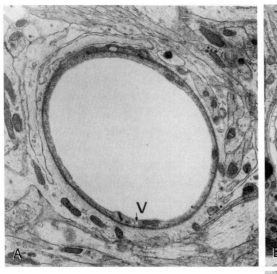

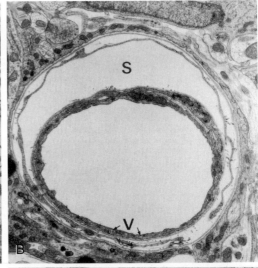

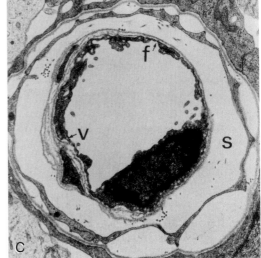

## Figure 1.43 CVO capillaries

**A.** Nonfenestrated capillaries, which are typical of ordinary neural tissue, are rarely seen in CVOs. **B.** A prominent pericapillary space (*S*) and vesicles or pits (*V*) are commonly found in CVO capillaries. **C.** This type of CVO capillary has not only pits and a pericapillary space but also fenestrations between the endothelial cells (*f*). (Reprinted with permission from Shaver et al. J Comp Neurol 1990:245.)

seems likely that there is a humoral regulatory system within the CNS that uses the CSF as its transport vehicle in much the same way that the endocrine system uses the bloodstream to transport hormones to distant targets. However, because the CSF is isolated from the bloodstream, these neuroactive peptides are restricted to CNS targets.

## S U M M A R Y

- **The nervous system is divided into several major regions.**

  The nervous system consists of the brain, brainstem, cerebellum, spinal cord, and peripheral nervous system. The brain consists of the cerebral hemispheres, basal ganglia, and thalamus. The brainstem consists of the mid-

brain, pons, and medulla. The cerebellum, spinal cord, and peripheral nervous system are not usually subdivided. The cerebral hemispheres are subdivided into the frontal, parietal, occipital, insular, and temporal lobes. The cerebral hemispheres are wrinkled into gyri and sulci. The cerebellar hemispheres are wrinkled into folia. This wrinkling greatly increases the surface area without greatly increasing the volume of the organ.

- **Most of the cranial nerves enter the brainstem.**

The brainstem receives all of the cranial nerves except the olfactory, optic, and accessory nerves. The olfactory nerve enters the brain directly, and the optic nerve enters the thalamus. The oculomotor and trochlear nerves enter the midbrain, and the trigeminal nerve enters the pons. The abducens, facial, and vestibulocochlear nerves all enter at the pontomedullary junction. The remaining nerves, except the accessory, enter the medulla; the accessory nerve, being a creature of the spinal cord, has an aberrant course into the cranium.

- **The spinal nerves are associated with the vertebrae.**

There are 31 pairs of spinal nerves, consisting of a merged dorsal and ventral root. The dorsal root is sensory and the ventral root, motor. Sensory nerves, both spinal and cranial, are mostly pseudounipolar and have ganglia associated with their roots. Exceptions include the olfactory and optic nerves and the mesencephalic branch of the trigeminal nerve (all discussed in later chapters).

- **The CNS is protected by several layers.**

The CNS is enclosed in a bony suit of armor that affords it considerable protection from external forces. It is further covered, from the outside in, by the dura mater, the arachnoid, and the pia mater. The dura mater also forms several septa that divide the brain into compartments. The falx cerebri, the largest, lies in the sagittal plane and separates the two cerebral hemispheres. The tentorium cerebelli separates the cerebral hemispheres from the cerebellum. The tentorial incisure is a hole in the union of these septa through which the brainstem passes. It can be a site of entrapment of the temporal pole in conditions that shift the intracranial contents. The arachnoid creates a space between the dura and the pia that contains cerebral spinal fluid. Where this space is very large, it is called a cistern. For the physi-

cian, the most useful cistern is the lumbar, from which CSF may be sampled.

- **Two pairs of arteries supply blood to all of the CNS except the spinal cord, which is supplied segmentally.**

The intracranial nervous system is supplied by only two pairs of arteries, the vertebral and internal carotid arteries. The carotid circulation gives rise to the middle cerebral and anterior cerebral arteries. Together they supply the major portion of the hemispheres. The vertebral arteries form the basilar artery of the pons, which in turn splits to form the posterior cerebral arteries. The circle of Willis consists of anastomoses between the basilar and carotid circulation. The posterior cerebral arteries supply the occipital pole of the brain and the inferior portion of the temporal lobes. The cerebellum is supplied by three arteries. The superior and anterior-inferior cerebellar arteries arise from the basilar artery, and the posterior-inferior cerebellar artery arises from the vertebral. The spinal circulation is derived from the dorsal and ventral spinal arteries and several radicular arteries. The spinal circulation is quite variable but richly anastomosed.

- **Blood is drained from the CNS through a network of sinuses and veins.**

In the spinal cord this system finds its way to the radicular veins in a straightforward manner. The intracranial veins collect as sinuses, specialized structures formed at the intersections of the external dura and the septa. The principal sinus, the superior sagittal, divides to form the two transverse sinuses, which eventually find their way to the internal jugular veins. Other sinuses drain other parts of the intracranial nervous system.

- **A hollow ventricular system within the CNS is filled with CSF.**

There are four ventricles: two lateral ventricles and one each of the midline third and fourth ventricles. The ventricles are filled with CSF secreted by the choroid plexus lining many of the ventricles. The CSF flows out of the ventricular system through two lateral foramina and one middle foramen in the fourth ventricle into the subarachnoid space with its cisterns. Eventually the CSF is reabsorbed into the bloodstream through the arachnoid villi, found mostly in the superior sagittal sinus. If CSF production exceeds reabsorption or if circulation among any of the CSF spaces is occluded, intracranial pressure increases (hydrocephalus). Pressure may also be increased by the growth of tumors or the seepage of blood into the epidural or subarachnoid space (hematoma).

- **The CNS has three biochemical compartments: the vascular compartment, the CSF compartment, and the neuronal extracellular space.**
  The blood-brain barrier and the blood-CSF barrier restrict passage of macromolecules between these compartments. Macromolecules have relatively free access between the CSF and the intercellular CNS space. The blood-brain barrier is specifically absent at certain regions of the brain, the circumventricular organs. At the circumventricular organs, hormones and large peptides can be exchanged among the blood, the brain, and the CSF.

## SUGGESTED READINGS

Augur AM, Lee MJ. Grant's Atlas of Anatomy. 10th ed. Baltimore: Lippincott Williams & Wilkins, 1999.

Daniels DL, Haughton VM, Naidich TP. Cranial and Spinal Magnetic Resonance Imaging: An Atlas and Guide. New York: Raven Press, 1987.

Haines DE. Neuroanatomy: An Atlas of Structures, Sections, and Systems. 4th ed. Baltimore: Williams & Wilkins, 1995.

Lundborg G. Nerve injury and repair. Philadelphia: Churchill Livingstone, 1988.

Martin JH. Neuroanatomy Text and Atlas. 2nd ed. Norwalk, CT: Appleton & Lange, 1996.

Nieuwenhuys R. Chemoarchitecture of the Brain. Berlin: Springer-Verlag, 1985.

Nieuwenhuys R, Voodg J, Van Huijzen C. The Human Central Nervous System. 3rd ed. Berlin: Springer-Verlag, 1988.

Parent A. Carpenter's Human Neuroanatomy. 9th ed. Baltimore: Williams & Wilkins, 1996.

Waddington M. Atlas of cerebral angiography with anatomic correlation. Boston: Little, Brown, 1974.

# The Microstructure of the Nervous System

The human nervous system is perhaps the most complicated structure ever to evolve on earth, yet its structural components are quite simple. Excluding the meninges and vasculature, the nervous system consists of only three fundamental cell types: **neurons**, **glia**, and **Schwann cells**.

Neurons are the principal cells of the nervous system. Although there are large numbers of morphologically different neuron cell types, the differences among them are derived from simple variations of cellular phenotype, not from major differences in cell metabolism, structure, or function. Neurons are unlike other cells of the body because they communicate among themselves through electrochemical contacts called **synapses** [G. *synapsis*, point of contact]. Although there are billions of synapses in the mammalian nervous system, most of these synapses have common chemical, structural, and functional features. It is important to understand that *the nervous system accomplishes its functions not by increasing the diversity of its components but by diversifying the connections among neurons.*

The glia and Schwann cells support neurons. They physically support neurons by supplying some firmness to the mass of the nervous system. They also provide the chemical milieu for the neurons. They are the only cells in intimate contact with neurons. Some supporting cells wrap themselves around axons, creating a structure known as the **myelin sheath** [G. *myelos*, marrow], which increases the speed with which electrical signals are propagated through out the nervous system.

The mammalian nervous system is divided into the **central nervous system (CNS)** and the **peripheral nervous system (PNS)**. Neurons are found in all parts of the nervous system. Within the CNS neuron cell bodies are organized into **nuclei**, and their axonal processes are collected into organized bundles called **tracts**. **Ganglia** are collections of neuron cell bodies in the PNS. The axons of ganglionic neurons and CNS neurons whose axons leave the CNS form the **peripheral nerves**. Of the supporting cells, the glia are found only in the CNS, while Schwann cells are found only in the PNS.

This chapter describes the cells that make up the nervous system, emphasizing the morphological and functional characteristics that establish their unique functional role in the nervous system. Chapter 3 discusses the electrical properties of neurons.

## THE NEURON

Estimates place the number of neurons in the human brain at about $10^{11}$, a number that is difficult to comprehend. To put it into perspective, assume for a moment that the average diameter of the neurons is 10 μm (a conservative estimate). If these neurons were placed side by side, they would form a chain 1030 km (roughly 650 miles) long. Traveling at the speed of sound (1229 kph), it would take nearly an hour to traverse this chain from end to end.

Neurons are cells and therefore have the characteristics common to all cells (Fig. 2.1).

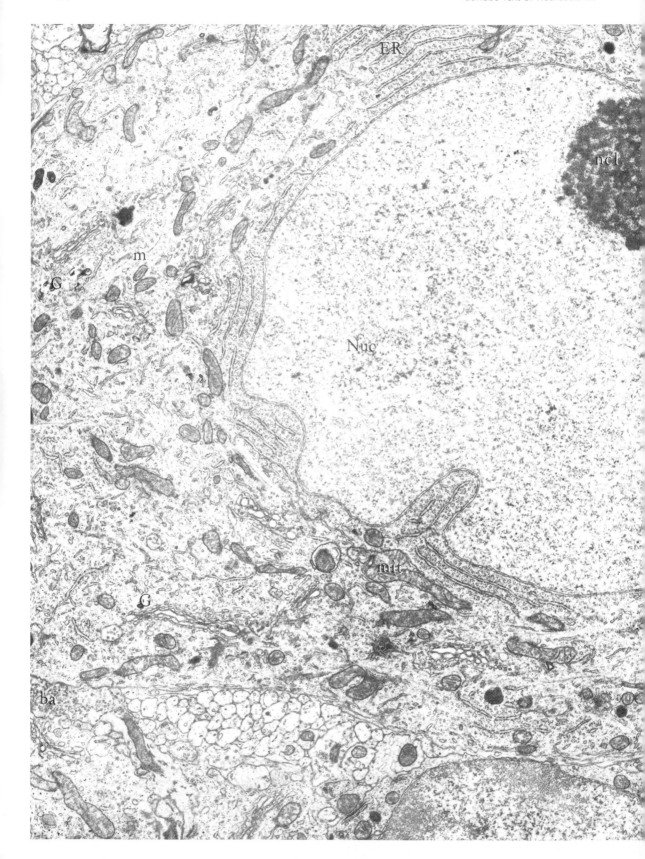

They are bound by a cell membrane. They have a nucleus and cytoplasm. The cytoplasm contains the usual complement of intracellular organelles: endoplasmic reticulum; Golgi bodies; mitochondria; peroxisomes; free ribosomes; and inclusion bodies such as lysosomes, lipofuscin bodies, and vesicles.

Typical neurons consist of three anatomically distinguishable regions: (*a*) the **soma** [G. *soma*, body] or cell body, (*b*) **dendrites** [G. *dendrites*, relating to a tree], and (*c*) a single **axon** [G. *axon*, axis]. The axons branch profusely. Each branch terminates as a specialized structure, the **synaptic bouton** [F. *bouton*, button] (Fig. 2.2).

Neurons are commonly classified according to the number of processes they exhibit. According to this traditional scheme, neurons with a single process are called **unipolar**; those with two processes, **bipolar**; and those with more than two processes, **multipolar**. For descriptive purposes this system is succinct and easily applied to light microscopic preparations.

Most neurons in the human nervous system are multipolar. The only truly bipolar neurons in the adult mammal are associated with the first, second, and eighth cranial nerves. The sensory neurons of the remaining cranial and spinal nerves have a single process that almost immediately divides into two. These neurons are called **pseudounipolar**. True unipolar neurons, while common in invertebrates, are not present in the adult mammalian nervous system (Fig. 2.3).

## The Soma

The soma of most neurons is compact and globular. It contains the ultrastructural organelles needed to carry out the metabolic functions of the cell. *Neurons are secretory cells that produce an extensive variety of proteins.* Consequently they have a large central nucleus with a very prominent nucleolus. Within the nucleus most of the DNA is in the extended form, making it readily available for transcription. It has been estimated that more than 20,000 proteins are produced by neurons, which is about twice the number found, for example, in a secretory cell in the liver.

Protein synthesis occurs on ribosomes. In keeping with the extraordinary amount and diversity of protein synthesis in neurons, the soma contains large numbers of ribosomes and a complex set of internal membranes (Fig. 2.4). This internal membrane complex is divided into several compartments: the **cell membrane**; the **nuclear membrane**; the **rough endoplasmic reticulum** [L. *reticulum*, little net] (rER); the **smooth endoplasmic reticulum** (sER); the **Golgi apparatus**; and **membrane-limited secretory granules**, such as **lysosomes** and **endosomes**.

One portion of the major membrane system, the rER, is so named because the cytoplasmic side of its membranes is decorated with ribosomes. The rER of neurons is so extensive that it is easily seen with light microscopy when the cells are stained with basic dyes. Displayed in this way, the rER of the neuron is called **Nissl substance**, named after the 19th-century cytologist who first described it.

Protein synthesis occurs on both free ribosomes and those bound to the membranes of the rER. Soluble proteins remain within the cell and are assembled on the free ribosomes in the cytosol. Secretory proteins are destined to leave the cell. They are assembled on the ribosomes of the rER as precursor polypeptides extruded through the membrane into the lumen of the endoplasmic reticulum. Further elabora-

---

**Figure 2.1   Ultrastructure of a typical neuron soma**

This electron micrograph of a typical neuron illustrates the various intracellular organelles mentioned in the text. Note the well-organized endoplasmic reticulum (*ER*). The Golgi apparatus (*G*) is well developed in neurons, and there are numerous mitochondria (*mit*). On the neuron is a synapse (*ba*), and adjacent to it are numerous dendrites from other cells. 15,000×. (Reprinted with permission from Peters A, Palay SL, Webster HD. The Fine Structure of the Nervous System. 3rd ed. New York: Oxford University, 1991.)

tion of the precursor polypeptide occurs in the rER and Golgi apparatus, where proteolytic enzymes cleave the functional proteins from the precursor. Membrane-bound vesicles containing the proteins and proteolytic enzymes are pinched off from the Golgi membrane. Further

elaboration of the peptides can occur within the vesicles as they are transported to various locations within the cell. Eventually the final protein product is secreted into the intercellular space by exocytosis or may be transported down the axon (Fig. 2.4).

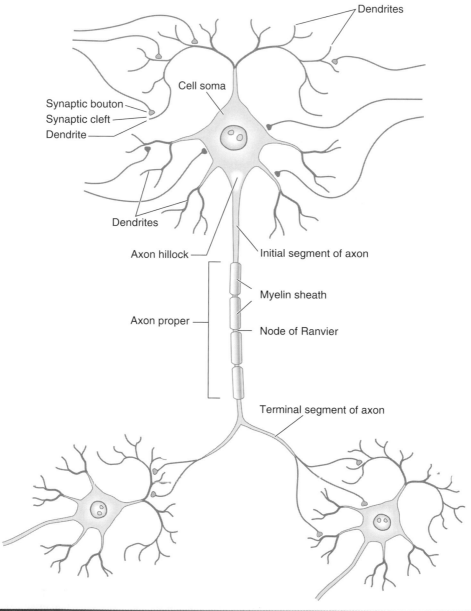

**Figure 2.2   Principal components of a neuron**

The major features and relations of neurons in the CNS of mammals. Dendrites branch close to the soma, while axons branch close to the distal end. One of the principles of neuroanatomy is that information from multiple sources *converges* on a single neuron that, in turn, distributes its information to multiple *divergent* targets.

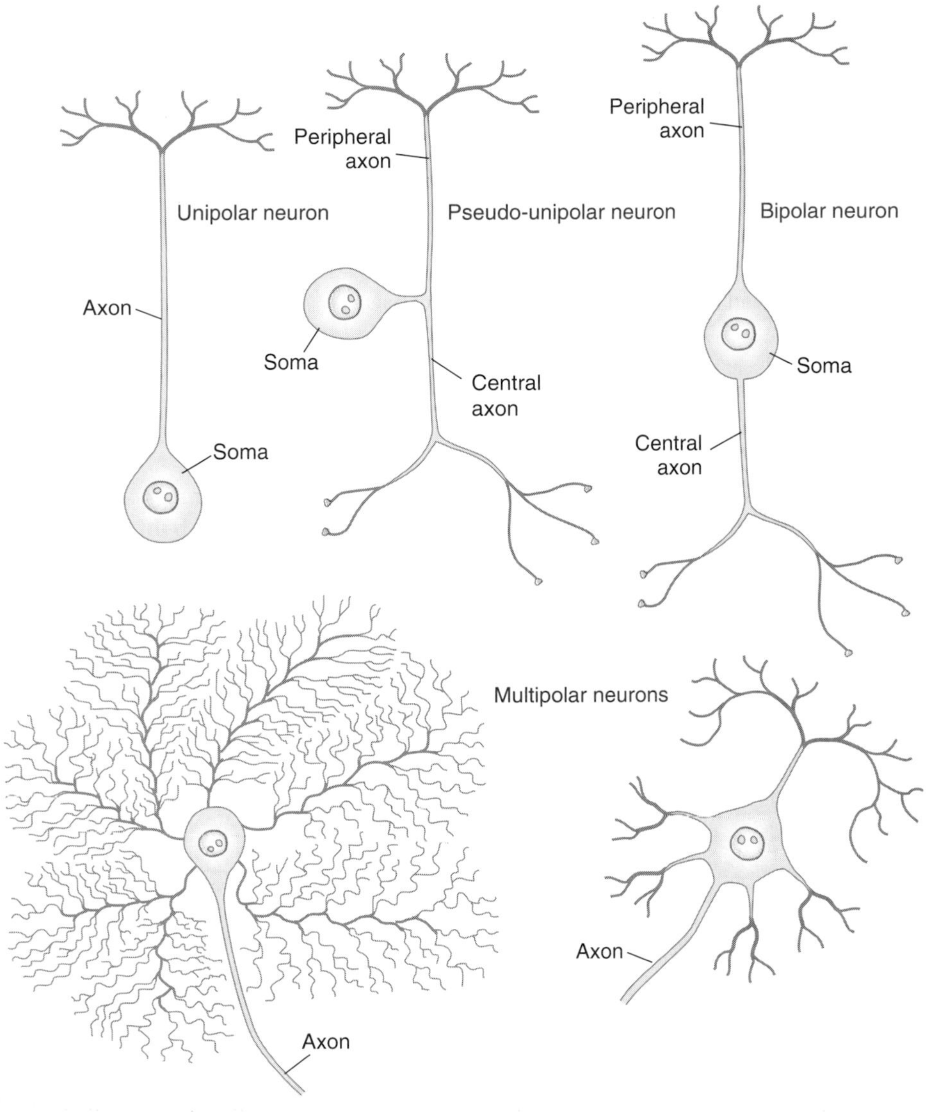

**Figure 2.3 Types of neurons**

Traditionally neurons are differentiated by their number of processes. Pseudounipolar neurons are found in most sensory ganglia. Bipolar neurons are associated only with cranial nerves I, II, and VIII. All other neurons in the mammalian nervous system are multipolar. Multipolar neurons can assume a number of forms.

**The Intracellular Matrix**

The cytoplasm of neurons contains a number of polymeric molecules that constitute the **intracellular matrix**. The principal structures formed by these molecules are **actin filaments**, **neurofilaments** (a subclass of the **intermediate filaments**), and **microtubules**. The intracellular matrix gives the cell its shape and

stiffness. It also provides the mechanisms by which cell growth and motility are achieved. The intracellular matrix also provides the internal network over which molecules and organelles are transported within the cell.

The molecules that constitute the intracellular matrix are dynamic polymers. They can lengthen or shorten simply by adding or sub-

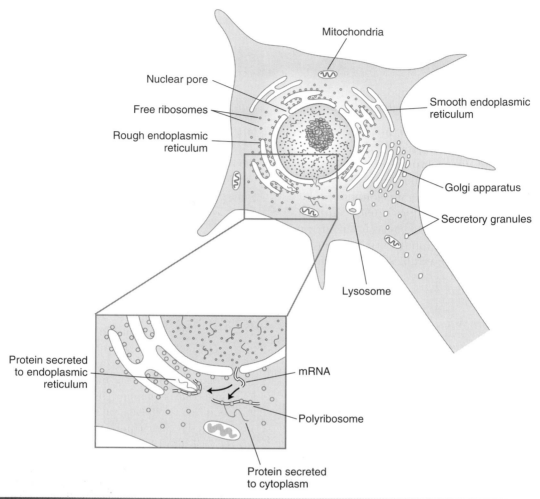

**Figure 2.4    The internal membrane system of neurons**

The internal membrane system of cells is in essence an extension of the extracellular space. The nuclear membrane and the endoplasmic reticulum (*ER*) are a continuous network within the cell. Proteins produced on the ribosomes take one of two routes within the cell. Proteins to be used in cellular metabolism enter the cytosol directly; those destined for export from the cell enter the space between the membranes of the ER. Portions of the ER separate to become the Golgi apparatus, within which proteins are further elaborated. Secretory granules bud off from the Golgi apparatus and migrate to the cell surface, where they may be secreted or in the case of neurons, transported down the axon.

tracting structural elements at either end of the parent molecule (Fig. 2.5). Depending on the balance between addition and removal, the strand extends or collapses its length. In some circumstances new elements can be added at one end of the molecule while others are removed from the opposite end. Known as **treadmilling**, this mechanism propels the structure and is an important source of mechanical energy. The dynamic properties of matrix molecules are important for changing the cell's shape and for cell motility. During growth and regeneration of the nervous system, they account for the extension of the growing axon and for the intracellular transport of macromolecules and organelles.

## ACTIN FILAMENTS

Actin filaments, with a diameter of only 5 to 8 nm, are the smallest of the intracellular matrix elements. An individual actin molecule is a small, globular, asymmetrical polypeptide associated with an adenosine triphosphate (ATP) molecule. The actin molecules poly-merize with the hydrolysis of the ATP to adenosine diphosphate (ADP). As the actin polymerizes, it forms a pair of filaments in a helix (Fig. 2.6). Within the cell actin filaments are closely associated with the cell surface. Through intermediate proteins, they can bind to the cell membrane and are responsi-

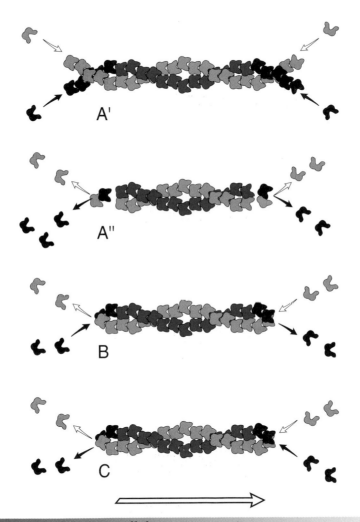

### Figure 2.5   Dynamics of the intracellular matrix protein structure

The intracellular structural proteins—neurofilaments, actin filaments, and microtubules—are polymeric structures built from monomers. The polymerized molecule can be in a state of flux. There are three types of instability: **A.** Dynamic instability occurs when monomer separation and attachment are unbalanced. As a result, the parent molecule rapidly expands (A') or contracts (A"). **B.** True equilibrium is achieved when the rate of monomer separation from the parent molecule is equal to the rate of monomer attachment. The separation and attachment may both occur at either end of the parent molecule, as shown here. **C.** Treadmilling occurs when monomer separation occurs at one end of the parent molecule as monomer attachment is taking place at the other end. The parent molecule maintains approximately the same size during the process but can move through the cytoplasm *(long arrow)*.

ble for developing and maintaining surface irregularities of cells. In neurons the most prominent of these surface irregularities are the **dendritic spines**, mushroomlike protrusions from the main shaft of the dendrite (Fig. 2.7). Actin filaments are particularly abundant in the tips of growing axons, the neural **growth cones**, where they play an important role in the mobility and plasticity of this structure.

## INTERMEDIATE FILAMENTS

The neurofilaments, vimentin-related filaments, and cytokeratin filaments constitute the group of cytoskeletal elements known as intermediate filaments. These subclassifications are based on the chemical nature of the protein forming the intermediate filament strands. Neurofilaments are found in neurons. Vimentin-related filaments are found in astrocytes as **glial fibrillary acidic protein (GFAP)** [G. *glia*, glue]. The cytokeratin filaments are not found in the nervous system but are abundant in epithelial cells. It appears that in all cells the intermediate filaments are the principal elements of the intracellular matrix giving cells mechanical rigidity.

In neurons, neurofilaments are the most numerous intracellular matrix proteins. Like all intermediate filaments, they are approxi-

mately 10 nm in diameter and consist of polymers of linear proteins. The central portion of the monomeric protofilament is an α-helix strand terminated at each end with a nonhelical segment. Pairs of monomers couple along the α-helical region to form a coiled-coil dimer. The dimers in turn align with each other to form a long tetrameric strand. The tetramer is the building block from which the intermediate filaments are constructed. Multiple tetrameric strands align end to end and twist together, much like a hemp rope but hollow, making an extremely strong filament (Fig. 2.8).

Within neurons, neurofilaments form long parallel arrays, especially in dendrites and axons. The parallel arrays are extensively cross-linked by bridges formed by the unusually long carboxyl terminus of the neurofilament monomers (Fig. 2.9). This arrangement gives axons considerable tensile strength. The GFAP filaments in astrocytes are also arranged in parallel arrays but are not so extensively cross-linked (Fig. 2.10). This arrangement imparts considerable firmness to neural tissue.

Normally neurofilaments are aligned in orderly parallel arrays. Under some circumstances this regular organization becomes disrupted. For example, neurofilaments increase in number in cells that have been exposed to

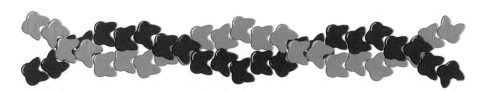

**Figure 2.6   Actin structure**

Actin filaments are composed of two strands assembled from protein subunits. The subunits are asymmetrical, which gives actin filaments directionality that is important in determining its motile characteristics.

**Figure 2.7   Ultrastructure of dendritic spines**

In this freeze-fractured specimen of a dendrite, several spines have been broken off at the neck during the fracture process (*arrows*). One spine (*t*) remains attached to the dendrite. It has a narrow neck and a large bulbous head that is partly hidden below the surface of this preparation. 76,000×. (Reprinted with permission from Peters A, Palay SL, Webster HD. The Fine Structure of the Nervous System. 3rd ed. New York: Oxford University, 1991.)

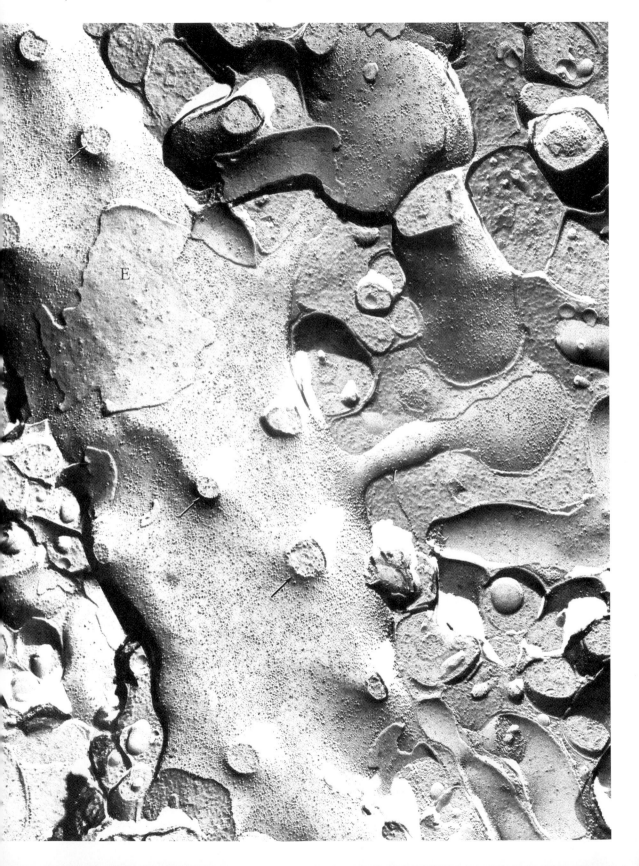

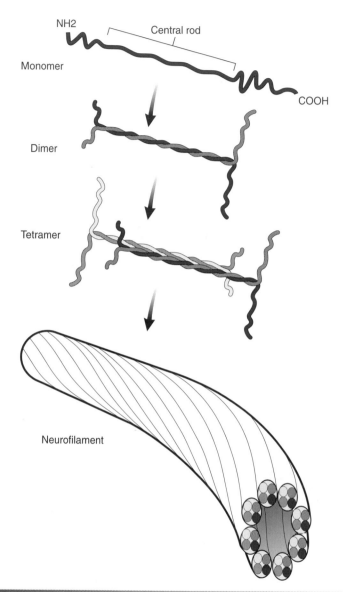

**Figure 2.8    Neurofilament structure**

Neurofilaments are complex structures formed from protofilaments. Pairs of monomer strands twist together at their central rod region to form a dimer. Two dimers align side to side to form a tetramer, the basic structural element of neurofilaments. Dimers attach side to side and twist together to make the fully assembled neurofilament, which is approximately 10 nm in diameter. The carboxyl end protrudes from the neurofilament to form cross-bridges with other matrix elements.

**Figure 2.9    Ultrastructure of neurofilaments and microtubules**

This freeze-etched micrograph of axoplasm illustrates mitochondria (*mit*), vesicles (*v*), microtubules (*m*), and thin neurofilaments (not labeled). Note the numerous cross-bridges (*arrows*) connecting neurofilaments to each other and to microtubules. These cross-bridges are probably the carboxyl end of the neurofilament monomeric strands. Bridges, presumably composed of kinesin, attach a vesicle to a microtubule. 250,000×. (Reprinted with permission from Peters A, Palay SL, Webster HD. The Fine Structure of the Nervous System. 3rd ed. New York. Oxford University, 1991.)

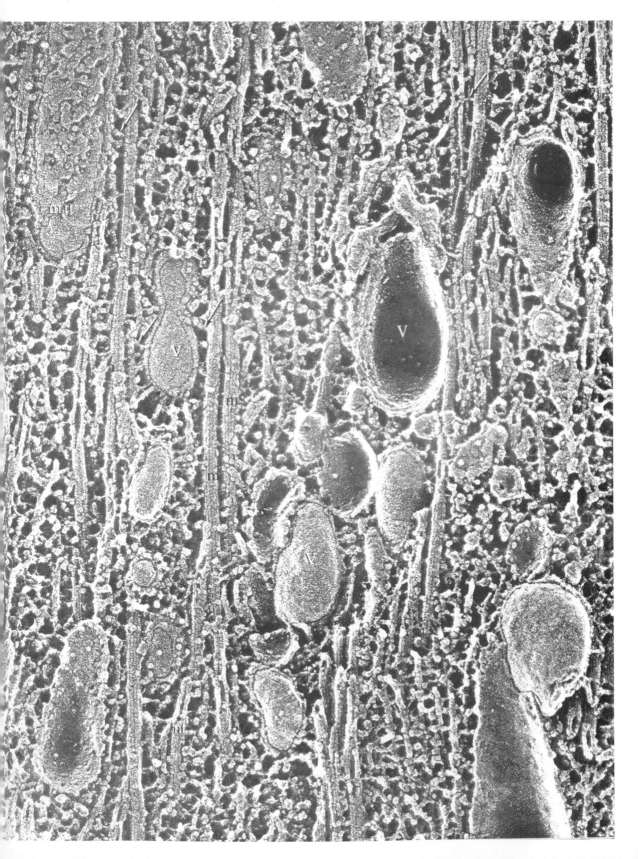

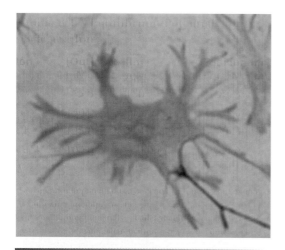

**Figure 2.10    GFAP filaments in astrocytes**

This light micrograph shows an astrocyte grown in cell culture. Antibodies to GFAP, which have a fluorescent tag, are attached to the filaments. The fluorescent tag emits visible light when illuminated with ultraviolet light, rendering the GFAP filaments visible.

aluminum salts, and they sometimes form dense, disorganized filamentous tangles. These knots of neurofilaments superficially resemble the intracellular neurofibrillary tangles that are one characteristic of Alzheimer's disease. Similarly disorganized neurofibrillary tangles are seen in neurons of patients with Down's syndrome and in some types of parkinsonism. These findings suggest that disorders of the intracellular matrix may play an important role in some neurodegenerative diseases.

## MICROTUBULES

The microtubules are the largest of the intracellular matrix proteins (Fig. 2.11). These complex structures are abundant in all cells. Each microtubule is formed by a hollow circular arrangement of 13 protofilaments. Each protofilament is assembled from alternating molecular subunits, α- and β-**tubulin**. Since the tubulin subunits are asymmetrical, the protofilaments formed from them are polar molecules. The protofilaments assemble in a strictly parallel mode so that the resulting microtubule is also polar. The so-called head end of the molecule is much more labile than

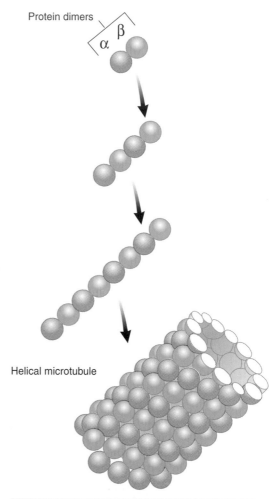

**Figure 2.11    Microtubule structure**

Microtubules are formed from parallel strands composed of alternating protein dimers (the α- and β-subunits). Thirteen strands are assembled to form the final tubular structure. Dimers can be added or removed primarily from the head end.

the tail, a property that gives directional growth to the molecule as it is assembled or disassembled. The assembled microtubule is about 25 nm in diameter and can be as long as 100 μm.

In most cells, microtubules are associated with the centrosome and are closely associated with the movement of internal cellular structures, especially during mitosis. Because mature neurons do not divide, neuronal microtubules are associated with more specialized functions. For example, microtubules form the kinocilia of specialized sensory cells of the olfactory epithelium and of the vestibular and auditory epithelia (Fig. 10.7). Microtubules also provide rigidity to neurons by cross-linking with neurofilaments and are essential in the transport of macromolecules and membrane-bound structures throughout the soma and along the axon (discussed later).

## Dendrites

Neurons have a number of processes. The most numerous, the **dendrites**, are extensions of the cell body. Large at their attachment to the soma, they branch repeatedly, forming a treelike structure whose shape is characteristic for different classes of neurons. As they branch, their diameter narrows (Fig. 2.3).

At the ultrastructural level, dendrites contain many of the structures commonly found in the soma. At the base of dendrites one usually finds rER and sER. All but the smallest dendritic branches have free ribosomes, mitochondria, microtubules, and neurofilaments (Fig. 2.12).

The principal function of dendrites is to increase the surface area of the cell. Accordingly, most of the synaptic connections received by a neuron occur on the dendrites. This principle is carried to an extreme in some cells, where dendritic spines cover the entire dendritic surface (Fig. 2.7). Numerous synapses occur on these spines. The spines are so important in certain cells of the cerebral cortex that mental function is closely correlated with the number of spines, and hence synapses, on the neurons.

The most characteristic morphologic feature of a multipolar neuron is the arrangement of its dendrites.[1] Considering that the dendrites provide almost all of the surface for synaptic contact from other neurons, it becomes apparent that the extent and diversity of these connections will be largely determined by the physical arrangement of the dendrites. Neurons with a small, compact, and sparsely branched array of dendrites will have few synaptic contacts. The number of cells

that can establish contact with such a sparse dendritic tree will also be limited. Neurons with large, extensively branched dendrites not only receive more synaptic contacts because of the large surface area but also receive contacts from a larger number of neurons due to the spatial arrangement of the tree (Fig. 2.13).

Some cells have odd-shaped dendritic fields (Fig. 2.14). For example, the dendritic arborization of the cerebellar Purkinje cell resembles a palm leaf. It has a large cross-sectional area, but it is thin, so the cell receives contact only from axons traveling perpendicular to its dendrites. Some cells, such as those found in the sensory ganglia, do not have dendrites at all. The synaptic contacts made by such neurons are extremely limited, being constrained to specialized axoaxonic synapses (discussed later).

## Axons

Neurons have a single specialized process called the axon. In general, axons are thinner than dendrites and considerably longer. Most neurons have quite short axons (less than 100 μm), but certain cells, such as motor neurons in whales, have axons as long as 10 m (about 30 feet). A few highly specialized neurons do not have an axon, but these are exceptional in mammals. The axon consists of three regions: (*a*) the **initial segment**, which is the transition zone from the soma to the axon proper; (*b*) the **axon proper**, which is the main extent of the axon; and (*c*) the **synaptic bouton**, which is the swollen tip that constitutes the terminus (Figs. 2.2 and 2.12).

Like dendrites, axons branch extensively, but unlike dendrites, the axons branch primarily at their distal end just before they terminate. Distal branching allows one axon to establish many synaptic contacts with a single cell or a small group of nearby cells (Fig. 2.15). Many axons divide into several major branches as they approach their targets. Each of these major divisions extends to a different group of cells before profusely branching prior to making the final synaptic contacts (Fig. 2.16).

---

[1] Scores of families of neurons have been described according to these patterns, but classification into a useful systematic nomenclature has not been possible.

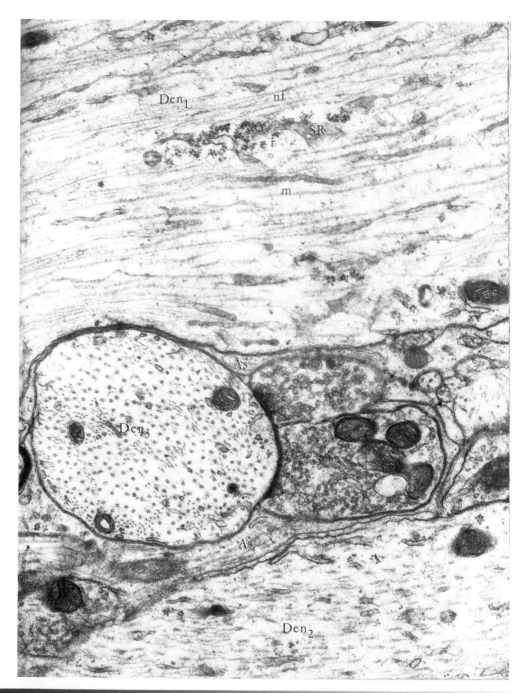

## Figure 2.12. Ultrastructure of dendrites

This electron micrograph shows three dendrites, two in longitudinal section (*Den₁* and *Den₂*) and one in cross-section (*Den₃*). In all three dendrites, neurofilaments (*nf*), microtubules (*m*), smooth endoplasmic reticulum (*SR*), and mitochondria are clearly seen. Free ribosomes (*r*) are also seen in Den₁ and Den₂. Two synapses with active zones make contact with Den₃. The upper synaptic bouton contains small spherical vesicles; the lower bouton contains small oval vesicles. 44,000×. (Reprinted with permission from Peters A, Palay SL, Webster HD. The Fine Structure of the Nervous System. 3rd ed. New York: Oxford University, 1991.)

Because of their great length, axons contain a significant proportion of the cytoplasm of the cell. For example, the average radius of a typical motor neuron soma with its dendrites is about 50 $\mu$m. Its axon would be approximately 10 $\mu$m in diameter and (in the human lumbar spinal cord) would be about 500 cm long. For such a neuron the volume of the soma would be $523 \times 10^3$ $\mu$m$^3$, and the axonal volume (assuming minimal branching) would be $39 \times 10^6$ $\mu$m$^3$, or 75 times the total cell volume. In extreme cases axonal volume can be as much as 10,000 times the cell volume.

## INITIAL SEGMENT

The soma of a large neuron contains a cone of cytoplasm that lacks free ribosomes and rER.

Because it lacks these structures, this area assumes a clear appearance in light microscopic preparations and is known as the **axon hillock**. In this region neurotubules and neurofilaments coalesce into long parallel bundles. They remain bundled for the initial 20 to 50 $\mu$m of the axon length. This portion of the axon is called the **initial segment.** It not only contains bundled neurotubules and neurofilaments but is lined with a dense membrane-associated undercoating of osmophilic material (Fig. 2.17). This undercoating may be the voltage-sensitive sodium gates (see Chapter 3) that are abundant in the initial segment and the internodal region of myelinated axons (discussed later). The initial segment ends at the first segment of the myelin sheath in myelinated axons.

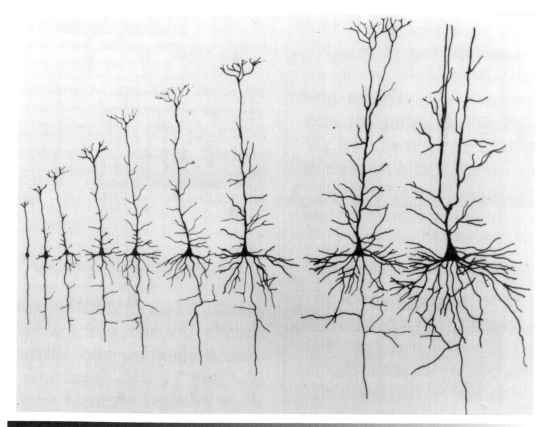

**Figure 2.13. Development of the neuron surface area**

The number of synapses that impinge on a neuron is critical to its function. Arborization becomes more complex during development. Pyramidal cells from humans of various ages are arranged in order, with fetal cells on the left and an adult pyramidal neuron on the right. The number of branches increases dramatically. (Figure courtesy of Dr. Pasko Rakic, Yale University, New Haven, CT.)

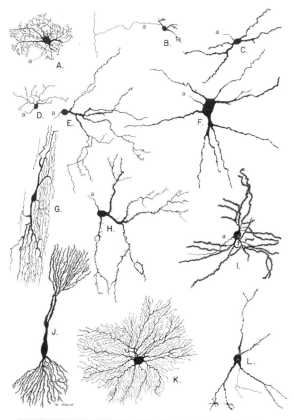

**Figure 2.14 Various shapes of dendritic fields**

(Reprinted with permission from Carpenter MB, Sutin J. Human Neuroanatomy. 8th ed. Baltimore: Williams & Wilkins, 1983.)

### The Axon Proper

The main body of the axon contains the usual collection of organelles, such as mitochondria, microtubules, neurofilaments, and sER. Conspicuously absent from the axoplasm of the main shaft are free ribosomes and rER (Fig. 2.18). Thus the axon does not have the necessary intracellular organelles required to manufacture proteins. These macromolecules must be continuously resupplied from the soma.

Many axons in both the CNS and PNS are covered by the myelin sheath, a dense structure consisting almost entirely of cell membranes layered one upon another with the intervening cytoplasm removed. The glia produce the myelin sheath in the CNS, and

Schwann cells produce it in the PNS. Not all axons are myelinated. However, separation between unmyelinated axons is maintained by intervening glia or Schwann cells. The elaboration and structure of myelin are discussed later.

### THE SYNAPTIC BOUTON

Neurons communicate with one another through **synapses**, specialized structures at the junction of two neurons. The synapse incorporates elements from both the presynaptic and the postsynaptic cell. In most synapses the presynaptic element is the synaptic bouton of the axon. It contains secretory vesicles containing a specific chemical, the **neurotransmitter**, that is released by exocytosis into the extracellular space under certain carefully regulated conditions (Figs. 2.12 and 2.17).

Although most synapses in the mammalian nervous system occur between axons and dendrites, synaptic contact can occur at any region of the neuron. For example, the somas of nearly all cells in the CNS receive synapses from axons. These synapses are appropriately called **axosomatic** synapses. The most common other arrangements are **axodendritic** (axon to dendrite) and **axoaxonic** (between axons) synapses. Dendrodendritic, dendrosomatic, and somatodendritic synapses have been described, although their number and distribution seem to be quite limited (Fig. 2.19).

Although these chemical synapses are the most common type found in mammalian systems, electrical synapses do occur in vertebrates and are quite common in invertebrates. Their neurological importance has yet to be established, and thus they are not discussed here. The mechanisms of chemical synaptic transmission are discussed in Chapter 3.

### The Transport of Proteins

The axon does not contain the intracellular organelles necessary for protein synthesis. Therefore, nearly all of the products of metabolism necessary for cell maintenance must be transported down the axon from the soma. In addition, materials from the environment

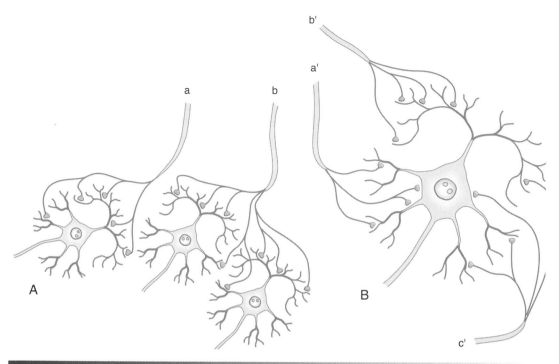

### Figure 2.15   Importance of the size and shape of neurons

The type and amount of information a neuron receives are largely determined by the size and shape of its dendritic field. Several small neurons receive tightly focused information from only a few afferent axons (*a* and *b*) (**A**). A large neuron receives convergent input from several axons (a', b', and c') (**B**).

taken up at axon terminals must be transported to the soma, where they can participate in the regulation of cellular metabolism.

Two transport mechanisms, one slow and one fast, operate in axons (Table 2.1). Matrix proteins and subcellular organelles are carried from the soma to the boutons (anterograde or forward [L. *antero*, in front, and *gradior*, go]) by **slow anterograde axoplasmic flow** [L. *plasma*, form or mold] at rates of 0.2 to 5 mm/day. Secretory proteins are carried away from the soma by **fast anterograde axoplasmic flow** at rates between 50 and 500 mm/day. Various materials are carried from the boutons to the soma (retrograde or backward [L. *retro,* in back]) by **fast retrograde axoplasmic flow** at rates of 200 to 300 mm/day.

### SLOW AXOPLASMIC FLOW

Two components constitute slow axoplasmic flow: slow component A ($SC_A$) and slow component B ($SC_B$). The slower component, $SC_A$, transports materials about 0.1 to 1 mm/day. Somewhat faster, $SC_B$ runs about 1 to 10 mm/day. The matrix proteins, $\alpha$- and $\beta$-tubulin, neurofilament proteins, and microtubule-associated proteins make up about 80% of the materials transported by $SC_A$. Actin, myosin, calmodulin, clathrin, and about 200 soluble proteins, including many cytosolic enzymes, are carried at the faster $SC_B$ rate.

The cytosol of the axon is structurally dynamic; its constituents are continuously being replenished by the matrix proteins freshly synthesized and assembled in the soma and transported along the axon by slow axoplasmic flow. This replenishment is especially evident during growth and regeneration of axons, which proceeds at about 1 mm/day. This rate roughly corresponds to the fastest $SC_A$ rate of axoplasmic transport. Since actin and myosin are carried by the $SC_A$ compartment, it is tempting to speculate that the mobility of the growing axon tip is based on these well known matrix proteins, although the actual mechanisms remain unclear.

## FAST AXOPLASMIC FLOW

Fast transport mechanisms carry the intracellular organelles that have membranes. These organelles include the mitochondria, secretory granules, and other membrane-bound

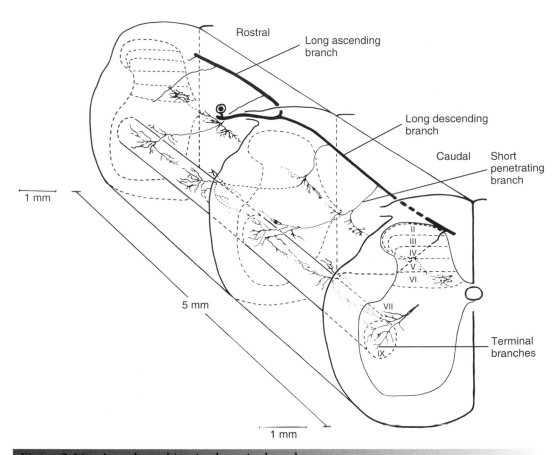

**Figure 2.16   Axon branching in the spinal cord**

This figure shows how a single primary afferent neuron is distributed within the spinal cord. The entering axon bifurcates into a long ascending and descending branch. Each long branch gives off several short penetrating branches that divide extensively, sending terminal branches among the dendrites of the neurons with which they eventually synapse. (Reprinted with permission from Brown AG. Organization of the Spinal Cord. New York: Springer-Verlag, 1981.)

**Figure 2.17   The axon hillock and initial segment**

The axon hillock (*AH*) of the neuron appears pale in the light microscope because of a diminution of Nissl substance. In this electron micrograph of a pyramidal cell, a small amount of rER (*ER*) remains in the axon hillock but does not extend into the initial segment of the axon. Ribosomes (*r*) are also plentiful in the perikaryon, but few enter the initial segment ($r_1$). Microtubules (*m*), neurofilaments, and mitochondria (*mit*) are prominent components. A number of synaptic terminals can be seen making contact with the initial segment ($At_i$). 23,000×. (Reprinted with permission from Peters A, Palay SL, Webster HD. The Fine Structure of the Nervous System. 3rd ed. New York: Oxford University, 1991.)

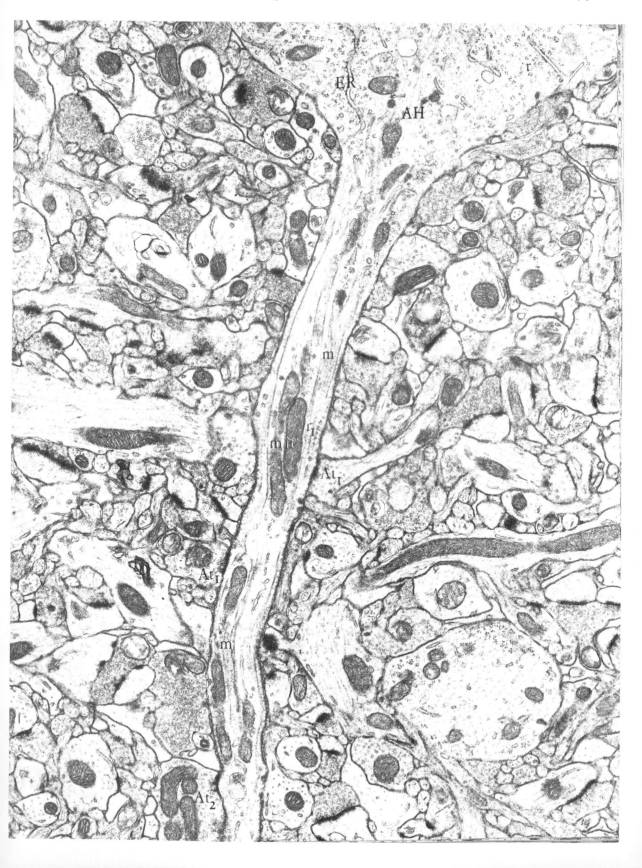

vesicles. The mechanism of fast transport involves two motor proteins, **kinesin** and **dynein**, both of which hydrolyze ATP. One end of these molecules apparently locks onto the organelle membrane. The other end forms temporary bonds to the tubulin of the microtubules and, by sequentially making and breaking these bonds, propels the organelle along the microtubule tracks (Fig. 2.20). Recall that tubulin is asymmetrical, having a head and a tail. Kinesin can move only toward the head end of tubulin, and dynein can move only toward the tail. Since most tubulin is oriented with the head toward the axon terminal, kinesin is responsible for anterograde flow and dynein is responsible for retrograde flow.

## Supporting Cells of the CNS: The Glia

The supporting cells of the CNS are collectively known as glia. Originally, the glia were not recognized as cells but were thought to be an amorphous intercellular matrix in which neurons were suspended. Early histologists coined the term glia because it seemed that this matrix glued the neurons together. The development of silver stains and the electron microscope have demonstrated that the glia are in fact individual cells. In general the glial cells are small but numerous, being approximately 10 times as abundant as neurons.

Three glial cell types are recognized. The most numerous are the **astrocytes** [G. *astron*, star, and *kytos*, hollow (cell)] and **oligodendro-**

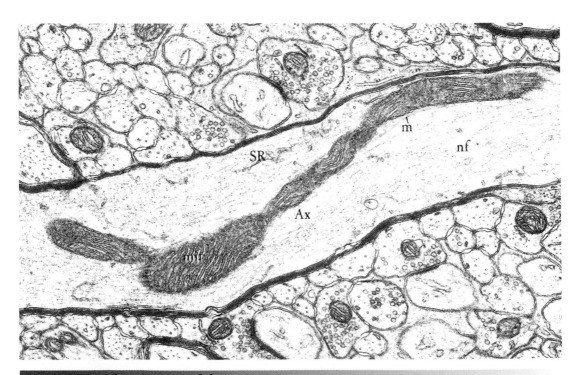

**Figure 2.18  Ultrastructure of the axon proper**

The axon contains numerous mitochondria (*mit*) and neurofilaments (*nf*) but only an occasional microtubule (*m*) and little sER (*SR*). 33,000×. (Reprinted with permission from Peters A, Palay SL, Webster HD. The Fine Structure of the Nervous System. 3rd ed. New York: Oxford University, 1991.)

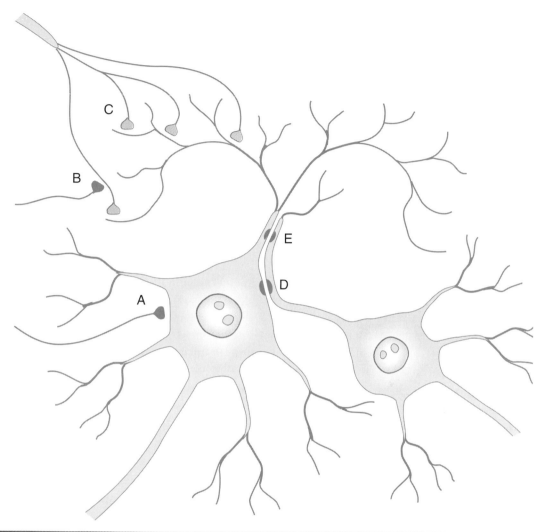

**Figure 2.19   Variety of synapse contacts**

Synapses can be formed between almost any neuronal structures. The most common sites for synaptic contact are between axon boutons and neuron somas (**A**), between two axons (**B**), and between axon boutons and dendrites (**C**). Much less common are synapses between dendrites and somas (**D**) and between two dendrites (**E**).

cytes [G. *oligos*, little]. The **microglia** are relatively rare. Because the microglia do not develop from ectoderm (see Appendix 1), some neuroscientists do not classify them as glia. However, since the microglia play an important physiological role in the nervous system, it is appropriate to consider them as one of the elements of glia (Fig. 2.21).

**Astrocytes**

Under the light microscope astrocytes are seen as star-shaped cells that fill the interneuronal spaces in the CNS. Two forms, **protoplasmic** and **fibrous**, are recognized (Fig. 2.21, *A* and *B*). Protoplasmic astrocytes are found in the gray matter, and fibrous astrocytes are found in the white matter. The names are derived

**Table 2.1   Summary of the Major Components of the Axoplasmic Transport Systems**

| Transport Component | Transport Rate (mm/day) | Transported Substances |
| --- | --- | --- |
| **Slow Transport** | | |
| Anterograde SC$_A$ | 0.1–1 mm/day | Cyoskeletal molecules (actin, myosin, tubulin) |
| Anterograde SC$_B$ | 1–10 mm/day | Soluble proteins and enzymes |
| **Fast Transport** | | |
| Anterograde (kinesin driven) | 50–500 mm/day | Membrane-limited vesicles, mitochondria |
| Retrograde (dynein driven) | 200–300 mm/day | Lysosomes, enzymes |

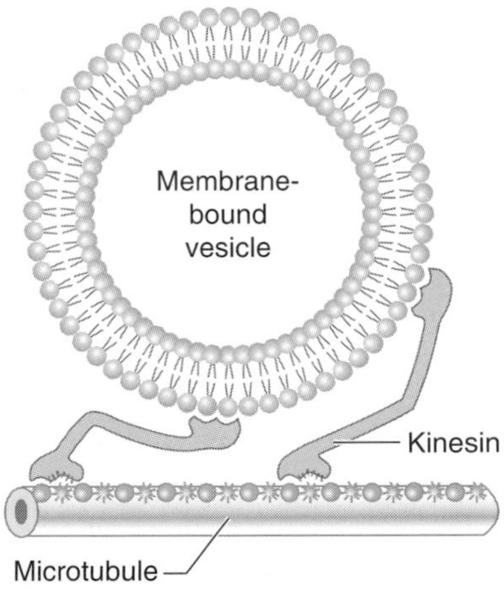

**Figure 2.20   Fast axoplasmic transport mechanism**

This schematic figure shows the presumed relations among the transported organelle, kinesin, and the microtubules. It is thought that the kinesis molecule flexes at a central hinge point and ratchets along the microtubule.

from the presence or absence of cytoplasmic fibers that can be discerned with light microscopy in appropriately stained material. Electron microscopy reveals that both types of astrocytes contain numerous fibrils 8 to 9 nm in diameter. These fibrils, though similar in appearance to neurofilaments, are composed of polymerized strands of **GFAP.** At the ultrastructural level the difference in the amount of GFAP fibrils in the two types of cells is a matter of degree (Figs. 2.22 and 2.23).

Astrocytes fill virtually the entire extraneuronal space in the CNS of mammals. In gray matter their processes are long and sinuous, wrapping around boutons, dendrites, and neuronal cell bodies and filling the tiniest crevasses between neuronal elements (Fig. 2.23). Where astrocytes are in apposition with one another or with oligodendrocytes, they frequently form **gap junctions**. These gap junctions are identical to the nexus of epithelial cells and smooth and cardiac muscle. Astrocytes also envelop capillaries and establish a boundary at the surface of the CNS. Here, astrocytes form a layer several micrometers thick between the pia mater and the neuronal elements, where a basal lamina and collagen are also present (Fig. 2.24). This layer of astrocytes is commonly called the **glial limiting membrane.**

A number of functions have been proposed for astrocytes. Since the GFAP fibrils within the astrocytes makes them fairly rigid cells, they provide gross support for the CNS by rendering some stiffness to the otherwise malleable neurons. Furthermore, astrocytes separate neurons from one another except at the points of synaptic contact. They also serve as reservoirs for potassium ions, buffering the extracellular potassium concentration. The significance of this function is made apparent in Chapter 3.

A special type of glia is important during development of the nervous system. Called **radial glia** because they span the distance between the ependyma and the surface of the developing brain like spokes in a wheel, these

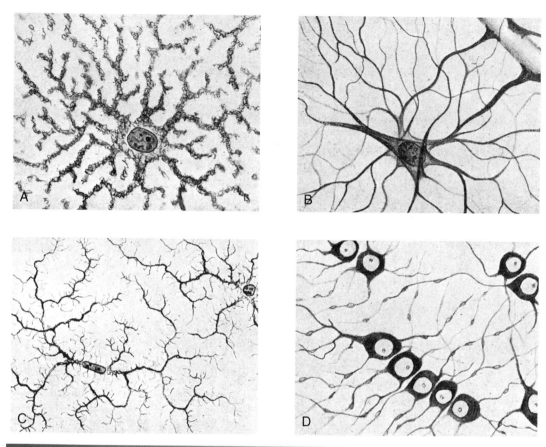

### Figure 2.21  Light macroscopic appearance of glia

The neuroglia are shown as they appear in silver-stained material in the light microscope. **A.** Protoplasmic astrocyte. **B.** Fibrous astrocyte. **C.** Microglia. **D.** Oligodendrocyte. (Reprinted with permission from Fawcett D, Raviola E. A Textbook of Histology. 12th ed. New York: Chapman and Hall, 1994.)

glia play a critical role in early CNS development by providing a pathway along which neuroblasts can migrate (Fig. 2.25). Neuroblasts are formed near the surface of the ventricle and must migrate to the surface, where they are located in the adult. This migration cannot proceed in an orderly manner without a guidance mechanism. Radial glia provide this function. Once the neuroblasts are in place, the radial glial cells differentiate into mature astrocytes.

The path-finding role that glia play during development seems to be lost in the adult mammal. For example, after CNS injury, astrocytes proliferate. They probably partici-pate in the phagocytosis of cellular debris, but more important, they form a glial scar by filling in and occupying the space created by the loss of CNS tissue, especially the loss of neurons. Following injury, damaged neurons attempt to reestablish their former connections by elaborating new axons. These regenerating axons are unable to penetrate this glial scar, and ultimately CNS regeneration fails. However, if an embryonic CNS graft is placed in an adult's CNS wound, the embryonic neurons frequently do survive and establish functional synapses. The embryonic astrocytes seem to play a critical role in this process, but the mechanisms are far from

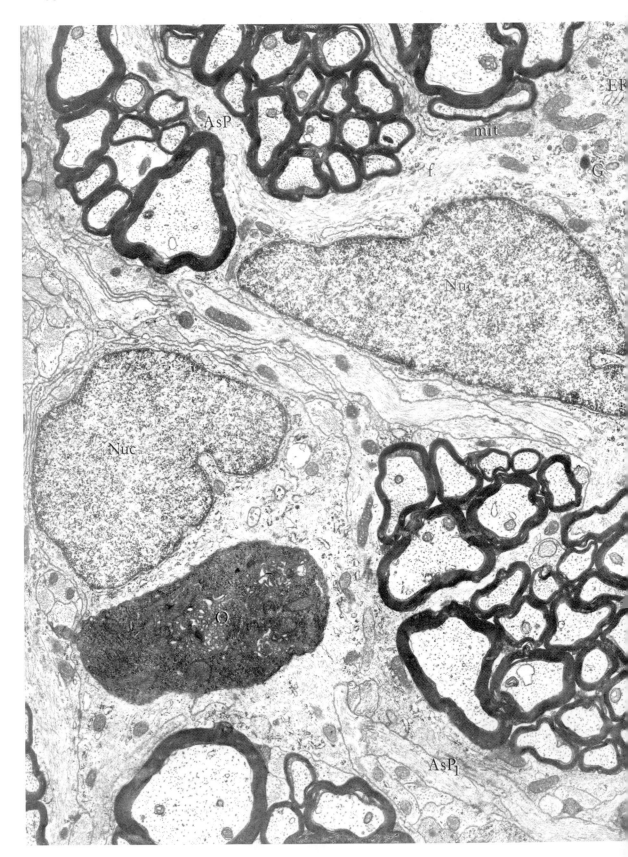

clear. What is clear is that *embryonic astro-cytes are different from mature astrocytes* and that difference is critical to neuronal growth, development, and regeneration.

## Oligodendrocytes

Oligodendrocytes are small glial cells; as their name implies, they have few processes (Fig. 2.21D). They are most commonly found in the white matter of the CNS, but they also exist in the grey matter. Oligodendrocytes produce myelin in the CNS.

## Microglia

Microglia are small cells with a few spindle-shaped processes. Although found in both white and gray matter, in normal tissue they are not abundant in either place. Only about 5 to 10% of the total glia population is composed of microglia (Fig. 2.21C). Microglia are proba-bly macrophages derived from bone marrow. They migrate to the CNS during development, where they become trapped after the blood-brain barrier forms. Microglia express both classes of the major histocompatibility com-plexes, MHC-I and MHC-II, but at much lower levels than do the macrophages in the periph-ery of the body. Despite their relatively weak MHC expression, microglia are probably the principal antigen-presenting cell in the CNS. Their weak expression of MHC may be due to their location within the CNS, where they are protected by the blood-brain barrier and are not stimulated by circulating antigens.

The microglia are normally quiescent but become active in response to antigenic stimu-lation. Once activated, they proliferate and mi-grate to the site of injury, where they bind to antigens by virtue of the MHC molecules on their surface. This antigen-MHC complex is then presented to T cells. Activated microglia also produce the cytokines interleukin I (IL-1) and tumor necrosis factor (TNF-$\alpha$), molecules that facilitate the interaction between T cells and the MHC-antigen complex. In the pres-ence of cytokines, microglia increase their ex-pression of MHC antigens, a positive feedback system that intensifies the immunological re-sponse and T-cell clonal expansion.

Activated microglia also engulf and phago-cytose cellular debris, myelin fragments, and injured neurons. When vascular injury or in-flammation accompanies brain injury, macro-phages from the bloodstream, as well as peri-cytes, invade the neural tissue and participate in the immune response and phagocytotic ac-tivity. *Under these conditions, microglia and macrophages are indistinguishable.* To acknowl-edge this ambiguity, the term *microglia* is usu-ally reserved for the resting microglial cells that are normal members of the ensemble of cells forming the CNS. Cells that respond to brain injury, whether microglia or macrophages, are simply called **phagocytes** [G. *phagein*, eat].

## SUPPORTING CELLS OF THE PNS: THE SCHWANN CELL

The PNS contains only one type of supporting cell, the Schwann cell. It performs all of the basic supportive functions in the PNS that are accomplished by the three types of glia cells in the CNS. For example, the Schwann cell en-closes and separates unmyelinated axons from each other, much as the astrocytes do in the CNS (Fig. 2.26). Like astrocytes in the CNS, Schwann cells reside in the interneuronal space between neuron somas. Like microglia, they can become phagocytes in the presence of inflammation or peripheral nerve injury. And,

**Figure 2.22 Ultrastructure of the fibrous astrocyte**

The large mottled nuclei of two fibrous astrocytes (*Nuc*) here stand in sharp contrast to the dark nucleus of the oligodendrocyte (*O*). The relation between the astrocyte processes (*AsP*) and the bundles of myelinated axons is apparent in the upper left corner of the figure. Numerous parallel fibrils are the most prominent feature of the cytoplasm of the fibrous astrocyte. 17,000×. (Reprinted with permission from Peters A, Palay SL, Webster HD. The Fine Structure of the Nervous System. 3rd ed. New York: Oxford University, 1991.)

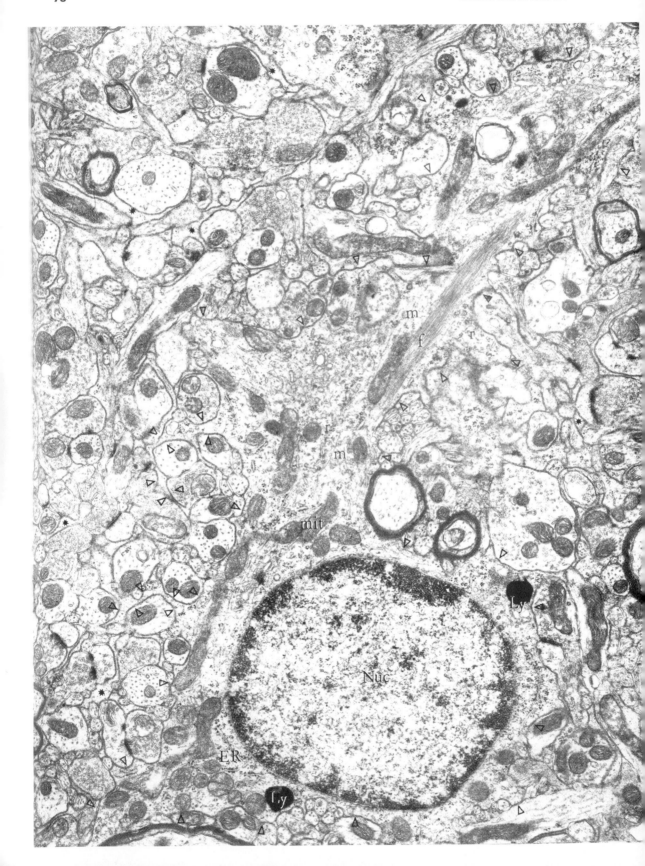

like oligodendrocytes in the CNS, they produce myelin for axons.

Schwann cells secrete **laminin, fibronectin, and collagen,** proteins that are the principal components of the neuronal **basal lamina** and **extracellular matrix.** Unlike the glia, Schwann cells secrete a basement membrane, or basal lamina, that surrounds the cell membrane. The extracellular matrix is found between the axons in nerve trunks, where it is a principal constituent of the epineurium.

Neurons in the peripheral ganglia are surrounded by a single layer of Schwann cells (formerly called satellite cells[2]). Much like the astrocyte in the CNS, they effectively isolate the neuron from the general extracellular environment. This investment of the neuron by the Schwann cells continues outside the ganglion and includes the entire axon. Most of the larger axons are enclosed by myelin, a product of Schwann cells. Unmyelinated axons, however, are simply nestled into a trough in the surface of the Schwann cell (Fig. 2.26). The lips of this trough extend around the axon until they meet to form a complete investment of the axon. By these mechanisms both the myelinated and the unmyelinated axons are isolated from the extracellular environment over most of their surface.

## MYELIN

Myelin [G. *myelos,* marrow], a dense laminated structure consisting of lipids and membrane proteins, is produced by oligodendrocytes in the CNS and by Schwann cells in the PNS. The cells wrap themselves around the axon so that their cell membranes form a multilaminated structure, the myelin sheath. The myelin sheath is arranged in segments along the length of an axon, the segments being separated longitudinally by **nodes of Ranvier** (Fig. 2.27). There are important differences between central and peripheral myelin based on the differences in the ways they are produced.

### Myelin Formation

Peripheral myelin is produced when Schwann cells become associated with bundles of developing axons in the nerve early in the development of the nervous system. Individual axons nestle in furrows along the margin of Schwann cells (Fig. 2.26). As the axons elongate, the Schwann cells associated with them proliferate by mitotic division to maintain a continuous covering for the axons.

As individual axons mature, many of them increase in diameter. When an axon exceeds approximately 1 μm in diameter, it leaves the bundle of immature smaller axons and attracts a number of individual Schwann cells, which begin to envelop it. As a result, a continuous series of Schwann cells becomes associated with a single axon along its entire length. As these Schwann cells mature, each develops a single myelin sheath segment for the axon. *Each Schwann cell produces one segment of myelin for a single axon.*

In the PNS, myelination is initiated when the axon nestles into a crevice of the Schwann cell and is completely enclosed (Fig. 2.28). The apposition of the two edges of the Schwann cell is called a **mesaxon** [G. *mesos,* middle]. One of these edges slides under the other, forming

[2] Satellite cells were originally thought to be an independent cell type. However, they are now recognized to be indistinguishable from Schwann cells.

**Figure 2.23    Ultrastructure of the protoplasmic astrocyte**

The nucleus of a protoplasmic astrocyte (*Nuc*) is characterized by a mottled appearance with condensed nuclear material lining its external limiting membrane. The protoplasmic astrocyte contains numerous filaments (*f*), mitochondria (*mit*), endoplasmic reticulum (*ER*), and occasional lysosomes (*Ly*). The cell insinuates itself between the other cellular elements of the CNS. In this way astrocytes occupy almost the entire extracellular space. The approximate outline of this astrocyte (*thin line* and *arrowheads*) illustrates this remarkable characteristic. 20,000×. (Reprinted with permission from Peters A, Palay SL, Webster HD. The Fine Structure of the Nervous System. 3rd ed. New York: Oxford University, 1991.)

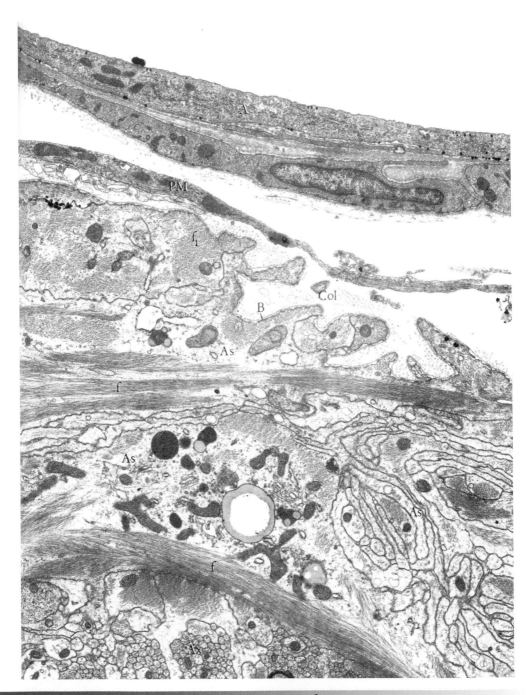

### Figure 2.24    Ultrastructure of the glial limiting membrane

The processes of numerous astrocytes form the glial limiting membrane. The wall of an arteriole (A) appears at the top of the figure with the pia mater (PM) immediately beneath it. A basal lamina (B) lies over the most extreme layer of astrocytes (As), which are conspicuously filled with numerous filaments (f). At the bottom of the figure are a number of small axons (Ax). 15,000×. (Reprinted with permission from Peters A, Palay SL, Webster HD. The Fine Structure of the Nervous System. 3rd ed. New York: Oxford University, 1991.)

an inner and an outer lip. The outer lip contains most of the cytoplasm and the nucleus of the Schwann cell. Current evidence supports the hypothesis that the inner cytoplasmic lip lengthens and slides under and around the outer stationary cytoplasmic lip. As the migration of the inner lip proceeds, the mesaxon necessarily elongates, eventually becoming layered upon itself. The cytoplasm is squeezed out of the diminishing intercellular space between the spiraled mesaxon membranes until only a compact membranous structure remains around the axon. Ultimately the Schwann cell cytoplasm and nucleus are relegated to a small peripheral band lying around the external perimeter of the developing myelin sheath and to cytoplasmic pockets at the edges of the segments of myelin sheath (Fig. 2.28).

The characteristic laminated appearance of the myelin sheath is determined by the asymmetrical nature of the cell membrane. Where the *outer surfaces* of the apposing Schwann cell membranes come in contact with one another at the mesaxon, an **intraperiod line** is formed. As the membranes spiral around the axon and the membranes meet again, the *inner surfaces* of the membranes meet and form a **major dense line**. The intraperiod line (outer surface apposition) appears *lighter* than the major dense line (inner surface apposition) in electron micrographs, giving myelin its characteristic laminated appearance (Fig. 2.29).

In the CNS, oligodendrocytes do not individually attach themselves to single axons during development. Rather, a single oligodendrocyte extends processes to several axons. Each process envelops a different axon and forms one segment of myelin (Fig. 2.30). *A single oligodendrocyte forms one myelin segment on 20 to 60 axons.*

Once an oligodendrocyte process has become associated with an axon, it envelops a mesaxon in essentially the same manner as in the PNS. However, axons of the CNS always have fewer spirals of myelin than peripheral axons of the same diameter. In addition, the cytoplasm of the oligodendrocyte is more completely extruded from the myelin than from myelin produced by Schwann cells. No

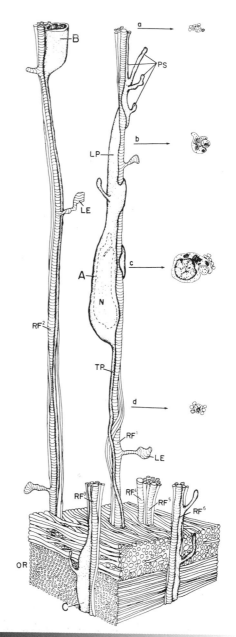

**Figure 2.25   Radial glia**

Radial glia form tracks along which neuroblasts migrate during development. Two radial glia are shown here with neuroblasts in different stages of migration (**A** and **B**). The leading process (*LP*) follows the radial glial fiber (*RF¹*) by sending out exploratory pseudopodia (*PS*). Note the trailing process (*TP*), which will become the axon. (Reprinted with permission from P. Rakic. In: Jacobson, Developmental Neurobiology, Plenum, 1978.)

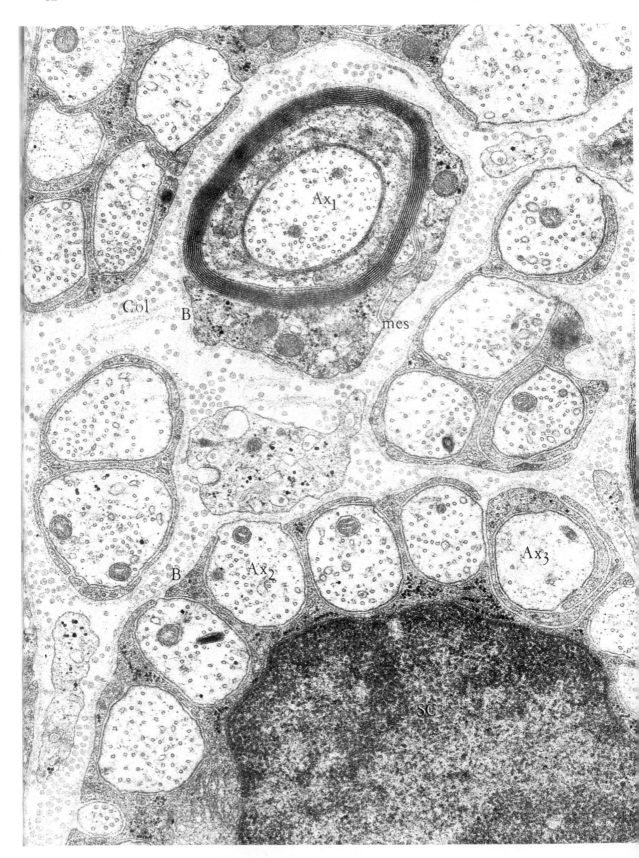

enveloping cytoplasmic blanket surrounds the myelin in the CNS; the remaining cytoplasm is reduced to a thin ridge running along the myelin surface and to pockets at the edges of the segment.

Axons in both the CNS and PNS are myelinated segmentally. The segments meet but do not join at nodes of Ranvier (Figs. 2.27 and 2.31). At the nodes the membrane separates at the major dense line to form a pocket of cytoplasm. There is a pocket at each wrap of the myelin membranes. Since the membrane

forming the myelin structure is continuous, the pockets formed at the ends of each major dense line are also continuous. The pockets spiral from the innermost layer near the axon to the surface of the myelin, where they meet with the cytoplasm of the Schwann cell or oligodendrocyte. Thus cytoplasmic continuity is maintained throughout the cell (Fig. 2.28F).

At the internodal space the axon is more or less directly exposed to the extracellular environment. A dense osmophilic undercoating can be seen in electron micrographs along the

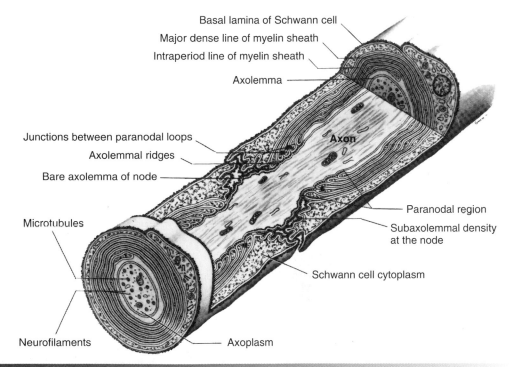

**Figure 2.27   Myelin and the node of Ranvier**

The principal structures of peripheral myelin are illustrated here. In the paranodal region, the Schwann cell cytoplasm is squeezed to the edges of the laminae, forming the paranodal loops. The cytoplasmic pockets in these loops are continuous, spiraling toward the surface, where they merge with the main cytoplasmic mass of the cell. (Figure courtesy of Dr. Kent Morest, University of Connecticut, Farmington, CT.)

**Figure 2.26   Ultrastructure of the Schwann cell**

In the peripheral nerve, a single Schwann cell forms one segment of myelin around a single axon ($Ax_1$). A single Schwann cell envelops a large number of unmyelinated axons. The basal lamina (B) surrounds the external surface of the Schwann cell. When the Schwann cell cytoplasm does not fully enclose an axon ($Ax_2$), the basal lamina extends over it. 48,000×. (Reprinted with permission from Peters A, Palay SL, Webster HD. The Fine Structure of the Nervous System. 3rd ed. New York: Oxford University, 1991.)

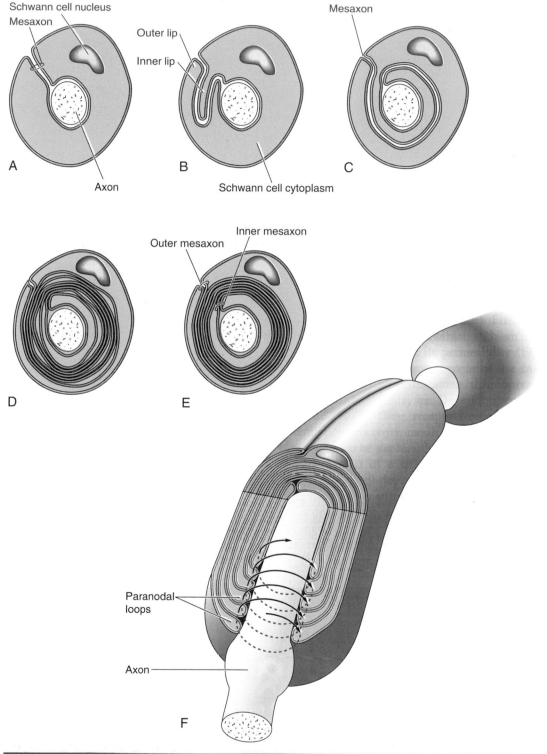

**Figure 2.28  Development of myelin**

The various stages of myelin formation are shown here. **A.** The mesaxon is formed by the apposition of two outer layers of the Schwann (or oligodendrocyte) cell membrane. **B.** The inner lip begins to wrap itself around the axon by invaginating the cytoplasm of the glial support cell. **C** and **D** show further elaboration of the myelin structure. **E.** The final form is achieved (for Schwann cells). **F.** A cross-section and longitudinal section show the paranodal loops.

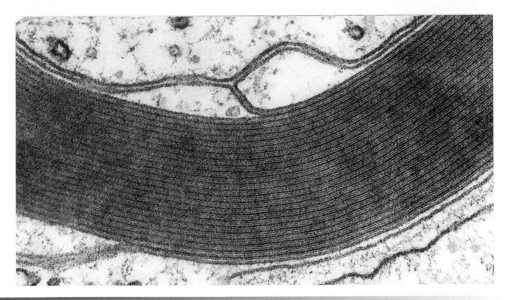

**Figure 2.29    Ultrastructure of myelin**

The relations among the various components of myelin are clearly shown in this electron micrograph. The inner and outer layers of the cell membrane are particularly well preserved. Within the myelin sheath the dark major dense line is formed by the apposition of the *cytoplasmic* side of the cell membrane, and the intraperiod line is formed by the apposition of the *extracellular* side of the membrane. (Reprinted with permission from Coggeshall RE. A fine structural analysis of the myelin sheath in rat spinal roots. Anat Rec 1979;194:201–211.)

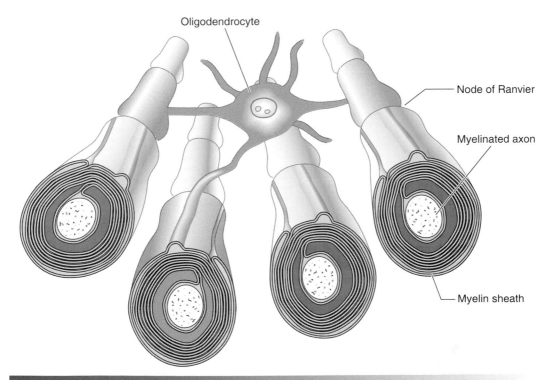

**Figure 2.30    The oligodendrocyte and CNS myelin**

The relation between a single oligodendrocyte and the number of axons it myelinates is shown in this schematic view. Like the Schwann cell, the oligodendrocyte myelinates only a single node on any given axon. Unlike the Schwann cell, the oligodendrocyte myelinates many axons. Myelin maintains its contact with the parent cell body by a long, thin process.

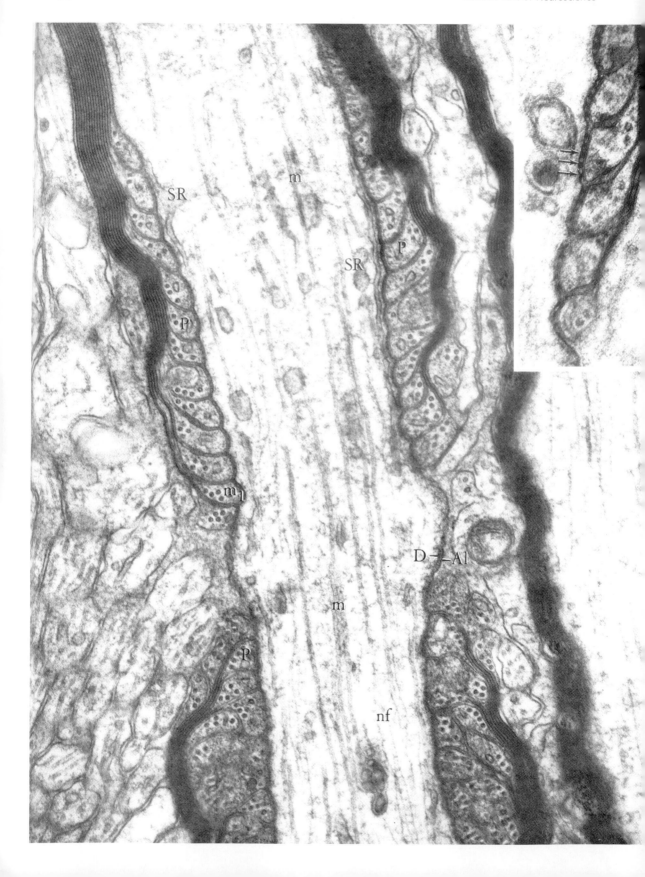

axon membrane at the node. This dense undercoating is similar to the one at the initial segment of the axon (Fig. 2.17). This density, like the density lining the initial segment of the axon, probably corresponds to the voltage-sensitive gates that are characteristic of excitable cells (see Chapter 3) visible in the electron microscope.

## The Chemical Structure of Myelin

Myelin is a chemically complicated structure. Approximately 70% of myelin is lipid, with the remainder composed of several proteins. Most of the lipid is cholesterol and cerebroside. Central and peripheral myelin do not appear to have important differences in lipid content.

Several proteins are important in myelin structure. To date, researchers have cloned seven genes that either produce the structural proteins of myelin itself or participate in regulating its formation. Three proteins are particularly important: **myelin basic protein (MBP)**, **proteolipid protein (PLP)**, and **protein zero ($P_0$)**.

MBP, which is common to both central and peripheral myelin, constitutes about 30% of the total protein in CNS myelin but no more than 18% in PNS myelin. It is a membrane-bound protein that resides entirely on the cytoplasmic face. MBP is essential for the adhesion of the CNS myelin structure at the major dense line (Fig. 2.32). This importance has been aptly demonstrated in certain mutant mice (called "shiverers") that synthesize defective MBP. The small amount of CNS myelin produced in these animals lacks major dense lines, although the intraperiod lines appear normal. Interestingly, the peripheral myelin appears to be normal in these animals even though it contains the same defective MBP.

PLP, a membrane protein found only in central myelin, accounts for about 50% of the myelin protein. It exists mostly on the extracellular surface of the membrane but has both cytoplasmic and intercellular domains. PLP is essential for the adhesion of myelin at the intraperiod line. It links the two intercellular layers together by linking with another PLP molecule from an adjacent membrane (Fig. 2.32).

The PLP gene is also subject to a number of mutations in various mammalian species including the "jimpy" mouse and humans, in whom it is responsible for **Pelizaeus-Merzbacher disease**. This disease is characterized at autopsy by an almost complete absence of CNS myelin but with normal peripheral myelin. PLP is also necessary for the normal development of oligodendrocytes. In both the "jimpy" mouse and humans, mature oligodendrocytes are absent from the CNS at autopsy. Another mouse with a PLP gene defect, the "rumpshaker," produces defective PLP and little CNS myelin but has normal-appearing oligodendrocytes. No human counterpart to the "rumpshaker" mouse has been described.

In addition to Pelizaeus-Merzbacher disease, a number of genetically determined diseases of CNS myelin are grouped simply as **leukodystrophies**. These progressive neurologic diseases are caused by metabolic errors of myelin. Some, like Pelizaeus-Merzbacher disease, are clearly genetic, with a recognized inheritance pattern and a known gene error, but most are simply unclassified; that is, their precise causation is unknown. All are relentlessly progressive and ultimately fatal.

$P_0$ is a membrane glycoprotein found only in peripheral myelin; it accounts for about half of the protein in peripheral myelin. Although it assumes the same role in peripheral myelin that PLP plays in central myelin, its structure is entirely different. Like PLP, $P_0$ is membrane spanning, and most of the mole-

---

**Figure 2.31 Ultrastructure of the node of Ranvier**

At the node of Ranvier the myelin thins as the inner layers terminate in the paranodal loops of cytoplasm (*P*). There is only a short distance between segments of myelin where the axon is exposed to the extracellular space. Here the dense undercoating (*D*) is apparent. 60,000×, inset 100,000×. (Reprinted with permission from Peters A, Palay SL, Webster HD. The Fine Structure of the Nervous System. 3rd ed. New York: Oxford University, 1991.)

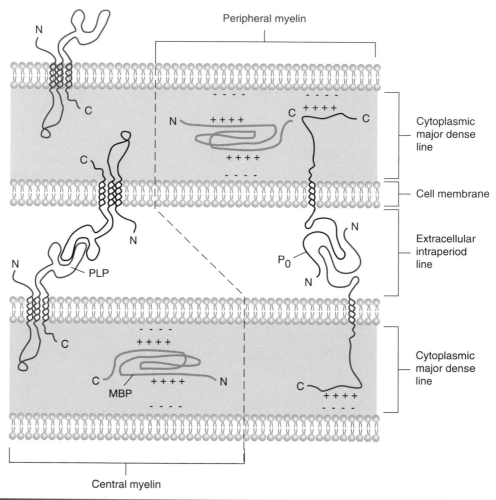

**Figure 2.32    Chemical structure of myelin**

This schematic drawing illustrates the molecular composition of myelin. Myelin basic protein (*MBP*) is common to both peripheral and central myelin and is the major adherent molecule that attaches the cytoplasmic surfaces of the membranes together. PLP is found only in central myelin. Multiple PLP molecules hold the extracellular surfaces together by attaching to sister molecules. $P_0$, the peripheral analog to PLP, holds the membrane together at the intraperiod line by self-adhesion. Self-adherence between $P_0$ also seems to play a role in forming the major dense line.

cule is on the extracellular side. A homophilic cell adhesion protein, $P_0$ plays a critical role in attaching the myelin membranes at the intraperiod line by linking to itself. However, unlike PLP, it also apparently plays a role in forming the major dense line, since peripheral myelin appears to be normal in the absence of functional MBP (Fig. 2.32). In the human, numerous single point mutations of the $P_0$ gene result in Charcot-Marie-Tooth 1b disease. All of these mutations result from a single amino acid substitution on the extracellular side of the $P_0$ molecule. This substitution results in defective membrane adhesion during myelin formation. The resulting hypomyelination causes slow peripheral nerve conduction and other lower motor neuron signs (see Chapters 3 and 6).

## Myelin As an Antigen

Myelin proteins are potent antigens. In rats two important autoimmune diseases can be initiated by immunizing the animals to their own myelin. If central myelin is used as the antigen, **experimental allergic encephalomyelitis (EAE)** develops. This disease is characterized by chronic relapsing episodes of CNS demyelination. Peripheral myelin is spared. Conversely, peripheral myelin can be used to induce a similar disease, **experimental allergic**

neuritis (EAN), which attacks only the myelin of peripheral nerves, leaving the central myelin unscathed. EAE and EAN bear a remarkable resemblance to two human diseases, **multiple sclerosis** and **Guillain-Barré syndrome**, respectively. Although no autoimmune cause has been conclusively established for either of these human diseases, immunological attack is clearly a major component of both disease processes. These important human diseases are discussed in subsequent chapters.

## S U M M A R Y

- **The nervous system is a complex structure that is divided into two regions, the CNS and PNS. This division is based on the cell types found in each region.**

  The CNS contains neurons, astrocytes, oligodendrocytes, and microglia; the PNS is composed of neurons and Schwann cells. In the CNS, neuron axons are myelinated by oligodendrocytes. The axons of the PNS are myelinated by Schwann cells. In the CNS, neuron cell bodies are collected as nuclei, and their axons form tracts. In the PNS, collections of neuron cell bodies are found in ganglia. Their axons and the axons of certain CNS neurons form the peripheral nerves.

- **Neurons are composed of a cell body (soma), dendrites, and a single axon.**

  The neuron soma contains a highly elaborated endoplasmic reticulum, rER, known as Nissl substance. Neurons are highly secretory cells, hence highly energy dependent. Most neurons have a large, highly branched dendritic tree, some with spines, that greatly increases the surface area of the cell. Dendrites, extensions of the soma, contain most of the same intracellular organelles found in the soma. Most synaptic contact is made on dendrites. Axons are thin elongations of the neuron with a specialized terminal called the synaptic bouton.

- **Neurons have an intracellular matrix that is composed of microtubules, intermediate filaments, and actin filaments.**

  The intracellular matrix determines the shape of the cell, provides an intercellular trans-

port mechanism for organelles and macromolecules, and renders some stiffness to the cells. The various filaments of the intracellular matrix are polymers, and subunits are continuously being added or removed from the parent structure.

- **Neurons have an elaborate intracellular transport mechanism that conveys organelles and macromolecules along the length of the axon, a process known as axoplasmic flow.**

  There are two types of axoplasmic flow, slow (0.1 to 10 mm/day) and fast (50 to 500 mm/day). The fast anterograde system, using the kinesis motor molecule, transports membrane-bound intracellular organelles; the slow anterograde system carries soluble proteins and intracellular matrix components. The fast retrograde system, using the dynein motor molecule, carries various materials from the bouton to the soma; there is no slow retrograde system.

- **Axons have three regions: the initial segment, the axon proper, and the terminal bouton.**

  The initial segment of the axon has a surface osmophilic density that probably corresponds to the specialized, voltage-sensitive gates essential for the initiation of the action potential. The axon proper contains most of the cytoplasm of most neurons. Axons branch near the area of termination. There is a synaptic bouton at the tip of each branch. The bouton contains specialized structures necessary for chemical synaptic communication with other cells. Axons can synapse on axons, dendrites, and somas.

- **There are four types of supporting cells in the nervous system: astrocytes, oligodendrocytes, microglia, and Schwann cells.**

In the CNS, astrocytes isolate neurons from one another and help regulate the extracellular milieu; oligodendrocytes form myelin; and microglia become phagocytes during inflammation or CNS infection. The Schwann cells are the only supporting cells in the peripheral nervous system. They perform all of the same functions as the three types of glia cells.

- **Many axons in both the central and peripheral nervous system are invested with a myelin sheath.**

The myelin sheath is segmented, and each segment is produced by a Schwann cell or oligodendrocyte. A Schwann cell produces a single segment of myelin for a single axon. An oligodendrocyte produces a single segment of myelin for a given axon but can form a segment of myelin for as many as 60 different axons. The space between each segment is called a node of Ranvier. The myelin sheath is composed of multiple layers of compacted cell membrane with all cytoplasm excluded from between the layers. A major dense line is formed between the cytoplasmic faces and an intraperiod line between the extracellular faces.

- **Myelin is formed from lipids and several proteins.**

The most important of the proteins are MBP, PLP, and $P_0$. MBP is common to both central and peripheral myelin. It is the principal molecule responsible for the adhesion of the cytoplasmic layers of the cell membranes (the major dense line). PLP is a component of CNS myelin. It attaches the intercellular side of the myelin membranes together, forming the intraperiod line. $P_0$, the corresponding protein for PNS myelin, spans the membrane and participates in adhesion of both the cytoplasmic and intercellular layers.

- **Myelin formation is subject to a number of genetically determined disorders.**

At autopsy these genetic diseases are characterized by severe hypomyelination and when associated with CNS myelin are classified as leukodystrophies. Some genetic diseases are associated with both CNS and PNS myelin.

- **The proteins in myelin are potent antigens, and the differences in the chemical composition of central versus peripheral myelin are important for understanding their immunogenic potential.**

Multiple sclerosis appears to be an autoimmune disease directed against central myelin, and Guillain-Barré syndrome seems to be an autoimmune disease directed against peripheral myelin.

## SUGGESTED READINGS

Alberts BB, Bray D, Lewis J, et al. Molecular Biology of the Cell. 3rd ed. New York: Garland, 1994.

Charcot-Marie-Tooth Disease, OMIM 118200, 1997.

Hall ZW. An Introduction to Molecular Neurobiology. Sunderland, MA: Sinauer, 1992.

Matthews JL, Martin JH. Atlas of Human Histology and Ultrastructure. Philadelphia: Lea & Febiger, 1971.

Myelin Basic Protein, MIM 159430, 1994.

Myelin Protein Zero, MIM 159440, 1997.

Online Inheritance in Man, OMIM. Baltimore: Johns Hopkins University.

Pappas G, Purpura D. Structure and Function of Synapses. New York: Raven, 1972.

Peters A, Palay S, Webster H. The Fine Structure of the Nervous System. 3rd ed. New York: Oxford University, 1991.

Proteolipid Protein, MIM 312080, 1997.

Siegel G, Agranoff B, Albers RW, et al. Basic Neurochemistry. New York: Raven, 1989.

Smith CM. Elements of Molecular Neurobiology. New York: Wiley, 1989.

# 3

# Electrochemical Signaling

Signaling within and between cells is essential for the development and survival of multicellular organisms. In complex organisms the signaling mechanisms are predominantly chemical. Intracellular signaling mechanisms direct the transcription of genes, the translation of proteins, and the distribution of proteins within the nucleus or the cytosol or to the cell surface, from which they may be secreted from the cell. Intercellular signaling mechanisms regulate the activity of adjacent cells through chemical synapses or distant cells by means of hormones. Even the behavior of entire organisms may be manipulated chemically at great distances by pheromones. Chemicals are probably the most omnipresent and diverse signaling mechanisms used by living systems.

The nervous system is the most complex signaling system to evolve from living matter. Neurons, unlike other cells, use two types of signaling mechanisms, chemical and electrical. *The transfer of information from one of these systems to the other allows for complex transformations of information not otherwise possible.* During this transfer, the information content of the signal can be modified; that is, the information is transformed. This modification of information is the mechanism by which the higher-order functions of the nervous system are accomplished. The basic mechanisms of electrical and chemical signaling within and among neurons are discussed in this chapter.

## ELECTROCHEMICAL POTENTIALS

In the mammalian nervous system *electrical signals are represented by changes in potential electrical energy across the neuron cell membrane.* The source of the potential electrical energy is the electromagnetic force[1] associated with **electrical charge.** Charge, as Benjamin Franklin discovered, exists in two forms: positive (+) and negative (−). The electromagnetic force acts on charge, causing like charges to be repelled and opposite charges to be attracted. Therefore, if opposite charges are physically separated, energy is expended and *work is performed on the system.* If these charges are released, they come together, returning to the system the energy that was expended separating them. Therefore, *separated charge is potential electrical energy.* This simple relation is expressed as:

$$\text{energy} = \frac{\text{work}}{\text{charge}} \qquad \text{(Eq. 3.1)}$$

or in the more formal terms of physics:

$$\text{volts} = \frac{\text{joules}}{\text{coulomb}} \qquad \text{(Eq. 3.2)}$$

### Membrane Permeability

To understand electrochemical potentials, one must understand the role that the cell membrane plays in separating charge. The lipid bilayer of the cell membrane is hydrophobic; if unaltered, the cell membrane

---

[1] In physics four forces are recognized: the strong force, the weak force, the electromagnetic force, and the gravitational force. In terms of scientific empiricism, the interactions of these forces and the measurement of their effects (temperature, length, mass, time, and charge) represent reality.

does not allow any hydrophilic substance, including ions, to cross it. The membrane's hydrophobic nature is greatly modified, however, by membrane-spanning proteins. Some of these proteins act as channels through which ions pass. Others act as pumps that actively transport ions (Fig. 3.1).

Ion channels are particularly important in neurons. They are composed of long sequences of amino acids arranged into six membrane-spanning helical domains. Interconnected by linear loops, these six domains aggregate to form a wedge-shaped structure. Four wedges associate to form the completed ion channel, which resembles an elongated doughnut. Like a doughnut, the ion channel has a central pore; through this pore ions can traverse the membrane (Fig. 3.2).

Ion channels are specifically permeable to particular ions; this specificity makes the cell membrane a **selectively permeable barrier.** Ion specificity is conferred by the linear sequence that connects the fifth and sixth helical domains. This linear sequence is folded so that it lies within the central pore of the ion channel. Since each wedge contributes one pore loop, four pore loops are present in a channel. These pore loops bestow the particular ion-selective characteristics on different types of ion channels.

### Single-Ion Systems

To visualize how a selectively permeable membrane allows charge separation to develop in a cell, imagine a hypothetical purely lipid membrane. Such a membrane has no protein channels, so it is impermeable to hydrophilic substances. Suppose that 10 mM of potassium chloride bathes one side of the membrane and 100 mM of potassium chloride bathes the other side (Fig. 3.3A). In each compartment all ions are paired with an electrically opposite partner. Electrical neutrality is maintained on both sides of the membrane. *There is no charge separation and consequently no membrane potential.* In addition, since the membrane lacks protein channels, ions cannot move across the membrane.

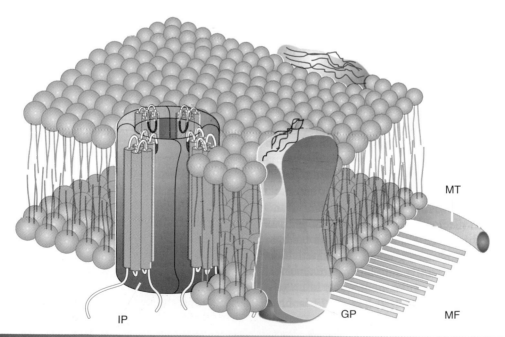

**Figure 3.1   Principal structures found in cell membranes**

The cell membrane's lipid bilayer is a matrix within which a number of other structures, mainly glycoproteins *(GP)*, reside. Ion channels *(IP)* are membrane-spanning proteins that form ion-selective channels through the membrane. Microfilaments *(MF)* are numerous at the internal surface along with a few microtubules *(MT)*.

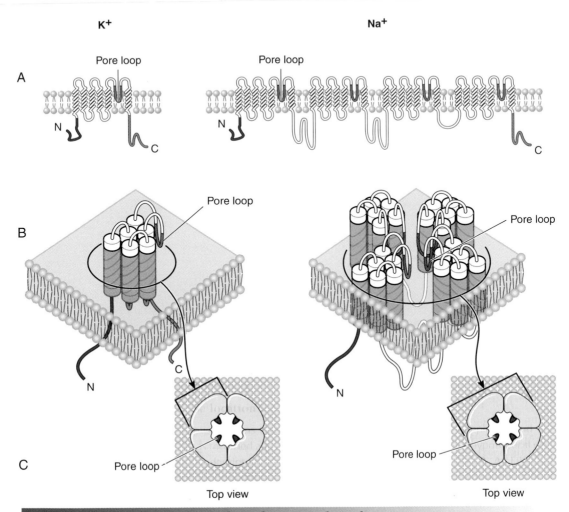

**Figure 3.2   Molecular structure of membrane ion channels**

Voltage-gated ion channels consist of assemblies of seven membrane-spanning segments (**A**). Four separate units aggregate to form the potassium ion channel, whereas the four substructures are synthesized as a single molecule of the sodium ion channel. The pore loop dips into the center of the ion channel (**B**) and gives the ion channel its voltage-sensitive properties. The assembly is shown from outside the cell in (**C**).

If nonselective pores were placed in the membrane, *pairs* of chloride and potassium ions would diffuse down their concentration gradients until equilibrium was established. The ions would move in pairs because the electromagnetic force that attracts opposite charges would hold them together. *Because the ions would move in pairs, electrical neutrality would exist at all times.* There would be no charge separation, and no electrical potential would develop across the membrane (Fig. 3.3B).

If the nonselective pores were replaced with potassium-specific ion channels, an entirely different situation would exist at equilibrium (Fig. 3.3C). Such channels allow only potassium ions to pass, excluding chloride ions. The force generated by the concentration gradient causes potassium ions to diffuse through the membrane channels. However, the chloride ions get stuck in the membrane, since they cannot pass through the potassium channel. With the potassium ions on one side of the membrane and the chloride ions on the

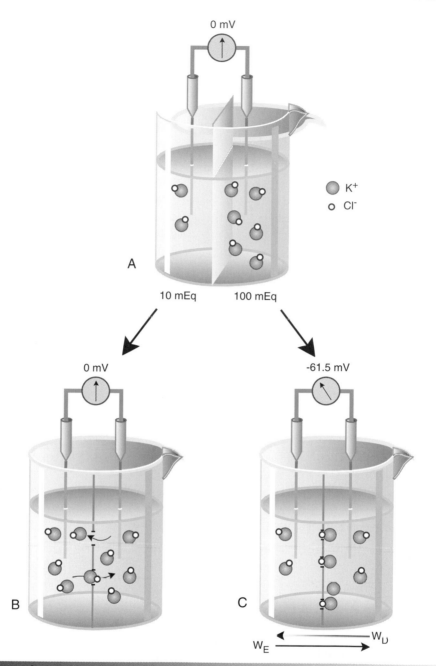

**Figure 3.3  Electrochemical equilibrium**

**A.** Two different concentrations of KCl are separated by an impermeable membrane. No electrical potential can be established across the membrane. Charge is balanced on each side of the membrane. **B.** When separated by a nonselective membrane, the ion *pairs* become evenly distributed on both sides of the membrane. There is no separation of charge, hence no membrane potential. **C.** When separated by a selectively permeable membrane, there is neither electrical nor chemical neutrality. A membrane potential exists across the membrane.

other side, a separation of charge is established across the membrane. One side of the membrane becomes negative with respect to the other. However, in this situation the potassium ions are not completely free to travel down their concentration gradient. The negative charge of the stuck chloride ions attracts potassium ions, restricting their movement.

Equilibrium is established when the diffusion force and the electrical force acting on an ion are equal; the **work of diffusion** is just balanced by **electrical work**. *At equilibrium, a residual concentration gradient and a residual charge separation exist across the membrane.* This phenomenon can be expressed quantitatively. The work of diffusion is equated to the diffusion gradient by the following expression:

$$W_D = RT \ln\frac{[K^+]_{OUT}}{[K^+]_{IN}} \quad \text{(Eq. 3.3)}$$

where $[K^+]_{OUT}/[K^+]_{IN}$ is the concentration gradient for potassium ions, **R** is the gas constant (8.3143 joules/mole degree), and **T** is the absolute temperature. Similarly, electrical work is equated to the separation of charge by:

$$W_E = V_m FZ \quad \text{(Eq. 3.4)}$$

where $V_m$ is the membrane potential measured in volts, **F** is Faraday's constant (96,487 coulombs/mole), and **Z** is the ionic valence.

At equilibrium these two forces are equal. Thus, equations 3.3 and 3.4 can be equated.

$$V_m FZ = RT \ln\frac{[K^+]_{OUT}}{[K^+]_{IN}} \quad \text{(Eq. 3.5)}$$

After rearrangement this equation becomes:

$$V_m = \frac{RT}{FZ} \ln\frac{[K^+]_{OUT}}{[K^+]_{IN}} \quad \text{(Eq. 3.6)}$$

Equation 3.6 is commonly known as the **Nernst equation.** It applies only to simple systems that are selectively permeable to a single ion species. At 37°C, **RT/FZ** reduces to the constant 0.0267 for univalent ions. In our example, the natural log of 10 mM/100 mM is −2.302, which, multiplied by the constant, predicts an equilibrium potential of −61.5 mV. A potential calculated in this way is the **equi-** librium **potential**, or **Nernst potential.** A Nernst potential is useful in determining the direction and magnitude of the forces acting on an ion. A comparison of Nernst potentials for various ions in a system determines the relative forces each ion can contribute to the system.

To establish an equilibrium potential, ion channels must exist for all pertinent ions. For example, if the potassium chloride on each side of the membrane of our hypothetical cell were replaced with sodium and chloride of equal concentration, *there would be no transmembrane potential* because the sodium ions could not pass through a membrane that contains only potassium-selective channels. The sodium and chloride ions would remain paired, and electrical neutrality would therefore exist on both sides of the membrane. For a membrane potential to develop with sodium ions, sodium-specific ion channels must be present in the membrane so that the sodium ions can be separated from the chloride ions.

### Multiple-Ion Systems

In physiological systems the interior and exterior cellular milieu contain many ions, and specialized ion channels exist for many of them. Axons, for example, have channels for sodium and potassium ions. Consequently, each of these ions, considered independently, is associated with an equilibrium potential, and each ion contributes to the resting membrane potential of neurons. Chloride ions do not contribute to the resting potential *in axons*[2] because they behave as if they were passively distributed across the axon cell membrane in response to whatever membrane potential is generated by the other ions. Table 3.1 summarizes the distribution of the physiologically important ions in the mammalian axon and the calculated equilibrium potential for each ion.

The membrane potential actually recorded from a cell is not the result of the action of a single ion. The physiological membrane potential is the sum of the potentials generated simultaneously by all the ions that can

---

[2] Chloride ions are important in the neuron soma and in the synaptic bouton but apparently have no physiological role in the axon.

| Ion | [Out] mM | [In] mM | Equilibrium Potential mV |
|-----|----------|---------|--------------------------|
| K⁺ | 5.5 | 150 | −88.3 |
| Na⁺ | 150.0 | 15 | +61.5 |
| Cl⁻ | 125.0 | 9 | −70.3 |
| Ca⁺⁺ | 100.0 | 0.0001 | +184.0 |
| A⁻ | — | 385 | a |

**Table 3.1  Equilibrium Potentials for Selected Ions**

[a] No equilibrium potential is associated with intracellular anions because they are impermeable.

The equilibrium potentials calculated at 37°C for the most important ions in mammalian neurons are presented here. These data are typical values for cat motorneurons. The concentration of internal calcium is an estimate of free $Ca^{++}$, since most intracellular calcium is sequestered in the smooth endoplasmic reticulum. (Data from Smith CU. Elements of Molecular Neurobiology. New York: John Wiley & Sons, 1989 and Partridge & Partridge. The Nervous System: Its Function and Its Interaction with the World. Cambridge, MA: The MIT Press, 1993.)

permeate the membrane. However, this sum is not calculated simply by adding all of the potentials, since each ion does not contribute equally to the membrane potential.

Consider another hypothetical cell (Fig. 3.4A) that initially has only potassium ion channels in the membrane. Chloride ions are freely permeable, and the ionic environment is given in Table 3.1. This natural environment includes intracellular proteins that carry a net negative charge. Potassium ions are driven out of the cell by the concentration gradient. The expulsion of potassium ions is opposed by the excess negative charge *carried by the cytoplasmic proteins*, which remain within the cell because they are too large to be permeable. Equilibrium develops when enough potassium has been expelled to establish a −97-mV membrane potential as predicted by the Nernst equation. Because they are freely permeable, chloride ions are simultaneously driven out of the cell until the chloride concentration gradient just balances the −97 mV membrane potential.

If sodium channels were also inserted into the membrane, sodium ions would be driven into the cell both by the concentration gradient for sodium and by the negative electrical charge inside the cell (Fig. 3.4B). If sodium ions could cross the membrane as easily as potassium ions, the exchange of sodium for potassium ions would be nearly equal, and the membrane potential would approach 0 mV. Normally, however, the membrane is about 100 times as permeable to potassium as to sodium ions. As a result, sodium ions have only a small—but measurable—effect on the membrane potential.

The effects on the membrane potential of variations in ionic permeability in multiple-ionic systems can be calculated with the **Goldman-Hodgkin-Katz (G-H-K) constant field equation:**

$$V_m = \frac{RT}{F} \ln \frac{p_K[K^+]_{OUT} + p_{Na}[Na^+]_{OUT} + p_{Cl}[Cl^-]_{IN}}{p_K[K^+]_{IN} + p_{Na}[Na^+]_{IN} + p_{Cl}[Cl^-]_{OUT}} \quad \text{(Eq. 3.7)}$$

where the different ionic permeability coefficients are represented by $p_K$, $p_{Na}$, $p_{Cl}$. This equation is essentially an expansion of the Nernst equation for univalent ions; the difference is that it includes permeability coefficients for each ion. The permeability coefficients represent the fraction of the membrane potential contributed by each ion species. Note that the valence term in the Nernst equation is missing. To account for the negative valence of chloride, the ratio is inverted.[3] In mammalian muscle the measured membrane potential is about −90 mV, close to the potassium equilibrium potential of −97 mV and quite close to the value predicted by the G-H-K equation (−89.5 mV) if sodium and potassium are both permeable at a ratio of 1:100. Chloride can be omitted from the equation for the purposes of muscle because there are no selective ion channels for it; chloride is freely diffusable through nonselective channels and therefore assumes a concentration gradient across the membrane in response to the membrane potential established for the other ions.

[3] Recall: $\frac{A}{B} = -\ln\frac{B}{A}$

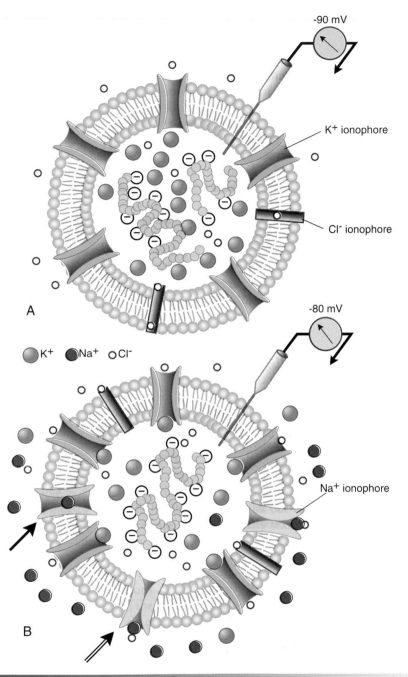

-90 mV

K⁺ ionophore

Cl⁻ ionophore

A

-80 mV

○K⁺  ●Na⁺  ○Cl⁻

Na⁺ ionophore

B

**Figure 3.4  Neuron membrane potential**

**A.** In a typical neuron that is permeable to potassium ions and chloride ions, potassium ions are driven out of the neuron because of the concentration gradient. Anions attached to large, impermeable proteins remain inside the neuron and make the interior negative. Chloride distributes itself passively across the membrane in response to the membrane potential because chloride channels offer essentially no resistance to the flow of chloride ions. The membrane potential is close to the Nernst potential for potassium ions. **B.** The addition of sodium-selective channels to the membrane has little effect on the membrane potential if the channels offer a high resistance to the flow of sodium ions (*double arrow*). The membrane is not totally impermeable to sodium ions (*single arrow*). In typical neurons the ratio of sodium to potassium flow is about 1:100, and the membrane potential is slightly more positive than the Nernst potential for potassium ions.

The absolute number of ions needed to establish the membrane potential is very small. The amount of charge separation needed to establish the membrane potential for an average-size neuron is only about $10^{-17}$ moles of univalent ions. An average neuron contains approximately $10^{-12}$ moles of potassium ions, about 100,000 times as much charge as is necessary to maintain the membrane potential. With such an excess of charge to draw on, *the small potassium and sodium currents associated with membrane potentials do not substantially affect the ionic concentrations within the cell.*

## The Sodium-Potassium Ion Transporter

In contrast to our hypothetical single-ion situation, real neurons exist in a multiple-ion environment. Because the membrane is not perfectly sealed, sodium ions continuously leak into the cell, driven by a large concentration gradient and a substantial electrical gradient (66 mV + −90 mV = 156-mV gradient). Similarly, potassium ions continuously leak out of the cell, because the diffusion gradient is not exactly balanced by the negative electrical potential inside the cell. If allowed to continue indefinitely, these small currents would eventually deplete their concentration gradients and, consequently, the transmembrane potential.

To counteract this slow leakage and therefore establish a steady state, a special transporter mechanism exists in the neuronal cell membrane. This transporter, the sodium-potassium-ATPase pump, is a transmembrane molecule. For every ATP (adenosine triphosphate) molecule it hydrolyzes, three sodium ions are removed from the cell and two potassium ions are inserted. The 3:2 ratio of ionic transport also makes the pump **electrogenic**, since more positive charge is removed from the cell than is returned to it. This property effectively adds about −3 mV to the membrane potential.

The rate at which sodium and potassium ions enter or leave the axon through their respective ion channels is about 100 times the rate at which they can be transported by sodium-potassium-ATPase pump. This dis-crepancy is not normally a problem for two reasons. First, as we shall presently see, the ion channels are open only very briefly, whereas the pump is continuously active. Second, the rate of pumping is partially determined by the membrane potential. The lower the potential (closer to zero), the faster the pump operates. Conversely, as the membrane becomes more polarized (more negative), the pump slows. Over long periods, this pumping action exactly counterbalances the slow, steady leakage of sodium and potassium.

## LOCAL MEMBRANE CURRENTS

The presence of an electrical potential implies that potential energy is available to do work. When that potential energy is released, electrical charge flows down a voltage gradient. The relation between electrical potential energy and current flow is expressed by Ohm's law:

$$E = I * R \qquad \text{(Eq. 3.8)}$$

where the potential electrical energy, **E**, is measured in volts; electrical current, **I**, is measured in amperes; and the resistance to current flow, **R**, is measured in ohms.[4] Resistance to current flow, a property of matter, varies from one substance to another.

The potential differences across the membrane can generate electrical currents. When (*a*) the relation of these currents to the membrane potential is accurately described by Ohm's law and (*b*) the energy is dissipated over short distances, they are called **local currents**.

Two membrane properties affect local currents. These properties, electrical resistance and capacitance, are called **passive properties** because they do not involve any structural (i.e., ion channels) or metabolic (i.e., ion pumps) alterations in the membrane.

Changes in charge across the membrane are reflected in changes in the membrane potential. These changes do not occur instantaneously, however, and the time it takes for the change in charge to be reflected in a change in membrane potential is described by the **time constant** ($\tau$). The changes in charge also do

---

[4] Expressed in this way, Ohm's law is in alphabetical order and easily remembered.

not cause an alteration of the membrane potential throughout the entire neuron. Instead, the membrane potential change is limited to a region very close to the stimulus. This distance is described by the **space constant** ($\lambda$).

## The Time Constant

Stimuli that generate small, rapid changes in membrane current cause similar changes in the membrane potential (Ohm's law), but the membrane potential changes more slowly than the stimulus. This observation seems to conflict with Ohm's law, which states that current and voltage are linearly related. However, membranes have a property known as **capacitance**. A capacitor consists of two conductors separated by an insulator and is used in electrical circuits to store charge. Charge accumulates on one of the conductive plates of a capacitor in proportion to the surface area of the plate, the applied current, and the resistance of the circuit. Opposite charge is attracted to the other plate. Larger plates can accumulate more charge than smaller ones, and circuits with low resistance can deliver charge to the plates faster than circuits with high resistance. Therefore the time required to fully charge a capacitor depends on both the capacitance (i.e., size of the plates, which determines how much charge is needed) and resistance of the circuit (which determines how rapidly the charge can be delivered). This relation is described by the **time constant** and is related to capacitance, $C$, and resistance, $R$, by the following simple expression:

$$\tau = RC \qquad \text{(Eq. 3.9)}$$

*Note that the time constant is independent of the applied stimulus current.* The time constant can be measured as the time required after the stimulus is applied for the potential to change $1 - 1/e$ (where $e = 2.718$), or a change of 63%

from the original steady-state value[5] (Fig. 3.5, A–C).

Membranes have the property of capacitance by virtue of the fact that the hydrophobic lipid portion of the membrane is an insulator that separates two conductive regions, the intra and the extra cellular fluid compartments. They also have resistance. Resistance to current flow through the axoplasm is called **axoplasmic resistance**, and resistance to current flow across the membrane is called **transmembrane resistance.**

The concept of the time constant as it relates to neuron membranes is best understood by considering an experiment in which an unmyelinated axon is isolated in a chamber filled with a balanced salt solution. Two electrodes are inserted into the midpoint of the axon; one electrode records the transmembrane potential and the other stimulates the axon by injecting current (Fig. 3.5A). A resting membrane potential of approximately $-70$ mV is recorded.[6] When a positive charge is instantaneously injected into the axon, the membrane **depolarizes**[7] (its potential becomes less negative) because the positive charge neutralizes some of the excess negative charge inside the axon.

A graph of the change in the membrane potential versus time reveals that the membrane potential changes more slowly than the stimulus but eventually reaches a plateau. When the stimulus is suddenly withdrawn, the membrane potential slowly returns to its original resting level (Fig. 3.5B). These slow changes follow an exponential curve. If several recordings are made, each with an increase in intensity of stimulus, a series of symmetrical membrane responses can be recorded, each showing a characteristic exponential response at the leading and trailing edges of the stimulus with a steady-state region between them. The symmetry of the response is maintained

---

[5] This concept can be confusing. $1 - 1/e = 0.632$ (63%), the change in membrane potential *from its initial state.*

[6] This is a reasonable value for the membrane potential of neurons. The actual membrane potential of a specific neuron is determined by a large number of variables and therefore not readily predicted. Most neurons have a resting membrane potential between $-60$ and $-80$ mV.

[7] It is unfortunate that most authors use the term **depolarize** in this situation. Strictly speaking, a depolarization of the cell membrane implies no separation of charge, hence no voltage across the membrane, which is rarely the case. The correct term, **hypopolarization**, describes precisely the actual event, a *decrease* in the membrane potential. The word depolarize should be reserved for the rare situations in which all membrane polarity is lost. However, since "depolarize" is commonly used for all cases of hypopolarization, it is used here.

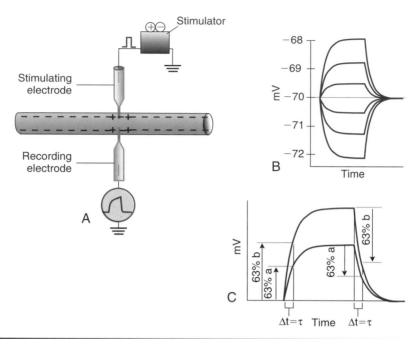

**A.** This figure shows how $\tau$ of a membrane can be measured. A small, rectangular current pulse is injected into the axon with one electrode, and the change in membrane potential is recorded with a different electrode. With good equipment the leading and trailing edges of the stimulus pulse change nearly instantaneously. **B.** The membrane response to stimuli of various strengths is illustrated. The rates of the rise and fall of the membrane response are not as fast as the stimulus (**A**). However, the shapes of the responses are fully symmetrical for stimuli of different intensities and polarities as long as the stimuli are subthreshold for the voltage-gated sodium channels. **C.** The time constant is the time it takes for the response to change to $1 - 1/e$ of the new steady state value. The time constant, $\tau$, is not affected by the intensity or polarity of the stimuli. The time constant varies only with physical properties of the membrane that affect membrane capacitance and resistance.

for both depolarizing and hyperpolarizing stimuli. The independence of the time constant from the stimulus can be demonstrated by measuring the time it takes the potential to change 63% of its initial value for each stimulus intensity (Fig. 3.5*B*).

**The Space Constant**

If we expand our experiment by inserting a series of recording electrodes into the axon at equally spaced intervals on either side of the stimulating electrode, we can determine the membrane potential simultaneously at various distances from the stimulus (Fig. 3.5*D*). Following a stimulus, the membrane responses at each of the recording sites along the length of the axon appear to be roughly the same as the re-

sponse close to the stimulus. However, closer inspection reveals that the farther from the stimulus the recording electrode is, the smaller the amplitude of the steady state response and the slower the rise time. If the *steady state response* is plotted against the *distance from the stimulus,* an exponential decline in the membrane steady-state response is revealed (Fig. 3.5*E*).

Since the axon membrane is not a perfect insulator, some of the injected current leaks across the membrane at sites close to the stimulus. Current also leaks out all along the axon, but in amounts diminishing with distance from the stimulus site (Fig. 3.5*D*). Because of this leakage, less current is available at distant recording sites than at more proximal sites. Some of the electrical energy is also dissipated

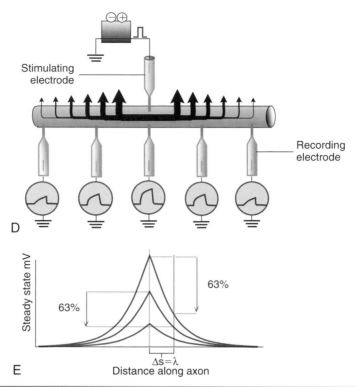

**Figure 3.5    Passive membrane properties—*continued***

**D.** The apparatus used to measure the space constant is the same as that used to measure τ. However, instead of recording the membrane potential at a single point, several recordings are made along the length of the axon. While superficially similar, the steady-state amplitude of the recordings diminish with distance from the stimulus site. Also, the rise and fall times become extended because τ increases with distance from the stimulus site. This increase in τ is due to the accumulation of membrane capacitance along the axon. **E.** The space constant is measured from a graph such as the one illustrated here, where the steady-state amplitude of each response (obtained from **D**) is plotted against distance from the stimulus site. Connecting the data points produces the curves illustrated. Each curve represents the steady-state membrane potential to stimuli of different intensities. The space constant, λ, is defined as the distance from the stimulus where the steady-state membrane potential has fallen by 1 − 1/e of the steady-state membrane potential at the stimulus site. This distance is the same for all three stimulus intensities.

by the resistance of the axoplasm. By Ohm's law, if less current is available, a smaller voltage is observed across a specific resistance. Since the transmembrane resistance for all practical purposes is the same along all parts of the unmyelinated axon, loss of this current results in a smaller observed voltage. *The effect of injecting current at one point in an axon is a steady decline in transmembrane voltage change with increasing distance from the source of the current.*

The measured *distance* from the current source to the point where the steady-state

transmembrane voltage has decayed by 63% of its peak value is λ, **the space constant** (Fig. 3.5E). The previous discussion indicates that if the axon's membrane resistance is increased, less current leaks across the membrane. Therefore, the effect of the stimulus extends farther along the axon, lengthening the space constant. Similarly, if the axoplasmic resistance decreases, for example because of an increase in the diameter of the axon, the space constant also increases because current can flow more easily down the length of the axon. The relation among the space constant, the membrane resistance, $R_m$, and the axoplasmic resistance, $R_a$, is approximately:

$$\lambda \simeq \sqrt{\frac{R_m}{R_a}} \qquad \text{(Eq. 3.10)}$$

The relevance of space constants and time constants to clinical medicine is not apparent to most students. However, the explanation of the way an action potential is propagated along an axon and how information integration occurs in neurons depends on understanding space and time constants. Furthermore, these principles help to explain how demyelinating diseases slow axon conduction and how the loss of synaptic contacts on pyramidal cells leads to dementia. Although space constants and time constants seem to be dry, arcane concepts, they are actually relevant and important to neurology.

## THE ACTION POTENTIAL

The preceding discussion about space and time constants deals only with leakage currents across the membrane, small currents that are generated by the small number of ions continuously passing through the membrane. Electrical signaling in neurons requires a class of ion-selective channels that alter the membrane's specific permeability *as a function of the transmembrane potential.* Such channels are called **voltage-gated channels.** Specific voltage-gated channels have been discovered for sodium, potassium, calcium, and chloride ions. Cells with voltage-gated channels can modulate their transmembrane potential.

The nervous system uses two types of electrical signals. **Action potentials** result from the action of voltage-gated ion channels. **Post-synaptic potentials** result from the binding of chemical ligands to specific receptors on neurons. *The action potential, a transient (less than 10 msec) reversal of the membrane potential, can be brought about by various stimuli. A postsynaptic potential is a longer (15 to 300 msec) alteration of the membrane potential that occurs in response to a chemical messenger. These mod-*

*ulations of the membrane potential are the electrical signals that constitute information in the nervous system.* Every sensation, every motor act, every thought an of organism is encoded by these electrical signals. The nature of the action potential is discussed here; postsynaptic potentials are discussed later in the chapter.

### Voltage-Gated Ion Channels

The tertiary structure of the voltage-gated ion channels is determined in part by the transmembrane voltage. The specific details of the way voltage affects the tertiary structure of ion channels is not known. However, it is well established that the shape of the channel protein is unstable. At resting potentials (about $-70$ mV) it flickers back and forth between two states, one state allowing passage of the ion and the other state preventing passage.

A probability function determines the shape of the protein, hence whether or not the ion channel is open or closed. The probability that the channel will snap from the closed to the open state diminishes as the membrane potential becomes more negative; conversely, it increases as the membrane potential becomes less negative. A second probability function, also a function of membrane potential, determines how long the channel remains in the open state. The less negative the membrane potential, the greater the probability that the channel will remain open once it has opened.

The opening and closing of the channel are nearly instantaneous (not more than 10 μsec) and discontinuous. In other words, the opened or closed state is an **all-or-nothing** phenomenon; there are no intermediate conditions (Fig. 3.6). At the normal resting potential for neurons, about $-70$ mV, the sodium and potassium channels are closed most of the time. When the channel is open, ions for which the channel is selective can cross the membrane, generating an electrical current. Each channel can pass only about $10^7$ ions/second, so the electrical current associated with each channel opening is small (about 2 pA)[8]. The current through an individual channel is determined by how often and how

---

[8]Picoamperes: $1 \text{ pA} = 10^{-12}$ amperes

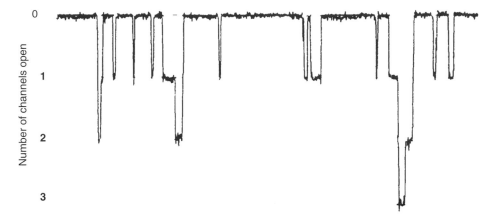

**Figure 3.6   Ion channel activity**

This is a recording of current flowing through as many as three separate ion channels. The ion channels snap open and shut almost instantaneously, and there are no intermediate states (all-or-nothing phenomenon). When more than one channel is open, the currents sum, giving the larger steps seen here. At any given membrane potential a channel flickers between the open and closed state. The time it remains open or shut is determined by a probability function that favors the open state as the transmembrane potential decreases.

long the channel is in the open state; integrated over time, it can be substantial.

## Sodium Current

The sequence of events that results in an action potential begins with any stimulus that causes a depolarization of the axon. If the stimulus is small, the membrane potential rapidly returns to its resting level. If the depolarization is large enough, however, the membrane potential rapidly diminishes to zero, reverses, and reaches a magnitude of about +30 mV. The membrane potential then rapidly returns to a magnitude that is greater than its original resting potential; that is, it becomes hyperpolarized for a brief time before finally returning to its original resting level (Fig. 3.7A).

The action potential is initiated by a small depolarizing stimulus. The depolarization slightly increases both the probability that individual ion channels will open and the average time they will remain open. When a few sodium channels open, sodium ions enter the axon, driven inward by both the sodium concentration gradient and the voltage gradient. This **inward sodium current** brings more pos-

itive charge into the cell, which depolarizes the cell further, increasing the probability that voltage-gated channels will open, which in turn further increases the inward sodium current (Fig. 3.7A; note sodium conductance curve). *When the inward sodium current becomes greater than the outward potassium current, the process is irreversible.* This point is called **threshold**. Once threshold is reached, more and more sodium channels open and the inward sodium current increases rapidly until the membrane potential reverses and becomes inwardly positive.

The opening of the sodium channels, called **sodium activation**, is a *positive feedback system*. In all positive feedback systems, a stimulus evokes a response that acts to reinforce the stimulus. Positive feedback systems must be terminated by mechanisms that are outside the feedback loop. For example, chemical explosions are positive feedback systems terminated by the consumption of the explosive material.

The process that terminates sodium activation is called **sodium inactivation**. The voltage-activated sodium channel behaves as if composed of an activation gate and an inactivation gate. The gates are arranged in series, so

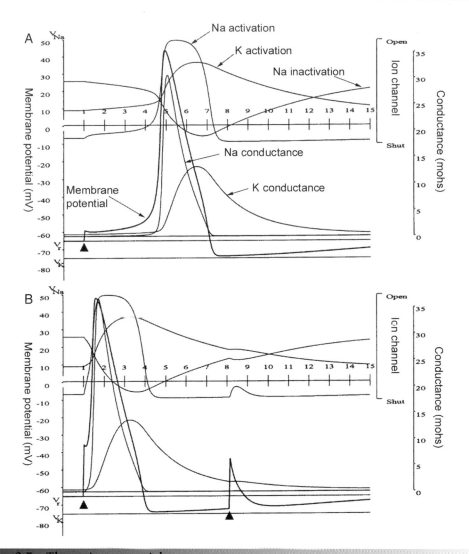

Figure 3.7   The action potential

In 1952 Hodgkin and Huxley published a mathematical model of the action potential. These graphs are a computer-generated solution of their model. **A.** The graphs illustrate the changes in the membrane potential, conductance changes for sodium and potassium ions, and representations of the state of the ion channels shown as sodium activation and inactivation and potassium activation during an action potential generated by a single 100-μA depolarizing pulse at the diamond. Time is in milliseconds. This stimulus is just above threshold. Initially the changes in membrane conductance are slow to develop, but at about 4.5 msec the sodium activation channel opens rapidly, generating the spike phase of the action potential. **B.** Here the axon is stimulated by two pulses of equal strength (500 μA) 7 msec apart. The stimulus, which is stronger than that in **A,** rapidly brings the axon to threshold, and an action potential is generated. The spike and recovery phases of the action potential are essentially identical to those in **A.** The second pulse, although equally strong, is unable to generate an action potential because the axon is refractory. Although the sodium activation channel has fully reset, the sodium inactivation and the potassium activation channels have not returned to their resting states at the time of the second stimulus.

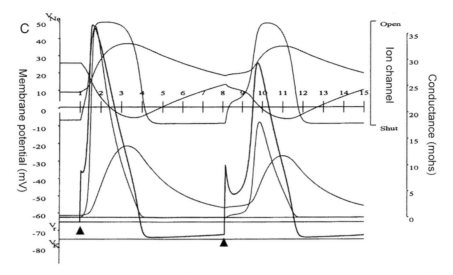

## Figure 3.7  The action potential—*continued*

**C.** The first stimulus is the same as that in **B,** but the second stimulus is set to 700 μA, which is sufficient to generate a second action potential. This graph demonstrates the relative refractory properties of the axon under these conditions. The second spike phase is attenuated with respect to the first action potential. Because the sodium inactivation gate was not fully reset to its resting state, the entry of sodium is reduced, as reflected in the attenuated change in sodium conductance. (Programming by J. Randall, R. E. Kingsley, and D. Turnock).

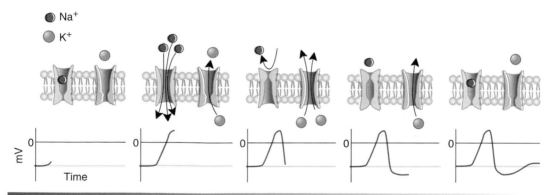

## Figure 3.8  Voltage-gated ion channels

The developing action potential is shown above in the schematic drawings of the gating of the sodium and potassium channels. Note particularly the sequence of sodium activation and inactivation gates.

both must be open for sodium to pass through the channel (Fig. 3.8). At rest the activation gate is closed and the inactivation gate is open, so ions cannot pass through the channel. As the membrane becomes depolarized, the activation gate rapidly opens and the inactivation gate slowly closes (Fig. 3.7, note activation curves). For a brief time both are open simul-

taneously, and sodium flows freely through the channel until the inactivation gate swings shut. Then the activation gate closes, followed by the opening of the inactivation gate.

Within the protein that constitutes the voltage-gated channel, the N-terminal linear chain represents the inactivation gate. It is physically separate from the fourth transmembrane domain, which represents the activation gate. The opening and closing actions are separate but linked processes. They do not act independently, and their opening and closing must proceed in the specific order described here. Consequently, the process that initiates activation cannot be reset until the inactivation is complete.

## Potassium Current

Depolarization also activates voltage-gated potassium channels. The probability that potassium channels will open is less than that for sodium channels for the same amount of membrane depolarization, and the potassium channels remain open longer. This results in a prolonged **outward potassium current** that removes positive charge from the cell (Fig. 3.7; note potassium conductance curve). This outward potassium current increases the membrane potential (makes it more negative), which decreases the probability that potassium channels will open. Consequently, this process is a negative feedback system that is inherently self-limiting. There is no need for a potassium inactivation mechanism.

Because of the difference in the time course of the sodium and potassium currents, the potassium current takes longer than the sodium current to reach its maximum, and it continues longer. Therefore, most of the potassium current flow occurs after sodium inactivation has reduced the sodium current to resting levels. Therefore, during the later stage of the action potential the increased potassium current is unopposed. This drives the membrane potential to a more negative value than its normal resting potential. This **afterhyperpolarization** may last for several hundred milliseconds in some cells.

## The Refractory Period

Once depolarization has reached threshold, it is more difficult to initiate another action potential until the membrane has been fully restored to its resting state. The membrane is **absolutely refractory** to further stimulation after threshold is reached but before the sodium inactivation mechanism is reset. The membrane is **relatively refractory** after the sodium inactivation mechanism is reset and before the end

of potassium activation. During this period the membrane can sustain another action potential, but only if the stimulus is more forceful than that required when the membrane is at rest (Fig. 3.7 *B* and *C*).

Three mechanisms account for the decreased sensitivity of the membrane to depolarizing stimuli during the refractory periods. First, once the sodium activation mechanism opens the channel, it is completely open, and further stimulation cannot open it further. Then, after the inactivation gate closes, no amount of stimulation can make it reopen until the activation gate resets. Sodium ions cannot flow through the channel. Thus the membrane is absolutely refractory to further stimulation.

Second, after the activation gate resets, the inactivation gate remains closed for about 2 msec, making any stimulation during this time ineffective. The opening of the inactivation gate has a long time constant. It does not snap open; it takes about 15 msec to reset completely. During this time it is partially impeding the flow of sodium ions, thereby contributing to the partial refractoriness of the membrane.

Third, the increased potassium current contributes to the relative refractory period. Recall that threshold is achieved when the inward sodium current becomes greater than the outward potassium current. During afterhyperpolarization, the outward-flowing potassium current is greater than normal, so a greater-than-normal inward depolarizing current is required to overcome it and bring the membrane to threshold. This **relative refractory period** lasts as long as the potassium current flow is greater than normal.

## PROPAGATION OF THE ACTION POTENTIAL

The action potential is limited in both time and space. An action potential exists for only a few milliseconds and at any given instant is localized to a few micrometers of the axon. To be an effective signaling device, the action potential must travel from one end of the axon to the other. Therefore, *the action potential must be capable of regenerating itself,* micrometer by mi-

**107**

crometer, in a continuously repetitive manner along the entire length of the axon.

### Conversion of Local Currents Into Action Potentials

At the peak of the action potential the membrane's polarity is reversed: the inside is positive with respect to the outside. This reversal exists over only a small segment of the axon. It results in a separation of charge *along the length of the axon* on either side of the region where the membrane potential is reversed.

This longitudinal charge separation generates local currents along the axon (Fig. 3.9A). The local currents generated by the action potential are depolarizing because positive charge is being delivered to the resting region of the membrane. These depolarizing local currents have very little effect on the proximal, most recently active portion of the axon, since that area is refractory. However, at the distal portion ahead of the action potential, these depolarizing currents can bring that region to threshold, renewing the action potential. In

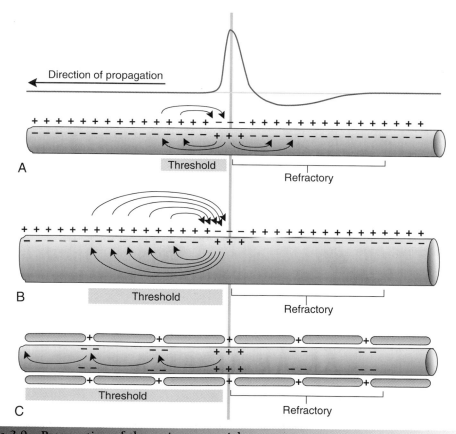

**Figure 3.9    Propagation of the action potential**

Local currents associated with the action potential are depicted for three types of axons. **A** and **B** are unmyelinated axons of different diameters. Because of the reduced axoplasmic resistance in the larger axon, the local currents extend farther down the larger axon (**B**) and are able to depolarize to threshold (*red box below axon*) more of the axon membrane than the local currents in the smaller axon. The axon in **C** is myelinated and the same diameter as the axon in **A**. The local currents can leave the axon only at the nodes of Ranvier. Therefore, the effective transmembrane resistance is increased in myelinated axons, which extends the depolarizing local currents farther along the myelinated axon. The effect of extending the influence of the local currents is to bring larger regions of axonal membrane to threshold and therefore to increase the velocity of propagation of the action potential. The action potential skips from node to node; this is saltatory conduction. Either decreasing the axoplasmic resistance or increasing the transmembrane resistance increases λ.

this manner the action potential regenerates itself. Since the action potential is regenerated de novo and continuously along the entire axonal membrane, *the amplitude of the action potential is not attenuated with distance.* Each patch of membrane sustains the complete action potential at that location and generates local currents that are the stimulus to renew the action potential at the adjacent location.

## Factors Affecting Conduction Velocity

The continuous regeneration of the action potential is a relatively slow process. Action potentials can be propagated up to 120 m/second. In contrast, electrical currents in copper wires travel about 300,000 m/second. Unlike electrical currents in wires, the conduction velocity of action potentials is greatly affected by the physical characteristics of the axon.

Adjusting the physical characteristics in any way that lengthens the space constant also extends the effective range of the local currents farther along the axon. Consequently, the region of depolarization is also extended, bringing a longer segment of the axon to threshold and thereby expanding the distance consumed by the action potential. Since each regeneration of the action potential consumes a greater length of the axon, the conduction velocity is increased. For example, increasing the diameter of the axon reduces the longitudinal resistance of the axon. A reduction in this resistance lengthens the space constant and increases the conduction velocity of the action potential (Fig. 3.9B). The relation between axon diameter and conduction velocity for unmyelinated axons is approximately 0.5 m/sec per $\mu$m.

Many animals use giant axons to increase conduction velocity, particularly the invertebrates, many of whose axons are several hundred micrometers in diameter. Giant axons are maintained at a cost, however, for the efficiency gained in conduction velocity is offset by the inefficiency in volume consumed by these large axons. As a nervous system becomes more complex, more axons are needed to meet the increased demand for information carriers, and volume efficiency becomes a critical factor.

Mammals have the most complex nervous systems, which are noted for their small axons. Mammalian systems typically have axons that range from 0.1 to about 10 $\mu$m in diameter. To achieve relatively fast conduction velocities, the mammals lengthen the space constant by increasing the axon membrane's resistance. The myelin sheath provides this additional membrane resistance because myelin is an effective electrical insulator.

The myelin sheath that envelops most mammalian axons increases the membrane's resistance so much that current leakage across the membrane is reduced to negligible levels. In effect, the only place where current can leave the axon is at the nodes of Ranvier (Fig. 3.9C). Furthermore, unlike unmyelinated axons, in which the voltage-gated channels are strewn along the entire axon, in myelinated axons sodium and potassium channels exist only at the nodes, hence the action potential can exist only at the nodes of Ranvier.

An action potential at a single node of Ranvier establishes local currents that extend along the axon. Typically, the space constant is long enough to include several adjacent nodes, which are all brought to threshold by the depolarizing local currents. Since action potentials are generated only at the nodes, the internodal segments of the axon are simply skipped. This phenomenon is frequently referred to as **saltatory conduction** [L. *salio*, dance, leap]. Myelinated axons conduct at approximately **6 m/Sec per $\mu$m**.

## THE SYNAPSE

Neurons exchange information at specialized structures called **synapses**. This transfer is not a simple process, and it requires special subcellular structures and highly refined physiological mechanisms. The transfer of information is usually one way, from the axon to the target cell. Under some circumstances, however, the transfer may be retrograde, from the cell to the axon. This section provides an overview of synaptic function. The interested student is encouraged to consult more detailed texts and articles in the Suggested Readings list.

In almost all synapses found in mammals, the transfer of information is accomplished by the passage of a chemical messenger from the neuron to the target cell. Neurons can chemically transmit signals in several ways, but not all involve synapses (Fig. 3.10). In **endocrine communication** the vascular system distributes the chemical signal. For example, neurons in the hypothalamus secrete a chemical messenger (hormone) directly into the bloodstream to be distributed throughout the body. **Paracrine communication** is a more restricted form of chemical signaling in which the messenger is distributed locally by diffusion through cells and the extracellular milieu. For example, ni-

tric oxide, a soluble gas, is produced by some neurons. Although highly diffusable, it has a short half-life. Therefore, it affects neighboring cells briefly but cannot be distributed throughout the organism. **Synaptic communication** is even more restricted in its effects because the signaling and the target cell are closely apposed. Diffusion of the chemical messenger is so highly restricted that signaling is usually limited to only one target cell. Synaptic communication is the principal method of intercellular signaling used by the nervous system.

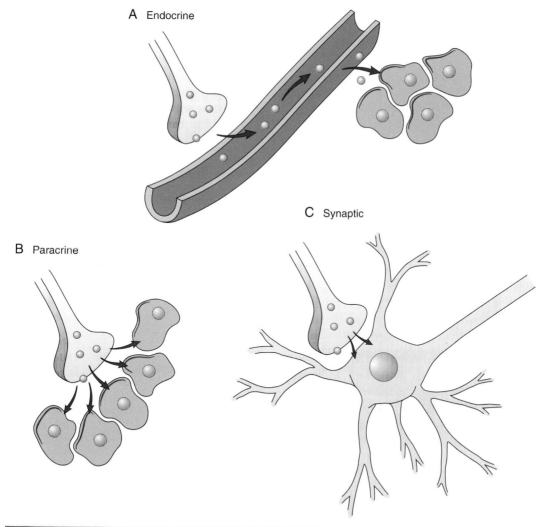

A  Endocrine

C  Synaptic

B  Paracrine

**Figure 3.10  Types of signaling**

**A.** An endocrine chemical messenger is distributed widely via the circulatory system. **B.** A paracrine chemical messenger is distributed locally by diffusion. **C.** A neurotransmitter chemical messenger is distributed only within or very close to the subsynaptic space.

The terminology of chemical messengers can be confusing. A **neurotransmitter** [G. *neuron*, nerve; L. *trans*, across, and *mittere*, to send] is a chemical messenger released at a synapse by a neuron. It binds to a specialized receptor in the target cell. Neurotransmitters are used in both synaptic and paracrine mechanisms. A **neuromodulator** is a chemical messenger that affects the release mechanisms of neurotransmitters or the function of the receptors. Some chemicals act as both neurotransmitters and neuromodulators.

A synapse requires two cells, one presynaptic and the other postsynaptic. Axons from the presynaptic neuron typically terminate in a bulbous structure, the **synaptic bouton**, that forms the presynaptic portion of the synapse. The postsynaptic element is the specialized patch of membrane that faces the synaptic bou-

ton (Fig. 3.11). Neurons make synaptic contact with other neurons, with muscle, and with glands. The structural details common to most chemical synapses are described in the following sections.

### Structures in the Synaptic Bouton

#### SYNAPTIC VESICLES

The synaptic bouton contains a large number of membrane-limited **synaptic vesicles** (Table 3.2). They are 40 to 60 nm in diameter and may have clear or dark centers as seen by electron microscopy. Found only in synaptic boutons, they are formed by endocytotic invagination from the synaptic bouton membrane. Their membranes are unique because they contain special membrane-spanning proteins. Four proteins—SV2, synaptophysin, synapto-

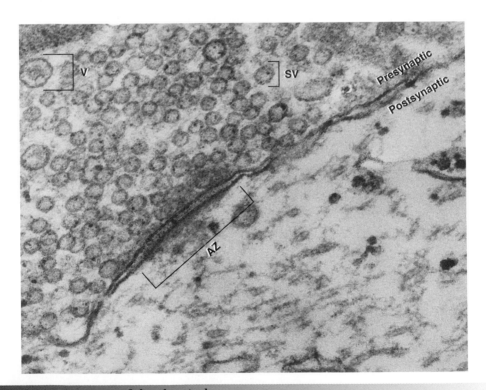

**Figure 3.11   Structure of the chemical synapse**

This electron micrograph illustrates some of the important ultrastructural features of chemical synapses, particularly the active zone *(AZ)*. Here the presynaptic thickening is quite evident, although the hexagonal structure of the docking complex is not shown with the stain used in this preparation. Structural elements can be seen within the synaptic cleft. The postsynaptic thickening is also visible, as are synaptic vesicles *(SV)* and a secretory vesicle *(V)*.

| Table 3.2 Classification of Synaptic Vesicles | | | |
|---|---|---|---|
| Size nM | Type | Appearance | Contents |
| 40–60 | Synaptic vesicle | Clear | Small molecule |
| 40–60 | Synaptic vesicle | Dark | Monoamines |
| 80–150 | Secretory vesicle | Dark | Neuropeptides |

tagmin, and synaptobrevin—have been described, but their exact physiological role is yet to be determined. Synaptic vesicles contain a low-molecular-weight chemical messenger that is rapidly released (about 0.5 msec) following depolarization of the synaptic bouton.

### SECRETORY VESICLES

Most synaptic boutons also contain a small number of **secretory vesicles**. These vesicles are also membrane-limited structures, but they are larger than synaptic vesicles (about 80 to 150 nm in diameter). Secretory vesicles contain peptides that appear dark in electron micrographs. The peptides are assembled in the endoplasmic reticulum–golgi membrane system found in the neuron soma. The secretory vesicles are pinched off from the Golgi apparatus and transported to the synaptic bouton by fast anterograde axoplasmic flow. Consequently, secretory vesicles can be found anywhere along the axon. The membranes of secretory vesicles do not contain the special membrane-spanning proteins found in synaptic vesicle membranes.

### DOCKING COMPLEX

Synaptic vesicles (but not secretory vesicles) can interact with the synaptic bouton membrane at specialized sites that appear in electron micrographs as small, electron-dense patches of membrane (Figs. 3.11 and 3.12). Although seemingly amorphous, these densities are actually a highly structured complex of proteins that forms a hexagonal grid. The size of the grid is matched to the size of synaptic vesicles. The

vesicles are nestled within this hexagonal structure and held close to but do not touch the synaptic bouton membrane. Because the vesicles are lined up like ships at a pier, the grid is known as a **docking complex**. It appears to be present in all chemical synapses.

### Postsynaptic Structures

### THE SYNAPTIC CLEFT

The **synaptic cleft** is a 10- to 20-nm space between the synaptic bouton and the postsynaptic cell (Figs. 3.11 and 3.12). The cleft is filled with 4- to 6-nm filaments that bridge the gap and help bind the two cells together. Both structural proteins and mucopolysaccharides have been identified within the cleft, but their function is uncertain. It is assumed that they play a role in cell recognition during development and may help determine the specificity of synaptic connections.

### THE POSTSYNAPTIC DENSITY

Like the docking complex, the membrane opposite the docking complex appears electron-dense in electron micrographs. This **postsynaptic density** is composed primarily of structural proteins, such as actin filaments and tubulin. Because its thickness is not consistent in all synapses, synapses can be described as either symmetrical or asymmetrical, depending on the relative thickness of the presynaptic and postsynaptic membrane specializations. There is little evidence that consistently correlates the relative thickness of these densities with differences in physiological function. In fact, there is a continuum of relative thicknesses between symmetrical and asymmetrical synapses that blurs this distinction, so classifying synapses in this way is not very useful. Nevertheless, the membrane densities are useful markers, because they indicate the places on cells where information transfer takes place. Therefore, considered together, the presynaptic and postsynaptic densities are called the **active zone** (Fig. 3.11). A single synaptic bouton may have several active zones associated with one or more cells. Neuron somas and dendrites may have tens of thousands of active zones.

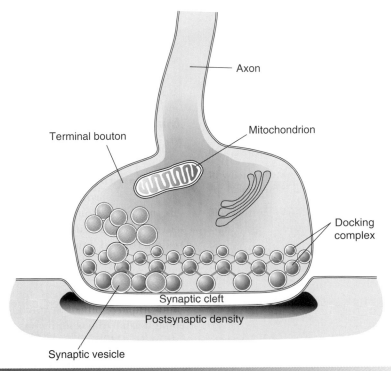

Axon

Terminal bouton

Mitochondrion

Docking
complex

Synaptic cleft

Postsynaptic density

Synaptic vesicle

**Figure 3.12    Docking complex**

This schematic drawing illustrates the synaptic bouton. The vesicles are shown locked into the docking complex but not fused with the presynaptic membrane. (Modified from Shepherd G. The Synaptic Organization of the Brain. 4th ed. New York: Oxford University, 1998.)

## SYNAPTIC TRANSMISSION

Chemical synaptic transmission, the passing of information from one cell to another, is a complex process. First, the action potential envelops the synaptic bouton, causing the synaptic vesicles to attach to the synaptic bouton membrane at the docking complex. Second, the vesicles fuse with the synaptic bouton membrane, releasing the neurotransmitter into the synaptic cleft, where it diffuses to the postsynaptic membrane. Third, the neurotransmitter combines with a receptor protein, initiating a response in the target cell. This response can be a change in membrane permeability or the activation of a second messenger system. Depending on the receptor and the second messenger system, a number of effects can occur, such as a conformational change in an ion channel that alters its specific ion permeability, protein phosphorylation, or the regulation of gene expression.

## Exocytosis of Synaptic Vesicles

The first step in synaptic transmission is the binding of the synaptic vesicles to the synaptic bouton membrane. This step is not easily accomplished because lipid bilayers do not fuse easily. Surface charges on the hydrophilic side of the membrane generate a repulsive force that keeps two membranes from touching, so energy must be supplied to the system to bring the membranes together. Once they are in contact, a hole or separation of the phospholipid molecules must develop before the membranes can fuse. Separating the phospholipids requires more energy. The mechanisms by which these energy barriers are overcome are not fully understood.

When the neuron is at rest, a few synaptic vesicles are held close to the synaptic bouton membrane by the docking complex. When an action potential envelops the synaptic bouton, the resulting depolarization opens **voltage-gated calcium channels**. These channels are probably incorporated into the structure of the docking complex. When these channels open, calcium ions rapidly enter the synaptic bouton very close to the synaptic vesicles. The result of this calcium influx is a very rapid increase in the local concentration of calcium ions (Fig. 3.13) that does not significantly alter their overall concentration in the synaptic bouton.

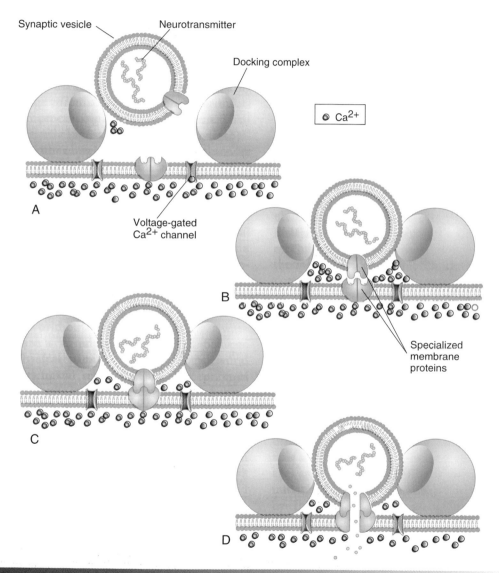

**Figure 3.13   The life cycle of synaptic vesicles**

The steps involved in the binding of synaptic vesicles with the presynaptic membrane are schematically illustrated. **A.** An undocked synaptic vesicle is brought into apposition with the synaptic bouton membrane by contact with the docking complex (**B**), where it is held in place awaiting the arrival of an action potential. This attachment is facilitated by calcium ions. **B.** The action potential opens voltage-sensitive calcium gates. **C.** The local increased concentration of calcium ions facilitates the contact of vesicles with the synaptic bouton membrane, which is facilitated by specialized proteins in the vesicular and bouton membranes. **D.** Once in contact with the membrane, the vesicular and synaptic bouton membranes fuse. This step cannot occur in the absence of calcium ions and may also require specialized membrane proteins as depicted here. Once fusion has taken place, the neurotransmitter is released into the synaptic cleft.

In the presence of this high local concentration of calcium ions, the synaptic vesicles already locked into the docking sites fuse with the synaptic bouton membrane. The calcium ions probably cause a conformational change in the proteins in the vesicular and synaptic bouton membranes that allows them to lock together. After these proteins lock together, the lipid bilayers fuse and the synaptic vesicle opens. The vesicle's contents empty into the synaptic cleft, where they diffuse onto the postsynaptic membrane. Simultaneously, the vesicle membrane is incorporated into the synaptic bouton membrane.

The continued presence of calcium ions in the region of the active zone facilitates the docking of new vesicles. However, calcium must be rapidly neutralized or the newly docked vesicles will immediately fuse with the

synaptic bouton membrane. The inactivation of calcium ions in the synaptic bouton is a complex, multistage process. Initially, the ions simply *diffuse* away from the docking complex. This diffusion prevents further vesicular fusion. After diffusion, the calcium ions are rapidly *sequestered* by cytosolic proteins. Also, special calcium *storage cisterns* in the synaptic bouton have transporter molecules in their membrane that rapidly pump calcium ions out of the cytosol. Finally, a calcium-sodium ion exchange transporter in the synaptic bouton membrane *transports calcium ions out of the synaptic bouton* cytosol into the interstitial space (Fig. 3.14). Calcium ions are exchanged among these systems until the normal intracellular concentration is restored.

The sequestering and removal of calcium ions are slow processes. Under some circum-

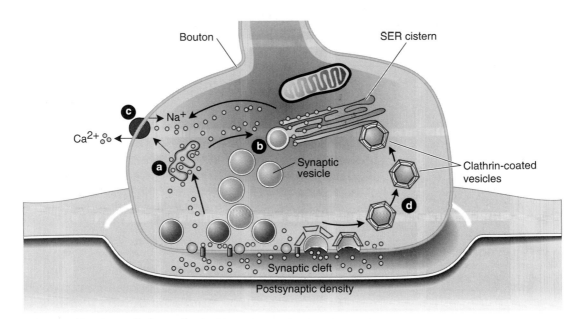

**Figure 3.14   Calcium sequestering and membrane recycling**

Calcium must be removed from the synaptic bouton or vesicle binding, and fusion will continue unabated. Three mechanisms account for this process. First, cytosolic proteins (*a*) can temporarily sequester calcium ions. Second, special transporters exist on the smooth endoplasmic reticulum (*SER*) that remove calcium ions from the cytosol so they can be isolated within the SER (*b*). Calcium ions are stored in the SER, where they can be made rapidly available. Ultimately calcium ions are returned to the extracellular space by special membrane transporters (*c*). Calcium can be exchanged among all three compartments. The vesicular membrane must be recycled. After a vesicle has fused with the synaptic bouton membrane, an invagination forms a clathrin coated pit (*d*). This invagination enlarges and separates as a clathrin-coated vesicle. This vesicle fuses with a cistern of the SER, within which new neurotransmitter is assembled. Synaptic vesicles filled with neurotransmitter separate from the SER and migrate to the docking complex.

stances action potentials can invade the synaptic bouton so quickly that the amount of calcium ions that enter the synaptic bouton is greater than the amount removed. As a result, an increase in the calcium ion concentration in the synaptic bouton causes a temporary increase in vesicle docking. Subsequent action potentials initiate a greater than normal release of the neurotransmitter because more vesicles are available for fusion. This process, called **posttetanic potentiation**, is an important physiological regulator of synaptic function.

## Endocytosis of Synaptic Vesicles

The fusion of the synaptic vesicle with the synaptic bouton is balanced by a system that recovers the vesicular membrane from the synaptic bouton. The first stage in this process occurs when **clathrin** molecules attach to the cytosolic surface of the synaptic bouton membrane. Clathrin is a triskeletal protein; that is, it has three legs. Individual clathrin molecules can interlink to form pentagonal and hexagonal substructures. As more clathrin molecules attach to the substructure, it begins to fold and bend into a ball that resembles a geodesic dome. As the clathrin dome assembles, it expands into the synaptic bouton, gathering a patch of membrane with it, forming a clathrin-coated pit. The pit eventually closes to become a **coated vesicle** within the synaptic bouton. The coated vesicle eventually fuses with a cistern of the smooth endoplasmic reticulum (sER). Within the cistern, the neurotransmitter is synthesized and inserted into pockets of membrane that are pinched off, forming new synaptic vesicles (Fig. 3.14).

## Exocytosis of Secretory Vesicles

The mechanism of exocytosis of secretory vesicles is quite different from that for synaptic vesicles. The primary difference is due to the larger size of secretory vesicles and their lack of specialized membrane proteins. Consequently, they are unable to associate with the docking complex in the synaptic bouton. They must fuse with the membrane directly, which is a more difficult process. Therefore, release of neuropeptides is considerably slower than the release of neurotransmitters. However, because they are freed from the requirement of a

docking complex, secretory vesicles can be released almost anywhere. In electron micrographs, secretory vesicles appear clustered in groups along axons and at the edges of synaptic boutons. They are never seen in association with the docking complex. Since they are not typically released into the confines of the synaptic cleft, neuropeptides are free to diffuse more widely. Thus, release of neuropeptides from secretory vesicles can effect both synaptic and paracrine types of signaling.

Unlike synaptic vesicles, secretory vesicles require a sustained train of action potentials to fuse with the membrane. One consequence of this requirement is that at low frequency stimulation only synaptic vesicles fuse with the synaptic bouton. Following a train of stimuli, both synaptic and secretory vesicles fuse.

Like synaptic vesicle membranes, secretory vesicle membranes are recycled, but the process is not well understood. Recycling probably involves clathrin, but given the large size of secretory vesicles, clathrin cannot form a complete cage around the developing vesicle because the cage structure of clathrin is too small. Therefore, secretory vesicle membrane recycling may occur in fragments, with small patches of membrane pulled from the outer limiting membrane.

## Neurotransmitters

In the nervous system, neurotransmitters are molecules released by neurons that interact with specific receptors located on target cells. Molecules that can interact with target receptors but are not produced or released by neurons are not considered true neurotransmitters. These false messengers, however, are often physiologically significant. These are the characteristics of true neurotransmitters:

1. They are *synthesized* by neurons.
2. They are *present* in presynaptic terminals.
3. They are *released* at the terminal as a result of electrical activity.
4. They *bind to a specific receptor* on the postsynaptic cell.
5. They are associated with a *specific mechanism of inactivation* at the synapse.

Not all substances thought to be chemical messengers in the nervous system meet all of these criteria. To date approximately 20 substances have been sufficiently characterized to be considered neurotransmitters. This list will surely grow.

### Neurotransmitter Inactivation

Once released, the neurotransmitter must be inactivated to limit the duration of its influence. An important characteristic of synaptic systems is the presence of mechanisms for the removal of the messenger (Fig. 3.15). The simplest of all mechanisms is *diffusion*. This passive mechanism is augmented in some cases by a specific *reuptake transporter* either in the synaptic bouton or in the adjacent astroglia. Reuptake has been specifically described for the catecholamines, glutamate, glycine, and γ-amino butyric acid (GABA). Alternatively, the neurotransmitter may be inactivated by *enzymatic degradation*. For example, acetylcholine (ACh) is rapidly destroyed by the enzyme acetylcholinesterase. This enzyme breaks ACh into inactive choline and acetate. Choline is subsequently returned to the synaptic bouton by a specific transporter molecule.

### RECEPTORS

Broadly speaking, there are two classes of receptors that interact with neurotransmitters, **ligand-gated ion channel receptors** and **G-protein–linked receptors.** A **ligand** is a small chemical messenger that binds to a large protein receptor molecule. At the synapse, ligand-gated ion channel receptors undergo a conformational change when a neurotransmitter (the ligand) binds to them. This structural change in the receptor selectively allows ions to pass into or out of the target cell through an ion channel in the receptor (Fig. 3.16A). The resulting altered flow of ions generates local currents, called **postsynaptic potentials**, that alter the membrane potential of the postsynaptic neuron.

The second class of receptors is linked with guanosine triphosphate (GTP) regulatory proteins (**G-proteins**) that float in the lipid membrane. These proteins initiate postsynaptic events by two principal mechanisms. First, the activated G-protein can interact with an ion channel directly to alter its permeability (Fig. 3.16B). Second, G-proteins can initiate a cascade of biochemical reactions that operate through a second enzyme. Depending on the enzyme system, these receptors can alter ion channel conductivity, modify cell metabolism, or regulate gene expression (Fig. 3.16C).

The action of a neurotransmitter on the postsynaptic cell depends on the nature of the receptor. Some neurotransmitters bind to more than one kind of receptor. In such cases a single neurotransmitter can initiate a number of different actions, depending on the receptor

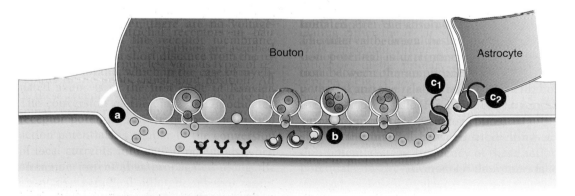

**Figure 3.15   Neurotransmitter inactivation**

Neurotransmitters are inactivated in three ways: by simple diffusion of the neurotransmitter away from the receptors into the intracellular space (*a*); by enzymatic degradation (*b*); and by specific membrane transporters that pump the neurotransmitter back into the synaptic bouton (*c₁*) or into adjacent astroglia cells (*c₂*).

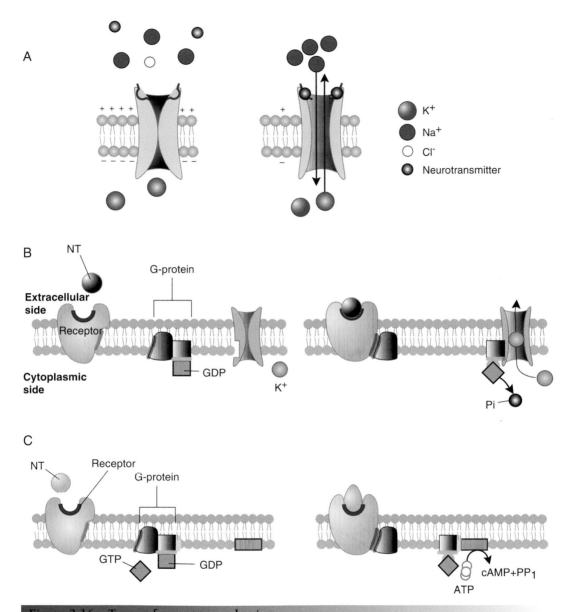

**Figure 3.16   Types of receptor mechanisms**

**A.** Ligand-gated ion channels directly regulate ion permeability. **B.** G-protein-gated ion channels require no intermediate enzyme to affect the ion channel. **C.** G-protein second messenger systems can regulate all aspects of cell metabolism through the action of an intermediate enzyme.

with which it interacts. Consequently, *neurotransmitters may have different effects at different synapses.*

## Ligand-Gated Ion Channel Receptors

In the presence of its neurotransmitter, a ligand-gated ion channel receptor protein opens its ion-selective channel. While the ligand is bound, the channel flickers between the open and closed state (Fig. 3.17), remaining in the open state for only a few milliseconds. The binding of the ligand to the receptor is tenuous, and the probability of dissociation is high. Once the ligand-receptor complex dis-

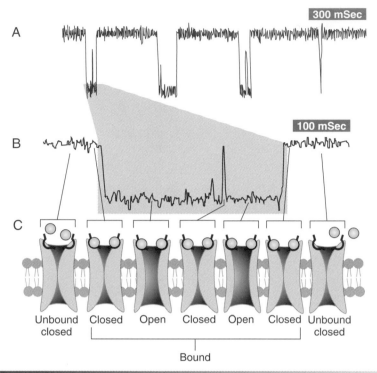

**Figure 3.17   Ligand-gated ion channel**

Many ligand-gated channels, when bound to their neurotransmitter, flicker between the opened and the closed state. **A.** Four separate receptor-ligand associations are recorded from a single channel in the presence of ACh. **B.** During the first association, which lasts 250 msec, the channel briefly closes, even though the ligand is still associated with the receptor. (Patch clamp data kindly supplied by D. Colquhoun, University College, London, and used with permission.) **C.** This schematic representation shows the state of the receptor during the 250 msec it is associated with ACh. (Modified from Hall Z. An Introduction to Molecular Neurobiology. Sunderland, MA: Sinauer, 1992.)

sociates, the channel closes. While the channel is open, ions enter or leave the postsynaptic cell in response to the electrical and diffusion forces acting on them, generating local currents that are recorded as postsynaptic potentials.

The release of neurotransmitter into the synaptic cleft is a quantum phenomenon. Each vesicle, with its cargo of neurotransmitter, is the minimal quantum unit of excitation or inhibition. Each vesicle produces one quantum of postsynaptic current. The integration of multiple quantum events, represented by the release of neurotransmitter from numerous synaptic vesicles, produces a postsynaptic potential (PSP) that extends throughout the entire postsynaptic cell. This PSP is a relatively

brief event, lasting about 15 msec. Its *amplitude*, unlike that of the action potential, is *variable*, and depends on the number of quanta, or packets of neurotransmitter, released at the synapse.

The dynamic behavior of ligand-gated ion channels is more complex than the dynamic behavior of voltage-gated ion channels. The time the channel remains open or closed is determined by separate rate constants for association and dissociation of the ligand-receptor complex. Each rate constant is subject to modification by a number of environmental factors, including other molecules that can attach to the receptor (i.e., neuromodulators). Therefore, the generation of PSPs is more complicated than the generation of action potentials.

The action potential is extinguished at the synaptic bouton. Its information is passed to the postsynaptic cell as the postsynaptic potential. The PSP can either depolarize (excite) or hyperpolarize (inhibit) the postsynaptic cell; that is, either increase or decrease the probability that its membrane potential will be brought to threshold. Neurons continuously receive thousands of PSPs that interact with each other. This interaction modifies the information content of each of the PSPs and ultimately determines the postsynaptic neuron's membrane potential. The following sections examine these issues in more depth.

### EXCITATORY SYNAPSES

One class of ligand-gated ion channels is specific only for cations ($Na^+$, $K^+$, and $Ca^{++}$), and it excludes anions (Fig. 3.16A). Postsynaptic neurons are excited (depolarized) by the activation of cationic channels because local currents are generated that depolarize the postsynaptic cell (Fig. 3.18). These local currents, called **excitatory postsynaptic potentials** (**EPSPs**), are the result of an increase in the transmembrane conductance[9] for cations.

If the conductance of sodium ions and potassium ions were to increases identically, there would be no alteration in the membrane potential because the inward ($Na^+$) and outward ($K^+$) current flows are balanced. However, because potassium is close to its equilibrium potential, only moderate forces drive it out of the cell. Sodium, on the other hand, is driven into the cell both by a strong diffusion gradient and by a substantial electrical gradient. Consequently, sodium conductance increases about 7.5 times as much as the increase in potassium conductance. As a result, more positive charge enters the cell than leaves it.

---

[9] Conductance is simply the reciprocal of resistance: $g = \frac{1}{R}$ The unit of conductance is the Siemen.

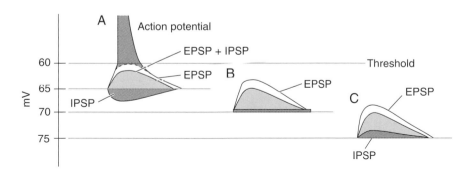

### Figure 3.18    Postsynaptic potentials

The shape of postsynaptic potentials is affected by the resting membrane potential and its relation to the equilibrium potential of the ions participating in the PSP. The EPSP is not affected significantly, since the resting membrane potential (about −75 mV) is usually quite far from the combined equilibrium potential for potassium ions and sodium ions (about 0 mV). The effect is dramatic in the case of the IPSP because the equilibrium potential of chloride is close to the resting potential of most neurons. **A.** An EPSP generates an action potential (*red line*) if the EPSP (*solid black*) exceeds threshold or fails if it is subthreshold (*broken black*). If the resting membrane potential is more positive than the equilibrium potential of chloride, the IPSP (*red area*) is a hyperpolarizing event. The temporal summation of an EPSP and an IPSP (*gray area*) decreases the amplitude of the EPSP over what it would be in the absence of the IPSP. In this case no action potential occurs. **B.** If the resting potential is equal to the equilibrium potential of chloride, the IPSP causes no change in the membrane potential (*red area*), but it still reduces the amplitude of an EPSP (*gray area*). **C.** If the resting potential is more negative than the chloride equilibrium potential, the IPSP is a depolarizing event (*red area*). Even so, the IPSP decreases the amplitude of a simultaneous EPSP (*gray area*). (Modified from Shepherd G. The Synaptic Organization of the Brain. 4th ed. New York: Oxford University, 1998.)

## INHIBITORY SYNAPSES

Ligand-gated channels that are selective for chloride ions also generate local currents. The chloride current can be either inward or outward, depending on the resting membrane potential. In most neurons the resting potential is about −60 mV and the chloride equilibrium potential is about −70 mV. In these neurons the opening of chloride channels causes an inward flow of chloride ions, since chloride is driven into the cell by both its concentration gradient and the chloride equilibrium potential (Fig. 3.18A). This inward chloride current hyperpolarizes the cell, making it more difficult to excite. Therefore, this current is called an **inhibitory postsynaptic potential (IPSP)**.

If the resting potential of the neuron is equal to the chloride equilibrium potential of −70 mV, which is the case in many neurons, the opening of the chloride channels causes *no increase in the inward flow of chloride ions* (Fig. 3.18B). This situation is still inhibitory, however, because the *potential* to increase chloride conductance exists. For example, any depolarizing event, such as an EPSP, allows positive charge to enter the cell. As the membrane potential becomes more positive, chloride ions are immediately drawn into the cell through the open chloride channels. These negative chloride ions neutralize the positive charge. Chloride enters the cell as long as the membrane potential is more positive than the chloride equilibrium potential. As the membrane potential approaches the chloride equilibrium potential, the net chloride current approaches zero. The membrane is said to be stabilized at the chloride equilibrium potential.

The IPSP can even be a depolarizing potential. If the resting potential of the neuron is −75 mV, a voltage quite within the normal physiological range, the opening of chloride selective channels causes an *outward* flow of chloride ions (Fig. 3.18C). The membrane potential becomes more positive, but as it approaches the chloride equilibrium potential, the net chloride current approaches zero. As in this example, the membrane potential tends to be stabilized at the chloride equilibrium potential.

## INITIATION OF THE POSTSYNAPTIC ACTION POTENTIAL

In the postsynaptic neuron action potentials are generated at the initial segment because voltage-gated ion channels are located only at the initial segment. Therefore, to trigger these voltage-gated ion channels, the depolarizing currents generated at excitatory synapses must reach the initial segment. Like all local currents, the postsynaptic currents generated at a synapse spread throughout the neuron and diminish with distance from the source. Consequently, the amplitude of postsynaptic potentials at the initial segment is determined by the *electrical distance* from the synaptic bouton and is best measured in space constants rather than metric units.

The electrical distance that separates a synapse from the initial segment dramatically affects both the amplitude and the shape of the PSP as recorded at the initial segment. The *amplitude* of the PSP is diminished in proportion to the space constant, λ, because of the leakage of current out of the cell. The *shape* is affected in proportion to the time constant, τ. The time constant increases with distance between the synaptic bouton and soma because of the greater membrane surface area, which increases membrane capacitance. The change in both shape and amplitude of an EPSP with increasing distance is illustrated in Fig. 3.19. The amount of synaptic current that reaches the initial segment has important consequences for the initiation of an action potential in the postsynaptic neuron.

Action potentials, of course, require the presence of voltage-gated channels. With few exceptions, the dendrites of neurons do not have voltage-gated channels in their membranes. Instead these channels are concentrated at the initial segment of the axon. Therefore, to be an effective trigger of action potentials, synaptic currents must have sufficient amplitude *at the initial segment* to affect the voltage-gated channels there. If depolarization at the initial segment is above threshold for the voltage-gated channels, an action potential is initiated. Once initiated, this action potential is conducted along the axon, as previously discussed (Fig. 3.20, *A* and *B*).

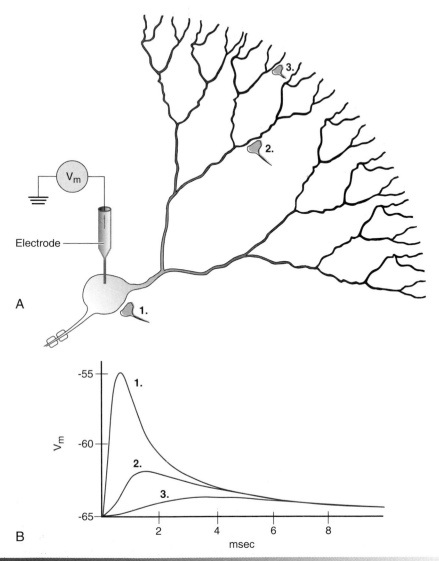

**Figure 3.19   Effect of dendrites on PSPs**

**A.** In this hypothetical dendritic tree with a simplified branching pattern, a recording site on the soma is indicated by the electrode. **B.** Recordings of EPSPs are based on computer simulations (Rall). The numbers correspond with the numbered synaptic boutons in **A.** The model calculates the resulting EPSP from a brief depolarizing event at the synaptic boutons indicated, and each is recorded at the soma. The amplitude and time course of the EPSP, as recorded in the soma, varies considerably with the location of the active synapse. (Data based on a model by Rall W. in Neural Theory and Modeling, R.F. Reiss, ed. Palo Alto: Stanford University Press, 1964:73-97.)

Most individual EPSPs are quite small at the initial segment (Fig. 3.19) because it is several space constants from the distal dendrites (Table 3.3). A single EPSP generated at a remote synapse generally cannot bring the neuron to threshold. However, the current from multiple EPSPs originating from various locations on the neuron combine at the initial segment. This **spatial summation** of EPSPs from many active synapses augments the amplitude of the depolarization and can bring the neuron to threshold (Fig. 3.20*C*). Similarly, **temporal summation** occurs when the current from multiple EPSPs collectively augment the

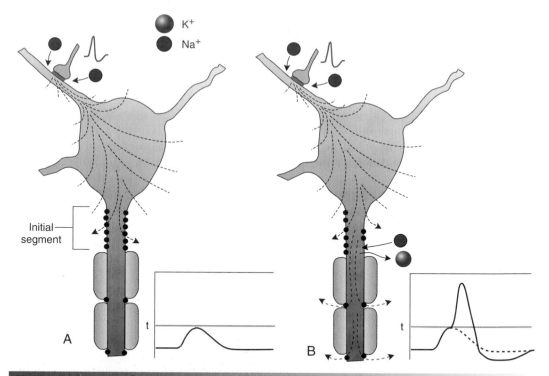

K⁺ → $K^+$
Na⁺ → $Na^+$

Initial segment

A

B

t

t

**Figure 3.20** **Spatial and temporal summation of PSPs**

The conversion of local postsynaptic currents into action potentials occurs at the initial segment. **A.** The depolarizing currents spread from the active synaptic bouton throughout the cell (*broken lines* and *arrows*). Voltage-gated sodium channels (*black dots*) at the initial segment can cause a secondary increase in inward current if the EPSP is above threshold. A subthreshold EPSP is shown (*solid black line*). **B.** If threshold is exceeded, the voltage-gated sodium channels open, and the regenerative process known as the action potential is initiated. This action potential in turn creates new local currents that spread down the axon, allowing the action potential to be propagated. The action potential is shown as a *solid black line;* the *dotted line* indicates the EPSP which is obscured by the action potential.

depolarization to bring the neuron to threshold (Fig. 3.20D). Spatial and temporal summation can, of course, occur simultaneously. The point is that for most neurons in the CNS, hundreds—if not thousands—of EPSPs from as many individual synapses are required to generate enough current to provoke a neuron into transmitting a *single* action potential.

## INTERACTION OF EPSPS AND IPSPS

Local currents, such as IPSPs and EPSPs, summate. The ebb and flow of synaptic currents follow the combined forces of the ionic equilibrium potentials, modifying the neuron membrane potential continuously in response to synaptic activity. At the initial segment this activity is translated into action potentials if the membrane potential reaches threshold (Fig. 3.21A). Therefore, any mechanism that controls the amount of current reaching the initial segment is important in controlling the activity of the neuron (Fig. 3.21B).

Synapses that produce IPSPs tend to be concentrated at the base of large dendrites and on the soma of neurons. Generally speaking, the excitatory synapses are more distal. Consequently, proximal inhibitory synapses have more influence on the membrane potential at the initial segment than the distal excitatory synapses. By providing a

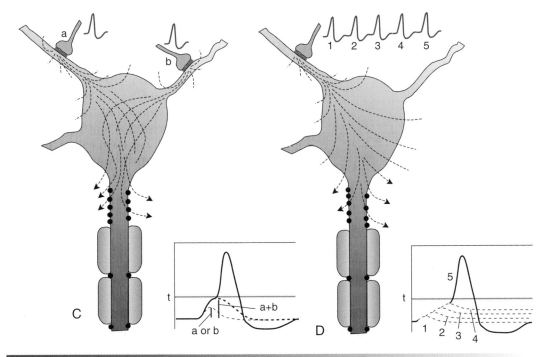

**Figure 3.20    Spatial and temporal summation of PSPs—*continued***

**C.** Spatial summation occurs when two nearly simultaneous EPSPs are produced by different synapses, here at *a* and *b*. Independently, each EPSP is subthreshold (*broken black lines*), but if they occur within an appropriate time-frame, their currents can summate at the initial segment and exceed threshold (*solid black line* leading to action potential). The active synaptic boutons may be derived from collateral branches of a single axon, or from different neurons. **D.** Temporal summation occurs when sequential action potentials invade a synaptic bouton. Each postsynaptic potential occurs before the effects of the previous postsynaptic potential have subsided. Therefore, their currents can sum as shown (*multiple broken lines*). Under physiological conditions temporal and spatial summation usually occur simultaneously and involve multiple EPSPs and IPSPs generated at numerous active synaptic boutons.

**Table 3.3    Equilibrium Potentials for Multi-Ion Systems**

| Condition | Permeability Coefficients | | | $V_m$ | | |
|---|---|---|---|---|---|---|
| | $P_{Na}$ | $P_K$ | $P_{Cl}$ | 0l | 2λ | 4λ |
| Rest | $1.0^{-8}$ | $1.0^{-7}$ | $1.0^{-8}$ | −54 | na | na |
| Peak of AP | $1.0^{-6}$ | $1.0^{-7}$ | $1.0^{-8}$ | 42 | −16 | −39 |
| After hypopolarization | $1.0^{-8}$ | $5.0^{-7}$ | $1.0^{-8}$ | −77 | na | na |
| Astrocytes | $1.0^{-8}$ | $1.0^{-6}$ | $1.0^{-8}$ | −82 | na | na |
| IPSP | $1.0^{-8}$ | $1.0^{-7}$ | $1.0^{-6}$ | −68 | −60 | −56 |
| EPSP | $7.5^{-7}$ | $1.0^{-6}$ | $1.0^{-8}$ | − 8 | −36 | −47 |

Equilibrium potentials computed using the Goldman-Hodgkin-Katz equation with the permeability coefficient shown. Potentials are shown to the right of the permeability coefficients at 0, 2, and 4 space constants removed from the hypothetical single point origin of the potential. (Permeability coefficients from Smith CU. Elements of Molecular Neurobiology. New York: Wiley, 1989.)

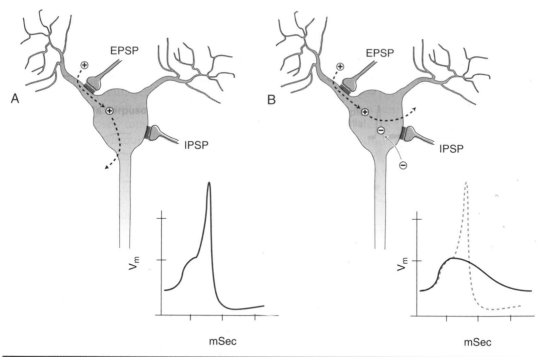

**Figure 3.21    Inhibition by IPSPs**

**A.** An unopposed EPSP generates enough depolarizing current to trigger an action potential at the initial segment. **B.** The same EPSP, paired with an IPSP, is insufficient to trigger an action potential because the depolarizing current is neutralized by the hyperpolarizing current generated at the IPSP (*inward arrow*). In effect, the active IPSP acts as a sink to drain the depolarizing current out of the cell.

low-resistance pathway, or sink, for electrical current to leave the cell,[10] the IPSP can short-circuit the positive currents generated by EPSPs (Fig. 3.22). An active IPSP at the base of a dendrite collapses the space constant for that dendrite by reducing its effective membrane resistance. *Inhibitory synapses in effect regulate the space constant of dendrites.* In this manner, a few well-placed inhibitory synaptic boutons can control the excitatory effectiveness of hundreds of excitatory synaptic boutons.

The smooth integration of excitatory and inhibitory events over time and space ultimately determines whether or not the postsynaptic cell initiates an action potential. This integration brings together information from diverse sources and at a single moment transforms this collective set of information into a single postsynaptic event, the action potential. *The summation of synaptic currents, both excitatory and inhibitory, at the initial segment of the axon is the fundamental decision-making process of the nervous system.*

## PRESYNAPTIC INHIBITION

The postsynaptic interplay between hyperpolarizing and depolarizing currents at the initial segment is not the only mechanism that regulates the excitability of a neuron. Presynaptic mechanisms *regulate the release of neurotransmitter* and thus modulate the amplitude of individual EPSPs and IPSPs. In contrast to postsynaptic regulation, which affects an entire neuron, presynaptic regulation is very specific, affecting only a single synaptic bouton. While

---

[10] When referring to current flow, it is customary to define its direction in terms of the flow of positive charge. Therefore, the inward negative chloride current associated with the IPSP is called an outward (positive) current.

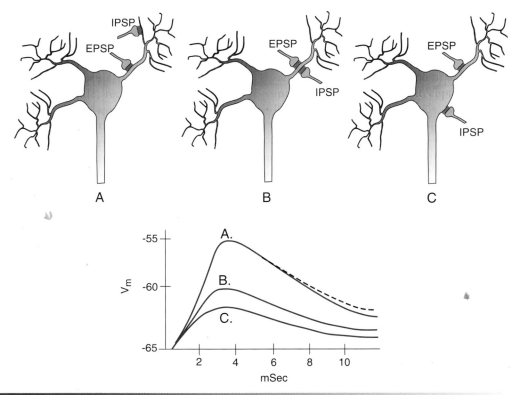

### Figure 3.22 Effect of synapse location

The physical relation between synaptic boutons that produce EPSPs and IPSPs affects the amplitude and time course of the postsynaptic potential as recorded at the soma of the neuron. In this illustration hypothetical computer-generated EPSPs at the base of a dendrite are calculated for three physical arrangements. **A.** An EPSP generated at the indicated site produces a response at the initial segment as shown by the *broken black line* in the graph. A simultaneous IPSP applied at a site distal to the EPSP hardly affects the amplitude or shape of the EPSP (*solid red line*). **B.** If the EPSP and the IPSP are simultaneously generated at the same site along the dendrite, the amplitude of the EPSP is diminished by about half and its time course is slowed. **C.** If the IPSP-generating synaptic bouton is between the recording site and the EPSP-generating synaptic bouton, the inhibitory effect is even more profound. (Data after a model by Rall W. in Neural Theory and Modeling, R.F. Reiss, ed. Palo Alto: Stanford University Press, 1964:73–97.)

both presynaptic inhibition and facilitation have been described in various species, only the presynaptic regulation of an EPSP, called **presynaptic inhibition**, has great significance in mammals.

Presynaptic regulation occurs when an axon synapses on the terminal synaptic bouton of another axon, which in turn forms a synaptic contact with a third neuron (Fig. 3.23). The presynaptic synapse contains vesicles, releases neurotransmitter, and triggers

ligand-gated events much as other chemical synapses do. Most mammalian presynaptic terminals secrete GABA, a neurotransmitter that when bound to the receptor, opens ligand-gated chloride ion channels. The chloride channels remain open for 100 to 150 msec, considerably longer than the 15 msec of a typical PSP. Since the chloride equilibrium potential is close to the axon resting potential, there is very little change in the synaptic bouton membrane potential (see page 120).

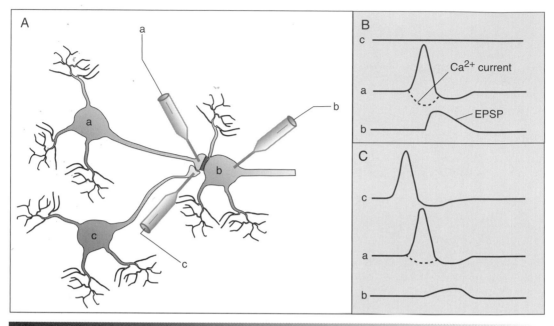

**Figure 3.23  Presynaptic inhibition**

**A.** In the physical arrangement between neurons that results in presynaptic inhibition, a synaptic bouton from neuron c terminates on the synaptic bouton of another neuron, a, that in turn synapses with neuron b. Neuron a is excitatory to b. Recordings from each cell correspond with the labeled electrodes. **B.** In the absence of activity from neuron c, an action potential enveloping synaptic bouton a opens calcium channels (*dotted line*), which in turn results in the release of neurotransmitter, causing an EPSP in neuron b. **C.** An action potential from neuron c diminishes the calcium current generated by a subsequent action potential arriving at synaptic bouton a (*dotted line*). As a result, fewer vesicles bind, and the EPSP in neuron b is diminished.

The open chloride channels, however, provide a large sink for positive current that diminishes the amplitude of any action potential that arrives at the synaptic bouton. The diminution of the amplitude of the invading action potential decreases the probability that voltage-gated calcium ion channels will open. Thus, fewer calcium ions will enter the synaptic bouton and fewer vesicles will fuse with the synaptic bouton membrane, resulting in the release of fewer quanta of neurotransmitter into the synaptic cleft. This reduced release of neurotransmitter ultimately results in a diminished EPSP in the postsynaptic cell.

## G-Protein–Linked Receptors

The second method by which neurotransmitters interact with postsynaptic cells is mediated through **G-protein** (guanosine nucleotide–binding protein) coupled second messenger systems. Although these systems can affect ion channels, the principal advantage is their ability to affect cell metabolism and to modulate the function of the postsynaptic receptor proteins themselves. In this latter role, they act as neuromodulators.

## ACTIVATION OF G-PROTEIN–LINKED SECOND MESSENGERS

All second-messenger-mediated synaptic responses are mediated by the action of a G-protein. This molecular complex freely floats within the lipid structure of the membrane. It randomly bumps into the receptor and other membrane proteins, but normally cannot react with them. However, when the neurotransmitter binds to the extracellular side of the receptor molecule, the receptor is altered so that it can bind to a G-protein if it happens to encounter one (Fig. 3.24). Once bound to

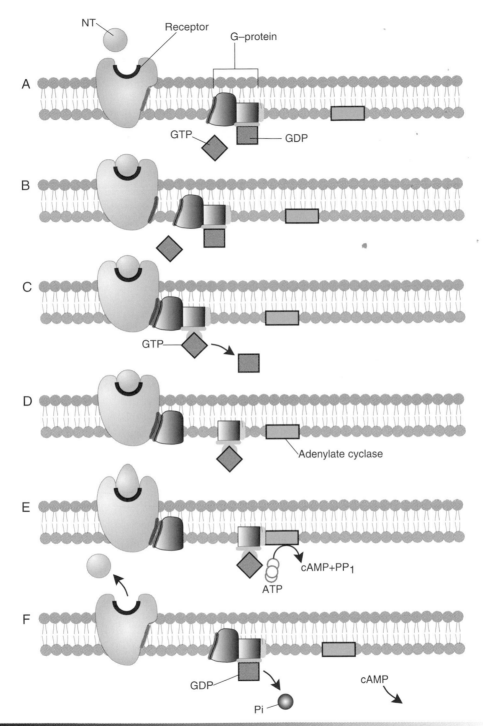

**Figure 3.24   G-protein-activated second messenger systems**

Collision-coupled systems are loosely coupled systems in which one or more components freely float within the matrix of the cell membrane. **A.** Initially the G-protein and receptor are dissociated. **B.** When a specific ligand (i.e., neurotransmitter, NT) is bound to the receptor, the conformation of the receptor changes, making it receptive to the G-protein. **C.** The G-protein attaches to the receptor when it bumps into it, and GTP replaces GDP on the G-protein. **D.** One subunit of the G-protein separates from the complex, becoming mobile within the membrane matrix. **E.** The subunit catalyzes the production of the second messenger with an appropriate enzyme (here, adenylate cyclase). **F.** With the dissociation of the ligand from the receptor, the G-protein can reunite.

the receptor, the G-protein is activated by the replacement of its guanosine diphosphate (GDP) with GTP. Now activated, the G-protein is released from the receptor and again freely floats within the structure of the membrane. Eventually it will encounter an appropriate target enzyme (e.g., adenylate cyclase) that stimulates the target enzyme to catalyze the formation of the second messenger. The process is self-limiting because the G-protein is itself an enzyme with GTPase activity. The GTPase eventually dephosphorylates the attached GTP and thus inactivates the G-protein. This cumbersome process is a **collision-coupled mechanism.**

## SECOND MESSENGERS

Although there are at least 12 G-proteins, only three second-messenger systems have been described in neurons. Each system uses reactions induced by a different intermediate enzyme. Three second messengers are closely associated with neurons: **adenosine 3',5'-cyclic monophosphate (cAMP), inositol 1,4,5-triphosphate (IP$_3$), diacylglycerol (DAG), and arachidonic acid** (Fig. 3.25). Each of these systems initiates a cascade of reactions that are specific to second messengers. These include the phosphorylation of proteins (cAMP), the liberation of calcium ions into the cytosol (IP$_3$ and DAG), and the production of arachidonic acid metabolites (arachi-

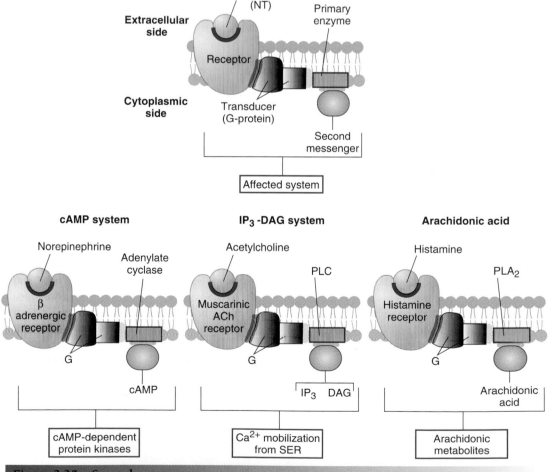

**Figure 3.25 · Second messenger systems**

G-protein-coupled systems fall into three classes that are defined by the nature of the enzyme that is catalyzed by the active form of the G-protein.

donic acid system). In addition, G-proteins can modify certain ion channels directly. Consequently, neurotransmitters that operate indirectly through second messengers have the potential to affect a much larger variety of cell functions than the direct ion channel systems.

For example, ACh in the central nervous system (CNS) acts through a muscarinic receptor to hyperpolarize the cell. This hyperpolarization is accomplished through the interaction of the receptor–G-protein–GTP complex with a potassium ion channel. This unusual ion channel is neither voltage-gated nor ligand-gated. It is a second-messenger-gated ion channel. When coupled with the G-protein complex, the potassium ion channel opens, increasing the conductance to potassium, which hyperpolarizes the cell (Fig. 3.16C). This process is not as straightforward as it seems, however, because at least four variations of the muscarinic receptor have been discovered in the CNS, and all respond somewhat differently to ACh.

Cell metabolism can also be regulated by second-messenger systems. Phosphatidyl inositol phosphates (PIP) are membrane phospholipids that are cleaved by phospholipase C (PLC). Only after it has been activated by a G-protein can PLC cleave PIP to form DAG and $IP_3$. $IP_3$ is water soluble, so it diffuses through the cytoplasm and binds to receptors on the endoplasmic reticulum, causing the release of calcium ions. Calcium ions in turn have a profound effect on the activation of protein kinases and are therefore a critical component in the regulation of most cell functions. DAG is not water soluble, so it remains in the membrane, where, when combined with calcium ions, it activates protein kinase C (PKC).

It is possible for neurotransmitters to regulate the expression of the genes themselves. Such regulation is accomplished through phosphorylation of transcriptional regulatory proteins via the protein kinase A (PKA) or PKC pathways. Genes have a coding and a regulatory region. Attached to regulatory regions are various transcription proteins that when phosphorylated, control the binding of RNA polymerase to the coding portion of the gene. By acting through second messengers, neurotransmitters can regulate the rate of RNA transcription by phosphorylating the regulatory proteins. For example, in some neurons synaptic activity causes the phosphorylation of the gene regulatory proteins that control the transcription of tyrosine hydroxylase, the precursor to the neurotransmitter norepinephrine, thereby regulating the synthesis of norepinephrine.

In addition to providing great variety to the ensemble of synaptic interactions that can occur between cells, second-messenger systems are extremely sensitive to low levels of neurotransmitter because the system greatly amplifies the signal. For example, one receptor can activate about 10 G-proteins. Each of these proteins in turn can activate about 10 adenylcyclase molecules, an amplification factor of 100.

The variety and sensitivity of function of second-messenger systems are accomplished, however, at the expense of speed. Directly ligand-gated ion channels respond within about 0.5 msec, and the response is usually complete in about 15 msec. Indirectly regulated systems may not respond for hundreds of milliseconds, and their effects may continue for hundreds of seconds. The effects on gene regulation may persist for days.

The chemical details of these second-messenger systems are beyond the scope of this book but may be found in standard biochemistry textbooks.

## COMMON NEUROTRANSMITTERS

Neurotransmitters, as we have seen, can be divided into several broad classes: **small-molecule neurotransmitters**, such as ACh; the **monoamines**; **neuroactive peptides**; and **gases**.

### Small-Molecule Neurotransmitters

The small-molecule neurotransmitters are the most common neurotransmitters in the CNS. Within this group, **glutamate** is the most pervasive excitatory neurotransmitter. There are two principal types of receptors for glutamate, the **AMPA** (α-amino-3-hydroxy-5-methyl-4-isoxazole propionic acid) and **NMDA** (N-methyl-D-aspartate) receptors. These strange names originate from the pharmacological studies that differentiated them and are not descriptive outside of that context. Both receptors are ligand-coupled ion channels. When bound to glutamate, the AMPA receptor is permeable to both sodium and potassium ions (Fig. 3.26*A*). The resulting current is a depolarizing EPSP. The activated NMDA receptor is permeable not only to sodium and potassium ions but also to calcium ions. However, the NMDA receptor, unlike its AMPA cousin, is highly sensitive to membrane potential. At normal resting potentials the NMDA receptor is blocked by magnesium ions and passes very little current when coupled with glutamate. However, at lower potentials (less negative), the blocking action of magnesium ions is released, and it passes significant ionic current, especially calcium current (Fig. 3.26, *B* and *C*). Since calcium can act as a potent second messenger, the NMDA receptor has many diverse effects. This complexity of the glutamate receptors offers a rich milieu for synaptic regulation. An appreciation of this milieu should dispel any notion that synapses are simple relay mechanisms designed to transfer action potentials from one cell to another.

Glutamate is also a potent neurotoxin. Its toxic effects are widespread because nearly every CNS neuron has glutamate receptors. The mechanisms of glutamate neurotoxicity are not known, but one hypothesis proposes that excessive extracellular concentration of glutamate acting at NMDA receptors prolongs the conductance of calcium ions into neurons. Since calcium is a potent regulator of intracellular metabolism, excessive amounts may inappropriately activate proteases, which can lyse the cell. Glutamate neurointoxication can occur in a number of conditions. For example, prolonged seizures may liberate an excessive amount of glutamate at the synapses of hyperactive cells and lead to neuron death. **γ-aminobutyric acid** (GABA) and **glycine** are the major inhibitory neurotransmitters in the mammalian CNS. GABA interacts with two types of receptors, **GABA$_A$** and **GABA$_B$**. The GABA$_A$ receptor is a ligand-gated chloride ion channel receptor, while GABA$_B$ is a G-protein–coupled potassium ion channel receptor. Both inhibit the postsynaptic cell.

The GABA$_A$ receptor is interesting because it has at least nine binding sites. GABA binds with low affinity to the primary site to open the chloride channel; the other sites are regulatory. Molecules that bind to the regulatory sites are generally ineffective in the absence of

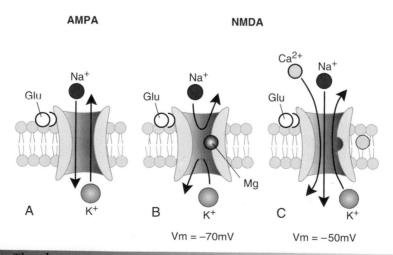

**AMPA**                    **NMDA**

A          K$^+$          B          K$^+$          C          K$^+$

Vm = −70mV          Vm = −50mV

**Figure 3.26   The glutamate receptors**

AMPA receptor (**A**) is a traditional ligand-gated ion channel that is selective to cations. The NMDA (**B** and **C**) receptor is a voltage-sensitive ligand-gated ion channel. At large membrane potentials (**B**) it is blocked by magnesium ions and does not change its permeability to cations, even when it is bound to its ligand. At low membrane potentials (**C**) it is unblocked and becomes freely permeable to cations, including calcium ions.

GABA. The *benzodiazepines* (e.g., Valium) bind with high affinity to one of these sites. Benzodiazepines increase the frequency with which the ion channel opens and closes when bound to GABA. As a result, the chloride current increases, enhancing the inhibitory effect. Hence these substances are an important class of pharmaceuticals that are used to increase CNS inhibition. They can be used to stop seizures, to facilitate muscle relaxation, and as tranquilizers. Another regulatory site binds *steroids*, which facilitate the action of GABA by increasing the open time of the ion channel. *Picrotoxin* is a potent neurotoxin that produces convulsions and death. It binds tightly to another regulatory site on the GABA$_A$ receptor. When bound, it alters the configuration of the ion channel in such a way that it blocks the passage of chloride ions.

The glycine receptor is similar to the GABA$_A$ receptor in that it is a ligand-gated chloride ion channel receptor, but it is not highly regulated by additional binding sites. It is blocked by strychnine, which explains the high potency of this neurotoxin.

**ACh** is a neurotransmitter that can bind to two receptors, the **nicotinic** and the **muscarinic.** These names are historical; they refer to the first agonists that were used to differentiate the two receptors. Acting through the nicotinic receptor, ACh is best known for its direct excitatory role at the neuromuscle junction. The binding of ACh to the nicotinic receptor opens an ion selective channel, which increases the permeability to both sodium and potassium ions. In cardiac muscle cells ACh is inhibitory and operates through muscarinic receptors that open only potassium ion channels acting via a second-messenger G-protein.

## Monoamines

Another large group of neurotransmitters are the monoamines. This group is divided into three classes, the **catecholamines, indolamines,** and **histamine.** All of the monoamines act through G-protein–coupled receptors and second-messenger systems. Several receptors are associated with each neurotransmitter, and most of these receptors have subgroups that usually act through different second-messenger systems. As a result, the actions of the monoamines are quite varied.

Unlike the ubiquitous small molecular neurotransmitters, the monoamines are produced by only a small number of cells that are confined to a few nuclei or nuclear groups in the CNS. Axons from these neurons branch extensively and are distributed to wide areas of the nervous system. Therefore, with a few specific exceptions, the monoamine systems do not seem to be involved in disseminating specific information among discrete nuclei but rather establish the general level of excitability of large regions of the CNS, especially the cerebral cortex and the forebrain. However, the specific functions of most monoamine systems are poorly understood.

**Norepinephrine** and **dopamine**[11] are the most important catecholamine neurotransmitters in the CNS. Norepinephrine is produced almost exclusively in the **locus ceruleus,** a small nucleus of the brainstem. Axons from these cells branch extensively to become distributed throughout the CNS (Fig. 3.27). The physiological role of this nucleus in CNS function is not known.

There are two principal classes of adrenergic receptors serving the catecholamines, $\alpha$ and $\beta$. Both are G-protein–mediated receptors, and each class is divided into subtypes. The $\alpha_1$-receptor functions through an IP$_3$ second messenger to open calcium ion channels, while the $\alpha_2$ receptor acts through cAMP to open potassium ion channels. Interestingly, the $\alpha_2$-receptors seem to be predominantly located on the synaptic bouton rather than on the target cell. Increasing conductance to potassium in the synaptic bouton hyperpolarizes it and increases the probability of vesicular binding in response to subsequent activity. The $\beta_1$-receptor functions through cAMP to increase potassium conductance in the target neuron.

Dopamine is produced by cells in two principal nuclei of the CNS (Fig. 3.28), the **sub-**

---

[11] Epinephrine, well established as a hormone, is also a CNS neurotransmitter. It is relegated to footnote status because its source and distribution are extremely small and its functions in the CNS are unknown.

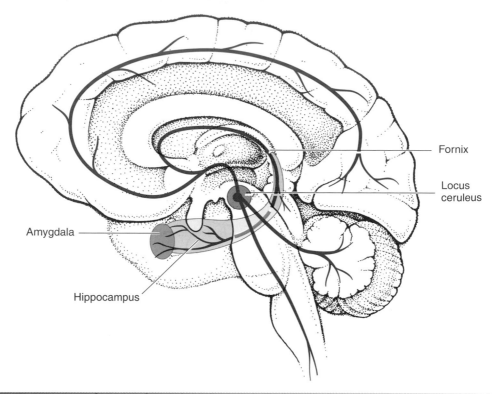

**Figure 3.27    Distribution of noradrenaline axons in the CNS**

Most of the noradrenaline-containing fibers in the CNS of mammals arise from the locus ceruleus in the brainstem. From there they are distributed fairly evenly throughout the CNS.

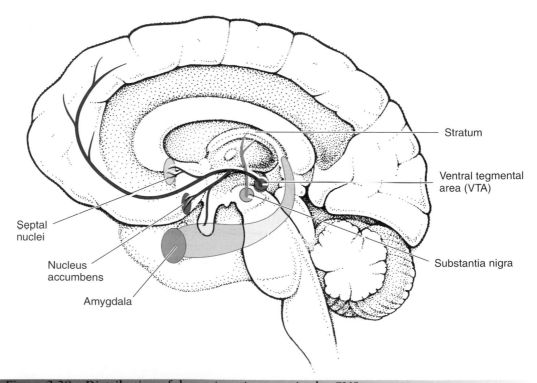

**Figure 3.28    Distribution of dopaminergic axons in the CNS**

Most of the dopamine-containing fibers in the CNS arise from two nuclei, the substantia nigra and the ventral tegmental area (VTA). The nigral system projects to the striatum. The VTA projects principally to the structures shown.

stantia nigra and the ventral tegmental area. The substantia nigra is located at the base of the mesencephalon and projects to the basal ganglia. This pathway is an essential component of the motor control system and is discussed in Chapter 8. The ventral tegmental area is also in the mesencephalon. It sends its axons into areas of the forebrain that play an important role in regulating behavior. The principal targets of these axons are the amygdaloid nuclei, septal nuclei, and the nucleus accumbens. This system is discussed in Chapter 14.

There are several dopamine receptors. The most common are designated $D_1$ and $D_2$. When bound to dopamine, the $D_1$-receptor increases the synthesis of cAMP, which subsequently increases the permeability of calcium and potassium channels. The $D_2$-receptor, however, acts to decrease the synthesis of cAMP, which reduces the permeability of the calcium and potassium channels. It is noteworthy that many antipsychotic drugs bind to and block the $D_2$-receptor, while amphetamine, a $D_2$-agonist, can produce paranoia and hallucinations. These effects are probably due to regulation of pathways associated with the amygdaloid, septal, and accumbens nuclei.

Serotonin (5-hydroxytryptamine, or 5HT) is the principal indolamine neurotransmitter of the CNS. Like the other monoamine systems, 5HT is produced in highly restricted areas of the CNS, specifically the raphe nuclei (Fig. 3.29). This nuclear group consists of small clusters of cells that lie in the midline of the medulla and pons. Axons from these cells project to all parts of the nervous system; most of their functions remain obscure. There are two receptors, $5HT_1$ and $5HT_2$. Both act through cAMP, but their properties are not well characterized in mammals.

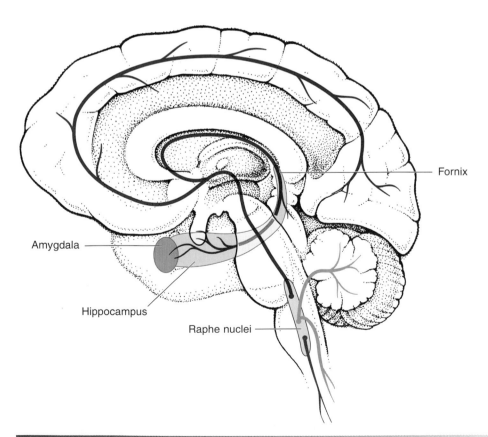

Fornix

Amygdala

Hippocampus

Raphe nuclei

**Figure 3.29    Distribution of serotonergic axons in the CNS**

Most of the serotonin (5-HT) containing fibers in the CNS arise from the raphe nuclei in the brainstem. They are distributed to all parts of the CNS.

## Neuropeptides

Neuroactive peptides form a large class of neurotransmitters. Although more than 100 peptides have been shown to affect the nervous system, only a few peptides have met a sufficient number of criteria (see page 115) to be classified as neurotransmitters. Neuropeptides are synthesized in the endoplasmic reticulum-Golgi complex of the neuron soma and packaged in secretory vesicles. More than 40 neuropeptides have been identified in the nervous system. Most of these neuropeptides are hormones, such as the hypothalamic-releasing hormones, pituitary hormones, neurohypophyseal hormones, and gut hormones. Although they play a role in communication between the nervous system and other physiological systems, their regulatory effects on the nervous system are limited.

A set of neuropeptides that play an important role in the function of the nervous system are the **opioid neuropeptides**. This group is distinguished by the ability to bind to receptors in the CNS that also bind morphine, a powerful analgesic purified from the poppy plant. About 18 endogenous peptides in this group have been identified. The most important members of this set are **met-enkephalin**, **leu-enkephalin**, **β-endorphin**, and **dynorphin**. Chemically, all begin with the sequence for *met-* or *leu-enkephalin* (Fig. 3.30). There are three principal receptors specific to the endogenous opioids, designated **μ**, **σ**, and **κ**. All of these receptors function by activating cAMP. The **μ** and **σ** receptors increase potassium and decrease calcium permeability, while the **κ** receptor decreases calcium permeability.

Another set of neuropeptides acts directly on the nervous system. Members of this heterogeneous group are not easily classified. Among these peptides are growth factors (e.g., **epithelial growth factor**), neuromodulators (e.g., **calcitonin gene–related peptide [CGRP]**), proteins with poorly understood actions (e.g., **galanin**), and neurotransmitters (e.g., **substance P**). Substance P, a small neuropeptide, probably is a sensory system neurotransmitter, which is discussed in a later chapter. Like most of the neuroactive peptides, substance P also has effects that are separate from its role as a neurotransmitter. For example, it induces cell division and is therefore a mitogen. As such, it may play a role in wound healing. Another neuropeptide, CGRP, can act through the cAMP system to phosphorylate certain ACh receptors, making them less responsive to the specific neurotransmitter ACh. In this case CGRP acts as a **neuromodulator** rather than a neurotransmitter because it regulates the function of the receptor protein.

## Gases

The gas **nitric oxide** appears to function as a neuronal chemical messenger. It is produced from L-arginine through the action of **nitric oxide synthase**, an enzyme that can be activated by an increased intracellular concentration of calcium ions (Fig. 3.31). Nitric oxide activates cytoplasmic guanyl cyclase to produce cGMP. This second messenger, like cAMP, can affect ion channels directly. It can also activate protein kinase G, which can cause protein phosphorylation. Nitric oxide can even regulate the synthesis of cAMP. Guanylcyclase is inhibited

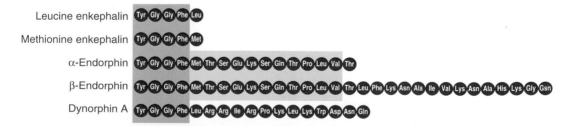

**Figure 3.30  Principal opioids**

The sequence of the principal endogenous opioids found in the CNS are shown here. They all begin with the sequence for either met- or leu-enkephalin.

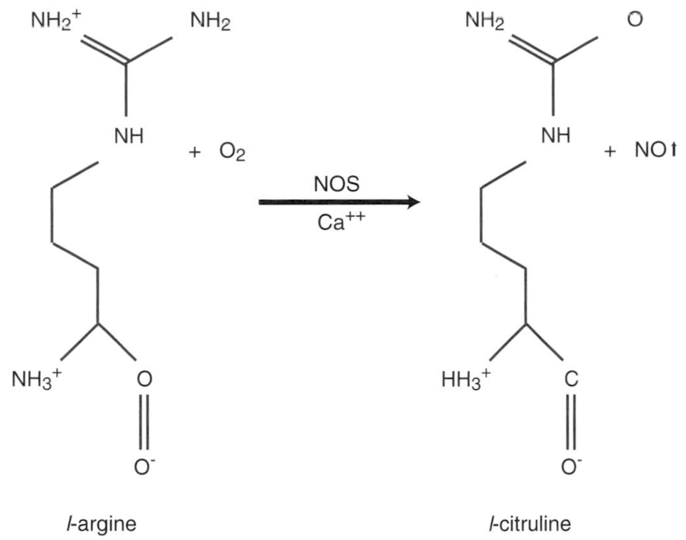

**Figure 3.31   Production of nitric oxide**

Nitric oxide is liberated from the conversion of L-arginine to L-citrulline by nitric oxide synthase in the presence of calcium ions.

by an increased intracellular concentration of calcium ions. Therefore, nitric oxide cannot be effective in the cell in which it is produced; rather, it must diffuse to other cells to be active. In this way it is thought to regulate the synaptic mechanisms in the synaptic boutons of the cells synapsing on the cell releasing the nitric oxide. Nitric oxide has a half-life of a few seconds at most, which limits its action to within a few micrometers of its release. Nitric oxide synthase is not distributed homogeneously in the CNS but is found primarily in the cerebellum and olfactory bulb. The physiological role of nitric oxide in the CNS is not known. In the periphery it is a potent vasodilator; it is released from endothelial cells and causes smooth muscle to relax.

## NEURAL PLASTICITY

Learning and memory are two essential properties of the nervous system. Early theories of learning often include a positive feedback system in self-sustaining oscillation. In theory, once activated, these feedback circuits remain active for long periods, even indefinitely in the case of permanent memory. Today, this theory seems naive.

Modern theories of learning focus on the synapse and mechanisms by which synaptic efficiency can be altered. One phenomenon of learning under intensive investigation is **long-term potentiation (LTP)**, which in the most general sense refers to the increased efficiency of a synapse following activity. For example, a signal entering a synaptic bouton of one cell and synapsing on a second produces an EPSP of a specific amplitude. Under controlled conditions this EPSP remains approximately the same amplitude each time the synaptic bouton is activated. However, if the activity on the synaptic bouton is paired with activity from another synaptic bouton, subsequent EPSPs are enhanced and remain enhanced for minutes to hours (Fig. 3.32). LTP can also be elicited following high-frequency trains of stimuli, whereas low-frequency stimulation over the same pathways fails to produce this effect. LTP is different from posttetanic potentiation, because the latter lasts for only a few hundred milliseconds at most. **Long-term depression (LTD)** is the converse of LTP.

Clearly, LTP and LTD involve some alteration of the synapse. This alteration may be presynaptic, involving enhanced release of

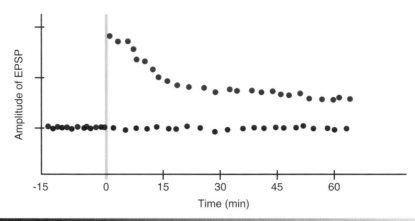

**Figure 3.32 Long-term potentiation**

This hypothetical experiment illustrates the alteration in the EPSP as a result of a constant stimulus (*black dots*) and the same stimulus following an event that alters the properties of the synapse and increases its efficiency (*red dots*).

neurotransmitter, or postsynaptic, involving alteration of the receptor function. And, of course, LTP and LTD may involve both presynaptic and postsynaptic changes. Our present understanding centers on three mechanisms that may account for LTP (Fig. 3.33).

First, high-frequency trains of action potentials are known to cause the release of neurotransmitters from both synaptic vesicles and secretory vesicles, whereas low frequency stimulation causes release from only the synaptic vesicles. Since proteins are released from the secretory vesicles, they could produce presynaptic and postsynaptic alterations by activating second messenger systems. As we have seen, second-messenger-mediated systems have the potential to regulate and modify all aspects of cell function.

Second, the NMDA glutamate receptor has the two important properties that are relevant to LTP. At large membrane potentials the NMDA receptor is blocked by magnesium ions. However, if the cell is moderately depolarized, the NMDA receptor is unblocked, and when bound to glutamate, calcium ion conductance is increased. Calcium, as we have seen, is an important second messenger that can initiate a number of metabolic events, some of which entail the activation of protein kinases.

The third mechanism relevant to LTP is the activation of nitric oxide synthase by intracellular calcium ions. A number of pathways lead to the liberation of intracellular calcium, including the activation of NMDA receptors, voltage-gated calcium ion channels, and $IP_3$-DAG activated systems. Therefore, it is not difficult to imagine that nitric oxide synthase is easily activated. The nitric oxide gas produced diffuses to the presynaptic bouton, where it generates cyclic guanosine monophosphate (cGMP) by activating guanylcyclase. Although the effects of cGMP in the presynaptic bouton are not known, it is a potent regulator of cell function. Nitric oxide synthase is not uniformly distributed in the brain. Two areas that strongly express it are the hippocampus and the cerebellum. These two structures display LTP and LTD, and certain forms of learning and memory take place in both structures. We are a long way from understanding how the nervous system stores information, but it seems likely that LTP and LTD are important features of this system.

## DISTURBANCES OF NEURAL FUNCTION

The complexity of chemical signaling between neurons creates many possibilities for malfunction. Consider the four criteria for neurotransmitter identification; each also presents an opportunity for synaptic failure. For example, genetic or metabolic dysfunction can lead to failure to synthesize the neurotransmitter. Disturbances within the voltage-gated calcium ion channels lead to diminished capacity to release neurotransmitter. False ligands can bind to the receptor in a way that blocks its physiological function, and methods of eliminating the neurotransmitter can be foiled. Many important neurological diseases can be understood in terms of failure of synaptic transmission.

## Myasthenia Gravis

Myasthenia gravis is a common disease with a prevalence of about 3/100,000. It is characterized by *fluctuating* that waxes and wanes throughout the day and also over longer periods. Frequently but not necessarily, episodes of weakness are correlated with exercise, and strength is regained with rest. The *distribution of weakness is asymmetrical,* involving the orofacial muscles more commonly than the limbs. This weakness almost always involves the ocular muscles. **Diplopia** (double vision), **ptosis** (eyelid droop), **dysphagia** (swallowing disorders), and **dysarthria** (speech slurring) are common symptoms. The other muscle groups

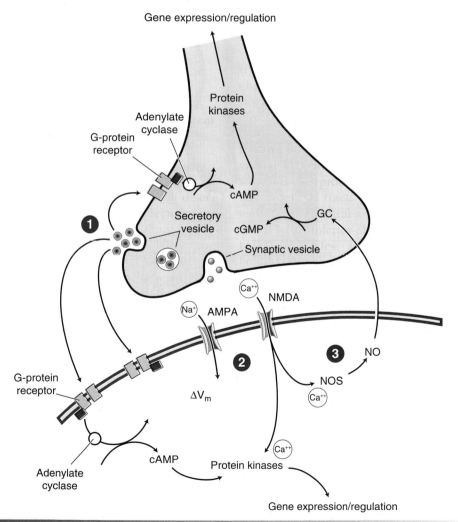

**Figure 3.33  Mechanisms of long-term potentiation**

Possible mechanisms of long-term potentiation are illustrated by (**1**) the release of neuroactive proteins from secretory vesicles, which can activate G-protein-mediated processes that eventually alter gene expression; (**2**) glutamate-NMDA-mediated calcium ion activation of other mechanisms that activate protein kinases; and (**3**) nitric oxide retrograde alteration of cGMP-mediated mechanisms (as yet unknown) that have the potential to alter presynaptic mechanisms.

of the body may be involved to varying degrees. Finally, strength improves dramatically if cholinergic agonist drugs are administered.

Myasthenia gravis is an autoimmune disease. Antibodies to the ACh receptor protein are almost invariably found in patients with this disease (see the case history later in the chapter). ACh receptor antibodies interfere with synaptic transmission at the myoneural junction in three ways. *First, the primary problem is the immunological destruction of the receptor.* In normal persons the ACh receptors are normally degraded and continuously replaced. In the myasthenic patient the receptors are destroyed faster than they can be replaced. As a result, the normal population of receptors is depleted. *Second, while bound to the receptor, the antibody interferes with the receptor's binding properties,* making it unable to bind to ACh. *Third, complement-mediated lysis of the end-plate membrane itself occurs,* which reduces its surface area. The loss of end-plate area further reduces the number of receptors at the end plate. Therefore, the patient has a subnormal number of ACh receptors and ion channels at the motor end plate. Those that remain are functionally deficient because of the direct action of the antibody. Together these deficiencies lead to a dramatic reduction in the effectiveness of the released neurotransmitter, hence to an abnormally small muscle end-plate potential (EPSP of the muscle). Many end-plate potentials do not reach threshold for the muscle, so fewer muscle fibers are activated and the compound muscle action potential is smaller than normal. Fewer muscle fibers participate in the contraction, and the patient is weak.

**Electromyography (EMG)** is used to record the compound muscle action potential (Fig. 3.34). Low-frequency repetitive stimulation (typically 3 Hz for 3 seconds) of the motor nerve produces a *decrementing response* in the amplitude of the compound muscle action potential in patients with myasthenia gravis, whereas in normal patients all of the muscle action potentials are of the same am-

plitude. This same decrementing response can be recorded in patients who have been given *d*-tubocurarine,[12] a drug that blocks ACh receptors. In both cases the release and enzymatic removal of neurotransmitter are unaffected.

### Eaton-Lambert Syndrome

Eaton-Lambert syndrome is also an autoimmune disease. Associated with carcinoma of the bronchus and only rarely seen in its absence, it is characterized by abnormal voltage-regulated calcium ion channels in the motor nerve terminals. It affects both muscarinic and nicotinic receptors. Most evidence suggests that the channels undergo immunological attack. The defective channels allow fewer calcium ions to enter the terminal bouton with each stimulus. As a result, an abnormally small number of vesicles bind to the active sites. Less neurotransmitter is released, which leads to a smaller end-plate potential and weakness of muscle contraction. In contrast to myasthenia gravis, repetitive stimulation of the motor nerve results in an *incrementing response* of the compound muscle action potential. This sign is probably caused by an accumulation of intracellular calcium ions in the presynaptic terminal. As the calcium ions build up with each succeeding stimulus, more vesicles are mobilized and fuse with the preterminal membrane. Therefore, more neurotransmitter is released with each stimulus (Fig. 3.34C).

### Neurotoxins

**Botulinum toxin,** produced by the spores of *Clostridium botulinum,* also acts on muscarinic and nicotinic muscle synapses by interfering with a calcium-dependent mechanism for the release of neurotransmitter. The exact mechanism is unknown, but since it interferes with known calcium-dependent processes, it is assumed that calcium channels are either destroyed or blocked. Its mode of action is similar to that of **tetanus toxin,** another potent

---

[12] A plant extract, curare is a natural toxin used by certain Indian groups to poison darts. The drug paralyzes the prey by blocking ACh receptors at the myoneural junction. In its purified form, *d*-tubocurarine chloride is used clinically to produce muscle relaxation during surgery.

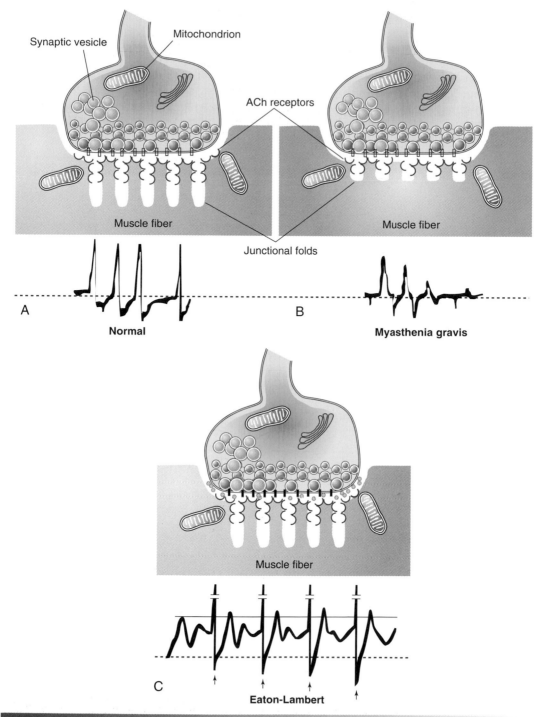

**Figure 3.34** **EMG of myasthenia gravis and Eaton-Lambert disease**

The myoneural junction is shown with EMG recordings below. **A.** The normal junction is characterized by an end plate with deep folds and ACh receptors. Repetitive electrical stimulation of the nerve produces muscle action potentials of equal amplitude. **B.** The disease process of myasthenia gravis reduces not only the number of ACh receptors but also the size of the postsynaptic folds in the motor end plate. In response to repetitive nerve stimulation, the EMG recordings show a decrease in the amplitude of successive muscle action potentials. **C.** Eaton-Lambert disease affects the calcium ion channels in the presynaptic synaptic bouton but not the myoneural junction. Neurotransmitter release is diminished, resulting in increments in the EMG on successive stimulation. Truncated spikes at arrows are shock artifacts of the stimulus.

microbial neurotoxin. The effects of botulinum toxin are similar to those seen in Eaton-Lambert syndrome, including the incremental response to repetitive stimulation. Botulinum toxin is one of the most potent poisons known. In the mouse it is lethal at 1 pg/kg. Extrapolated to an 80-kg human, only 80 pg is required for a lethal dose.

**Black widow spider venom** ($\alpha$-latrotoxin) is also a presynaptic poison. This unusual toxin binds to specific receptors in the presynaptic motor nerve terminal, where it is incorporated into the membrane. It then acts as a continuously open ion channel that allows sodium, potassium, and calcium ions to enter the cell. The result is both membrane depolarization and a massive influx of calcium ions that leads to inappropriate vesicle binding and rapid depletion of neurotransmitter. Since the incorporation of the toxin into the membrane is essentially irreversible, vesicle recycling is impossible because the intracellular calcium concentration can never be restored. Clinically, victims of this spider's bite first manifest spasms and rigidity, followed by flaccid paralysis. Death is uncommon (about 4%, mostly children), probably because this small spider is unable to inject a large amount of venom.

## CASE HISTORIES

The case histories given in this and the following chapters are presented in standard clinical style. In the earlier chapters much of the material reported in the histories has not yet been presented. Do not worry about it. Each case emphasizes principles presented in the corresponding chapter. For the cases through about Chapter 6 you should pay close attention to the history of present illness, the presentation of sensory findings, and the commentary. You should also familiarize yourself with the contents of Appendix 2, paying particular attention to the sensory examination. As you progress through the book, continue to refer to Appendix 2 and the cases presented in previous chapters until you can appreciate all elements of the case.

# C A S E   H I S T O R Y

## THE CASE OF THE INTERMINABLE MEAL

### HISTORY OF PRESENT ILLNESS

Mr. S. B. is a 65-year-old man who went to the neurology clinic complaining of trouble swallowing, slurred speech, and double vision for the past week. His trouble swallowing occurred with both liquids and solids. It took him an hour to eat a meal because he had to rest after each bite. His speech became unintelligible after talking with the examiner for about 2 minutes. Early in the morning and after his afternoon nap he could talk and swallow almost normally for about 30 minutes. He noticed no weakness of his arms or legs. He is taking diltiazem, a calcium channel blocker, for his blood pressure. He has no allergies. His only medical problem is hypertension. He has no family history of neuromuscular disease.

### PHYSICAL EXAMINATION

Mr. S. B. is in good physical health for a man of his age. His blood pressure was 135/85.

### NEUROLOGICAL EXAMINATION
#### Mental Status
Mr. S. B. was alert and knew who he was, where he was, and why he had come to the clinic for evaluation. He gave a coherent and concise his-

tory. He could name the presidents in order back to Franklin D. Roosevelt. At the end of the examination he remembered the three items he was asked to memorize.

### Cranial Nerves

All cranial nerve functions were normal except the following:

CN III: On examination he had moderate bilateral ptosis. He could look up for only 5 seconds without his eyelids falling.

### Station and Gait

His gait was balanced, smooth, and on a narrow base.

### Motor Systems

STRENGTH: His neck flexor strength was 3/5. After exercise his arms retained their strength (5/5), but his ptosis became worse and his speech became markedly slurred.

TONE: There was no spasticity or rigidity.

BULK: Appropriate and symmetrical for a man of his age.

ABNORMAL MOVEMENTS: None observed.

### Sensory Systems

He could perceive light touch to cotton and pinprick in all extremities, including the face. Proprioception was intact at the fingers and toes. He was stable on a narrow base with eyes open and closed (normal Romberg test) (see Chapter 5).

### Reflexes

Muscle stretch reflexes (MSRs) were present and normal at all extremities. Toes were down going.

### Coordination and Control

Finger-to-nose and heel-to-shin tests were accomplished without difficulty. Rapid alternating hand slapping and finger touching were easily done.

### Parietal Functions

Optokinetic reflex (OKN) was present in both directions. There was no aphasia or atavistic signs.

### ANCILLARY STUDIES

An edrophonium[13] test showed no improvement in his ptosis following injection of the substance in syringe A. His ptosis resolved and he could speak normally for about 7 minutes following injection of the substance in syringe B. The nurse confirmed that edrophonium was in syringe B, indicating a positive edrophonium test result. His acetylcholine receptor antibody titer was 1.3 (normal < 0.5). EMG showed a 30% decrement in motor action potential amplitude at 3 Hz comparing the first and fourth action potential. Chest computed tomography (CT) showed an involuted thymus.

### SUBSEQUENT COURSE

Mr. S. B. was prescribed pyridostigmine 60 mg four times a day. His symptoms persisted. He was hospitalized and prednisone 10 mg/day was added to his drug regimen. His weakness immediately worsened, and he soon developed respiratory failure and required ventilatory support. Plasmapheresis was performed every other day for 2 weeks, and prednisone was increased to 60 mg a day. At the end of 2 weeks he was removed from the ventilator and was doing well, with only mildly slurred speech after talking for an hour. He was sent home with prescriptions for pyridostigmine 90 mg four times a day and prednisone 60 mg/day.

### COMMENTARY

The clinical picture presented by this patient is typical of myasthenia gravis. The presenting symptoms are weakness exacerbated by exercise and alleviated, at least partially, by rest. His weakness was restricted to the cranial nerve distribution, sparing the extremities, a pattern that is typical in older men. Ptosis is a common sign associated with myasthenia gravis because the levatores palpebrae are constantly active while the person is awake and thus are subject to fatigue.

---

[13] Edrophonium is the generic name for Tensilon. This test is often called the Tensilon test.

The edrophonium test is performed when myasthenia gravis is suspected. This drug is a short-acting acetylcholinesterase (AChE) inhibitor. Blocking the action of AchE, the enzyme that deactivates ACh, prolongs activation of the receptors at the myoneural junction. Therefore, if weakness is caused by receptor failure at the myoneural junction, injection of edrophonium temporarily relieves the symptoms. Since in the office the measurement of strength is subjective, a double-blind procedure is followed. A nurse prepares two syringes, one containing edrophonium and the other containing saline, and labels them without informing the physician or the patient of their contents. Only after the physician has recorded the effect of each injection are the contents of the syringes revealed. A positive response to edrophonium is considered diagnostic for myasthenia gravis.

Mr. S. B.'s treatment followed a stormy course. Because the initial dose of pyridostigmine did not alleviate his symptoms, the corticosteroid prednisone was begun. As in this case, prednisone can precipitate a **myasthenic crisis,** severe muscle weakness that often leads to respiratory arrest. The crisis usually resolves within about 2 weeks with proper respiratory management. Myasthenic crisis is most common in patients who have dysarthria, dysphagia, or documented weakness of the respiratory muscles, like Mr. S. B.

Plasmapheresis is a procedure in which the patient's blood plasma is dialysed to remove high-molecular-weight proteins in an effort to reduce the plasma antibody titer. After dialysis the blood is returned to the patient. This process is often remarkably successful in reducing an autoimmune crisis. It is noteworthy that antibody titers do not correlate with the patient's symptoms. Mr. S. R.'s antibodies were only slightly elevated, yet he did not respond to pyridostigmine. Patients with few symptoms who respond well to pyridostigmine may have antibody titers as high as 400.

## FURTHER APPLICATIONS[14]

3.1.  **Explain how pyridostigmine acts therapeutically.**

3.2.  **Does the use of pyridostigmine attack the cause of the disease, as antibiotics do in the case of infection? What about plasmapheresis?**

3.3.  **Since antibody titers do not correlate very well with the severity of the patient's symptoms, what is the value of measuring antibody titers in myasthenia gravis?**

3.4.  **Myasthenia gravis is only one of many autoimmune diseases that affect the nervous system. Consider the various roles of plasmapheresis, corticosteroids, and thymectomy in the treatment of this class of diseases and myasthenia gravis in particular.**

---

[14] These questions are intended to provoke thoughtful reflection on the clinical aspects of the material in the chapter. Answers to these questions are not necessarily provided in the chapter. While brief answers are provided at the back of the book, students are encouraged to consult standard neurology texts, Online Mendelian Inheritance in Man (OMIM), or other convenient sources for fuller explanations.

# S U M M A R Y

- **The nervous system uses both chemical and electrical processes to generate and transmit signals.**

  In the nervous system, electrical signaling processes are used for intracellular signaling, transmission along axons, and at the synapse, where the postsynaptic signals are electrical (PSPs). Chemical signaling is used for intercellular transmission and synapse, endocrine, and paracrine signaling.

- **The energy for electrical signaling comes from ion imbalances across a selectively permeable cell membrane.**

  The ion imbalances cause ions to move through the membrane down their concentration gradient. If the membrane is not permeable to one species of charged molecules, charge is separated by the membrane and an electrical gradient is established. When the force of diffusion is just balanced by the electrical force of the separated charge, equilibrium exists. The electrical potential at equilibrium is the equilibrium potential, or Nernst potential. If a membrane has several ion channels that select different ions, each ion contributes to the equilibrium potential in proportion to its relative permeability. The membrane potential of a cell is the equilibrium potential established by several ions.

- **The membrane potential can be manipulated by altering the permeability coefficients for the various ions.**

Neuron membranes contain membrane-spanning proteins that alter their permeability in response to the transmembrane potential. These voltage-gated ion channels create the action potential, a brief modulation of the membrane potential, by altering the membrane permeability to sodium and potassium ions in response to changes in membrane potential.

- **In contrast to action potentials, local currents are not associated with dynamic changes in membrane permeability but are simply the passive distribution of current throughout the neuron.**

The potential associated with local currents diminishes with distance from the current source in proportion to the membrane resistance and the cytoplasmic resistance. Local currents associated with action potentials are distributed along axons and supply the depolarizing stimulus needed to propagate the action potential along the axon. Local currents associated with synaptic events are distributed along the dendrite and soma and supply the depolarizing stimulus at the initial segment where action potentials are generated.

- **Axons terminate as complex structures known as synapses.**

At most synapses in the mammalian nervous system, presynaptic action potentials are converted to chemical signals that in turn are converted into electrical signals at the postsynaptic cell. The presynaptic action potential opens voltage-gated calcium channels, allowing calcium ions to enter the synaptic bouton.

In the presence of calcium ions, vesicles containing the neurotransmitter bind to the synaptic bouton membrane and release their contents into the subsynaptic space. The neurotransmitter diffuses across the space and combines with a membrane-spanning receptor protein on the postsynaptic cell.

- **There are two recognized types of receptor proteins: those that are ion-selective ion channels and those that initiate collision-coupled second-messenger biochemical cascades.**

The association of neurotransmitter and receptor with the former group opens ion channels in the postsynaptic cell. The postsynaptic potentials that are associated with the ionic currents resulting from these channel openings can be either hyperpolarizing or depolarizing. At the initial segment, the forces of all postsynaptic potentials are integrated in proportion to their electrical distance from each synapse, and action potentials are generated if threshold is exceeded.

- **Receptor proteins that initiate collision-coupled reactions operate through G-proteins that activate one of three second-messenger systems.**

Cell metabolism can be altered by cAMP systems acting through protein phosphorylation or by DAG- $IP_3$ systems that regulate intracellular calcium ions. A third second messenger, arachidonic acid, can also be invoked by neurotransmitters acting through specific receptors.

- **There are four principal groups of neurotransmitters.**

The small-molecule neurotransmitters are packaged and secreted from synaptic vesicles. Typical members of this group are acetylcholine (ACh), γ-aminobuteric acid (GABA), glycine, and glutamate. The monoamines (catecholamines, indolamines, and histamine) form a second large group of neurotransmitters. The third group consists of neuropeptides, and the fourth is the gases.

- **The function of CNS synapses can be modified by their own activity.**

Long-term potentiation (LTP) and long-term depression (LTD) are two mechanisms by which the function of synapses can be modulated by synaptic activity in a neuron. The special properties of the magnesium ion block in the NMDA glutamate receptor and make magnesium ions a candidate for synaptic modulation. Finally, since nitric oxide appears to act as a paracrine messenger and cannot effect changes in the cell in which it is liberated, it probably plays an important role in the modulation of CNS functions.

- **Synaptic function can be disrupted in several clinically relevant ways.**

Neurotransmitter receptors can be destroyed by the immune system to produce disease (myasthenia gravis and Eaton-Lambert syndrome). Synaptic vesicle release can be disrupted by toxins (e.g., botulinum and tetanus toxin) that interfere with the voltage-gated calcium channels in the synaptic bouton. Receptors can be blocked by false ligands (e.g., curare) that bind more tightly than the natural ligand but do not activate the receptor's function.

## SUGGESTED READINGS

Clements JD. Neurotransmitter time course in the synaptic cleft: its role in central synaptic function. Trends Neurosci 1996;19:163–170.

GENESIS. A neurostimulation program (UNIX OS) available from: http://www.bbb.caltech.edu.

Hall ZW. An introduction to molecular neurobiology. Sunderland, MA: Sinauer, 1992.

Hölscher C. Nitric oxide, the enigmatic neuronal messenger: its role in synaptic plasticity. Trends Neurosci 1997;20:298–302.

Murphy S, Grzybicki D. Glial NO: normal and pathological roles. Neuroscientist 1996;2:90–99.

NEURON. A neurostimulation program (Windows OS) available from: http://neuron.duke.edu.

Rowland LP. Merritt's Textbook of Neurology. 9th ed. Baltimore: Williams & Wilkins, 1995.

Shepherd G. Foundations of the Neuron Doctrine. New York: Oxford University, 1991.

Shepherd G. The Synaptic Organization of the Brain. 4th ed. New York: Oxford University Press, 1998.

Shepherd G. Neurobiology. 3rd ed. New York: Oxford University, 1994.

Siegel GJ, Agranoff BW, Albers RW, et al. Basic Neurochemistry. Molecular, Cellular, and Medical Aspects, 6th ed. Baltimore: Lippincott Williams & Wilkins, 1999.

Smith CU. Elements of Molecular Neurobiology. 2nd ed. New York: Wiley, 1996.

Wu L, Saggau P. Presynaptic inhibition of elicited neurotransmitter release. Trends Neurosci 1997; 20:204–212.

Zufall F. Cyclic nucleotide-gated channels, nitric oxide, and neural function. Neuroscientist 1996; 2:24–32.

# Principles of Sensory Transduction

The mammalian nervous system is an information processing organ. Information by itself is sterile unless given meaning by association with objects and processes that are significant to the organism. The energy forces of the external world (heat, light, sound, and so on) are represented as electrochemical events in the nervous system. The process of converting energy from external world events into an internal representation creates meaningful information. This chapter shows how elements of the external world are transduced and represented as local currents and action potentials in the internal world of the brain.

There is an important distinction between the **physical stimuli** that the external world presents to our senses and our **perception** of these stimuli. In our everyday lives we behave as if the relation between stimulus and perception is both accurate and tightly linked. This is not always the case. Everyone has experienced an optical illusion (Fig. 4.1), a familiar situation in which our perceptions do not match reality. All of our senses are capable of deceiving us.

To understand the relation between **physical stimuli**, that is, sensations, and conscious **perception**, one must understand the nature of **transduction** [L. *trans*, across, and *duco*, lead] and **representation** in the nervous system. Transduction is the process by which the energy of a physical stimulus is detected and converted to a form of energy used by the nervous system. Representation is the way information is encoded and organized as an **analogue** of the stimulus within the structure of the nervous system.

## TRANSDUCTION

The process of transforming the energy content of an environmental stimulus into coded action potentials is called **sensory transduction.** The transduction occurs at a specialized area of neuronal membrane called the **receptor.** The transduction process has two steps. First, the physical stimulus is converted into a **receptor potential,** a small, brief alteration in the membrane potential. Second, the receptor potential is converted into **action potentials.** Because receptor potentials are local graded responses that diminish in amplitude with distance from the receptor membrane, this second conversion is required for the transport of the information represented by the receptor potential to the central nervous system (CNS).

### Ionic Mechanisms

The mechanisms by which changes in membrane permeability produce receptor potentials are similar to those associated with voltage- and ligand-gated systems. The process of initiating a receptor potential is best illustrated by the **mechanoreceptors** in the terminal membrane of certain sensory axons. Mechanoreceptors convert mechanical energy into receptor potentials. The specialized terminal axon membrane contains ion channels that are sensitive to mechanical deformation of the membrane (Fig. 4.2). Unlike voltage- or ligand-gated channels, these channels are linked to the cytoskeleton in such a way that mechanical distortions of the receptor membrane open the channels. These channels are simultaneously selective for sodium and potassium ions, so that when they open, the axon terminal becomes depolarized.

The depolarization caused by the opening of the ion channels is the receptor potential. *The receptor potential is simply a local current* that displays all of the properties of local currents. Its *amplitude* is proportional to the number of open ion channels; that is, it is a graded potential and its *duration* is approximately as long as that of the stimulus. These properties make the receptor potential an **analogue** [G. *analogos*, according to ratio, proportionate] of the stimulus (Fig. 4.3), so the receptor potential follows the stimulus more or less accurately in intensity and duration.

## Information Coding

At the receptor, the energy content or **intensity** of the stimulus is represented by the *amplitude* of the receptor potential. In the case of the mechanoreceptor, the degree to which mechanical energy deforms the receptor membrane determines the number of ion channels that open, which in turn determines the amount of depolarization of the nerve ending. Since the amplitude of the receptor potential varies in time with the intensity of the stimulus, the receptor potential is **amplitude modulated (AM)**.

The receptor potential, like all local currents, degrades in amplitude with distance from the

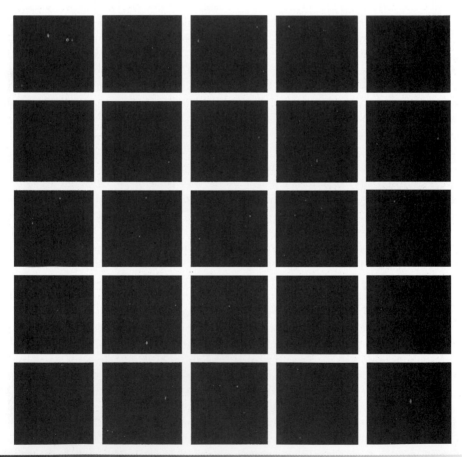

**Figure 4.1   Perception versus reality**

The gray spots seen at the intersections of the white lines are not "real." The true physical stimulus at the intersections is the same as at the middle of the white lines. The perception of gray is caused by neuronal interactions in the retina.

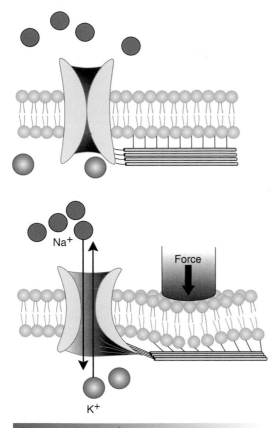

### Figure 4.2   Mechanoreceptors

Mechanoreceptor membranes are mechanically coupled to ionophores. They are normally closed (*top*), but if the membrane is deformed (*bottom*), they open because of their linkages with the cytoskeleton. When open, they allow both sodium and potassium ions to cross the membrane.

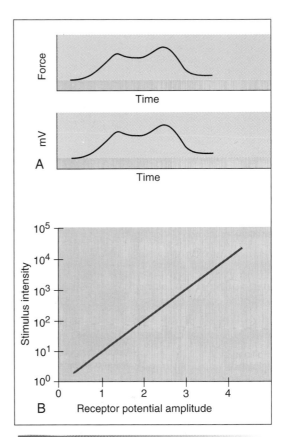

### Figure 4.3   Representation of AM

A perfect transducer creates an analogue signal that is identical to the stimulus in amplitude and time course. **A.** *Top,* force versus time of an arbitrary signal. *Bottom,* the idealized receptor potential that represents the stimulus as (mV) versus time and follows the amplitude and time course of the signal exactly. This receptor potential is a voltage analogue of the mechanical stimulus. **B.** The log relation between the amplitude of the stimulus and the amplitude of the receptor potential.

current source. This degradation is in proportion to the space constant, $\lambda$, of the membrane. Therefore, transmission of the information content of the receptor potential to the CNS must be transformed into action potentials.

Action potentials all have the same amplitude; they are in effect binary signals, either present or absent. Since stimulus intensity cannot be represented by the amplitude of the action potential, it must be represented by the interval between action potentials. The inverse of the interspike interval is **frequency**, that is, the number of action potentials per second (Fig. 4.4). Since the number of action potentials

varies over time with the intensity of the stimulus, the associated series of action potentials is **frequency modulated (FM)**. Consequently, the internal representation of the intensity of the stimulus is both amplitude modulated (receptor potential) and frequency modulated (action potentials).

As Chapter 3 shows, action potentials are produced by voltage-sensitive ion gates in the

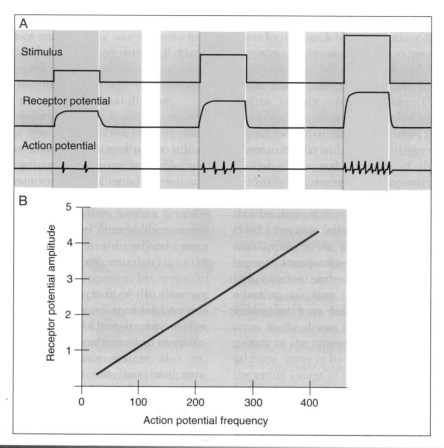

**Figure 4.4    Representation of FM**

Frequency modulation is a form of representation. **A.** An idealized receptor potential is plotted below the stimulus that produced it. Below each are shown the resulting action potentials. The interspike interval decreases with increasing amplitude of the receptor potential. **B.** The amplitude of the receptor potential is plotted against the frequency of action potentials.

membrane. However, there are no voltage sensitive gates in the receptor membrane. They first appear a short distance from the receptor membrane, which in the case of myelinated axons is at the first node of Ranvier. The conversion of the amplitude-modulated receptor potential into frequency-modulated action potentials is similar to the conversion of local currents into action potentials when an action potential is propagated along the axon. The principal difference is that receptor potentials vary in amplitude. If the receptor potential has large amplitude, it continues to depolarize the voltage-sensitive membrane above threshold after the initial action potential recovers. Thus another action potential is

initiated after the absolute refractory period. The interval between the first and second action potential is determined by the interaction between the amplitude of the receptor potential and the relative refractory period of the action potentials (Fig. 4.5). The larger the amplitude of the receptor potential, the shorter the interval between succeeding action potentials. The frequency of these action potentials is the inverse of the interspike interval:

$$f_{Hz} = \frac{1}{\Delta t_{sec}} \qquad \text{(Eq. 4.1)}$$

where $f$ is the frequency in hertz and $t$ is the interspike interval.

## Conversions Between AM and FM

The conversion of intensity information from AM to FM occurs in several critical places in the nervous system. As we have seen, external stimuli are initially transduced as an AM signal (the receptor potential). This AM signal is immediately transformed into an FM signal (action potentials) at the distal portion of the axon, which is the first node of Ranvier in myelinated axons. The action potential produces local currents that are necessary for the propagation of the action potential along the axon (see Chapter 3). Action potentials invading the bouton are converted to the calcium current, an AM signal. The calcium current initiates vesicle binding and subsequent release of neurotransmitter from the bouton. Interaction between the neurotransmitter and the postsynaptic membrane receptors generates AM postsynaptic potentials (PSPs) in the postsynaptic neuron. Finally, the PSPs are converted into action potentials, a FM signal, at the initial segment in the postsynaptic cell.

Why does the nervous system use these complex conversions between AM and FM signals to carry information? These modulations represent different forms of the same information. Each type of modulation has advantages in certain situations.

Action potentials can transmit information over long distances, in some cases several hundred centimeters. In large animals, such as whales and giraffes, the distance can be measured in meters. Local currents degrade with distance and over the course of a few microm-

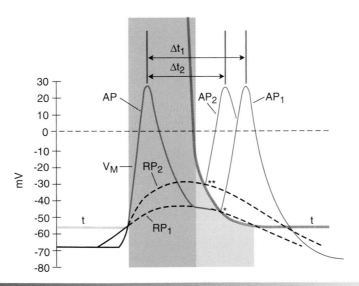

### Figure 4.5 AM to FM conversion

The relation between the receptor potential amplitude and the interspike interval of the generated action potentials. Example 1: A low-amplitude receptor potential (*RP₁*) reduces the membrane potential to threshold (*t*), at which time an action potential (*AP*) is produced. From this point until sometime during the repolarization of the action potential, the membrane is absolutely refractory (*dark pink area*). During the subsequent relative refractory period (*light pink area*), threshold is high but declining (*t* after spike). When threshold declines and meets the recovering membrane potential (*\**), a second action potential is initiated (*AP₁*). Example 2: Given a larger receptor potential (*RP₂*) that initiates an identical action potential (*AP*), the recovering membrane potential meets the declining threshold level sooner (*\*\**) than in Example 1, initiating a second action potential (*AP₂*). The interspike interval $\Delta t_2$ is shorter than $\Delta t_1$, resulting in faster firing. In both examples, during the action potential the receptor potentials are indicated by *broken lines*. In normal recordings, the receptor potentials are masked by the action potential during this time and cannot be visualized directly.

eters diminish to the point of extinction. They cannot carry information over the distances required without being regenerated along the way. By harnessing the potential energy of the membrane potential and creating new local currents, the action potential renews the local currents. *The regenerative interplay between the action potential and the local current along the axon continually restores the signal.* This regeneration allows information to be transmitted over axons for indefinite distances with *no loss of signal quality.*

In contrast to the action potential, local currents can easily combine and interact with one another. The speed and fluidity of local current interactions is essential to the function of the nervous system. Interaction of local currents occurs predominantly in the soma and dendrites of neurons, where information is represented by the amplitude of PSPs (one form of local current). The addition and subtraction of PSPs in the neuron and the subsequent generation of the action potential at the initial segment are the mechanism by which computation (that is, transformation of information) is performed by the nervous system.

## REPRESENTATION

We are accustomed to perceiving several sensory inputs simultaneously. If our nervous system is intact, we can hear, see, taste, touch, and smell our environment, all at once. We also have sensations for heat, cold, and **proprioception** [L. *proprius*, one's own, and *capio*, take], the ability to sense the position of our limbs. The various forms of perception are called **modalities.** *Each modality is closely coupled with forms of energy that can be described in terms of physics and chemistry.* Furthermore, each of these physical stimuli has specific receptors that are most sensitive to that form of energy. Under normal circumstances a specific receptor is affected by only one stimulus modality, the **adequate stimulus.**

Receptors are the starting point of a chain of neurons that ascend the nervous system. Each chain carries only one sensory modality and is therefore **line labeled.** In other words, the information in each chain of neurons is interpreted by central structures *according to the modality of the receptors connected to the origin of the chain in the periphery.*

## Types of Receptors

There are five classes of receptors: photic, chemical, mechanical, thermal, and noxious (Table 4.1). Each class is closely coupled to a distinct form of energy and is most efficient in transducing that form of energy into neuronal signals. **Photoreceptors** exquisitely respond to energy in the form of photons. **Chemoreceptors** are cells with specific membrane proteins that recognize various steric classes of molecules. **Mechanoreceptors** give rise to the sensations we generally call *touch;* **thermoreceptors** account for our perceptions of *temperature;* and **nociceptors** detect tissue damage that we perceive as *pain.* The last three receptors are collectively called **somatosensory receptors** because they are found in the skin,

| Table 4.1 Classes of Sensory Receptors | | |
|---|---|---|
| **Receptor Type** | **Stimulus** | **Perceptions** |
| Photoreceptors | Photons | Light |
| Chemoreceptors | Specific molecules | Taste, smell |
| Thermoreceptors | Temperature | Heat, cold |
| Mechanoreceptors | Mechanical force | Touch, proprioception, sound, etc. |
| Nociceptors | Chemicals associated with tissue damage | Sharp pain, dull pain, burning pain, etc. |

muscles, joints, and viscera. **Proprioceptors** are a special class of mechanoreceptors in muscles and joints that allow us to perceive the *position of our limbs* (see Chapter 6). Photoreception is discussed separately in Chapter 12.

## CHEMORECEPTORS

Chemoreceptors are transducers at the terminals of olfactory and gustatory axons, which mediate the sensations of smell and taste, respectively. Chemoreceptors have specific **binding sites** for certain molecules that we associate with olfaction and taste. When the binding site is occupied by an appropriate molecule, the chemoreceptor is activated. Binding specificity is based on the steric relation between the receptor molecule and the molecule to be bound. A number of binding sites have been identified in both the taste and olfactory epithelia. When stimulated in isolation, it appears that each binding site evokes a separate sensation. Stimulation of multiple sites by complex odors creates new perceptions that are not directly attributable to a single binding site, much as many hues are perceived from the multiple stimulation of only three primary color receptors in the retina (see Chapter 12). In this way a great variety of tastes and smells can be encoded by a small number of binding sites.

There are several mechanisms by which chemoreceptors cause epithelial cell membranes to depolarize (Fig. 4.6). In the simplest mechanisms the chemoreceptor and the ionophore are the same molecule. For example, hydrogen ions can directly block certain potassium ion channels, reducing the potassium current and depolarizing the membrane. Other chemoreceptors act indirectly through G-protein-coupled membrane receptors. Gustatory and olfactory systems do not play a major role in neurology, so chemoreception is not considered further in this text. The student with a special interest in this subject should consult the suggested readings at the end of this chapter.

## MECHANORECEPTORS

Mechanoreceptors are sensitive to mechanical energy. The basic transducers for mechanical

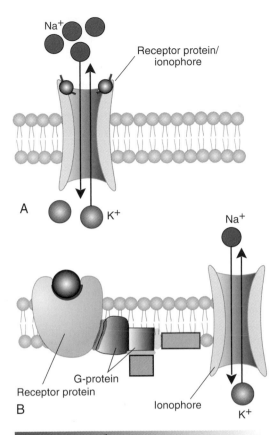

**Figure 4.6   Chemoreceptors**

There are two principal types of chemoreceptors, direct and indirect. Direct chemoreceptors combine the ionophore and the receptor mechanism in the same molecule (**A**), so that binding of the receptor directly affects the permeability of the ion channel. The indirect chemoreceptors (**B**) act through G-protein second-messenger systems.

energy are mechanically sensitive ionophores. However, since there are many forms of mechanical energy (touch, sound pressure, muscle tension), secondary structures have evolved that allow the basic mechanoreceptor membrane to respond to these various forms of energy presentation. In other words, different ionophores are *adapted by external structures* to be most sensitive to a specific form of mechanical energy (Table 4.2).

Mechanoreceptors make the skin an exquisitely sensitive sensory organ. Hairless, or **glabrous, skin** [L. *glaber*, smooth] contains two types of specialized mechanoreceptors,

**Table 4.2   Subtypes of Mechanoreceptors**

| Modality | Location | Specialized Receptors |
|---|---|---|
| Touch intensity | Skin | Merkel disks |
| Touch velocity | Skin | Meissner's corpuscle |
| Touch acceleration | Skin | Pacinian corpuscle |
| Hair movement | Hair shafts | Peritrichal receptors |
| Proprioception | Joints, muscles | Joint receptors[a] |
| Muscle dynamics | Muscle | Muscle spindle[a] |
| Muscle tension | Tendons | Golgi tendon organs[a] |
| Sound | Cochlea | Cochlear hair cells[b] |
| Head acceleration | Vestibular apparatus | Vestibular hair cells[c] |

[a] see Chapter 6.
[b] see Chapter 11.
[c] see Chapter 10.

Meissner's corpuscles and Merkel disks (Fig. 4.7A). They are differentiated by the elaborations that surround the mechanically sensitive receptor membrane. The location of these specialized mechanoreceptors between the epidermis and the dermis makes glabrous skin extremely sensitive to touch. Hairy skin contains special receptors at the base of the hair shafts that are exquisitely sensitive to mechanical displacement of individual hairs. The dermis of both hairy and glabrous skin contains another set of touch-sensitive mechanoreceptors, Pacinian and Ruffini corpuscles.

The **receptive fields** of touch receptors are not the same size. For example, the receptive fields of Meissner's corpuscles and Merkel disks in glabrous skin are very small, whereas the Ruffini and Pacinian corpuscles, which lie deep in the dermis, have large receptive fields (Fig. 4.7B). Furthermore, these somatosensory receptors are not evenly distributed over all parts of the body. In the fingertips they are very close together. One can perceive two points of contact on the fingertips that are only 1 or 2 mm apart. Two separate points of contact on the skin of the back cannot be discriminated until they are about 40 to 50 mm apart.

## NOCICEPTORS

Pain does not arise from the overactivation of the other somatosensory receptors. Rather, the perception of pain is elicited by the action of nociceptors [L. *noceo*, to injure], a specific class of sensory receptors associated with the free nerve endings of small myelinated (Aδ fibers) and unmyelinated (C fibers) axons. Under ordinary conditions nociceptors are inactive, that is, they do not have a resting background activity.

Nociceptors are high-threshold receptors activated by strong stimuli associated with tissue damage. In the case of direct trauma to axons, the breakdown of the axon membrane produces action potentials at the stump of the injured axon. The loss of membrane integrity depolarizes the axon directly. Axons can also be directly activated by potassium ions that are released from ruptured cells following trauma. What sets nociceptors apart from a simple naked axon is that they contain specific receptors that induce depolarization of the axon terminal when bound by specific molecules. Notable among these molecules are **bradykinin**, **histamine**, **serotonin**, and the **prostaglandins**, especially $PGE_2$. These molecules are released into the extracellular space following tissue damage.

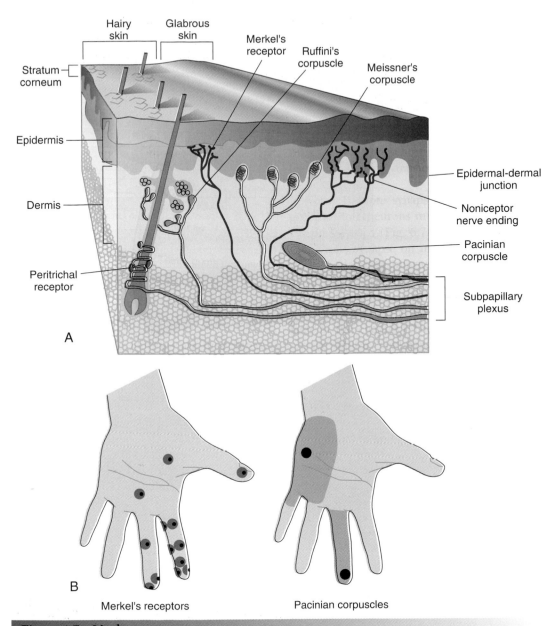

**Figure 4.7  Mechanoreceptors**

**A.** Skin contains a variety of mechanoreceptors. Most receptors in glabrous skin are at the junction of the epidermis and the dermis. This means that the slightest deformation of the skin is transmitted to the receptor. Peritrichal receptors at the base of hair shafts are also situated so as to ensure exceptional sensitivity. The receptors deep in the dermis are much less sensitive to light touch. The highly branched naked nerve endings infiltrate the interstitial spaces in the epidermis and are the principal nociceptors. **B.** The receptive fields of various mechanoreceptors. The *black dot* indicates the point of greatest sensitivity; the *pink* indicates the total receptive area. The size of the receptive fields is highly correlated with the location of the receptor in the layers of the skin. Receptors at the most superficial layers of the skin have the smallest receptive fields (*left*). Receptors deep in the dermis have larger receptive fields (*right*). (**B** Adapted from data in Johansson RS, Vallbo ÅB. Tactile sensory coding in the glabrous skin of the human hand. Trends Neurosci 1983;6:27–32.)

Stimulation of the nociceptor's highly branched sensory axons sends action potentials not only to the CNS but to all the terminal branches of the sensory axon as well (Fig. 4.8). The terminals are invaded by action potentials traveling **antidromically** [G. *anti*, against, opposite, and *dromos*, running] toward the peripheral end of the axon. When the action potential reaches the sensory terminus, a number of substances, including neuroactive peptides, are released from the axon. This process is called an **axon reflex**. Therefore, the terminal arborizations of sensory axons act as both sensory and motor (i.e., secretory) fibers.

Two particularly important neuroactive peptides, **substance P** and **calcitonin gene—related peptide (CGRP)**, are released from

sensory axons by axon reflex. Both peptides are potent vasodilators, so they actively participate in evoking the inflammatory response associated with tissue injury. Substance P in particular increases capillary permeability, which promotes the release of blood-borne sensitizing agents such as histamine, a potent nociceptor stimulant. Substance P also acts directly on the axon terminal, sensitizing it to decrease its threshold to subsequent stimuli.

## THERMORECEPTORS

Two skin receptors that respond to thermal stimuli have been discovered. One set, the **heat receptors**, has a linear relation between the firing rate of their axons and temperature over a range between approximately 32 and 45° C. Between about 45 and 50° C the firing

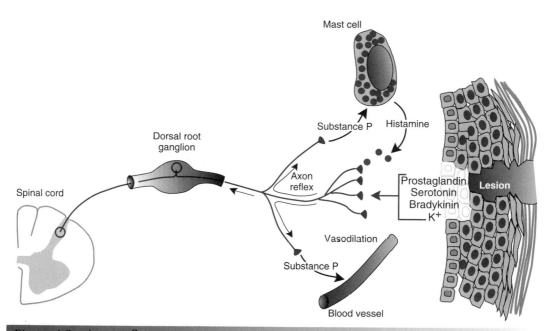

## Figure 4.8 Axon reflex

Bradykinin, histamine, and serotonin, as well as potassium ions leaking from disrupted cells, are potent nociceptive stimulants that directly affect the naked nerve endings. Axons terminating as nociceptors branch copiously in the epidermis. If one axonal branch is stimulated (*central axon*), action potentials generated there are carried to the spinal cord directly and antidromically to other branches of the parent axon. The antidromic conduction is called an axon reflex, although it is not a true reflex. At the antidromically excited terminal, the neuroactive peptide substance P is liberated, which causes mast cells to release histamine. Histamine intensifies the nociceptive stimulation. Substance P also causes vasodilation. (Modified from Jessell TM, Kelley DD. Pain and analgesia. In: Kandel ER, Scwartz JH, Jessell TM, eds. Principles of Neural Science. 3rd ed. Norwalk, CT: Appleton & Lange, 1991;387.)

rate of these receptors rapidly drops to zero (Fig. 4.9). Below about 45° C the perception of heat correlates with temperature, but above 45° C the perception of heat rapidly changes to pain because nociceptors begin to respond to the products of tissue damage. **Cold receptors** are sensitive to skin temperatures from about 24 to 34° C. Paradoxically, cold receptors also respond to temperatures between about 45 and 55° C because of the activation of nociceptors above this temperature.

## Secondary Properties of Somatosensory Receptors

Since the internal representation of a sensory stimulus is an analogue of that stimulus, it is tempting to suppose that the analogue corresponds to the original stimulus in every detail. However, this correspondence is not possible. A physical stimulus has many descriptive properties. For example, a touch on the skin may be described in terms of intensity (pressure), location, duration, and modality (hair movement or skin touch). Furthermore, each sensory modality has many properties, particularly properties associated with the dynamic aspects of the stimulus. For example, the **location, intensity, velocity,** and **acceleration** have to be encoded if a stimulus is to be represented with reasonable accuracy. Receptors encode the location of a stimulus according to the size of the receptive field and the location of the receptor on the body. Most receptors also encode some intensity and some dynamic (velocity and acceleration) information as well, but each type of somatosensory receptor most accurately detects and encodes only one of the principal properties of the mechanical stimuli. Therefore, sensory receptors do not accurately encode all of the properties of a stimulus into a single signal. Being incomplete, *the analogue representation in the CNS is distorted with respect to the original signal.*

## DYNAMICS

When presented with a constant stimulus, the response of most receptors diminishes with time. This is **adaptation.** Receptors are classified as rapidly or slowly adapting, ac-

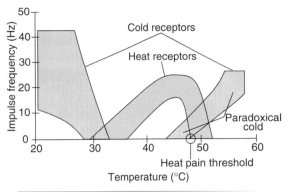

### Figure 4.9  Thermal receptors

Heat (*pink area*) and cold (*gray area*) receptor stimulus response curves. The neuronal response to heat rapidly diminishes to zero above 45°C. Cold receptors have a bimodal response, firing paradoxically above about 45°C.

cording to their response to a steady-state signal (Fig. 4.10).

**Slowly adapting receptors,** like the Merkel disk, generate receptor potentials that are approximately proportional to the amplitude of the signal (Fig. 4.10A). The amplitude of the receptor potential does not change much during the duration of the signal. Within the brief physiological time-course of most signals, the receptor potentials from slowly adapting receptors may be considered nonadapting. Slowly adapting receptors are thought to be the principal receptors that encode intensity of the stimulus.

**Rapidly adapting receptors,** like the Meissner corpuscle, respond primarily to the dynamic properties of the signal. They produce large receptor potentials, called the **on-response,** at the beginning of a stimulus. If the stimulus is maintained at a steady state, the receptor potential rapidly diminishes. When a constantly applied signal ceases, many rapidly adapting receptors generate a potential that signals another transition in the stimulus, the **off-response** (Fig. 4.10E). Rapidly adapting receptors do not encode intensity well. Their activity helps define the temporal boundary conditions of the signal.

Generally speaking, adaptation is not a property of the receptor membrane itself but is

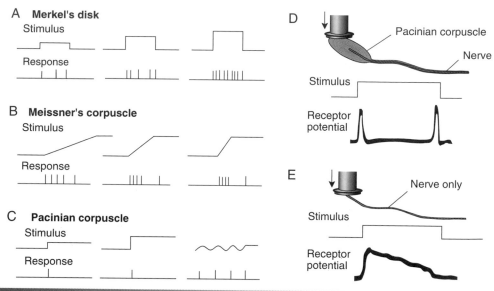

Receptors can be classified according to their rate of adaptation. **A.** Slowly adapting receptors (e.g., a Merkel disk shown here) respond in proportion to the *intensity* of the stimulus and maintain the receptor potential during the entire stimulus. **B.** Rapidly adapting receptors respond primarily to *changes* in the intensity of the stimulus. The Meissner corpuscle shown here responds approximately in proportion to the velocity of the stimulus application, not its intensity. **C.** The most rapidly adapting receptors respond approximately to the *acceleration* of the stimulus. The Pacinian corpuscle shown here is typical. It responds only to a very rapid application of the stimulus, especially rapid vibration (*far right*). **D.** The Pacinian corpuscle responds both to the onset and termination of a stimulus. The very rapidly adapting receptor potential is shown in the middle trace, with the stimulus shown at the bottom. **E.** If the external connective tissue structures are removed from the Pacinian corpuscle, the native response of the receptor membrane is revealed. The lowest trace is the receptor potential of the naked axon ending, showing relatively little adaptation. This trace shows that the mechanical characteristics of the capsule are important to the response characteristics of the receptor membrane. (**D** and **E** modified from Partridge LD, Partridge LD. The Nervous System: Its Function and Its Interaction with the World. Cambridge, MA: MIT Press, 1993:86).

provided by the elaborated structures attached to it. In the case of mechanoreceptors, these elaborations are simple encapsulations, such as those seen in Pacinian or Ruffini corpuscles.

The principal teleological reason for adaptation is to extract the dynamic information, *velocity* and *acceleration,* from the signal (Fig. 4.10, *B* and *C*). For example, the slowly adapting Merkel disk is a somatosensory receptor that responds to the *steady-state* pressure of the stimulus without significant adaptation. It encodes *intensity* and *duration.* The rapidly adapting Meissner corpuscle, by contrast, responds almost exclusively to the *velocity* of the

applied pressure. Finally, the Pacinian corpuscle, a very rapidly adapting receptor, detects *acceleration.* All of these receptors have an axon membrane with mechanically sensitive ion channels. They are differentiated from one another by the external apparatus covering the naked axon that modifies the way the stimulus affects the receptor membrane.

## INTENSITY

The physiologically significant range of intensity that most stimuli present to the nervous system covers six to eight orders of magnitude. Encoding such a wide range of intensity into neural signals cannot be accomplished directly because amplitudes of receptor potentials and frequencies of action potentials cannot accommodate this range. Action potentials (FM) have a dynamic range of about three orders of magnitude; receptor potentials (AM), only about two. Two peripheral mechanisms overcome this shortcoming.

First, different receptors within the same class (e.g., Merkel disks) have different thresholds. If two receptors have the same dynamic range (e.g., two orders of magnitude) but the threshold of one is two orders of magnitude higher than the other, together they can encode an intensity range of 4 orders of magnitude (Fig. 4.11). Given receptors of overlapping thresholds, the entire range of intensity information can be accommodated.

Second, the relation between the stimulus intensity and the receptor potential is usually not linear. For most systems this nonlinear re-

lation can be approximated by the following expression:

$$R \propto \log(S) \qquad \text{(Eq. 4.2)}$$

where R is the receptor potential and S is the intensity of the stimulus. Receptors with nonlinear response characteristics, such as cold receptors, encode a greater range of intensity at the expense of resolution.

## LOCALIZATION

Somatosensory information can be localized to specific anatomical sites because *the spatial relation between the tactile receptors distributed over the body surface is maintained in the anatomical organization of the CNS neurons that receive information from those receptors.* Therefore, the physical arrangement of CNS neurons and their axons is in fact a representation of the body, a **somatotopic map.** The various maps throughout the nervous system are not limited to the somatosensory system. The body is mapped, for example, in the ascending sensory tracts in the spinal cord and at each synaptic level in a chain of neurons within the CNS, up to and including the cerebral cortex. Similar maps for the motor systems and the special sensory systems exist. The representation in the nervous system of the anatomical arrangement of the body, a fundamental feature of the nervous system, greatly affects its function.

Spatial discrimination of sensory stimuli is enhanced by synaptic interactions within the sensory nuclei as information is transmitted from one set of neurons to another. The most common form of synaptic interaction is a process known as **lateral inhibition.** Briefly, within the nuclei of the CNS some neurons (transmission cells) send long axons that project to distant nuclei and short recurrent collateral axons that terminate locally on inhibitory interneurons. The interneurons in turn terminate on adjacent transmission cells within the same nucleus (Fig. 4.12). Through the activity of the interneuron, each transmission cell can inhibit the activity of its neighbor. The most active neurons diminish the activity of adjacent, less active neurons. Since the organization of the central tracts is

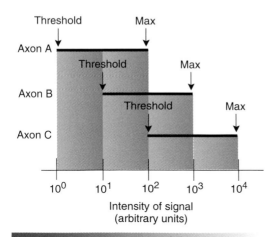

### Figure 4.11   Extension of dynamic range

A wide dynamic range of information can be carried by multiple information channels of narrow dynamic range if each channel carries a subset of the information. In this example each axon is limited to two orders of magnitude. *Axon A* carries intensity information from 1 to $10^2$ arbitrary units; *axon B* carries intensity from 10 to $10^3$; and *axon C* carries intensity information from $10^2$ to $10^4$. Together the three axons can convey intensity information of four orders of magnitude, even though each axon is limited to only two orders of magnitude.

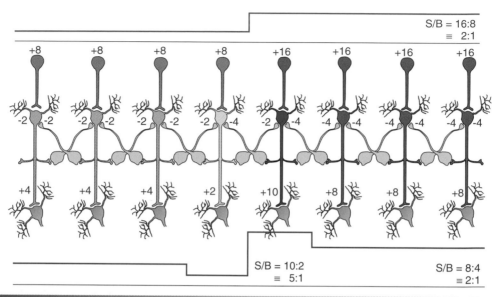

**Figure 4.12   Lateral inhibition**

The mechanism of lateral inhibition is schematically illustrated and highly simplified here. A stimulus with an arbitrary intensity of 8 units on one side of a boundary and 16 units on the other side is presented to a set of receptors (*top, dark red neurons*). The receptors synapse with a corresponding set of sensory neurons, providing the same arbitrary units of excitation to the sensory neurons. The axons of each sensory neuron provide recurrent collateral fibers that synapse with interneurons (*light gray neurons*) that inhibit adjacent sensory neurons by 25% of the stimulus intensity. The final level of excitation, the simple sum of inhibition and excitation, is indicated at the boutons of the sensory neurons. The signal intensity ratio of the stimulus is 2:1. After passing through this simple neural network, the signal ratio is still 2:1 except at the boundary, where the ratio has increased to 5:1. Thus, lateral inhibition incurs no overall loss of signal contrast over most of the stimulus field and enhances the signal contrast at the boundary condition, making it more prominent. While greatly oversimplified, the principles illustrated by this neural network have been verified in numerous neuronal systems. *S/B*, signal intensity ratio.

mapped to the surface of the skin, the effect of lateral inhibition is to restrict the ability of sensations arising from the immediately surrounding regions of a punctate stimulus to reach higher levels in the CNS. Favoring the most active neurons and suppressing less active neurons enhances boundary contrasts.

## INTERPRETATION OF SENSATIONS

Receptors can respond to more than one type of energy. The sensitivity of a particular receptor to a specific form of energy may be increased both by *restricting the energy forms* that normally arrive at the receptor and by *creating* *specialized receptor mechanisms* for receiving that energy. In most cases, however, the specific sensitivity of receptors is not absolute. If the intensity is great enough, receptors can generate neuronal signals even if they are stimulated by forms of energy for which they were not specifically adapted. Photoreceptors, for example, can be stimulated mechanically by pressing on the eye. One's *perception* is light, not pressure, because the structures within the brain that receive the information *interpret* any signals received from the visual pathways as light. *The brain has no mechanism for distinguishing the absolute nature of the stimulus.* Similarly, under laboratory conditions when isolated cold receptors are stimulated above 45°C, the subject reports the perception of cold, not warmth or pain. Just as in the case of pressing on the eye, *the brain interprets the information it receives according to the receptor from which it originated as projected through the nervous system along a specific line-labeled chain of neurons.* If the temperature stimulus were applied over a larger region of the skin so that nociceptors were also stimulated, creating a more complex, information-rich signal, the brain would interpret the stimulus as local pain.

All sensory modalities are closely coupled with energy forms that can be quantified in terms of physics and chemistry, because specific receptors have adapted to detect these forms of energy. Each modality is presented to our consciousness as an **objective sensation**. We also have **subjective sensations**, which we can perceive but for which we have no specific receptors. The feeling of wetness is one example. We have no hydrologic receptors that sense the presence of water on our skin, yet we are aware of being wet. Itch, tickle, and pain are other examples.

These subjective sensations are *derivative perceptions* that arise from complex neuronal activity. They represent specific combinations of objective sensations that are interpreted by our nervous system as unique. Our perceptions of hue are derived from various combinations of photons presented to three primary photoreceptors that have overlapping color sensitivities. We do not have a specific color receptor for each hue we perceive. Most of our perception of hues is the result of neuronal interactions resulting from the reception of the primary color information received from specific photoreceptors.

# C A S E  H I S T O R Y

## THE CASE OF THE WRETCHED WRENCH

### HISTORY OF PRESENT ILLNESS

Mr. S. M. is a 21-year-old architecture student who was in good health until June 16. He was repairing his motorcycle when a wrench slipped off a nut, causing his right hand to smash into the handlebar. In great pain he came to the student health center thinking he had broken his thumb.

### PHYSICAL EXAMINATION

Unremarkable

### NEUROLOGICAL EXAMINATION

**Mental Status**
Normal

**Cranial Nerves**
All normal

**Station and Gait**
Normal

**Motor Systems**

STRENGTH: 5/5 in all groups tested

BULK: Symmetrical and appropriate for a young man

TONE: Normal resting tone; no spasticity or rigidity

## Figure 4.13. Cutaneous radial nerve distribution

The normal distribution of the superficial radial cutaneous nerve to the hand. Note how crushing the lateral division can cause the lack of sensation noted by Mr. S. M. (Modified from Grant JCB. Grant's Atlas of Anatomy. 5th ed. Baltimore: Williams & Wilkins, 1962;plate 83.)

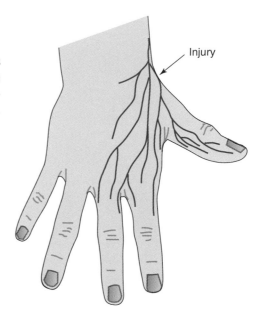

ABNORMAL MOVEMENTS: None noted

### SENSORY SYSTEMS
The patient was able to perceive pinprick and light touch from all extremities except for a total anesthesia of the dorsal surface of the right thumb, sparing the palmar surface and the dorsal surface of the hand. Detailed examination revealed that there was no feeling to light touch or pinprick from the dorsal surface of the thumb (Fig. 4.13). Light pressure near the point of injury produced paresthesias (abnormal, unpleasant sensations) at the most distal portion of the thumb, on the dorsal surface, and near the thumbnail.

### Reflexes
Muscle stretch reflexes (MSRs) were symmetrical and judged to be normal. Toes were down going.

### Coordination and Control
Not tested.

### Parietal Functions
Not tested.

### ANCILLARY STUDIES
Radiographs of the hand revealed no fractures.

### SUBSEQUENT COURSE
No follow-up. Uneventful recovery is anticipated.

### COMMENTARY
Mr. S. M.'s thumb struck the handlebar at the base of the metacarpal near the insertion of the *abductor pollicis longus.* Superficial cutaneous branches of the radial nerve pass over this point before being distributed to the mediodorsal surface of the thumb and hand. Although radiographs showed that no bones were fractured, apparently the bar crushed the lateral branch of the nerve, producing total anesthesia of the skin served. Light pressure at the point of injury could be expected to stimulate the crushed axons *at the point of injury,* sending action potentials to the CNS. The signals so received would be localized to the receptors normally attached to those axons. This accounts for the patient's perceived sensations from the anesthetized areas of the thumb.

# C A S E   H I S T O R Y

## A REACH TOO FAR[1]

### HISTORY OF PRESENT ILLNESS

Mrs. M. W. is a 68-year-old moderately obese woman who came to the emergency room after falling from a ladder while reaching for some blankets. She landed on a tile floor, injuring her right arm. She called the paramedics, who splinted the arm, abducted 90° to her body, before transporting her to the hospital. She is alert and in mild pain.

### MEDICAL HISTORY

She has a history of chronic obstructive pulmonary disease.

### PHYSICAL EXAMINATION

Unremarkable except for expiratory wheezes. There is a palpable defect in the right shoulder joint. The overlying skin is intact. There is a strong bilateral radial pulse, and capillary refilling in the digits is rapid bilaterally.

### NEUROLOGICAL EXAMINATION

**Mental Status**
Normal

**Cranial Nerves**
All Normal

**Station and Gait**
Normal

**Motor Systems**

STRENGTH: The patient displays full movement and normal strength of her right fingers and wrist. The right shoulder and arm could not be tested without inflicting pain. The other extremities were not tested.

BULK: Symmetrical and normal for a woman of her age.

TONE: Normal resting tone; no spasticity or rigidity.

ABNORMAL MOVEMENTS: None observed.

**Sensory Systems**
The patient has decreased light touch sensations over the first three digits of the right hand and over the region of the right deltoid. Pinprick was not tested.

**Reflexes**
MSRs were symmetrical and within normal limits. Toes were down going.

**Coordination and Control**
Not tested

**Parietal Functions**
Not tested.

### ANCILLARY STUDIES

Radiograph of the right shoulder revealed an anterior inferior dislocation of the right humeral head.

### SUBSEQUENT COURSE

The dislocation was reduced with gentle traction. Following reduction, the patient was unable to abduct her arm. Strength of the deltoid was rated zero (see Appendix 2). The lack of sensation over the deltoid remained. The sensory perception was restored in the right hand. The patient was told that she had injured the nerve to a muscle in her arm, which was causing the weakness and numbness. She was told that with rest its function might be restored but that it was possible that full function would not return.

---

[1] This case was kindly supplied by Dr David Halpern, M.D.

## COMMENTARY

Peripheral nerves do not normally lie close to the surface; they are deep, protected by the surrounding muscle and bone. There are specific locations, however, where peripheral nerves are relatively unprotected and commonly injured. Determining the distribution of paresthesias or sensory loss over the skin and specific muscle weakness is often the best diagnostic clue. For example, in this case there is sensory loss over a small area of the shoulder combined with weakness of the deltoid muscle. The muscle is supplied by the axillary nerve, and its cutaneous branch supplies the superficial skin. Therefore, one can conclude that this nerve was crushed during the accident. The numbness in the fingers is referred to the distribution of the median nerve. Pressure was probably placed on this nerve by the dislocated humerus, which blocked conduction. Reduction of the dislocation relieved the pressure on the nerve and restored median nerve function. The crush injury to the axillary nerve will require regeneration of the axons. Nerve regeneration and the principles of peripheral nerve distribution are considered further in Chapter 5.

## FURTHER APPLICATIONS

4.1. Peripheral nerves are particularly prone to injury in a number of places because of their superficial course. Using your knowledge of gross anatomy, identify these sites and the nerves in jeopardy.

4.2. Why was special note taken of the movements of the fingers and wrist?

4.3. What patterns of sensory and motor losses would you expect to observe after nerve injury of the posterior cord of the brachial plexus; the radial nerve after the axillary nerve has separated; the radial nerve distal to the elbow?

4.4. The function of peripheral nerves can also be affected by simple compression that does not actually crush the nerve. What neuronal mechanisms would be affected by compression?

4.5. Compression syndromes frequently affect the carpal tunnel and ulnar nerve at the wrist. What is unusual about the anatomy of this region that places the nerves passing through the wrist particularly at risk?

4.6. How can repetitive movements of the fingers and wrist exacerbate this situation?

4.7. What patterns of sensory and motor dysfunction would you expect to ob-

## S U M M A R Y

- Physical stimuli are received by sensory receptors and converted to internal signals that are the basis of conscious perceptions.

Transduction is the process by which the energy of the stimulus is converted to an energy form appropriate for the nervous system. Representation is the manner in which the neuronal energy is organized as an analogue of the stimulus. Specific receptors convert the energy of a stimulus into an AM receptor potential. The receptor potential is itself converted into a series of FM action potentials.

- Our sensations are divided into modalities that correspond to objective physical stimuli.

The modalities have specific receptors and segregated neuronal pathways (line labeled). There are five classes of receptors: photic, chemical, mechanical, thermal, and noxious. The last three are collectively called somatosensory receptors. Somatosensory receptors usually adapt to constant stimuli, a property that makes them sensitive to velocity and acceleration. The dynamic range of receptor sensitivity is expanded by nonlinear transformation of the stimulus into the receptor potential. This transformation extends the range of response at the expense of sensitivity. The physical organization of somatosensory receptors is maintained in the CNS, a process called mapping. Maps are maintained at all levels of the CNS.

- **The brain has no independent way of interpreting information arriving on the sensory pathways.**

Any form of energy that can stimulate a receptor or the nerve causes the brain to perceive a stimulus appropriate to the receptor. The sensory modalities are closely linked to objective physical forms of energy for which there are specific receptors. Derivative sensations are not associated with specific receptors. These sensations arise from neuronal activity that represents certain combinations of objective stimuli. While not real in the objective sense, these perceptions are real to the conscious awareness of the organism.

## SUGGESTED READINGS

Augur AM, Lee MJ. Grant's Atlas of Anatomy. 9th ed. Baltimore: Lippincott Williams & Wilkins, 1999.

Bach FW. Beta-endorphin in cerebrospinal fluid: relation to nociception. Dan Med Bull 1997; 44:274–286.

Campbell WW. Diagnosis and management of common compression and entrapment neuropathies. Neurol Clin 1997;15:549–567.

García-Añoveros J, Corey DP. The molecules of mechanosensation. Annu Rev Neurosci 1997;20: 567–594.

Sidall PJ, Cousins MJ. Neurobiology of pain. Int Anesthesiol Clin 1997;35:1–26.

Szabo R, Steinbert D. Nerve entrapment syndromes in the wrist. J Am Acad Orthopaed Surg 1994;2:115–123.

# The Somatosensory System

The brain receives information about the environment by means of its sensory systems, which in humans include the olfactory, taste, hearing, visual, and somatosensory [G. *soma,* body, and L. *sensorium,* the seat of the senses] systems. This chapter describes the somatosensory system, a collection of receptors, tracts, and nuclei that convey the sensations of light touch, proprioception, temperature, and nociception [L. *nocere,* injure; *capio,* take] to consciousness. Somatosensory receptors inhabit the skin, muscles, joints, and viscera, a distribution that makes the somatosensory system the largest and most varied of the sensory systems. While chiefly sensory, it also plays a critical role in motor control by providing appropriate feedback to the motor system about joint position, muscle tension, velocity of muscle contraction, and contact of the body with external surfaces. It is therefore appropriate to begin our examination of the function of the nervous system with this sensory system.

## ANATOMICAL ORGANIZATION OF SOMATOSENSORY SYSTEMS

The gross and microscopic features of the nervous system are discussed in Chapters 1 and 2. This chapter addresses the intermediate structures, the tracts and nuclei. Before the sensory pathways can be presented, it is necessary to describe the relations of the prominent sensory tracts and nuclei at the various levels of the nervous system. The description that follows focuses on the sensory components within the central nervous system (CNS). The

motor tracts and nuclei are discussed in Chapters 6 to 9. Finally, the cranial nerve nuclei are described in Chapter 10. Therefore, three trips through the neuraxis are required to describe the internal structure of the nervous system.

### The Peripheral Nerves

The peripheral nerves consist of bundles of axons. Two nomenclature systems describe axons (Fig. 5.1). The system that groups axons by diameter labels them A, B, and C; the largest axons, which are myelinated, belong to group A, and the smallest axons, which are unmyelinated, belong to group C. The A group is further divided into four subgroups, $\alpha$, $\beta$, $\gamma$, and $\delta$. The B group contains the myelinated preganglionic axons of the autonomic nervous system (see Chapter 13). The B classification is now seldom used.

The second system classifies certain sensory axons according to their origin, function, and conduction velocity. This system is used to describe afferent axons originating in muscles, tendons, and joints. Axons are designated by roman numerals as I, II, III, and IV in decreasing conduction velocity; group IV contains unmyelinated axons. Since diameter and conduction velocity are related, the two systems overlap. Unfortunately, since the two systems were developed independently, the overlap is not exact. Both nomenclatures are in use, and it is easy to become confused.

### The Spinal Cord

The **spinal cord** is organized into a central gray area surrounded by white matter. In fresh, un-

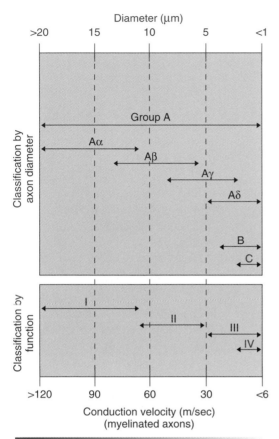

**Figure 5.1    Classification of axons**

The classification schemes of peripheral axons are correlated with their diameters and conduction velocities. Axons indicated in *red* are unmyelinated.

fixed material it appears gray because it is composed mostly of neuron cell bodies. The white matter obtains its color from the myelin that covers most of the axons found there. Cell bodies are not found in white matter.

It is convenient to divide the gray matter of the spinal cord into a series of layers, or **laminae**, that extend its entire length. These laminae transcend the segmental divisions imposed upon it by the spinal nerves. The spinal cord gray matter was divided into 10 laminae by Rexed, who used strictly cytoarchitectural methods to distinguish the laminae (Fig. 5.2).

Over the years it has been recognized that certain physiological properties correlate with the lamina. These observations have given Rexed's system practical use.

The laminae are labeled I through X. They form nearly flat ribbons that lie parallel to the long axis of the spinal cord. The dorsal horn is composed of laminae I through VI, which receive the primary afferent axons from the dorsal root and contain **interneurons** and **projection neurons.** Interneurons have short axons that form synapses within a few hundred micrometers of their soma. Projection neurons have long axons that transmit information to relatively distant locations in the CNS. The somatic motor neurons, the principal source of axons that leave the CNS, are in lamina IX, and the autonomic motor neurons (see Chapter 13) are in lamina VII. Interneurons associated with motor reflexes are in lamina VIII. Lamina X, which surrounds the central canal, includes the ependyma and a thin layer of gray matter. Cells in lamina X are important to the perception of visceral pain.

The white matter of the spinal cord can be separated into three regions according to its relation to the gray matter (Fig. 5.3). The **dorsal columns** lie dorsal and medial to the dorsal horns. Caudal to the midthoracic levels, the **fasciculus gracilis** [L. *fasciculus,* small bundle, *gracilis,* thin, slender] fills the entire dorsal column space. In the cervical and upper thoracic spinal cord, the dorsal columns are divided by the **dorsal intermediate sulcus** into the fasciculus gracilis and the **fasciculus cuneatus** [L. *cuneo,* wedge shaped].

The **lateral white columns** lie lateral to the gray matter and between the dorsal and ventral horns. They contain several motor tracts that are described in Chapter 6. The region medial and ventral to the ventral horns is occupied by the **ventral white columns.** The most important sensory tract in the ventral white columns is the **anterior lateral system** (ALS[1]). A small but important collection of axons interconnecting the two halves of the

---

[1] Do not confuse the abbreviation ALS as used here to signify a CNS tract with the same abbreviation used to designate the neurological disease amyotrophic lateral sclerosis.

spinal cord, the **ventral white commissure,** crosses the midline just ventral to the central canal.

## The Brainstem

Descriptions of brainstem structures are based on their relation to the fourth ventricle and cerebral aqueduct (Fig. 5.4). The principal mass of neuronal tissue ventral to the fourth ventricle is the **tegmentum** [L. *tego,* cover]. The tegmentum can be further described as the medullary tegmentum, pontine tegmentum, and tegmentum of the midbrain. The **tectum** [L. *tego,* cover, roof] lies dorsal to the ventricle. In the midbrain the tectum is composed of the corpora quadrigemini. In the pons the roof is the cerebellum. There are no neuronal structures of the roof in the adult medulla.

A large collection of axons commonly called the **basis** lies ventral to the tegmentum. In the midbrain the basis consists of the **cerebral peduncles** [L. *pes,* foot]. The basis is greatly enlarged in the pons and contains considerable gray matter, the **basal pontine nuclei.** The **medullary pyramids** form the basis of the medulla.

Most of the brainstem tracts and nuclei are in the tegmentum. Long ascending sensory and descending motor tracts traverse the entire brainstem. Shorter tracts connect brainstem structures with the cerebellum or establish intrinsic connections among cell groups within the brainstem. Most of the nuclei of the brainstem are associated with the cranial nerves or the cerebellum. With a few exceptions, the remaining cells in the tegmentum are considered part of the **reticular formation** [L. *reticulum,* little net], an area of diffusely organized groups of cells. The following brief description of brainstem structures is not complete. It does emphasize the structures associated with the somatosensory system.

## THE MEDULLA

The transition between the spinal cord and the brainstem, which occurs over a few millimeters, is marked by changes in the pattern and location of certain structures in the spinal cord

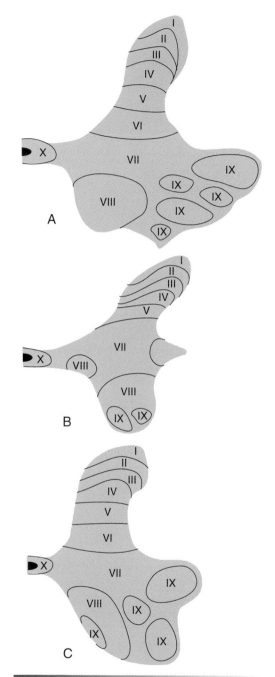

**Figure 5.2   Laminae of Rexed**

**A.** Cervical. **B.** Thoracic. **C.** Lumbar. The laminar system is best applied to the dorsal horn. In the ventral horn the motor neuron nuclei (lamina IX) can be considered discrete nuclei, segregated according to the muscles they innervate.

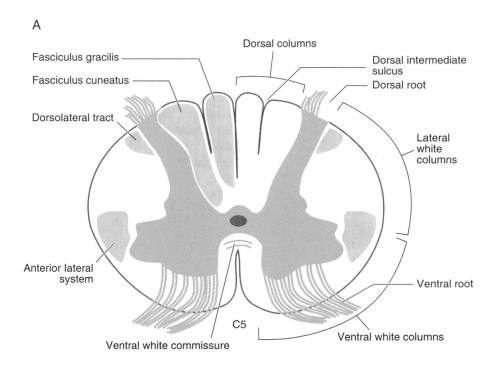

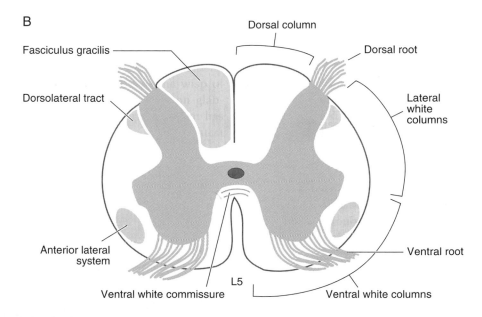

**Figure 5.3 Cross-sections of the spinal cord**

**A.** Cervical. **B.** Lumbar. The principal ascending sensory tracts are shown in *gray.* The gray matter and dorsal and ventral roots are shown in *pink*.

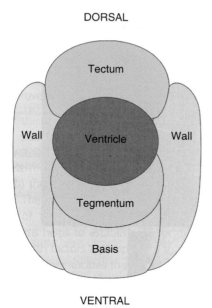

DORSAL

VENTRAL

**Figure 5.4   Organization of the brainstem**

(Fig. 5.5A). The ventral horns become disorganized rostral to the level of the **decussation of the corticospinal tracts** [L. *decussatus*, X shaped] and are no longer distinguishable. The rapidly diminishing ventral horn becomes incorporated into the **medullary reticular formation**. At about the same level the dorsal horn enlarges and moves dorsolaterally, separating from the central mass of gray matter and forming a separate nucleus, the **spinal trigeminal nucleus**. This nucleus is an important landmark that can be followed throughout the medulla and into the pons. Immediately lateral to the spinal trigeminal nucleus lies the **spinal trigeminal tract**. It contains primary afferent axons from the trigeminal nerve (cranial nerve [CN] V) that synapse in the spinal trigeminal nucleus.

At the transition from the spinal cord into the medulla the dorsal columns are gradually replaced by two pairs of nuclei, the **nucleus gracilis** and **nucleus cuneatus**, respectively. The fasciculus gracilis, fasciculus cuneatus, and spinal trigeminal tract all lie toward the surface of their respective nuclei. Together these three pairs of tracts and their associated

nuclei occupy approximately the dorsal half of the caudal medulla. While the spinal trigeminal nucleus and tract are constant features of the medulla, the dorsal column nuclei and their tracts extend rostrally to approximately the level of the obex.

The **medial lemnisci** [G. *lemniskos*, a woolen fillet] are a pair of tracts that occupy the central region of the medulla. In cross-section they appear as a pair of cigar-shaped structures that lie perpendicular to the long axis of the medulla on either side of the midsagittal plane (Fig. 5.5B). The medial lemnisci, another constant feature of the brainstem, are readily identified throughout its length.

The obex divides the caudal from the rostral medulla. At this transition, the medulla changes from a round to a rhomboid shape (Fig. 5.5, C and D). The fourth ventricle begins at the obex and extends the length of the rostral medulla and pons. In the rostral medulla, the **inferior olivary nuclei**, which lie ventral laterally on either side of the brainstem, become prominent. The spinal trigeminal nuclei and tracts lie at the lateral margin with the ALS ventral to them and immediately dorsal to the inferior olives. The **inferior cerebellar peduncles**, also called the restiform body, occupy the dorsolateral corners.

THE PONS

The basis of the pons is its most conspicuous feature (Fig. 5.5, E and F). In addition to massive fiber tracts, it contains a large amount of gray matter, the **basal pontine nuclei**. Axons from neurons in the basal pontine nuclei cross the midline and form the **middle cerebellar peduncles**, also called the brachium pontis. Since the axons of the middle cerebellar peduncles lie in the plane of cross-section of the pons, they are *cut in longitudinal section*, which makes them readily identifiable. The remaining axons are part of the corticobulbospinal tracts (see Chapter 6), which course the pons rostrocaudally. These axons are *cut in cross-section*.

The area between the basis of the pons and the fourth ventricle is the pontine tegmentum, which contains the nuclei associated with the cranial nerves of the pons, the pontine reticular formation, and various other fiber tracts. In

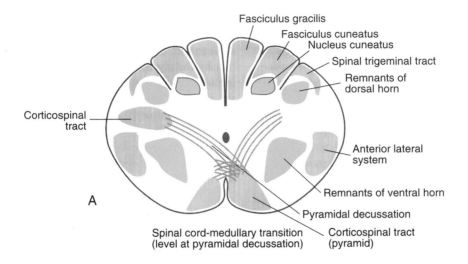

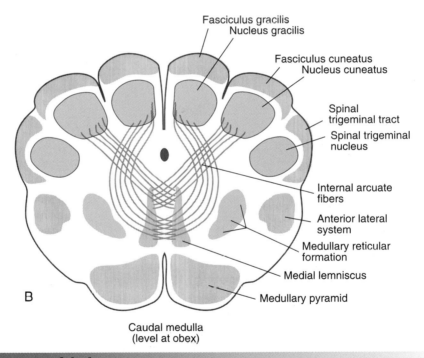

**Figure 5.5    Sections of the brainstem**

**A.** Cross-section of the caudal medulla (pyramidal decussation).
**B.** Cross-section of the caudal medulla at the obex.

the caudal pons (Fig. 5.5E) the medial lemnisci form a pair of oval structures on either side of the midline at the junction of the basis and tegmentum. As one moves rostrally, the medial lemnisci become more horizontal. They continue to move laterally to the most rostral end of the pons, where they form a thin ribbon at the extreme lateral half of the junction of the basis and tegmentum (Fig. 5.5F). The ALS occupies a constant position at the ventral lateral margin of the pontine tegmentum. Throughout the length of the pons the medial lemniscus becomes more laterally placed until, at the rostral pons, it joins the ALS.

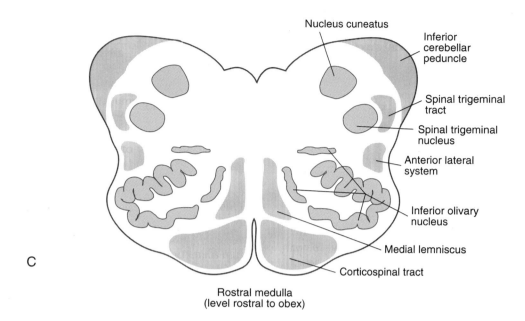

C

Rostral medulla
(level rostral to obex)

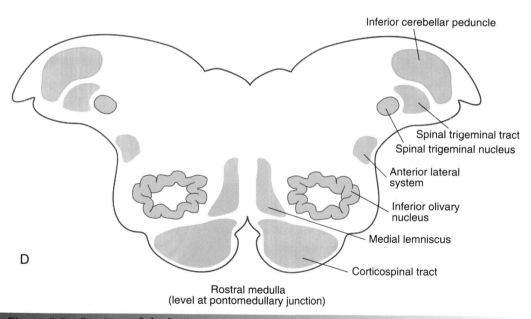

D

Rostral medulla
(level at pontomedullary junction)

**Figure 5.5    Sections of the brainstem—*continued***

**C.** Cross-sections of the rostral medulla rostral to the obex. **D.** Cross-section
of the rostral medulla (pontomedullary junction).

The **superior cerebellar peduncle,** also called the brachium conjunctivum, is a prominent structure of the rostral pons, forming part of the walls of the rostral pons and midbrain. As one moves from the pons into the midbrain, the superior cerebellar peduncles descend from their superolateral position toward the center of the midbrain tegmentum, where they decussate (Figs. 5.5*E, F,* and *G*).

THE MIDBRAIN

The fourth ventricle narrows to form the **cerebral aqueduct** in the midbrain (Fig. 5.5*G*). Immediately surrounding the aqueduct is a

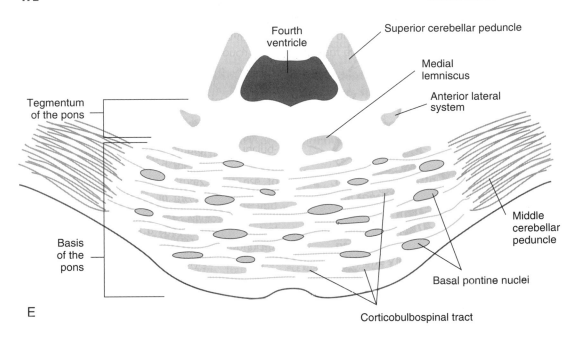

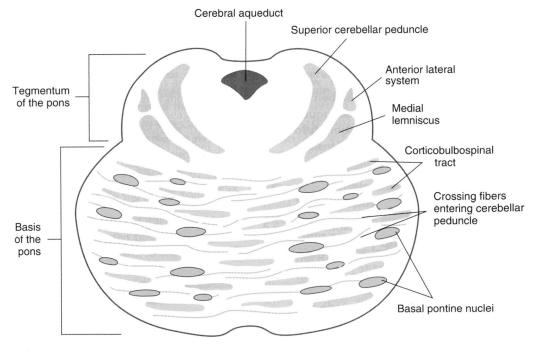

**Figure 5.5    Sections of the brainstem—*continued***

**E.** Cross-section of the caudal pons. **F.** Cross-section of the rostral pons.

prominent core of gray matter, the **periaque-ductal gray** (PAG). An imaginary line passed horizontally through the aqueduct separates the midbrain tegmentum (ventral) from the tectum (dorsal), the latter consisting of the superior and inferior colliculi (corpora quadrigemini). The medial lemniscus and the ALS maintain their extreme lateral position.

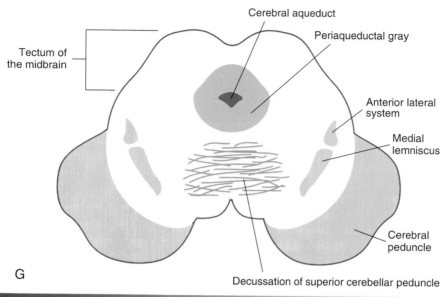

G

Cerebral aqueduct

Periaqueductal gray

Tectum of
the midbrain

Anterior lateral
system

Medial
lemniscus

Cerebral
peduncle

Decussation of superior cerebellar peduncle

**Figure 5.5  Sections of the brainstem—*continued***

**G.** Cross-section of the midbrain.

## The Thalamus

As the midbrain blends into the thalamus [G. *thalamos,* chamber], the cerebral aqueduct lengthens dorsoventrally to become the third ventricle (Fig. 5.6), which divides the thalamus at the midline. However, in many persons an **interthalamic adhesion**, a small mass of gray matter, connects a small part of the two halves of the thalamus.

Each half of the thalamus is an egg-shaped body that is divided into many nuclei. For convenience these nuclei can be organized into five groups that are partly defined by a band of white matter, the **internal medullary lamina** (Figs. 5.6 and 5.7). The anterior pole of the thalamus is split by the lamina, which forms a pocket. The nuclei in this pocket belong to the **anterior nuclear group**. The remainder of the thalamus is divided by the internal medullary lamina into medial and lateral areas. Medial and dorsal to the internal lamina lies the **medial group**. Lateral and ventral to it is a collection of nuclei, the **lateral group**. Within the internal medullary lamina are scattered cells and one prominent nucleus, the **centromedian (CM)**, that constitute the **intralaminar group**. An **external medullary lamina** surrounds the main body of the thalamus, and external to it lies a thin

band of cells, the **reticular group**. The remaining parts of the thalamus are described in later chapters.

The posterior thalamus contains three nuclei, the **pulvinar**, the **lateral geniculate** [L. *geniculare,* to bend the knee], and the **medial geniculate**. The pulvinar and lateral geniculate nuclei serve the visual system, and the medial geniculate serves the auditory system. These nuclei are discussed in later chapters.

The thalamus is a complex structure serving many sensory, motor, and cognitive functions. With the exception of olfaction, all sensory information must pass through the thalamus before reaching the cerebral cortex. Similarly, motor command information must pass through the thalamus before a motor act can be initiated (see Chapter 8). Given this heterogeneity, the thalamus is considered in several parts of this book.

A feature of all thalamic nuclei is their reciprocal connections with the ipsilateral cerebral cortex. Some nuclei are connected to very small parts of the cortex (**specific thalamic nuclei**); others have widespread connections (**nonspecific thalamic nuclei**). The specific thalamic nuclei associated with somatosensory function are subdivisions of the lateral

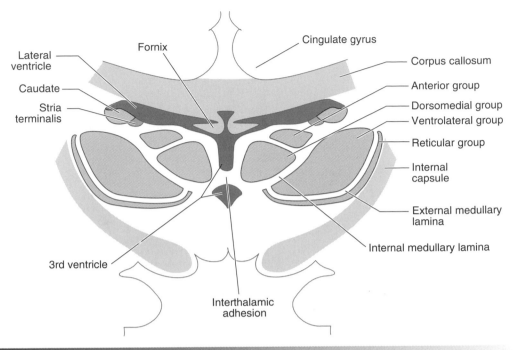

**Figure 5.6    Cross-section of the thalamus**

group (Fig. 5.7A). This large group is subdivided into ventral and lateral divisions. Within the ventral division lies the **ventrobasal complex,** a set of four nuclei, the **ventral posterior medial** (VPM), the **ventral posterior lateral** (VPL), the **ventral posterior superior** (VPS), and the **ventral posterior inferior** (VPI). Within the intralaminar group are the nonspecific nuclei associated with somatosensory function. The intralaminar group consists mostly of scattered cells within the white matter of the internal medullary lamina, but one collection—the **centromedian** (CM)—is large enough to be named.

### The Cerebral Cortex

The cerebral cortex is composed of a 2- to –4-mm-thick superficial layer of gray matter with an underlying mass of white matter. The gray matter is divided into six horizontal layers designated by roman numerals in ascending order from the surface (Fig. 5.8) and defined by histological criteria. While all neocortex exhibits this six-layer organization, the neo-

cortex is not totally homogeneous. Differences lie mostly in the thickness of the various layers and the size and number of many of the cells. It is these differences that Brodmann used to subdivide the cerebral cortex into 50 numbered areas (see Fig. 1.13).

### HISTOLOGY OF THE CEREBRAL CORTEX

The principal cell type found in the cerebral cortex is the **pyramidal cell,** named for its triangular soma (Fig. 5.9). Found in all but the most superficial layer of the cerebral cortex, pyramidal cells have an apical dendrite that extends from the peak of the triangle and rises toward the surface of the cortex, crossing several layers. Basal dendrites extend parallel to the surface from the base of the soma. A single axon projects into the white matter. The pyramidal cell is the only type to extend axons out of the cortical gray matter. All other cell types in the cerebral cortex are interneurons.

Input to the cerebral cortex comes from three areas: other parts of the cerebral cortex, the thalamus, and specialized subcortical nuclei.[2] Association fibers from other parts of the cortex penetrate and synapse in all layers. Fibers from the specific nuclei of the thalamus synapse primarily in layer IV. Both corticocortical association fibers and specific thalamocortical fibers terminate within a single cortical column (discussed later in the chapter). Fibers from the nonspecific thalamic nuclei and from the specialized subcortical nuclei

synapse in all layers. Most of the nonspecific fibers branch extensively and terminate in very large areas of the cerebral cortex.

Output from the cerebral cortex is only from pyramidal cells and is classified according to the projection of the axon. **Short association fibers** project to adjacent gyri or gyri within the same lobe. **Long association fibers** interconnect lobes in the same hemisphere. **Callosal**

---

[2] These nuclei are the locus ceruleus in the brainstem and the basal nucleus of Meynert in the basal ganglia.

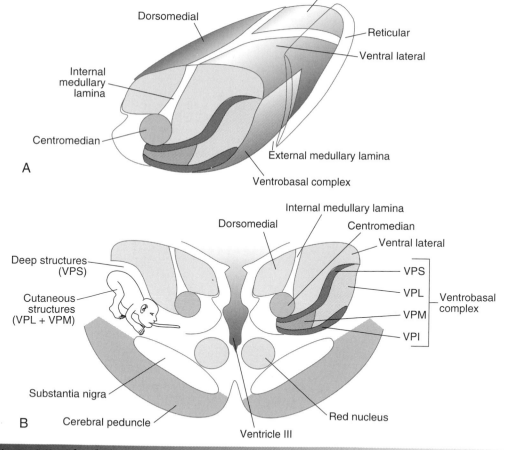

**Figure 5.7   The thalamic nuclei**

**A.** In this posterior view of the right thalamus, the internal medullary lamina divides the thalamus into three main groups, the anterior, dorsomedial, and ventral lateral. Within the internal medullary lamina lie scattered cells and one large nucleus, the centromedian. The structures within the internal medullary lamina constitute the intralaminar nuclear group. External to the external medullary lamina lies the reticular nuclear group. **B.** This transverse section through the thalamus shows the location of the ventrobasal complex (*pink*) and its division into four nuclei. The homunculus (*left*) shows the somatotopic arrangement of the VPL and VPM nuclei.

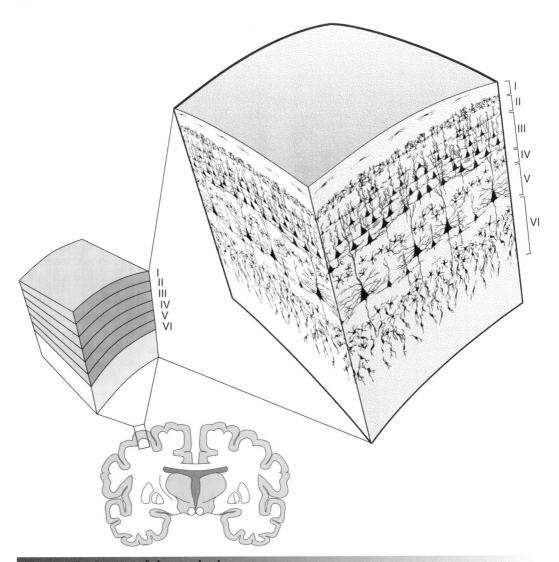

**Figure 5.8    Layers of the cerebral cortex**

**fibers** cross the midline in either the anterior commissure or the corpus callosum. The cell bodies of association and callosal fibers are found primarily in layers II and III. **Projection fibers** originate from pyramidal cells of layers III, V, and VI (Fig. 5.9). They leave the cortex and innervate subcortical structures such as the basal ganglia, thalamus, brainstem, and spinal cord. No pyramidal axons leave the CNS.

Projection fibers are the only pyramidal axons that leave the cerebral cortex. They collect as bundles in the subcortical white mat-

ter, forming the **corona radiata** (see Fig. 1.14). As they pass deeper into the core of the telencephalon, they concentrate into a massive bundle, the **internal capsule**. The internal capsule passes through the caudate nucleus, then passes between the thalamus (dorsomedial) and the globus pallidus (ventral lateral) as it progresses through the diencephalon. Many of these fibers terminate in the thalamus and basal ganglia. The remaining fibers become the cerebral peduncles of the midbrain.

## CORTICAL COLUMNS

Approximately 300 to 600 cells of the neocortex are interconnected vertically to form a local functional unit, a **cortical column**. Although there are billions of columns, they are not obvious in histologic preparations. The columns are arranged horizontally across the cortex. The vertical organization of cells within a column is superimposed on the horizontal organization of the columns across the cerebral cortex. Individual axons originating in the specific thalamic nuclei terminate in a single cortical column. This arrangement imparts regional functional specificity to the column. For example, within a single sensory column in area 3a, all of the cells respond only to a stimulus of a single modality from a specific location (Fig. 5.10). An adjacent column responds to a different modality but from the same location on the skin. This pattern repeats in an organized manner across the cortex.

A current hypothesis proposes that *the cortical column is the principal computational unit of the cerebral cortex*. According to this concept, the columns are quasi-independent processing units that act in parallel. The independence of the column is established by the distinct input-output relation that each column has with the thalamus and with other cortical and subcortical structures. Although each column is relatively independent, it is not isolated. The columns are richly interconnected with adjacent columns in the same cortical area and with neighboring areas, gyri, and lobes. The manner in which these functional columns are interconnected determines the ultimate function of various areas of the cerebral cortex. The concept of the cortical column is developed further in later chapters.

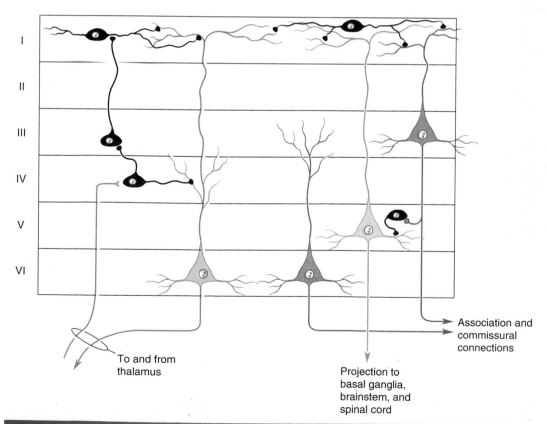

To and from thalamus

Projection to basal ganglia, brainstem, and spinal cord

Association and commissural connections

I
II
III
IV
V
VI

**Figure 5.9   Simplified input-output relations of the cortical layers**

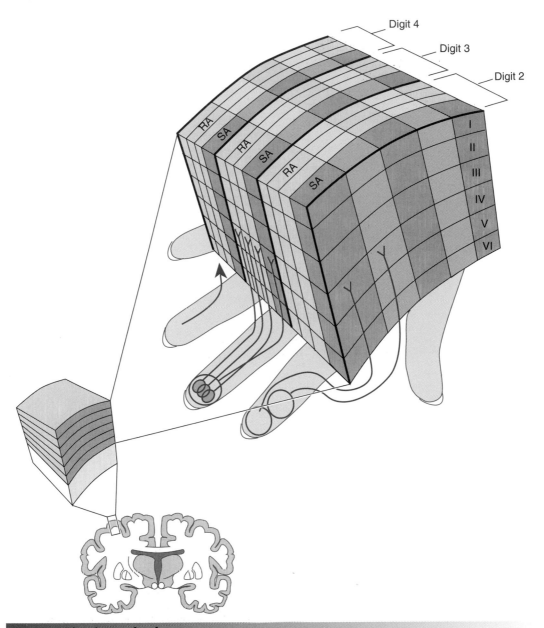

## Figure 5.10   Cortical columns

Each sensory cortical column receives signals derived from one specific sensory modality from one specific anatomical site (for clarity, the intervening spinal and thalamic circuits are not shown here). The neurons within a column synapse primarily with other neurons in the same column. The columns are arranged like a map of the body surface. The *large circles* on the fingers represent slowly adapting mechanoreceptor receptive fields; the *small circles,* rapidly adapting mechanoreceptor receptive fields.

## THE SOMATOSENSORY PATHWAYS

There are two somatosensory pathways. One pathway, the **dorsal column system**, consists of large-diameter myelinated fibers that convey

*fine tactile, vibratory,* and *proprioceptive* (joint and limb position) sensations. The receptors associated with this system have low thresholds and very small receptive fields. Therefore, the dorsal column system is **epicritic** [G. *epi,* on, and *krino,* separate, judge], because it provides the ability to distinguish between two separate but simultaneous touches to the skin, a property called *two-point discrimination.*

The second pathway is the ALS, which consists of small-diameter myelinated and unmyelinated fibers. It is **protopathic** [G. *protos,* first, and *pathos,* suffering] because it conveys *nociceptive* and *temperature* sensations. Because the receptors associated with the ALS have large receptive fields, the spatial representation within this system is not highly specific. In the absence of the

dorsal column system, it can convey a gross, poorly localized sense of touch.

These two systems have much in common. Both convey information from the peripheral receptor to the cerebral cortex over a core pathway consisting of only three neurons (Fig. 5.11). The first neuron of the pathway is the **primary afferent axon.** Its specialized peripheral termination is the sensory receptor. The soma is in the dorsal root or cranial nerve ganglion, and it makes synaptic connections in the ipsilateral gray matter of the spinal cord or

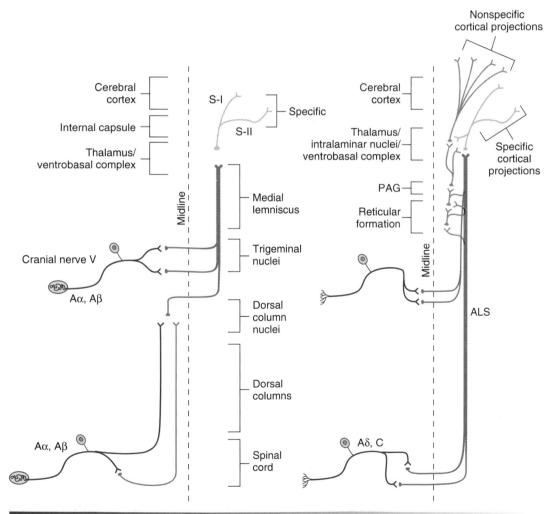

**Figure 5.11   Ascending sensory pathways**

The somatosensory ascending pathways (dorsal column, epicritic on the left; ALS, protopathic on the right). Both the ALS and the dorsal column systems share the basic three-neuron structure: primary (*dark pink*), second-order (*medium pink*), and third-order (*light pink*) neurons. The ALS has an extensive parallel path to the thalamus through the reticular formation (*gray*). The ALS also has a heavy projection into the nonspecific intralaminar nuclei, which the dorsal column system lacks.

medulla. The primary afferent axons entering the dorsal root segregate by size as they enter the spinal cord. Large, myelinated Aβ axons form the **medial division of the dorsal root,** and small, myelinated Aδ and the unmyelinated C axons form the **lateral division.**

The **secondary neuron,** a projection neuron, receives synapses from the primary afferent axon. Its soma is ipsilateral to the side of entry of the primary afferent neuron. The secondary axon *crosses the midline* and terminates in the thalamus contralateral to the stimulus. The cell body of the **tertiary neuron** is in the thalamus. Its axon passes through the internal capsule and terminates in the cerebral cortex ipsilateral to its origin but contralateral to the origin of the stimulus.

With the single exception of the olfactory system, all sensory systems are based on this three-neuron pattern. Although quite useful, this description of the pattern is an oversimplification. Each sensory system also expresses elaborations of this basic structure. Learning is simplified, however, if one first identifies the three-neuron core and later adds the elaborations.

## The Dorsal Column System

The axons in the dorsal columns are the primary afferent axons of a rapidly conducting sensory system, appropriately called the **dorsal column system** (Fig. 5.12). Fine tactile sensations and two-point discrimination arise from the encapsulated receptors in glabrous skin and the peritrichal receptors in hair shafts, while vibratory sensations are ascribed to the Pacinian corpuscles. Various types of receptors in the joints signal joint position. All of these receptors convey information to the spinal cord over large, myelinated Aβ axons.

### PRIMARY AFFERENT NEURONS

After entering the spinal cord, the primary afferent axons divide. A *short local branch* enters the gray matter of the spinal cord, and a *long ascending branch* enters the dorsal columns,

within which it ascends to the medulla. The *short local branch* bifurcates close to the point of entry to the spinal cord. One branch ascends and the other descends one or two segments along the spinal cord close to the gray matter of the dorsal horn. These short branches give off collaterals that penetrate the dorsal horn, within which they synapse in laminae III, IV, and V (Fig. 5.13).

The shape and location of the terminal fields of these axons differ somewhat, depending on the sensory modality they convey. The terminations of some axons, such as those derived from hair follicle receptors, terminate in overlapping fields, forming a continuous, rostrocaudal projection field in the dorsal horn. Other axons, such as those from some slowly adapting receptors, terminate in discontinuous fields that form ball- or balloon-shaped patterns in the dorsal horn. In general, they terminate in the intermediate laminae of the dorsal horn, more or less continuously throughout the entire extent of the spinal cord.

The *long ascending branch* ascends the ipsilateral dorsal column and terminates in the dorsal column nuclei of the medulla (Fig. 5.12). Axons that enter the spinal cord below approximately the midthoracic level ascend in the fasciculus gracilis and terminate in the nucleus gracilis. Those that enter above midthoracic levels ascend in the fasciculus cuneatus and terminate in the nucleus cuneatus.

The primary afferent axons enter the fasciculus gracilis or fasciculus cuneatus from the lateral aspect. As the tract ascends, more axons are added in the lateral position, increasing the size of the fasciculus. In this manner the axons in the dorsal columns are organized according to their somatic origin. Axons from the leg are most medial, and those from the arm are most lateral. **Somatotopic** [G. *topos,* place] arrangements are carefully preserved at all levels of the nervous system.

Somatosensory information from the face enters the CNS over primary afferent axons in cranial nerves V (trigeminal), VII (facial), IX (glossopharyngeal), and X (vagus)[3] (Fig.

---

[3] The cranial nerves VII, IX, and X innervate only a small area of skin near the external auditory meatus and the pinna. Their central connections follow those of the trigeminal nerve (see Chapter 10).

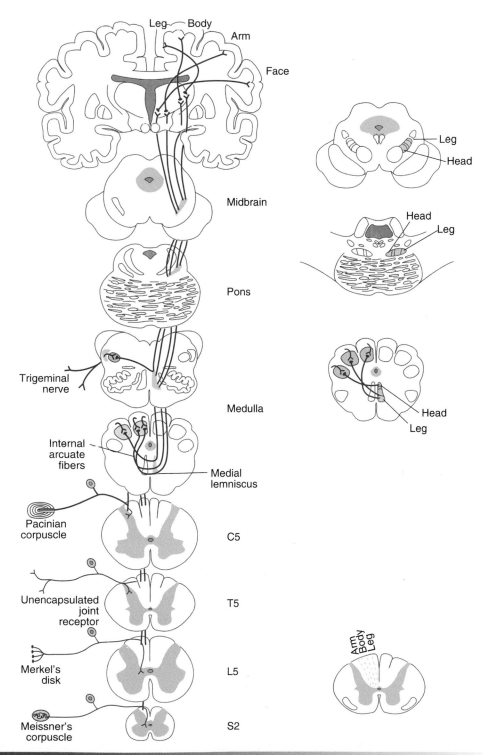

**Figure 5.12  The dorsal column (epicritic) pathways**

*Left,* the anatomical location of the principal elements of the dorsal column system. *Right,* the somatotopic arrangement of the fibers at the various levels. The types of epicritic receptors are found at all levels, not just those shown in the figure.

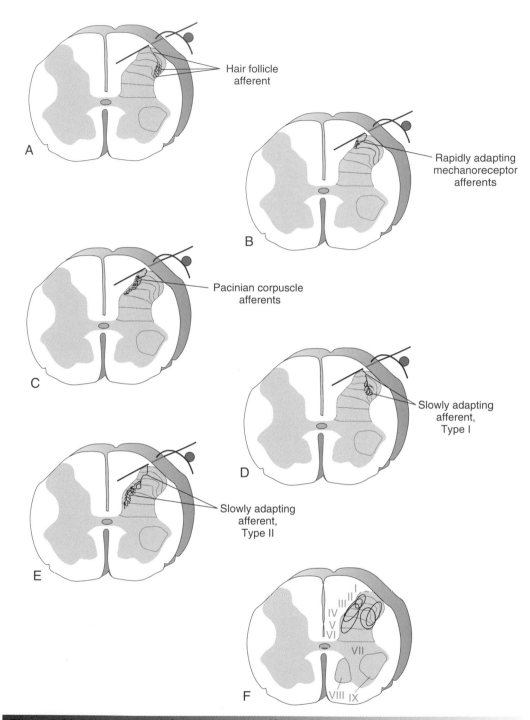

Hair follicle
afferent

Rapidly adapting
mechanoreceptor
afferents

Pacinian corpuscle
afferents

Slowly adapting
afferent,
Type I

Slowly adapting
afferent,
Type II

## Figure 5.13  Termination of some primary afferent axons

The distribution of the short local branch of the large-diameter afferent axons in the dorsal horn. These figures are based on three-dimensional reconstructions of individually labeled and identified axons. All of the afferent axons share a pattern in which the afferent axon divides after entering the spinal cord and sends an ascending branch up and a descending branch down the spinal cord. The branches send collaterals deep into the dorsal horn gray matter, where they further collateralize into a terminal arborization. The axons here represent different sensory modalities that terminate in specific locations in the dorsal horn with a characteristic pattern. **F** identifies the laminae and summarizes the figures shown in **A–E**. (See Chapter 4 for a discussion of receptor types.)

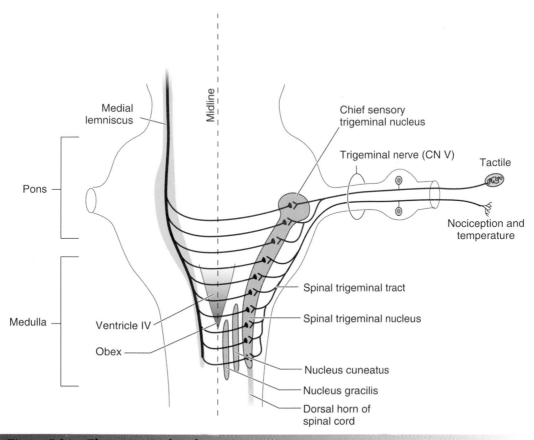

**Figure 5.14    The trigeminal pathways**

The nociceptive and thermal afferent axons terminate primarily in the caudal two-thirds of the spinal trigeminal nucleus. Fine tactile and proprioceptive afferent axons terminate mostly in the chief sensory trigeminal nucleus and the rostral third of the spinal trigeminal nucleus.

5.14). Just as in the spinal cord, the somatosensory primary afferent axons in the cranial nerves form two groups, one composed of large-diameter Aβ axons and the other composed of small-diameter Aδ and C fibers. The large-diameter axons enter the brainstem and bifurcate. One branch descends into the medulla, coursing in the spinal trigeminal tract. These axons send collateral branches into the rostral third of the spinal trigeminal nucleus, where they synapse. A short ascending branch terminates in the **chief sensory trigeminal nucleus.**

## SECOND-ORDER NEURONS

The second-order neurons in the nucleus gracilis and nucleus cuneatus receive synaptic contact from the primary afferent axons of the fasciculus gracilis and fasciculus cuneatus respectively. Axons arising from neurons within these nuclei leave their place of origin, course ventral medially, and cross the midline (Fig. 5.12). At this point they make an abrupt 90° turn and begin to ascend the brainstem. Where they arc across the medulla, these axons are known as the **internal arcuate fibers.** After they cross the midline, they are known as the **medial lemniscus.** The internal arcuate fibers and the medial lemniscus both contain axons that arise from the dorsal column nuclei. The axons have different names to distinguish their different locations. Second-order neurons from the spinal trigeminal nucleus and the chief sensory trigeminal nucleus send axons across the midline to join the medial lemniscus at its medial margin (Fig. 5.14).

The axons in the medial lemniscus are arranged in a somatotopic pattern that is maintained at all levels of the brainstem (Fig. 5.12). Near the origin of the medial lemniscus in the lower medulla, fibers from the nucleus cuneatus enter the dorsal portion of the tract, and axons from the nucleus gracilis form the ventral portion. At this level the medial lemniscus is a vertical structure in transverse sections of the medulla. Therefore, the fibers are arranged in a head-up position. In the lower pons the medial lemniscus begins to tilt horizontally, so that the fibers from the head are dorsomedial and those from the lower extremity are ventral lateral. In the midbrain, the medial lemniscus is nearly horizontal and occupies an extreme lateroventral position in the tegmentum. The leg area occupies the most lateral portion of the medial lemniscus; the head area occupies the most medial portion.

The medial lemniscus enters the thalamus and terminates in a precise somatotopic manner in the **ventrobasal complex** (Fig. 5.7). Signals originating from mechanoreceptors terminate primarily in VPL and VPM; the axons of trigeminal origin enter VPM, and those of spinal origin enter VPL. VPS receives strictly proprioceptive signals.

## THIRD-ORDER NEURONS

Third-order axons arising from neurons within the ventrobasal complex project into the ipsilateral cerebral cortex after passing through the posterior limb of the internal capsule (Fig. 5.12). The axons terminate primarily in **Brodmann's areas 3a, 3b, 1, and 2** (see Fig. 1.13) of the **postcentral gyrus**. The association between this area of the cerebral cortex and somatosensory information processing is so specific that this cortical area is frequently called **the primary somatosensory cortex, or S-I.**

The somatotopic arrangement that is so characteristic of the dorsal columns, the medial lemniscus, and the ventrobasal complex of the thalamus is preserved in the S-I cortex (Fig. 5.15). Here, projections carrying infor-

mation from the lower extremity terminate along the superomedial aspect of the postcentral gyrus. The representation of the upper extremity descends across the surface toward the lateral fissure. The face and internal surfaces of the mouth and throat are represented at the most inferolateral portion.

The surface area of the body is not proportionally represented in the somatotopic organization of the cerebral cortex. The upper extremity and thorax occupy about as much cortical surface area as the hand, and about a third of the hand area is taken up by the thumb. The face area is about the same size as the hand area, with about a third of it occupied by the lips. The map of somatotopic representation in the cerebral cortex corresponds quite closely with a map depicting the resolution of two-point discrimination, the areas with finest discrimination having the largest cortical representation.

The S-I cortex is not functionally or anatomically homogeneous. The four Brodmann areas that constitute the primary sensory cortex do not receive thalamic projections equally. For example, about 70% of the thalamic axons from VPL and VPM terminate in areas 3b and 3a; the remaining 30% are divided between areas 1 and 2 (Fig. 5.16A). Furthermore, the thalamic projections into the cortex are divided by modality. Area 3a receives information originating primarily from muscle stretch receptors (see Chapter 6), and 3b receives input from cutaneous receptors. Information from rapidly adapting cutaneous receptors goes to area 1, and deep pressure receptors project to area 2. *Each of these modalities is separately mapped, creating parallel somatotopic cortical maps.*

Cortical areas have cascading reciprocal connections (Fig. 5.16B). For example, area 3a sends short association fibers to areas 3b, 2, 4, and 6 (areas 4 and 6 serve motor functions; see Chapter 7). Area 3b projects to areas 1 and 2. All four primary somatosensory areas send projection axons to a small area of the operculum at the lateral sulcus that serves as a second, complete sensory cortex, **S-II.** The S-II projection is also somatotopically arranged.

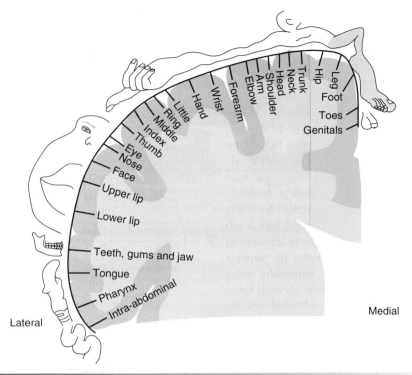

**Figure 5.15    The human sensory cortex**

A somatotopic map of the human S-I based on studies of awake, alert persons undergoing cortical stimulation during brain surgery. The *pink* area is supplied by the anterior cerebral artery. The remainder of the S-I is supplied by the middle cerebral artery. (Adapted from Penfield W, Rasmussen T. The Cerebral Cortex of Man: A Clinical Study of Localization of Function. New York: Macmillan, 1950.)

Although S-II receives direct thalamic projections, chiefly from VPI and with a lesser contribution from VPL and VPM, it cannot process sensory information independently of S-I. The S-II cortex may play an important role in pain perception.

The stimulus-response characteristics of cortical neurons differ in the various cortical areas. For example, neurons in areas 3a and 3b respond best to simple punctate stimuli appropriate to the receptive field of the cell. Neurons in areas 1 and 2, however, respond only to more complex stimuli. Most are *motion sensitive,* that is, an object must be moving across the skin before the cell will respond. Other cells are *direction sensitive;* that is, the cell preferentially responds to objects moving only in one direction, such as left to right across the hand but not right to left.

As the cortical areas become synaptically more removed from direct thalamic input, the response characteristics of the cortical neurons are more and more abstracted from the initial stimulus. *Motion, direction, texture, and object shape are not properties of the stimulus that are encoded by single, individual receptors; they are an abstracted feature of the stimulus.* The ability to develop these abstract properties from a single stimulus is unique to the cerebral cortex. Spinal, brainstem, and thalamic neurons do not have these properties. The ability to process abstract information is essential to **stereognosis** (the ability to recognize objects by tactile shape alone), **graphesthesia** (figure writing on the skin), and fine coordinated movements, especially of the fingers. Cortical lesions to the postcentral gyrus cause loss of these functions.

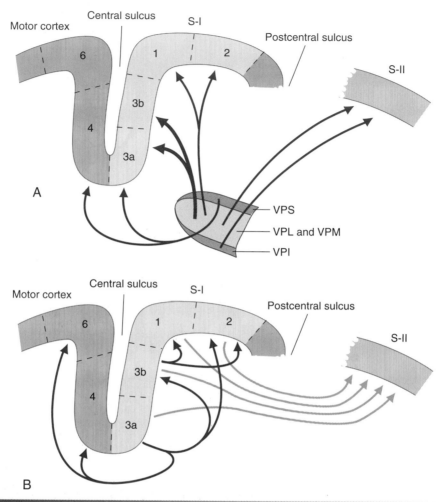

**Figure 5.16  Extrinsic and intrinsic connections of S-I**

**A.** The relations between the ventrobasal complex of the thalamus and the subdivisions of the somatosensory areas of the cerebral cortex. About 70% of the thalamic projections are from VPL and VPM to areas 3A and 3B **B.** Short association fibers interconnect the various regions in a series of cascades. All four subdivisions of S-I project to the secondary sensory area, S-II, in the parietal operculum.

## VISCERAL SENSATIONS

Sensations arising from the viscera are also carried in the dorsal columns. Primary afferent C fibers carrying nociceptive information from visceral organs enter the spinal cord and synapse on neurons in the dorsal horn. Secondary neurons form a polysynaptic projection into laminae III and X from which projection neurons send axons that ascend in the most ventral medial aspect of fasciculus gracilis (Fig. 5.17). Although lying within the dorsal columns, this visceral pain path appar-

ently carries only protopathic information from the viscera. The axons synapse in the nucleus gracilis. The pathways by which this nociceptive information is carried beyond the medulla are not known. However, selective interruption of these fibers in the dorsal columns dramatically reduces the perception of pain from the viscera.

### The Anterior lateral System

The ALS is named for the fiber tract in the ventral lateral aspect of the spinal cord. This tract

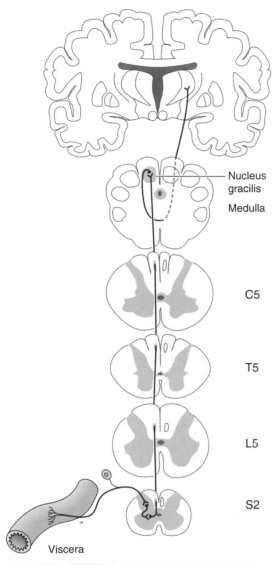

Figure 5.17   **Visceral nociceptive pathways**

the spinothalamic tract because it follows the three-neuron model of sensory systems.

## PRIMARY AFFERENT NEURONS

Primary afferent axons contributing to the ALS are A$\delta$ and C fibers. They enter the spinal cord in the lateral division of the dorsal root and immediately bifurcate, forming an ascending and a descending branch (Fig. 5.18). These branches travel for one to three segments in the **dorsolateral tract**, also known as Lissauer's tract. Collateral fibers from these branches leave the dorsolateral tract to enter the dorsal horn, where they synapse. The A$\delta$ fibers synapse primarily in laminae I and V, and the C fibers synapse principally in laminae II and I.

## SECOND-ORDER NEURONS

Neurons with cell bodies in laminae I, IV, V, and VI send second-order axons to the contralateral thalamus. These axons cross the midline in the ventral white commissure at approximately their level of origin. On the contralateral side they collect in the ventral lateral funiculus, where they make an abrupt 90° bend before ascending (Fig. 5.19). Somatotopic organization is established as new axons join this tract at the medial margin, creating a laminar structure.

The second-order axons of the ALS maintain their ventral lateral position the entire length of the spinal cord and medulla, lying ventral to the spinal trigeminal tract in the caudal medulla and between the inferior olive and the spinal trigeminal tract in the rostral medulla. They maintain their ventral lateral position throughout the pontine tegmentum. In the rostral pons the medial lemniscus is lateral enough to meet the ALS, and from that point onward the axons travel juxtaposed into the thalamus. Axons originating in lamina I terminate primarily in VPL and VPI. Those originating in the base of the dorsal horn in laminae IV to VI project primarily to the intralaminar group, especially CM. Only the axons that terminate in VPL and VPI maintain a somatotopic organization in the thalamus.

consists of secondary projection neurons that originate in the spinal cord and terminate primarily in three areas of the brain—the **brainstem, thalamus,** and **hypothalamus**—and related regions. Most of the axons in the ALS terminate in the thalamus (the **spinothalamic tract**), the brainstem reticular formation (the **spinoreticular tract**), or the mesencephalon (the **spinomesencephalic tract**). It is easiest to begin consideration of the ALS by describing

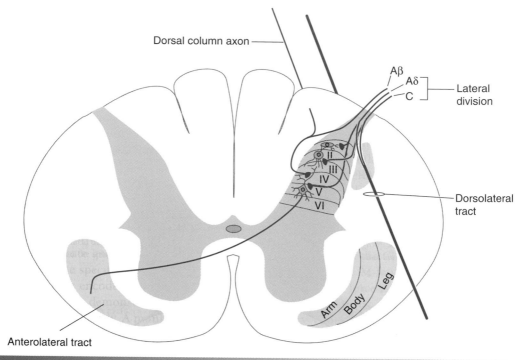

**Figure 5.18   Somatic nociceptive input to the spinal cord**

## THIRD-ORDER NEURONS

At the thalamus the dorsal column system and the spinothalamic division of the ALS share the same third-order neurons from VPL and VPI to the cerebral cortex. Although the dorsal column system and the ALS share the VPL and VPI thalamic nuclei, information from the dorsal column system dominates this pathway. Without dorsal column input, protopathic information is poorly localized.

## TRIGEMINAL CONTRIBUTIONS TO THE ALS

Primary afferent Aδ and C fibers originating in the face follow pathways that are quite similar to those described for the Aβ fibers that enter the spinal cord (Fig. 5.14). These fibers enter the brainstem in the trigeminal nerve, descend into the medulla in the spinal trigeminal tract, and give off collaterals that terminate in the caudal two-thirds of the spinal trigeminal nucleus. From this nucleus secondary neurons send axons across the midline and join the medial lemniscus, eventually terminating in

VPM of the ventral basal complex of the thalamus. From there, tertiary neurons ascend to the cerebral cortex.

## ELABORATIONS OF THE ALS

Not all fibers in the ALS ascend directly to the thalamus. Many, perhaps most, terminate in the medulla and midbrain. These fibers do not follow the three-neuron pattern but elaborate the principal spinothalamic pathway.

Axons in the spinoreticular division of the ALS, as the name of this division implies, ascend to the reticular formation from the spinal cord. Most terminate in the nucleus **gigantocellularis** of the medullary reticular formation. Neurons in laminae I and V contribute to the spinomesencephalic division and project to the **locus ceruleus** and the PAG in the midbrain.

Another set of axons with no specific name contributes to the ALS. These axons project to the **hypothalamus, amygdaloid nuclei, nucleus accumbens,** and the **septal nuclei**. These regions of the brain are important in determining one's subjective feelings and emotional

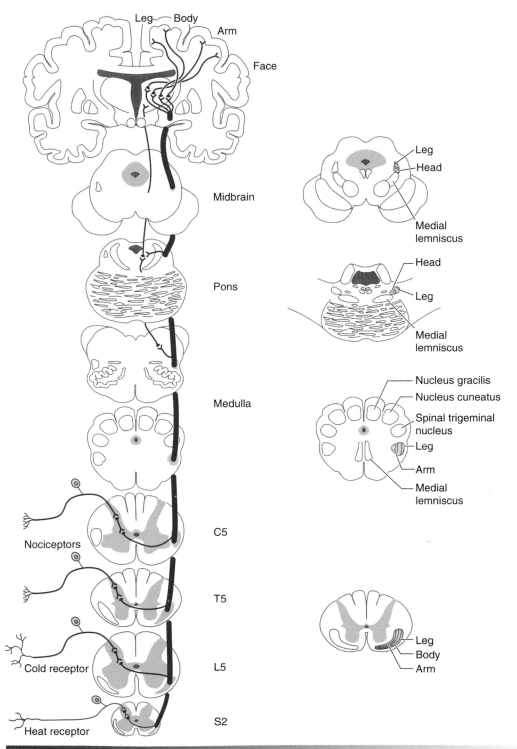

**Figure 5.19   The anterior lateral system pathways**

reaction (the psychological affect) to sensory stimuli (see Chapter 14).

## PAIN

*Pain is the affective perception of nociceptive stimulation.* Pain is not a sensation in the same sense that warmth, cold, touch, and sound are sensations; it is a complex experience derived from nociception, much in the same way that vision is a complex experience derived from light sensations. However, pain differs from vision because pain carries with it a disturbing **affect** [L. *affectus,* state of mind] (the emotional feeling or mood attached to perceptions and thoughts), which vision ordinarily does not.

Pain is an abstraction of nociception. Under some circumstances nociception and pain can be dissociated. For example, it is common for patients with pain who are given morphine to describe the nociceptive sensations, yet they also report that the emotionally disturbing affect of pain is absent. Patients with certain thalamic lesions have the opposite experience: they may have total numbness on half of the body yet report excruciating pain "from somewhere."

The mechanisms and pathways by which nociceptive sensations are interpreted as emotionally disturbing and painful are not completely understood. The pathways almost certainly involve the projections to the hypothalamus and amygdaloid, accumbens, and septal nuclei. Recent advances in our understanding of the anatomy and physiology of nociceptive systems are beginning to yield rational and effective treatments for a variety of pain syndromes. The following section addresses some of the clinically relevant aspects of pain as a basis for understanding this phenomenon.

### Types of Pain

Two clinical states of pain are recognized: **physiological (nociceptive) pain** and **neuropathic (intractable) pain**. Physiological pain results from the direct stimulation of nociceptors and is conveyed to the CNS over A$\delta$ and C fibers. Physiological pain is the pain we associate with simple pinpricks, cuts, and minor burns. Experimental stimulation of A$\delta$ fibers produces a sharp and highly localized pain of relatively short duration. Stimulation of C fibers produces a dull, burning, or aching pain that persists long after the stimulus is removed.

Acute or chronic inflammatory pain is physiological pain that has been intensified by peripheral mechanisms (**peripheral sensitization**). It results from a long-term modification of nociceptors. As discussed in Chapter 4, nociceptive stimuli enhance inflammation by an axon reflex, which causes the release of substance P and calcitonin gene related peptide (CGRP). Evidence suggests that inflammation also alters the type and number of membrane receptors on free nerve endings, lowering the overall threshold to nociceptive stimuli. The mechanisms are not clear, but the alteration in nociceptive receptors may be caused in part by the recruitment of second-messenger systems by inflammatory agents (bradykinin, histamine, and so on). This positive feedback system increases and prolongs physiological pain.

Physiological pain can also be intensified by changes in the spinal cord. For example, most nociceptive projection cells in laminae IV to V are silent; they do not display spontaneous activity. When stimulated for long periods, such as by inflammation, they can become spontaneously active. The exact mechanism is not completely understood. The development of spontaneous activity requires both A$\beta$ and C-fiber stimulation; C-fiber stimulation alone is not sufficient. Apparently the postsynaptic neurons become depolarized to the extent that the magnesium ion block is released from the NMDA receptors (see Chapter 3). As a result, the neuron is further depolarized, making it hypersensitive. Known as **central sensitization**, this hypersensitive state can last for minutes to hours after the stimulus stops. *It does not result in permanent changes in the CNS.*

Peripheral and central sensitization are normal physiological responses related to specific injury. They perform protective functions. Simple physiological pain causes reflex withdrawal of the affected region from the stimulus (the flexion reflex; see Chapter 6). Pain intensified by peripheral and central mechanisms helps to provoke behavioral modifications that protect the affected area during healing, as when one limps with a sprained ankle.

Neuropathic (intractable) pain is maladaptive and serves no known useful function. It results from *injury to the nervous system that causes permanent changes in the CNS connections.* For example, peripheral axons attempt to regenerate after an injury. Regeneration is usually incomplete; small fibers are less likely to survive and regenerate than large fibers. Therefore, the long-range consequence of peripheral nerve injury is likely to be a greater loss of small-diameter A$\delta$ and C fibers than of large-diameter A$\beta$ fibers. During regeneration, the central axons of the surviving A$\beta$ fibers sprout new terminal branches that invade lamina II. The branches of the A$\beta$ fibers make synaptic contact on the neurons vacated by the lost C fibers. Thus, previously innocuous signals reaching the CNS over A$\beta$ fibers from peripheral mechanoreceptors make inappropriate contact with pain circuits in the dorsal horn. *When stimulated, primary afferent fibers serving innocuous normal sensations facilitate transmission pathways associated with nociception.* The altered pattern of neuronal activity associated with this activity is interpreted as noxious, thereby *making previously nonpainful stimuli severely painful and disturbing.* This change from innocuous to noxious perception is called **allodynia** [G. *allos,* other, and *dynamis,* force].

Neuropathic pain is often associated with amputation of extremities. Such sensations are not directly associated with injury to the body but seem to the patient to come from the missing extremity. Because of the discrepancy between obvious injury and the location of the sensations, this type of pain is called **phantom pain.**

Lesions that cause phantom pain can be either peripheral or central. **Peripheral lesions** affect both small- and large-diameter primary afferent axons. In addition to amputations, peripheral lesions can also follow severe nerve lacerations that do not include loss of an extremity. This same type of pain can accompany entrapment lesions, in which whole peripheral nerves become irritated and inflamed by constant pressure or intermittent insult. For example, the median nerve is frequently injured at the flexor retinaculum (**carpal tunnel syndrome**), an injury that often results in pain affecting not only the hand but the entire arm. The pain extends far beyond the territory of the nerves injured at the carpal tunnel. While the mechanism is probably the same, the neuropathic pain associated with entrapment lesions is not usually called phantom pain.

**Central lesions** that produce neuropathic pain are usually found in the ventrobasal complex of the thalamus following vascular insult such as a stroke (**thalamic pain syndrome**). Like phantom pain, such pain is perceived in the absence of specific injury to the body. After receiving either central or peripheral lesions, patients usually describe the psychological affect of the pain as unlike and more excruciating than any previous pain.

## SPINAL MECHANISMS MODULATING PAIN

The transmission of pain information from the spinal cord can be modulated by spinal afferent axons. The **gate-control hypothesis** proposes that in addition to the connections already described, large-diameter primary afferent axons (A$\beta$ fibers) make excitatory synaptic contact with interneurons in the dorsal horn (Fig. 5.20). These interneurons also receive inhibitory synapses from the small-diameter afferent axons A$\delta$ and C. When activated, the interneurons suppress primary afferent C fibers by presynaptic inhibition. Thus, the hypothesized interneuron acts as a gate, controlling the transmission of pain stimuli conveyed by C fibers to higher centers.

This hypothesis predicts that if small-fiber activity predominates, the interneuron will be inhibited, opening the gate. If large-diameter fiber activity predominates, the interneuron is excited, closing the gate. The gate-control hypothesis offers an interesting explanation of the universal behavior associated with pain—the rubbing or otherwise innocuous stimulation of an injured area. Such behavior increases tactile sensations carried by large fibers, closing the gate on the C-fiber activity and thereby lessening nociceptive input.

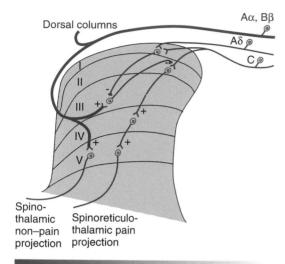

Spino-thalamic non–pain projection    Spinoreticulo-thalamic pain projection

**Figure 5.20    The gate-control hypothesis**

Although the detailed synaptic interrelations suggested by the gate-control hypothesis have yet to be proved, its essential correctness has been demonstrated clinically. Electrodes placed on the dorsal columns to antidromically (backward conduction) stimulate the large-diameter primary afferent axons can reduce or eliminate previously intractable pain. **Transcutaneous electrical neural stimulation (TENS)** is a less invasive procedure based on the gate-control hypothesis. In TENS, electrodes are placed on the skin over a peripheral nerve. Large-diameter axons can be preferentially activated by transcutaneous stimulation because they have the lowest threshold to electrical stimulation. TENS devices have been successfully employed in the treatment of some types of intractable pain.

## DESCENDING SYSTEMS MODULATING PAIN

Some descending pathways modulate pain perception. They are closely linked with endogenous opioid systems. The most prominent of these pathways originates in the PAG and descends into the medulla, where it synapses (Fig. 5.21). The medullary neurons project into the spinal cord, where they synapse in the dorsal horn and inhibit nociceptive pathways. A number of nuclei and

neurotransmitters are associated with this pathway.

PAG neurons send axons into the **nucleus raphe magnus (NRM)** and the **nucleus reticularis paragigantocellularis (NRPG)** in the medullary reticular formation, where they make excitatory synaptic contacts. Neurons from the NRM and NRPG send axons into the spinal cord. These reticulospinal axons travel in the dorsal aspect of the lateral white column and synapse in the dorsal horn, probably laminae II and III.

Most of the neurons from the NRM release serotonin at their spinal synapses and excite interneurons in the spinal cord. These interneurons apparently presynaptically inhibit primary afferent C fibers by secreting enkephalin. Neurons from the NRPG also descend in the dorsal lateral white column, but they secrete noradrenaline on interneurons of the dorsal horn. Activation of these interneurons inhibits the thalamic projection neurons of lamina V through a nonopioid polysynaptic pathway. This descending control system exerts a strong analgesic effect. This knowledge has been used successfully to treat patients suffering from intractable pain by exciting PAG neurons with indwelling electrodes.

Neurons in the PAG of the mesencephalon can be activated by many parts of the brain. The PAG receives ascending sensory projections from the spinomesencephalic division of the ALS. It also receives descending projections from the hypothalamus and many parts of the cerebral cortex. PAG neurons have μ-receptors that can be activated by circulating or medically administered opioids or opioids secreted by axons synapsing in the PAG. The thalamic and cortical projections into the PAG provide a potential explanation for the suppression of pain during periods of high stress and anxiety, a phenomenon that has frequently been reported by soldiers wounded in battle and civilian accident victims.

### Surgical Intervention

The ALS is anatomically important for pain perception. Stimulating the ALS causes severe pain that is localized to the contralateral side of the body. This fact suggests that intractable

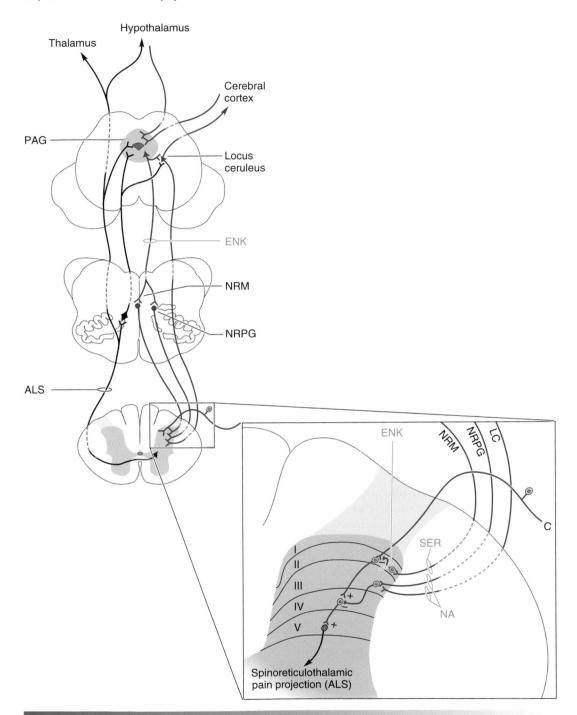

**Figure 5.21   Descending pain modulating systems**

The descending control pathways are shown in *pink;* the ascending nociceptive pathways, in *black. ALS,* anterior lateral system; *LC,* locus ceruleus; *PAG,* periaqueductal gray; *NRM,* nucleus raphe magnus; *NRPG,* nucleus reticularis paragigantocellularis; *ENK,* enkephalinergic synapse; *NA,* noradrenergic synapse; *SER,* serotonin synapse.

pain might be alleviated by cutting the dorsal roots (**rhizotomy**) or the ALS (**tractotomy**) in the spinal cord. After such operations the patient usually has prompt and profound relief. Unfortunately, the relief is usually transitory. The pain almost always returns and is usually more intense and unmanageable than before surgery. This relapse is not surprising in light of recent findings showing that axotomy causes synaptic reorganization of the central deafferented structures, which can lead to "wind-up" (increased inappropriate activity in neurons carrying protopathic signals) and neuropathic pain. The inference is that the abnormally active neurons are the source of the pain signals. With time the nervous system may adapt somewhat, but some residual intractable pain and/or allodynia is common.

Therapeutic lesions to the thalamus also have only questionable clinical value. Ablation of the ventrobasal complex usually decreases sensations from the contralateral side of the body. However, the affect of pain remains, leaving the patient more miserable than before. A lesion to the intralaminar group supposedly relieves pain without altering sensation, but the results have been unpredictable.

Therapeutic lesions of the cerebral cortex designed to alleviate intractable pain provide a special challenge to the surgeon because *there is no cortical representation for pain*. Direct stimulation of the cerebral cortex results in a variety of sensations, including feelings of numbness, tingling, or pressure and visual or auditory perceptions, but it does not elicit pain. This remarkable fact allows neurosurgeons to operate on the brains of conscious persons. It also means that simple, local cortical ablations cannot be used to eliminate pain. Various ablations have been directed at nonsensory parts of the cerebral cortex in an effort to eliminate the psychological affect of pain. These operations are extremely controversial and have been difficult to evaluate dispassionately.

## CLINICAL EXAMINATION OF SENSORY SYSTEMS

Examination of sensory systems presents a special challenge to the physician because it is

the only part of the neurological evaluation that requires the full, honest participation of the patient. A successful sensory examination begins with communicating to the patient exactly what is expected. If the patient cannot understand and follow the instructions or attempts to lie about the results, the sensory examination may be invalid, but the physician has gained significant insight about the patient and the problem.

### Patterns of Sensory Loss

In assessment of somatosensory systems it is frequently necessary to differentiate between lesions within the CNS, lesions to the spinal roots, and those affecting the peripheral nerves. Making these distinctions is facilitated by noting the *distribution* of sensory derangements projected on the body surface and the *modalities* affected. These distinctions are possible because of the way the various components of the somatosensory system are organized.

### PERIPHERAL LESIONS

*Complete lesions to spinal or peripheral nerves elicit sensory losses involving all sensory modalities and motor functions* because all modalities are represented in the axons of these structures. Occasionally pressure insults and other conditions affect the largest axons first. In these cases fine tactile, vibratory, and proprioceptive sensations may be compromised with pain and temperature sensations left relatively intact. These latter sensations are aberrant, however, because their affect depends partly on signals transmitted by the large-diameter fibers. Nearly everyone has had a nerve pressure palsy after sitting in an awkward position that places pressure on a major peripheral nerve. In such cases we say that the affected extremity is "asleep." Light touches to the skin cannot be perceived and proprioception is absent. Walking may be hazardous if the sciatic nerve is affected. This difficulty in walking is due not to paralysis but to the lack of proprioceptive feedback, which makes controlling the limb impossible. Painful tingling sensations are present and pinpricks are readily felt, although they feel unnatural.

The distribution of sensory losses due to peripheral injuries is quite characteristic. The pattern is based on the segmental organization of the embryo established during development. *As the embryo expands and develops, the skin carries its segmentally derived innervation with it.* Thus embryonic segmentation is reflected in the segmental organization of the adult spinal cord and is preserved in the distribution of sensory axons to the skin. The area of skin supplied by the axons from a single dorsal root is a **dermatome.** The distribution of dermatomes over the limb buds is modified somewhat by growth, but not as much as one might think. The essential segmental pattern remains in the adult; it is simply stretched to fit the extruded extremity (Fig. 5.22).

The development of the nerve plexus complicates the innervation of the extremities. Each trunk, cord, division, and peripheral nerve stemming from a plexus contains varying sets of axons from several adjacent spinal roots (Fig. 5.23). In the adult extremities, *individual peripheral nerves contain axons that arise from several spinal roots* and, conversely, *various peripheral nerves contain axons that arise from the same root.* The practical result of this organization is that after peripheral nerve injuries, the pattern of sensory denervation on the skin is strikingly different from the pattern that follows spinal nerve injuries.

*When a spinal root is damaged, the sensory loss is revealed over the entire dermatome.* Conversely, when the peripheral nerve is damaged, the sensory loss extends to the area of skin supplied by a subset of axons from one or more adjacent spinal roots. Hence, only a part of the dermatome for each contributing root is affected. *Therefore, the peripheral nerve pattern consists of fragments of adjacent dermatomes.* It is important that the physician have a mental picture of the dermatomes and peripheral nerve patterns so that sensory losses can be tested in a methodical and useful way. The most diagnostic patterns are found on the hands and feet. The student is advised to memorize them (Table 5.1).

**Peripheral neuropathy** is a general loss of sensory and motor function of peripheral nerves. Because peripheral neuropathy is commonly caused by toxins or metabolic disturbances, the most metabolically active neurons are usually affected first. These neurons usually include those with the longest axons; therefore, symptoms usually begin at the distal portion of the extremities, producing a **stocking-and-glove** pattern of sensory loss (Fig. 5.24A).

## CENTRAL LESIONS

*Central lesions are commonly characterized by dissociations of functions.* Motor functions can be affected, with sparing of sensory functions in the same area and vice versa. Pure sensory dissociations, in which only some of the sensory modalities are lost over an affected part of the body, can also occur. Sensory dissociation is possible because the dorsal column system crosses the midline in the brainstem, whereas the ALS crosses at the spinal cord. For example, hemisection of the spinal cord (**Brown-Sequard syndrome**) produces sensory losses below the level of the lesion (Fig. 5.24B). Fine tactile, proprioceptive, and vibratory sensations are lost from the side of the body *ipsilateral* to the lesion because the dorsal columns carry primary afferent axons that have not yet crossed the midline. Nociception and temperature sensations are lost on the contralateral side because the ALS contains secondary axons that have already crossed the midline.

Lesions to the brainstem or cerebral cortex that involve sensory structures produce a deficit in all somatosensory modalities on the entire side of the body *contralateral* to the lesion (Fig. 5.24C). If the lesion is in the brainstem, usually the cranial nerves are also involved (see Chapter 10). Knowing these basic patterns is essential to neurological diagnosis.

Many other spinal cord lesions produce characteristic patterns of combined sensory and motor losses that are diagnostic once the underlying anatomy is understood. One of these characteristic patterns is caused by a spinal syrinx; it is reported in the case of Ms. J. R. later in the chapter. Description of other classic spinal cord lesions is deferred until after the motor systems are discussed.

PERIPHERAL NERVES

SPINAL (RADICULAR)
DERMATOMES

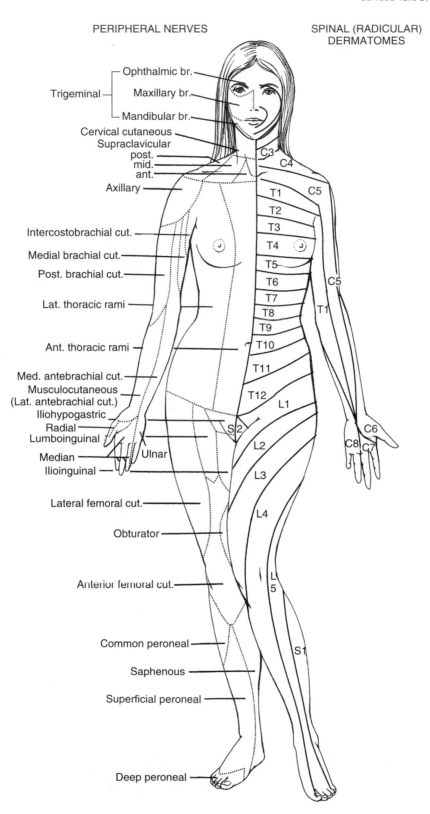

Ophthalmic br.

Trigeminal

Maxillary br.

Mandibular br.

Cervical cutaneous
Supraclavicular
post.
mid.
ant.

C3
C4

Axillary

C5

Intercostobrachial cut.

T1
T2
T3
T4
T5
T6
T7
T8
T9
T10
T11
T12

C5

Medial brachial cut.

Post. brachial cut.

C5

Lat. thoracic rami

T1

Ant. thoracic rami

Med. antebrachial cut.
Musculocutaneous
(Lat. antebrachial cut.)
Iliohypogastric
Radial
Lumboinguinal

L1

S2

L2

C6

Median
Ilioinguinal

Ulnar

C8 C7

Lateral femoral cut.

L3

L4

Obturator

Anterior femoral cut.

L
5

Common peroneal

Saphenous

S1

Superficial peroneal

Deep peroneal

SPINAL (RADICULAR)
DERMATOMES

PERIPHERAL NERVES

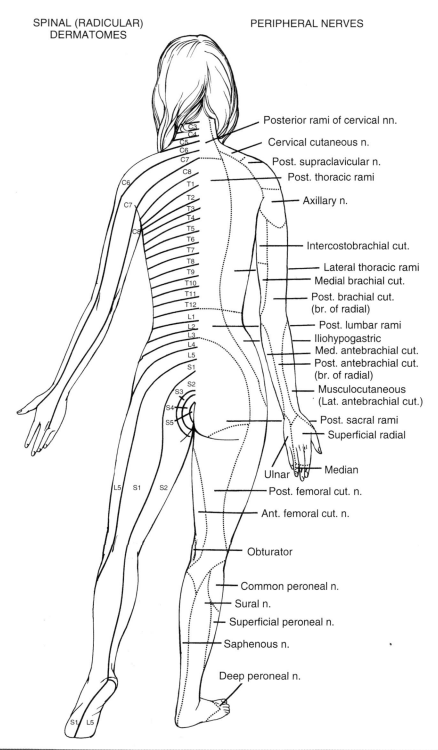

Posterior rami of cervical nn.

Cervical cutaneous n.

Post. supraclavicular n.

Post. thoracic rami

Axillary n.

Intercostobrachial cut.

Lateral thoracic rami

Medial brachial cut.

Post. brachial cut.
(br. of radial)

Post. lumbar rami

Iliohypogastric

Med. antebrachial cut.

Post. antebrachial cut.
(br. of radial)

Musculocutaneous
(Lat. antebrachial cut.)

Post. sacral rami

Superficial radial

Median

Ulnar

Post. femoral cut. n.

Ant. femoral cut. n.

Obturator

Common peroneal n.

Sural n.

Superficial peroneal n.

Saphenous n.

Deep peroneal n.

**Figure 5.22  Dermatome and peripheral nerve patterns**

The peripheral nerve patterns are on the *right side* of the model, the dermatomes on the *left side.*

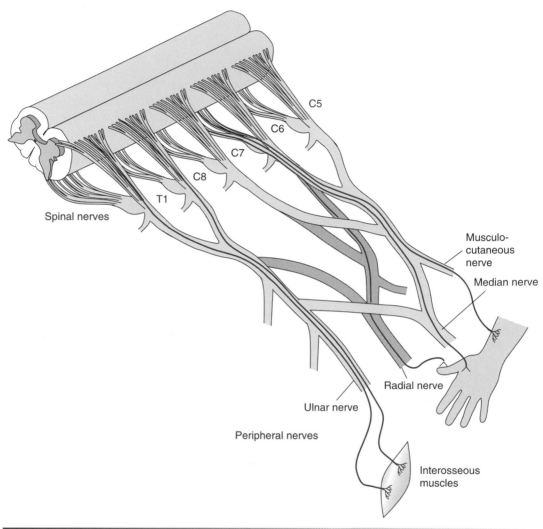

**Spinal nerves**

C5
C6
C7
C8
T1

Musculo-
cutaneous
nerve

Median nerve

Radial nerve

Ulnar nerve

**Peripheral nerves**

Interosseous
muscles

**Figure 5.23    Distribution of axons in a plexus**

A segment of the brachial plexus shows how a single spinal nerve may contribute to several peripheral nerves and how a single peripheral nerve may receive axons from more than one spinal nerve.

**Table 5.1    Spinal Nerve Innervation of Surface Landmarks**

| Root | Diagnostic Pattern |
|------|--------------------|
| C6 | Thumb |
| C7 | Index and middle fingers |
| C8 | Ring and little fingers |
| T4 | Nipples |
| T10 | Umbilicus |
| L4 | Patella and large toe |
| L5 | Middle three toes and sole of foot |
| S1 | Little toe and lateral aspect of foot |

## REFERRED PAIN

Sensations arising from the viscera are not only painful and poorly localized but are often *inappropriately perceived as arising from surface structures*. This phenomenon is called **referred pain**, since the pain is referred from the viscera to surface structures. After entering the spinal cord, visceral pain afferent fibers presumably excite both the epicritic and protopathic transmission pathways. Alternatively, the mixing of epicritic somatic and protopathic visceral information may occur at second-order neurons in the nucleus gracilis. In either case, *the vis-*

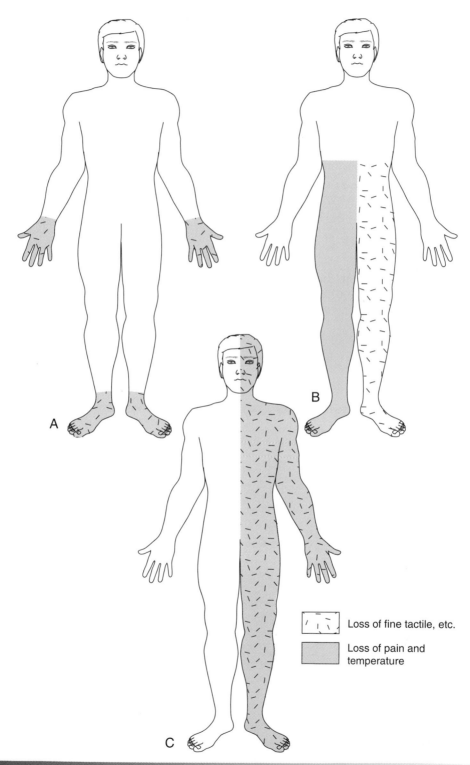

Loss of fine tactile, etc.

Loss of pain and
temperature

**Figure 5.24  Important patterns of sensory loss**

**A.** The stocking-and-glove pattern is characteristic of peripheral neuropathies. **B.** The harlequin pattern is characteristic of a spinal hemisection. **C.** The division of the body along the midsagittal plane is characteristic of lesions to the brainstem or cerebral cortex.

*ceral and somatic sensations are simultaneously facilitated.* Since the viscera are not mapped separately within the CNS, the brain interprets visceral signals to be somatic, and visceral pain is mistakenly perceived to be from the body surface.

The body area to which visceral pain may be referred is not necessarily near the affected organ. Like the skin, the viscera carry their embryonic innervation with them during development. Many of the viscera migrate great distances from their embryonic origin. Visceral migration does not necessarily follow somatic migration. Therefore, pain referred from viscera may be remote from the actual site of the stimulus. For example, blood from abdominal bleeding can irritate the diaphragm, causing pain. The pain is not localized to the abdomen; it is referred to the scapular area because the diaphragm originates from cervical myotomes. Table 5.2 lists some important organs and the dermatome to which pain from that organ is referred.

## Performing the Somatosensory Examination

The dorsal column system can be tested by lightly touching the skin with a fine wisp of cotton. This test is equally effective on glabrous as on hairy skin. The normal patient has no difficulty perceiving even the slightest touch of the cotton; the only exception is heavily callused hands or feet. As another test

### Table 5.2 Principal Dermatomes for Referred Pain and Visceral Origin

| Somatic Projection | Visceral Organ |
| --- | --- |
| C3–C4 | Diaphragm |
| T1–T8 | Heart |
| T10 | Appendix |
| T10–T12 | Testes, prostate |
| T10–T12 | Ovaries, uterus |

of the dorsal column system, the base of a 128-Hz tuning fork can be firmly placed on a bony protrusion, such as the fibular or tibial malleolus, the patella, the styloid process of the radius, or the olecranon of the ulna (Fig. 5.25A). The normal patient has no difficulty perceiving the vibration of the tuning fork. As a test of the patient's veracity, while shielding the patient's vision, grasp the tines while still pressing the base of the tuning fork on the bony protrusion and ask the patient to report when the vibration stops.

The proprioceptive component of the dorsal column system can be tested by holding the patient's finger or toe and ever so slightly bending one of the joints (Fig. 5.25B). The normal person perceives the slightest motion. A patient with a severe lesion may not sense any joint movement, no matter how gross. The **Romberg test** is a valuable test of proprioception from the lower extremities. The patient is asked to stand with the feet together. If the patient is steady and does not fall, the patient is directed to close the eyes. If the proprioceptive sense is lost, the patient falls. (Be prepared to catch!) In such cases the patient can stand with eyes open because the visual sense detects and compensates for the slight unsteadiness we all have when standing on a narrow base. The patient falls if deprived of vision when the sense of joint position is missing from the lower extremities.

The ALS can be independently tested by sharply poking the skin with a pin[4] (Fig. 5.25C). If the ALS is damaged, the patient may perceive the touch of the pin, but it is dull and not annoying. The normal patient perceives the pin as a sharp, painful prick. Since perceptions of sharpness and pain vary, it is best to compare one side of the body with the other. For example, prick the arm at the C8 dermatome on the left and then at the same dermatome on the right. Ask the patient if the two pinpricks seem about the same. Alternatively, one can circumscribe the extremity, crossing dermatomes. The patient with a

---

[4] Because blood is frequently drawn during this examination, it is important to discard used pins in an appropriate container and to use a new pin for each patient. In the hospital, one can always identify neurologists because of the number of safety pins attached to their medical bags.

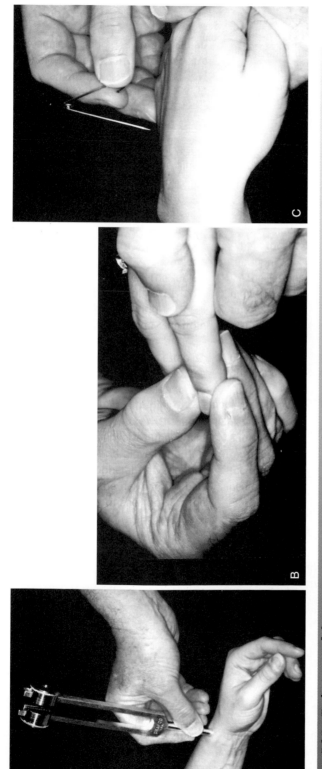

**Figure 5.25    Techniques of the sensory examination**

**A.** Proper placement of the 128-Hz tuning fork on the styloid process of the radius. **B.** Proper position for testing proprioception at the second phalangeal joint. The proximal end of the joint is stabilized by one hand and the joint is manipulated by the other. The distal end of the phalange is held by the side to avoid placing upward or downward pressure on the skin when manipulating the joint. **C.** Proper technique for testing pinprick sensation. By holding the safety catch of the pin between the fingers, one can repeatedly strike the skin with a nearly constant force.

lesion reports a definite demarcation between sharp and dull sensations. The ALS can be further tested by placing a cold instrument (e.g., the side of the nonvibrating tuning fork) on the skin at various locations and asking the patient whether it feels warm, cold, or neutral. Normal patients report that the instrument feels cold.

The somatosensory examination rarely reveals absolute anesthesia because of the considerable overlap of the terminal fields of the primary afferent axons in the dorsal horn of the spinal cord. What a patient feels is a *change in the perception* of the stimulus as it passes from a normally innervated area to one that has been denervated. This change in perception is especially obvious if the lesion involves a spinal root. Therefore, it is important to ask the patient to compare the sensations presented at two areas, either by stimulating the two extremities in turn or by crossing dermatomes on a single extremity.

# C A S E  H I S T O R Y

## A CASE OF STOICISM

### HISTORY OF PRESENT ILLNESS

Ms. J. R. is a 67-year-old previously healthy black woman who came to the emergency department complaining of swelling and decreased mobility of her right arm. She states that 5 days ago she noticed a burning sensation under her right axilla and weakness in her right arm that has persisted to the present. She has no pain.

### MEDICAL HISTORY

In the past she has had bilateral ear surgery (diagnosis not stated) and bilateral carpal tunnel surgeries. She began using a cane about a year ago because she developed a limp.

### PHYSICAL EXAMINATION

Temperature was 95.2, heart rate 80, respirations 20, and blood pressure 152/82. She was in good spirits and showed no signs of discomfort or distress. A burn scar was noted on her left shoulder which she said was the result of using a heating pad 10 years ago. She no longer uses heating pads. Her left elbow joint was greatly enlarged and deformed.

### NEUROLOGICAL EXAMINATION

**Mental Status**
Ms. J. R. was oriented to place, person, and time. She gave a coherent history.

**Cranial Nerves**
No abnormalities in cranial nerve function were noted.

**Station and Gait**
She walked with a slight limp, favoring the right side. She was steady on her feet. Deep knee bends and hopping on one foot were deferred.

**Motor Systems[5]**

STRENGTH: The strength in the patient's legs was equal bilaterally (5/5). Weakness (3/5) and lack of mobility in the right upper extremity were noted. The left hand grip was weaker than right.

TONE: No spasticity or rigidity was noted.

BULK: Wasting of the interosseous muscles of the left hand was noted.

[5] Defer consideration of motor systems and reflexes until after reading Chapters 6 through 8.

ABNORMAL MOVEMENTS: None observed.

### Sensory Systems

There was a bilateral decreased perception of pin-prick and temperature from the base of her neck to 2 cm above the umbilicus. Perception of wisps of cotton stroked across her skin was appreciated equally from all four extremities and from her torso. She was able to stand unassisted with her eyes open and closed (normal Romberg test).

### Reflexes

Muscle stretch reflexes (MSRs) were absent bilaterally from the biceps, triceps, and brachioradialis muscles. MSRs were increased (+) bilaterally from the quadriceps and gastrocnemius muscles. Babinski's sign was present bilaterally.

### Coordination and Control

Heel-to-shin and finger-to-nose (left arm) were accomplished.

### Parietal Functions

No aphasia was noted. Atavistic signs and the optokinetic reflex were not tested.

### ANCILLARY STUDIES

1. Radiographs revealed a displaced fracture of the distal head of the right humerus and severe degeneration of the left elbow and right shoulder joints (neurotrophic joint).
2. Magnetic resonance imaging (MRI) of the brain and spinal cord revealed an Arnold-Chiari malformation and syringomyelia of the spinal cord from the cervicomedullary junction to the midthoracic level (Fig. 5.26).

### COMMENTARY

**Syringomyelia** [G. *syrinx*, tube, and *myelos*, marrow], as the name implies, is a cavitation of the spinal cord of unknown etiology. In most cases the central canal of the spinal cord becomes filled with fluid and enlarges. The cavity usually communicates with the fourth ventricle. The deformity frequently begins in the cervical spinal cord and gradually expands. It may extend into the thoracic cord, as in the present case, or into the medulla, in which case it is called **syringobulbia.** In this case the cavity has spontaneously decompressed, which accounts for the distorted shape of the spinal cord in the MRI. Spontaneous decompression is unusual.

The cavity first appears near the center of the spinal cord, where its expansion destroys the secondary fibers of the ALS where they cross in the ventral white commissure. *Consequently, the ini-*

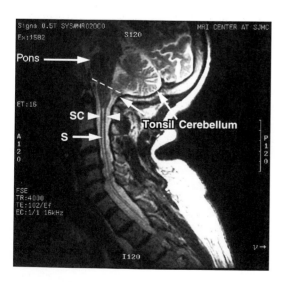

### Figure 5.26   MRI of Ms. J. R.

A T2-weighted MRI in the midsagittal plane from Ms. J. R. (case study) reveals a large syrinx (*S*) that extends from the cervicomedullary junction to midthoracic levels. The full extent of the syrinx cannot be seen in this image because it passes out of the plane of section in the upper thoracic region. In this T2-weighted MRI the CSF is light and neural tissue is dark. The spinal cord (*SC*), delineated by a pair of *facing arrows,* is very narrow and much smaller than normal, leaving a very large subarachnoid space in the cervical region. These findings suggest that the syrinx was at one time much larger and spontaneously ruptured into the subarachnoid space, causing the spinal cord to collapse. Ms. J. R. also exhibits a very mild Arnold-Chiari malformation, an extension of the cerebellar tonsils into the opening of the foramen magnum. Here the tonsils are pointed downward and extend below the base of the skull (*broken line*). This finding is incidental in this case. (MRI courtesy the Magnetic Imaging Center, South Bend, IN.)

*tial symptom is bilateral loss of pain and temperature with the preservation of light touch, proprioception, and vibratory sensations over the upper extremities.* The pattern follows several dermatomes, depending on the rostrocaudal extent of the cavity.

As the circumference of the cavity expands, other structures become compromised, including the ventral horns and the lateral columns. Compromise of these structures gives rise to lower motor symptoms in the upper extremity and upper motor symptoms in the lower extremity (see Chapters 6 and 7). Involvement of the dorsal columns leads to loss of proprioception and fine tactile and vibratory sensations that may involve all four extremities, depending on the extent of the expansion. Since the expansion may not be symmetrical, involvement of these structures may be capricious.

As shown in the present case, syringomyelia is commonly associated with Arnold-Chiari malformation and neurotrophic joint disorders. Arnold-Chiari malformation is characterized by protrusion of the cerebellar tonsils into the foramen magnum. Neurotrophic joints are a trophic enlargement and malformation of the joint associated with certain neurological diseases, particularly syringomyelia and neurosyphilis. The joints are malformed by repeated stress injuries that are not guarded against because of the loss of pain sensations from the joint. The interested student is referred to the suggested readings.

## FURTHER APPLICATIONS

Loss of pain and temperature following lesions to the ALS is dramatically illustrated by Ms. J. R., who despite a fractured humerus, was in no par-

ticular discomfort or pain. Her case illustrates important diagnostic principles.

5.1.   Identify the level of involvement of the spinal cord from the pattern of anesthesia to pinprick. Make a sketch, illustrating the pattern of sensory losses. How closely does this agree with the MRI evaluation?

5.2   It is important to be able to identify the specific tracts and parts of the gray matter of the spinal cord that are involved in the lesion. How does the preservation of fine tactile sensations limit one's hypotheses about the scope of the lesion? Draw a cross-section of the spinal cord at the C8 level and color areas you know to be lesioned and areas you know to be intact.

5.3   What is the significance of the results of Ms. J. R.'s Romberg test? How does this information help you color your spinal cord drawing?

5.4   How does the fact that Ms. J. R. burned herself on a heating pad affect your understanding of the time course of the disease and the veracity of the patient?

5.5   Can the diagnosis of syringomyelia be made in this case without the use of MRI? Explain.

5.6   The initial symptom of syringomyelia is anesthesia. Later in the course of the disease, some patients develop intractable pain from the previously insensible areas. How can you explain this observation?

# C A S E    H I S T O R Y

## THE CASE OF THE PERSISTENT PHANTOM

### HISTORY OF PRESENT ILLNESS

Mr. H. D. is a 40-year-old white man who injured his right brachial plexus in a bicycle accident 20 years ago. He had immediate total motor and sensory loss to his entire right arm. Since the accident he has had continuous, severe, burning pain from the right arm. Four years after his accident, his right arm was amputated, a procedure that provided no pain relief. Ten years ago, chronic electrodes were placed on the dorsal columns between C2 and C5. Dorsal column stimulation was maintained for six months but produced no relief from pain.

Four years ago, Mr. H. D. submitted to another surgical procedure designed to ablate the right dorsal horn from C5 through C7. At the time of the operation a cervical laminectomy (removal of the dorsal laminae of the vertebrae) from T1 through C5 revealed complete avulsion of both the dorsal and ventral roots. After identifying the former dorsal root entry zone, the surgeon inserted an electrocautery needle about 3 to 4 mm into the right spinal cord at an angle of about 20°. After passing a brief electrical current sufficient to cauterize a sphere of tissue about 1 to 2 mm in diameter, the surgeon removed the needle. This process was repeated 15 times between C5 and C7.

Immediately on recovery from anesthesia, for the first time in 20 years, Mr. H. D. had significant (subjectively 50% reduction) relief from the pain in his right arm. In addition, he had some slight weakness in his right leg. There was normal response to pinprick from all parts of his body, but he had decreased appreciation for light touch (cotton wisp) and vibration in his right leg. He sometimes reported a burning sen-

sation in response to vibration stimuli. These difficulties cleared in 2 weeks.

### COMMENTARY

Dorsal root avulsion (in which the roots are ripped out of the cord) frequently results in intractable phantom pain because of neuropathic changes in the spinal cord following deafferentation. These changes cause spontaneous activity in protopathic projection neurons in the dorsal horn. This activity is interpreted by higher centers as pain referred to the phantom limb. Avulsion is more likely to produce phantom pain, according to this theory, than simple amputation because the primary afferent neuron is totally destroyed. Simple amputation leaves the dorsal root and the dorsal root ganglion intact. It is possible in such cases for the cell body in the dorsal root ganglion to survive, and if it does, the central connection of the primary afferent may be maintained, reducing the potential for abnormal spontaneous activity to develop.

### FURTHER APPLICATIONS

5.7   Explain why amputation of the arm did not alleviate chronic phantom pain in this case.

5.8   Explain why it was predictable that dorsal column stimulation would be ineffective in this case. Would TENS be more likely to be successful? Explain.

5.9   What is the rationale for coagulating the dorsal horn to alleviate chronic phantom pain? What is the important difference between this procedure and ALS tractotomy? Would you expect the procedure described here to provide more permanent relief from

chronic phantom pain than ALS tractotomy? Explain.

5.10 Sketch the dorsal horn. Indicate the
needle track and fill in the area of the
surgical lesion. Label the adjacent
structures and predict the possible
complications of this type of surgery if
the lesion is not placed accurately.

Color the area where postoperative
edema might be expected.

5.11 Refer to your drawing and explain the
postoperative sensory findings in this
case. Which findings are the direct result of the coagulation of neural tissue
and which are secondary to edema?

## S U M M A R Y

- All sensory systems except olfaction convey information from the receptor to the
cerebral cortex over a three-neuron pathway. This pathway can be generally summarized as follows:

(a) The primary afferent axon enters the
CNS over a dorsal root or cranial nerve and
synapses ipsilateral to its point of entry;
(b) the secondary neuron receives synaptic input from the primary afferent axon; its axon
crosses the midline and terminates in the thalamus; (c) the third-order neuron leaves the
thalamus, and its axon traverses the internal
capsule and terminates in S-I ipsilateral to its
thalamic origin but contralateral to the side of
the body from which the information it carries
originated. Important elaborations of the core
pathways are described in the main text.

- Two CNS systems, the dorsal column (epicritic) system and the protopathic ALS,
carry somatosensory information from the
periphery to consciousness in the cerebral
cortex.

For clinical purposes epicritic information
is considered to be fine tactile (light touch),
two-point discrimination, vibratory perception, and proprioception. Epicritic information can be highly localized to the source of
the stimulus. Protopathic information is nociception (pain) and temperature perception.
Protopathic information cannot be well localized in the absence of the epicritic pathways.

- The dorsal column (epicritic) system is as
follows:

The primary axons are large-diameter Aβ
fibers that ascend in either the fasciculus gra-

cilis or fasciculus cuneatus. On reaching the
medulla, they synapse in the nucleus gracilis
or nucleus cuneatus, depending on their origin. Secondary neurons from these nuclei send
axons that cross the midline as internal arcuate fibers and ascend the brainstem as the medial lemniscus. They terminate primarily in
the thalamic nuclei VPL and VPS. Axons carrying fine tactile and proprioceptive information from the face enter the CNS over the
trigeminal nerve and synapse in the chief sensory trigeminal nucleus and the rostral third of
the spinal trigeminal nucleus. Secondary axons from these nuclei cross the midline, join
the medial lemniscus, and terminate in VPM
and VPS. Third-order axons pass from the
thalamus through the posterior limb of the internal capsule to terminate in Brodmann's areas 3a, 3b, 1, and 2, also known as the primary
somatosensory cortex, or S-I.

- The ALS (protopathic) system is as follows:

The primary axons are small-diameter Aδ
(myelinated) and C (unmyelinated) fibers that
enter the spinal cord and synapse in the dorsal
horn. Secondary neurons arise from several areas of the dorsal horn, cross the midline in the
ventral white commissure, and ascend to the
thalamus as the ALS. They synapse in VPL,
VPI, CM, and the intralaminar nuclei. From
the face, similar small-diameter primary afferent axons enter the CNS over the trigeminal
nerve and synapse in the caudal two-thirds of
the spinal trigeminal nucleus. Secondary axons cross the midline, join the medial lemniscus, and synapse in the thalamic nuclei VPM,

VPI, CM, and the intralaminar nuclei. From the thalamus, nociceptive and thermal information reaches S-I via third-order neurons that traverse the internal capsule.

- **Nociception from the viscera takes an unusual route.**

A small subset of fibers in the fasciculus gracilis convey nociceptive information from the viscera to the nucleus gracilis. This appears to be the only protopathic ascending pathway for visceral pain.

- **A precise somatotopic relation is maintained at all levels for the epicritic and protopathic systems.**

The fiber tracts for both systems are highly organized in a somatotopic manner throughout their course in the spinal cord and brainstem. VPL and VPM in the thalamus also reflect this precise organization. The cerebral cortex has multiple somatotopic maps that are organized by modality, although pain is conspicuously absent. The separately mapped areas are connected to one another in a series of cascades by short cortical association axons. Cortical neurons respond to more and more specific stimuli as one follows these cascades away from the principal thalamic synapses in the cortex. The response characteristics of cortical neurons become more abstracted from the stimulus with distance from direct thalamic input.

- **The nervous system abstracts the perception of pain from nociceptive and tactile information.**

Nociceptors, which reside on the free nerve endings of $A\delta$ and C fibers, respond to specific molecules associated with tissue injury. Nociceptive stimuli are brought to consciousness via the principal ALS pathways. Pain, the psychological affect response to nociception, is associated with the concurrent activation of the nonspecific thalamic nuclei, hypothalamus, amygdala, and septal nuclei. These areas are activated by spinoreticular and spinomesencephalic divisions of the ALS.

- **Pain perception can be enhanced by PNS activity.**

Temporary enhancement can be promoted by local inflammation, which can produce sustained stimulation of primary afferent $A\delta$ and C fibers. This stimulation produces spontaneous activity in spinal neurons that are normally quiescent (central sensitization, or "wind-up"). Inflammation can be enhanced by axon reflex.

- **Permanent enhancement of pain can be produced by injury to the nervous system.**

Loss of $A\delta$ and C fibers leads to a synaptic reorganization in the spinal cord that can also produce central sensitization. Synaptic reorganization can produce the perception of pain in the absence of objective nociceptive stimuli (phantom pain). Surgical ablations at the level of the spinal cord, thalamus, and cerebral cortex have not proved to offer long-term relief of intractable pain.

- **Pain perception can be diminished by CNS activity.**

The local gate-control mechanism causes inhibition of $A\delta$ and C fiber activity by simultaneous $A\beta$ activity. Descending systems modulate the activity of the ascending ALS pathways. The best-studied system originates in the PAG and synapses in the medullary reticular formation (NRM and NPGC). These reticular nuclei send axons into the spinal cord in the dorsolateral funiculus, where they can suppress thalamic transmission neurons through both opioid and nonopioid polysynaptic pathways.

- **Dermatomes indicate the pattern of distribution of spinal nerves on the skin.**

Because peripheral nerves are composed of some axons from one or more spinal nerves, when injured, they leave patterns of sensory loss that are composed of fragments from adjacent dermatomes whose spinal roots contribute to the peripheral nerve. Recognizing the patterns of sensory losses following lesions to spinal and peripheral nerves is essential to neurology.

- **Understanding the dermatomes also helps to explain referred pain, the localization of painful visceral stimuli to the body surface.**

Visceral pain is localized to the dermatomes that correspond to the embryonic origin of the visceral organ, not to its adult position in the body (referred pain).

- **The object of the sensory part of the neurological examination is to establish the pattern and modality of any sensory losses. The patterns are important for localizing the lesion.**
  Peripheral lesions are characterized by a pattern of sensory loss affecting all modalities. Spinal nerve injuries produce patterns of loss that follow dermatomes, whereas peripheral nerve lesions produce patterns that are composites of fragments of adjacent dermatomes. Central lesions frequently produce somatosensory dissociations or loss of all modalities over half of the body.

## SUGGESTED READINGS

Brown AG. Organization in the Spinal Cord: The Anatomy and Physiology of Identified Neurons. Berlin: Springer-Verlag, 1981.

Melzack R, Wall PD. The challenges of pain. 2nd ed. Harmondsworth: Penguin, 1996.

Melzack R, Wall PD, eds. The Textbook of Pain. 3rd ed. Edinburgh: Churchill Livingstone, 1994.

Sacks O. Phantoms. In: Sacks O. The Man Who Mistook His Wife for a Hat. New York: Harper & Row, 1987.

Schaible H. On the role of tachykinins and calcitonin gene-related peptide in the spinal mechanisms of nociception and in the induction and maintenance of inflammation-evoked hyperexcitability in spinal cord neurons (with special reference to nociception in joints). In: Kumazawa T, Kruger L, Mizumura K, eds. Progress in Brain Research, vol 113. New York: Elsevier, 1996.

Willis WD. Neuroanatomy of the pain system and of the pathways that modulate pain. J Clin Neurophysiol 1997;14:2–31.

Willis WD, Coggeshall RE. Sensory Mechanisms of the Spinal Cord. 2nd ed. New York: Plenum Press, 1978.

# Motor Systems I: Spinal Mechanisms of Motor Control

Locomotion is one of the most important attributes of living things because it liberates an organism from some of the constraints imposed on it by the environment. Improvement in motor skills is one of the hallmarks of the evolution of animals. The survival value of improved motor performance, it appears, was a major factor driving the elaboration and development of the nervous system. In mammals more than half of the nervous system is directly involved in motor performance, so damage to the nervous system almost always results in a degradation of motor skills. Therefore, assessment of the motor system is central to the clinical examination of the nervous system.

There are three types of motor acts: (a) autonomous motor functions, such as the beating of the heart and peristalsis of the gut; (b) reflexes, which are automatic responses to external stimuli, such as the startle reflex in response to an unexpected loud noise; and (c) voluntary motor acts, such as talking. Some gray areas, of course, such as breathing or swallowing, have both voluntary and involuntary components. Nevertheless, it is useful to consider motor control in terms of these three divisions.

These divisions are reflected in the anatomical and physiological organization of the nervous system. Within autonomous functional units such as the heart and gut are numerous internal connections between neurons or nervelike elements. Connections outside the functional unit are minimal, and thus it can still function fairly well if those connections are severed. The ability of the heart to function independently makes heart transplants possible.

Most motor functions in mammals, however, do require the full participation of the central nervous system (CNS). These functions are described in the next three chapters. Because the disruption of motor control mechanisms is the most common manifestation of disease in the nervous system, the principal goal of these chapters is to illustrate how motor acts are regulated and controlled.

The spinal cord and brainstem contain the circuitry that implements reflex coordination around joints and between extremities. The basal ganglia and cerebral cortex are the major command centers that initiate and plan motor acts, and the cerebellum refines motor acts as they occur. This chapter presents the fundamental regulatory mechanisms in the spinal cord. These mechanisms affect the motor neurons directly. Subsequent chapters present higher-order systems that are more indirectly involved in initiating and regulating motor activity.

## MUSCLE SENSORY RECEPTORS

Accurate movement of an extremity from one place to another necessitates that the motor control system have information about the current position and orientation of that extremity and the length of the muscles that control it. The muscle sensory receptors [L. *musculus*, little mouse; *sensus*, feeling; and *receptor*, a receiver] supply this information. As a motor act progresses, the system must also have continuous information about the state of the muscles (length, tension, velocity of contraction); the position of the extremity; and the velocity of the extremity's movement toward its target. Much of this information is made available by specialized receptors in muscle, tendons, and joints. Because muscle spindles and Golgi tendon organs (GTOs) have been studied extensively, their role in the regulation of motor activities is reasonably well understood. The joint receptors have not been so extensively studied,

and therefore information about their physiological role in motor control is sparse.

### The Muscle Spindle

The principal specialized sensory receptor in muscle is a complex encapsulated receptor, the **muscle spindle apparatus**, that contains both sensory and motor elements. Its name is derived from the shape of the capsule, which resembles the spindle of a spinning wheel. The spindle apparatus is small, consisting of 2 to 14 specialized muscle fibers called **intrafusal muscle fibers** [L. *fusus*, a spindle] (meaning inside the spindle apparatus) that are enclosed within a connective tissue capsule (Fig. 6.1). Surrounding the muscle spindle apparatus are the main contractile muscle fibers, the **extra-**

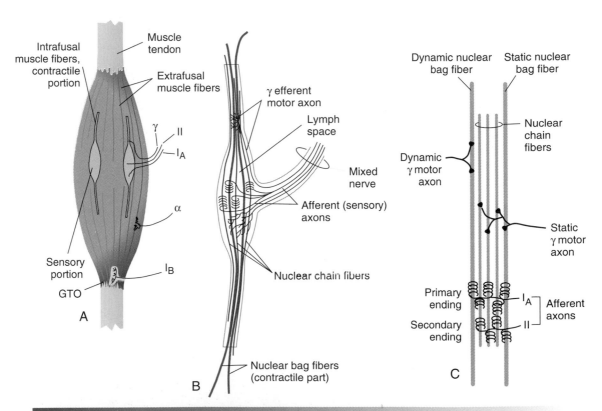

### Figure 6.1   Anatomy of the muscle spindle apparatus

**A.** The muscle spindle apparatus arranged in parallel with the main contractile elements (extrafusal fibers) of the muscle. The GTOs are arranged in series. The sensory elements are enlarged for clarity. **B.** The isolated muscle spindle apparatus. The receptor is innervated by a mixed nerve, which contains both sensory and motor fibers. Note how the afferent (sensory) axons branch before terminating and how they innervate more than one sensory fiber. The efferent (motor) axons are of the γ-type. **C.** The typical arrangement of afferent and efferent axons.

fusal muscle fibers, which make up the bulk of the muscle. Every striated muscle contains large numbers of muscle spindles.

There are two kinds of intrafusal fibers, named after their histological appearance. One type, called the **nuclear bag**, is composed of a modified, multinucleated, muscle fiber. The central, sensory portion of the fiber forms a non-contractile, baglike structure. The two types of bag fibers, **dynamic** and **static**, differ in their response to muscle stretch. The other intrafusal fiber type is called the **nuclear chain** because its central portion contains a number of nuclei arranged in a chainlike series along the length of the fiber. The distal portion of both types of intrafusal fibers consists of striated muscle that has contractile properties. A typical muscle spindle apparatus contains two bag fibers, one of each type, and about five chain fibers.

## INNERVATION OF THE MUSCLE SPINDLE

The spindle apparatus is innervated by two kinds of afferent axons (Table 6.1) that make contact with the central, receptor portion of the intrafusal fibers (Fig. 6.1). Group $I_A$ myelinated axons (12 to 20µm) innervate the sensory portion of bag and chain fibers. Because it has multiple terminal branches, a single $I_A$ axon can innervate all of the intrafusal fibers of a muscle spindle. The most distal portion of each branch of the $I_A$ axon spirals around the central part of an intrafusal fiber before leaving the capsule. The peripheral terminals of the $I_A$ axons are called the **primary** or **annulospiral** receptors. Smaller, **group II** myelinated axons (4 to 12µm) innervate static bag fibers and all of the chain fibers. None innervate dynamic bag fibers. The terminals of group II axons are called **secondary** or **flower spray** receptors.

Muscles receive innervation from two sets of motor neurons (Table 6.2). One set of efferent axons to the muscle, the **α-motor neurons**, innervate only extrafusal muscle fibers. These large, myelinated axons (8 to 13µm) initiate movement through extrafusal muscle contraction.

The other set of efferent muscle fibers, **γ-motor neurons**, innervate only intrafusal muscle fibers. For this reason they are often called **fusimotor neurons**.[1] The γ-motor neurons have small (3 to 8µm), myelinated axons that innervate only the distal, contractile portion of intrafusal muscle fibers. *Contraction of the intrafusal muscle fibers places tension only on the central, sensory portion of the intrafusal muscle fiber; it does not directly cause movement of the joint to which the extrafusal muscle is attached.*

Fusimotor neurons can be further categorized on the basis of their innervation of dynamic and static fibers. Dynamic γ-motor ax-

### Table 6.1  Classification of Muscle Afferent Axons

| Receptor | Axon | Size | Conduction Velocity |
|---|---|---|---|
| Primary muscle spindle | $I_A$ | 12–20 µm | 72–120 m/sec |
| Secondary muscle spindle | II | 4–12 µm | 24–72 m/sec |
| GTO | $I_B$ | 12–18 µm | 72–108 m/sec |

### Table 6.2  Classification of Muscle Efferent Axons

| Motor Neuron | Target | Size | Conduction Velocity |
|---|---|---|---|
| α-Motor neuron | Extrafusal muscle | 8–13 µm | 44–78 m/sec |
| γ-Motor neuron, dynamic | Intrafusal muscle; dynamic bag, static bag and flower spray | 3–8 µm | 18–48 m/sec |
| γ-Motor neuron, static | Intrafusal muscle; static bag and flower spray | 3–8 µm | 18–48 m/sec |

---

[1] A third hybrid class of efferent axons, the **β-motor neurons**, innervate both the intrafusal and extrafusal muscles. While all vertebrates have muscle spindles, the separate innervation of the intrafusal and extrafusal muscles occurs only in mammals. In other animals all motor neurons are in the β-class.

ons innervate only the dynamic bag intrafusal fibers. Static γ-motor axons innervate the static bag and all the chain fibers, but they do not innervate the dynamic bag fibers.

## STIMULATION OF THE MUSCLE SPINDLE RECEPTOR

Appreciating the relation between intrafusal and extrafusal muscle fibers is critical to understanding how spinal motor mechanisms function. The main mass of the muscle consists of extrafusal muscle fibers. The muscle spindles lie within the extrafusal muscle mass. Tendons attached to the intrafusal muscle fibers merge with the tendons or fascia of the adjacent main contractile elements of the muscle (Fig. 6.1). Thus the entire spindle apparatus lies *in parallel* with the extrafusal muscle fibers. In contrast, the receptors of the nuclear bag and chain are *in series* with the intrafusal muscle fibers. The series-parallel arrangement is the key to understanding how this system works.

The sensory portion of the intrafusal muscle fibers is sensitive to tension. Because the intrafusal muscle fiber and the receptor lie in series, tension can be applied to the receptor simply by lengthening the intrafusal muscle fiber. This can be done by stretching the entire muscle (both intrafusal and extrafusal fibers), because the intrafusal and extrafusal fibers are arranged in parallel. Physiologically, therefore, tension can be applied to the receptor by *lengthening the extrafusal muscle.* Increasing the tension in the receptor depolarizes the receptor membrane and initiates action potentials in the group $I_A$ and II axons.

Tension can also be applied to the sensory portion of the muscle spindle apparatus by *stimulating the contractile portion of the intrafusal muscle.* Since the intrafusal muscle is incapable of causing movement of the entire muscle mass, tension brought about by intrafusal muscle contraction cannot be relieved by joint movement. Therefore, the tension is transferred directly to the receptor, depolarizing it.

### The Golgi Tendon Organ

Contrary to its name, the **Golgi tendon organ (GTO)** is rarely found in tendons. Rather, most GTOs are in the aponeurotic sheaths of muscle attachments. GTOs are encapsulated sensory receptors consisting of collagen fibers intertwined with the naked nerve endings from large-diameter **Group $I_B$** (12 to 18μm) myelinated axons (Fig. 6.2). Applying tension to the collagen fibrils squeezes and distorts the bare axon membrane, depolarizing it and triggering action potentials along the $I_B$ axon.

GTOs are arranged *in series* with extrafusal muscle fibers, an arrangement that ensures that tension on the muscle is transferred to the GTO. Because approximately 10 extrafusal muscle fibers are attached to a single GTO capsule, tension from only a few motor units[2] is applied to an individual GTO. The CNS connections that take advantage of this arrangement are described on page 218.

## PHYSIOLOGICAL RESPONSES OF MUSCLE RECEPTORS

Muscle sensory receptors can sense the steady-state length of the muscle as well as dynamic changes in muscle length, tension, and the velocity with which muscle length changes. The static (steady-state length) and dynamic (velocity) properties of the muscle receptors can be studied in nerve-muscle preparations in which all of the connections that the muscle nerve makes with the CNS have been severed. Under these isolated conditions, stretching (lengthening) the entire muscle mass or stimulating either the α- or γ-motor neurons reveals important differences in the response properties of the primary and secondary receptors (Fig. 6.3A). The isolated response properties of muscle sensory receptors are briefly discussed in the following sections. Understanding these properties is necessary to appreciate how the integrated system participates in motor control.

### Passive Muscle Stretch

When a muscle is stretched and held steadily (passive stretch), both the group $I_A$ (primary receptor) and group II (secondary receptor)

---

[2]A motor unit is all of the muscle fibers innervated by the collateral branches of one α-motor neuron.

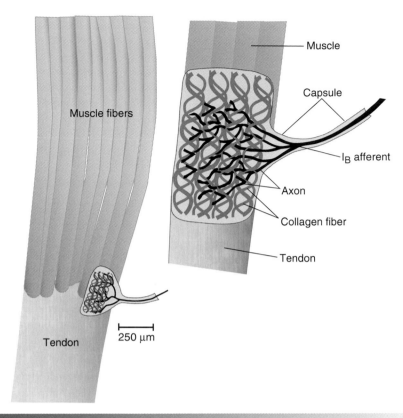

Muscle

Capsule

$I_B$ afferent

Axon

Collagen fiber

Tendon

Muscle fibers

Tendon

250 µm

**Figure 6.2   The Golgi tendon organ**

*Left.* The GTO associated with a muscle fiber. *Right.* The axon endings
entwined with the collagen fibers of the tendon.

axons fire at an increased rate that is proportional to the new length of the muscle (Fig. 6.3B). This proportional axon firing is a static property of the receptors, because their response remains more or less constant as long as the muscle length remains constant. The group II axon that arises from static bag and chain fibers displays only static responses. The group $I_A$ axon, however, in addition to displaying static properties, also displays dynamic properties, since it responds with a burst of activity during the initiation of the stretch.

The dynamic properties of the primary receptor are best revealed during small-amplitude oscillating stretches of the muscle that apply alternating stretches and relaxations to the muscle (Fig. 6.4A, *left*). During this type of stimulation, the $I_A$ axon fires only when the muscle is lengthened, and it ceases to fire when the muscle is allowed to shorten by passive elastic relaxation. No steady-state response occurs during this type of stimulus.

## Isotonic Contraction

In isolated muscle preparations it is possible to stimulate only the α-motor neurons to generate an **isotonic** contraction (constant load) of the extrafusal muscle. In this artificial condition the γ-motor neurons and their associated intrafusal muscle fibers remain unstimulated. When the whole muscle mass shortens, the muscle spindle apparatus passively shortens because of its intrinsic elastic properties (Fig. 6.3C). As the intrafusal fibers in the spindle shorten, the firing rates of both group $I_A$ and II axons are *reduced* because tension in the central, receptor portion of the intrafusal fibers is relieved. During an isotonic contraction, the overall tension on the extrafusal muscle is unchanged because the load remains constant. Therefore, because the

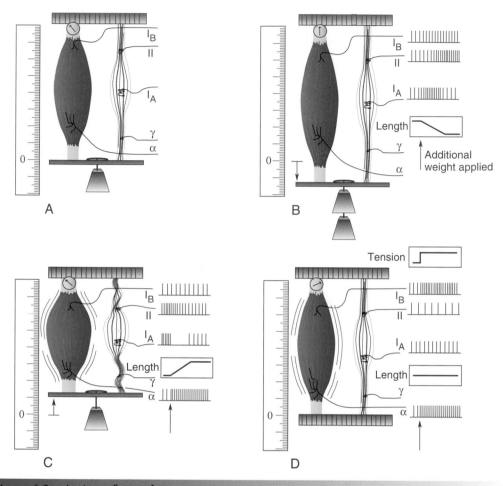

## Figure 6.3   Action of muscle receptors

**A.** Resting state. A typical muscle is shown with the muscle spindle apparatus separated from the extrafusal muscle to emphasize that they are parallel. The *weight symbol* is used to indicate a constant steady resting load on the muscle. The *hash marks* symbolize a fixed reference platform. Action potentials from the various axons are indicated to the right. Muscle length and tension are also indicated where appropriate. **B.** Linear stretch. The extra weight symbol indicates that the muscle has been stretched from its initial state (**A**) and is under slightly greater tension (gauge in the tendon). **C.** Isotonic contraction. Stimulation of the α-motor neuron makes the muscle contract. Note particularly that the overall tension on the muscle is the same as in **A**. **D.** Isometric contraction. The weight at the bottom is replaced with a fixed platform so that the muscle cannot shorten during α-motor neuron stimulation.

GTOs are not subjected to any changes in tension, the firing rates of the $I_B$ axons remain constant.

### Isometric Contraction

If the α-motor neuron is selectively stimulated in a muscle that is firmly fixed at both ends, tension in the muscle increases, but its length remains constant. This type of contraction is called an **isometric** (same length) contraction. Since the muscle length remains constant, the length of the intrafusal muscle fibers and the tension on their receptors are unchanged. Consequently, no change in the firing rate of the $I_A$ and II axons occurs (Fig. 6.3D). Instead, all of the tension is transferred to the GTOs,

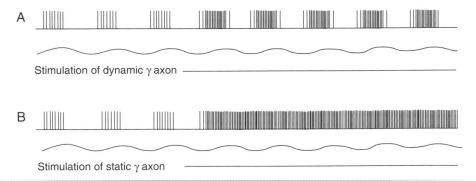

**Figure 6.4    Effects of gamma stimulation**

This recording from a $I_A$ afferent axon shows the effects of stimulation on dynamic γ-axons (**A**) and static γ-axons (**B**). The muscle was stretched with a sinusoidal pattern (1 mm peak to peak). The *horizontal bars* indicate stimulation of the γ-efferent axons. Stimulating the dynamic γ-axon (**A**) increases the rate of $I_A$ firing only during the stretching phase of the sinusoid. In sharp contrast, stimulation of the static γ-efferent axon (**B**) increases the overall firing rate of the $I_A$ axon, in this experiment masking the increase in firing during stretch. (Reprinted with permission from Crowe A, Matthews PBC. Further studies of static and dynamic fusimotor fibres. J Physiol [Lond] 1964;174:132–151.)

since they are in series with the extrafusal muscle fibers. Therefore, the firing rate of the $I_B$ axon increases.

### Fusimotor Stimulation

*The CNS can adjust the sensitivity of the primary and secondary receptors by stimulating g-motor axons.* Stimulation of γ-motor neurons causes the contractile elements of the intrafusal muscle fibers to shorten. Since these tiny muscle fibers are too weak to cause the whole muscle mass to contract, *γ-motor neuron stimulation, in effect, is an isometric contraction of the intrafusal muscle* (Fig. 6.5). Tension rapidly rises on the central, sensory element of the fiber, depolarizing it and triggering action potentials along the group $I_A$ and II sensory axons.

The dynamic and static γ-systems are independently regulated. Stimulation of the dynamic γ-motor neurons enhances the response observed on the $I_A$ axon only during muscle lengthening. In other words, the sensitivity of the $I_A$ fiber to the *rate of stretch* is enhanced, while its response to the absolute spindle length is only slightly changed. This phenomenon is best observed during low-amplitude oscillatory stretching of an isolated

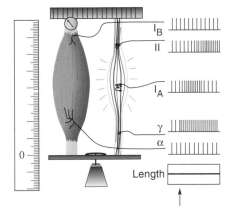

**Figure 6.5    Response of muscle receptors to gamma stimulation**

Activity on the γ-motor axon increases tension on the intrafusal fibers and the firing of $I_A$ and II axons but does not directly affect the tension on the extrafusal fiber.

muscle (Fig. 6.4A). In contrast, stimulation of the static γ-motor neurons enhances the sensitivity of the $I_A$ fiber to *absolute changes in spindle length*. Stimulating static γ-motor neurons is analogous to turning up the volume of a radio (Fig. 6.4*B*).

## REFLEX PATHWAYS

A number of local circuits within the spinal cord regulate the coordinated action of the muscles connected to the spinal cord through the afferent and efferent axons in the dorsal and ventral roots. The simplest of these connections are **reflexes** [L. *reflexus*, bent back]. A reflex pathway has five components: (*a*) a sensory receptor, (*b*) an afferent path to the CNS, (*c*) one or more synapses within the CNS,[3] (*d*) an efferent path, and (*e*) an effector (Fig. 6.6). Several clinically relevant reflexes involve muscle sensors. Although their salient features are presented here, their full clinical significance cannot be fully developed until more details of the motor system are described.

### The Muscle Stretch Reflex

As its name implies, the **muscle stretch reflex** (MSR) is invoked by rapidly stretching a muscle. The stretch depolarizes the nuclear bag and chain fibers in the muscle spindle, causing an increase in the firing rate of the $I_A$ and group II axons. This activity travels to the spinal cord, where it facilitates the α-motor neurons that innervate the *same muscle* (called the **homonymous muscle** [G. *homonymous*, same name]. The $I_A$ also facilitates α-motor neurons that facilitate synergist muscles (**heteronymous muscles** [G. *heteronymous*, different name]) and inhibits the α-motor neurons that innervate the antagonist muscles acting on the same joint (Fig. 6.6).

### GROUP I AFFERENT AXONS

The $I_A$ axon synapses in three functionally distinct areas in the spinal cord gray matter: the motor neuron pools of lamina IX, interneurons in lamina VII, and dorsal horn interneurons in laminae V and VI (Table 6.3). First, $I_A$ axons synapse with α-motor neurons in lamina IX of the ventral horn (Fig. 6.7A).

---

[3]To avoid labeling all CNS activity as reflexes, it is customary to limit the number of CNS synapses to those involving not more than two or three neurons. This restriction is not universally accepted, however, and many authors consider some types of complex behavior, involving perhaps thousands of synaptic links, to be reflexes.

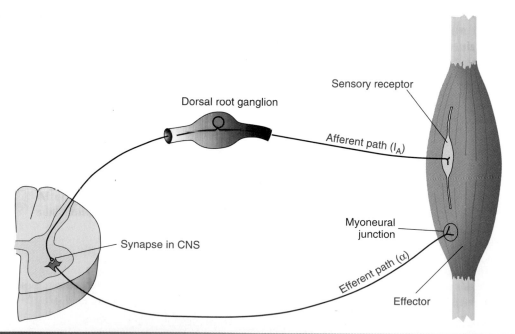

Dorsal root ganglion

Sensory receptor

Afferent path ($I_A$)

Synapse in CNS

Myoneural junction

Efferent path (α)

Effector

**Figure 6.6   The anatomy of the muscle stretch reflex**

The five elements of the MSR.

**Table 6.3    Termination of Muscle and Cutaneous Axons in the Spinal Cord**

| Afferent Axon | Laminae of Termination | Target Neuron Pool |
|---|---|---|
| **Muscle afferents** | | |
| $I_A$ | IX | Motor neurons |
| | VII | Inhibitory neurons |
| | V–VI | Mixed interneuron pools |
| II | IX | Motor neurons |
| | IV–VI | Mixed interneuron pools |
| $I_B$ | V–VII | Inhibitory interneurons |
| **Cutaneous afferents** | | |
| FRAs (II–IV) | III–VII | Mixed interneuron pools |

Two sets of α-motor neurons are innervated: those that innervate the homonymous muscle and those that innervate heteronymous synergist muscles.

A single $I_A$ axon forms synapses, with about 80%[4] of the motor neurons innervating the homonymous muscle from which it originated and about 60% of the neurons innervating heteronymous synergists *acting on the same joint.* These synapses produce very large—about 100 μV—EPSPs that strongly facilitate the homonymous group and somewhat weaker EPSPs (about 70 μV) that facilitate the heteronymous synergists.

If stimulated above threshold, the α-motor neurons fire and send action potentials back to the homonymous and synergistic muscles, causing them to contract and thus shorten. Thus *muscle stretch causes a reflex muscle contraction to oppose the stretch.* The connections that constitute this reflex pathway involve a single synapse, the $I_A$ afferent on the α-motor neuron. For this reason the MSR is also known as the **monosynaptic reflex** [reflex having only one synapse].

Second, muscle spindle afferent axons make excitatory synapses with interneurons in lamina VII (Fig. 6.7A). These interneurons

make inhibitory synapses on α-motor neurons. Like the synapses discussed earlier, these connections are quite specific. The α-motor neurons that are inhibited by this pathway all serve antagonist muscles, that is, muscles having opposite action *on the same joint* from which the initial stretch originated. Depolarization of α-motor neurons decreases the number of action potentials reaching the muscle, lessening the tension on the antagonist muscle.

Third, $I_A$ axons synapse on a heterogeneous group of interneurons in laminae V and VI of the dorsal horn (Fig. 6.7A). Some of these interneurons synapse on motor neurons; others synapse on other interneurons. They also receive additional sensory input from sources other than the muscle. (These additional inputs are the basis for the flexion reflex discussed later in the chapter.) These interneurons also receive motor commands from supraspinal sources. These connections are discussed in Chapter 7. Not all of the connections of these interneurons are known. It is important to recognize, however, that the interneurons of laminae V and VI form the major motor integrating center of the spinal cord. They participate in a wide variety of complex motor functions that transcend the simple reflex.

### GROUP II AFFERENT AXONS

Group II afferent axons from secondary muscle spindle receptors also synapse in the spinal cord and influence α-motor neuron activity. Since the secondary receptors are poorly stimulated by rapid stretch, their influence is minimal during the MSR. However, their static characteristics help determine the overall level of excitability of the motor neuron pool. Group II axons terminate primarily in two areas in the spinal cord (Fig. 6.7B). Like the group $I_A$ axons, group II axons synapse monosynaptically on α-motor neurons in lamina IX. These synapses are less potent than those from $I_A$ afferents, producing EPSPs with an amplitude of about 24 μV. Their distribution is also less pervasive; they synapse on only about 50% of the homonymous and 20% of the het-

---

[4]Some authors report 100%.

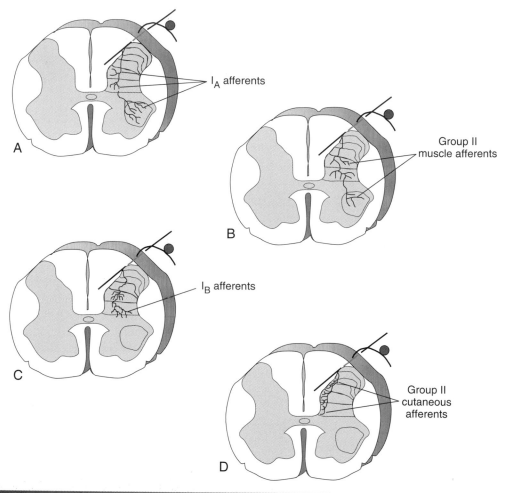

## Figure 6.7    Terminal fields of sensory fibers

Terminal fields in the spinal cord of the principal sensory afferent fibers affecting the MSR are shown here. Although only one slice through the spinal cord is shown for each axon group, the distribution of terminal fields extends for several segments (See Chapter 5). (Based on data from Brown AG. Organization in the Spinal Cord: The Anatomy and Physiology of Identified Neurons. Berlin: Springer-Verlag, 1981.)

eronymous synergist motor neurons. Group II axons also terminate in laminae IV through VI of the dorsal horn, and like the group IA axons, they excite interneurons.

### GROUP I$_B$ AFFERENT AXONS

The group I$_B$ primary afferent axons from GTOs terminate in laminae V through VII in the spinal cord (Fig. 6.7C). There they make excitatory synapses on interneurons that subsequently inhibit homonymous and heteronymous synergist α-motor neurons while facilitating the antagonists. Like group I$_A$ axons,

group I$_B$ axons exert their primary influence on motor neurons that affect movement around the same joint.

When contraction of a muscle is initiated by a general facilitation of the motor neuron pool innervating that muscle, certain motor units within that pool inevitably carry more of the tension than others. Under physiological conditions the GTOs play an important role in adjusting tension among the various motor units so that each carries approximately the same load. These adjustments are accomplished by inhibiting α-motor neurons to motor units that carry a disproportionate amount of the load. Because only a limited number of muscle fibers are attached to an individual GTO capsule, each GTO measures the tension developed only by those motor units (Fig. 6.8). The $I_B$ afferent axon originating in a GTO primarily inhibits the α-motor neurons that innervate the same motor units attached to the GTO capsule. However, since this $I_B$ inhibition mostly affects the motor units under the most tension, those motor units relax slightly. *Therefore, the primary physiologic role of IB inhibition is to regulate α-motor neuron excitability to distribute tension evenly among motor units.*

## The Clasp Knife Reflex

The **clasp knife reflex** is evoked by attempting to stretch a muscle during an isometric contraction. The attempted stretch causes the tension in the muscle to increase rapidly, eliciting a massive discharge from the GTOs and consequent inhibition of the homonymous and synergistic α-motor neurons. The inhibition is evoked rapidly at high tension and quickly collapses the limb, much like closing the blade on a jackknife; hence the name, clasp knife reflex. Power weight lifters sometimes have this reflex if they try to lift too heavy a load. Muscle tension increases rapidly during the lift. If the tension is too great, partway through the lift the muscles suddenly lose power for no apparent reason, and the bewildered weight lifter drops the load. A variation of the clasp knife reflex is the basis for testing for spasticity, which is discussed later in this chapter.

## The Flexion Reflex

The flexion reflex [L. *flexio*, bending] produces a general flexion of the entire limb in response to noxious stimuli. For example, stepping on the sharp point of a thumbtack with a bare

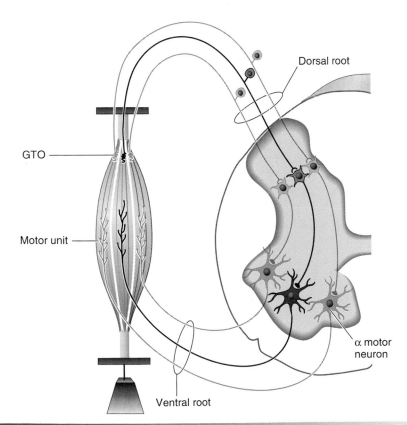

### Figure 6.8 Distribution of force among motor units

The GTO in a motor unit inhibits the α-motor neurons innervating that motor unit, relaxing it and ensuring that the load is evenly distributed among all active motor units.

foot makes one reflexively withdraw the foot by flexing all the joints in the leg.

Cutaneous afferents belonging to axon groups Aβ, Aδ, and C fibers carry sensations from nociceptors, tactile receptors, and joint receptors. The Aβ cutaneous axons[5] terminate in laminae III through VII, where they make excitatory synapses on interneurons (Fig. 6.7D). Normally, stimulation of the Aβ, Aδ, and C fibers, acting through interneurons, facilitates flexor motor neurons innervating the ipsilateral extremity and inhibits the extensor antagonists (Fig. 6.9). For this reason, this

group of afferent axons is commonly called **flexion reflex afferents (FRAs)**. Unlike the MSR and clasp knife reflex, in which the effects are limited to muscles acting on the same joint, the effects of FRA stimulation are distributed over the entire limb.

In the intact animal, stimulation of FRAs normally produces flexion of the entire limb, even though only a small area of skin may have been stimulated. The interneurons that mediate this FRA reflex also send collateral axons across the midline of the spinal cord, where they facilitate additional interneurons

[5] Because of the technical difficulties in marking individual axons, the terminal fields of single-group Aδand C cutaneous axons have not been mapped within the spinal cord. It is probable that these axons terminate in roughly the same laminae as the Aβcutaneous axons.

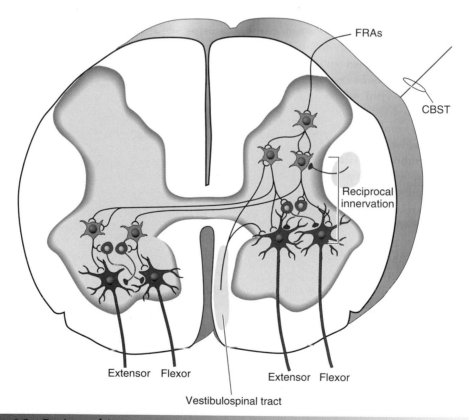

**Figure 6.9   Reciprocal innervation**

Reciprocal innervation is implemented by the anatomical arrangement of interneurons in the spinal cord. Sets of interneurons, when activated, produce opposite effects on motor neuron pools innervating antagonist muscle groups—for example, excitation of flexor motor neurons and inhibition of extensor motor neurons. *FRAs* initiate complex polysynaptic reflexes in the spinal cord. The simplest connections shown here illustrate the basic pattern. The effects of FRA stimulation are widespread, involving synergistic muscle groups in an entire limb and their contralateral counterpart. The axon labeled CBST represents supraspinal control elements (see Chapter 7).

that ultimately facilitate the extensor motor neurons and inhibit flexors (Fig. 6.9). This crossed extension reflex makes sense if one considers our hapless barefoot wanderer. When the stimulated leg is reflexively withdrawn to remove the foot from the tack, the weight is transferred to the contralateral leg. A reflex facilitation of extensors contralateral to the noxious stimulus is obviously desirable to avoid having that leg collapse as the body weight shifts to it.

## Reciprocal Innervation

In all of these afferent pathways, interneurons provide a means by which one pool of motor neurons is facilitated while its antagonist pool is inhibited (Fig. 6.9). This anatomical arrangement is known as **reciprocal innervation** [L. *reciprocus*, alternate; *in*, into; and *nervus*, nerve]. Its utility is obvious, since it is often desirable to relax the antagonist of a contracting muscle so that smooth joint movement is facilitated. This inhibition is automatically accomplished by the connections of interneurons, which minimizes the need for detailed central motor commands.

## SPINAL INTEGRATION OF MOTOR COMMANDS

Except for local spinal reflexes, all motor commands are initiated in supraspinal structures and sent to the spinal cord over the descending motor tracts. These descending control systems exert their influence indirectly through interneurons and to a lesser degree, directly through motor neurons. The direct activation of $\alpha$-motor neurons has certain advantages, such as increased speed and precision of movement (see Chapter 7). Reflecting these evolutionary advantages, the number of directly activated $\alpha$-motor neurons has increased with phylogeny. However, most motor control, even in the most evolutionarily derived mammals, is exerted through interneurons, a process that capitalizes on the intrinsic coordinating circuitry in the spinal cord. This approach relieves higher centers from the task of computing all the details of a motor act.

Group II muscle afferents facilitate two parallel interneuronal paths; one path facilitates flexors and the other facilitates extensors (Fig. 6.9). This apparently irrational anatomical arrangement makes sense if it is understood that neither path can be effective without continual subliminal facilitation from supraspinal systems. By facilitating one of the two antagonistic parallel pathways in the spinal cord, these higher descending control systems can regulate the balance between flexor and extensor muscle groups with simple generic commands. At rest, this balance normally favors the antigravity muscles, the extensor muscles in the lower extremity. Activity on FRAs produces the characteristic flexion response because these afferent axons provide more activity to the flexion pool of interneurons.

## Coactivation of $\alpha$- and $\gamma$-Motor Neurons

As noted previously, $\alpha$-motor neurons innervate only extrafusal muscle fibers. When the muscle contracts, the muscle spindle apparatus within it is unloaded (i.e., the tension on the spindle is released). Consequently, fewer action potentials are returned to the spinal cord over the group $I_A$ and II axons from the muscle spindle (Figs. 6.3C and 6.10A). The decrease in action potentials disfacilitates the $\alpha$-motor neuron and relaxes the muscle, restoring its overall length. This negative feedback system works well to maintain a constant muscle length under varying loads, but it interferes with the execution of commands intended to alter muscle length.

This problem can be overcome if $\alpha$- and $\gamma$-motor neurons are facilitated simultaneously by higher-center command signals. In this way the intrafusal muscle shortens at the same time that the extrafusal muscle contracts, and steady tension on the muscle spindle receptors is maintained (Fig. 6.10B). $I_A$ facilitation of the motor neurons does not decline during active muscle contraction. In the intact animal, $I_A$ facilitation is maintained so precisely that during voluntary movements, $I_A$ activity remains almost constant as the muscle contracts.

The problem can also be solved by using the gamma system to establish a new baseline

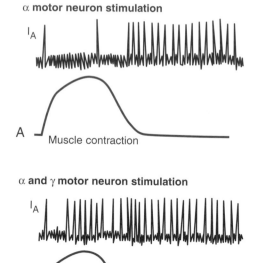

**α motor neuron stimulation**

$I_A$

A ⎤ Muscle contraction

**α and γ motor neuron stimulation**

$I_A$

Muscle contraction

B          200 ms

**Figure 6.10    Effects of α- and γ-motor neuron stimulation**

**A.** Effect of α-motor neuron stimulation on $I_A$ activity in the intact animal. **B.** Effect of simultaneous α- and γ-motor neuron stimulation on $I_A$ activity. (Reprinted with permission from Hunt CC, Kuffler SW. Further study of efferent small-nerve fibers to mammalian muscle spindles. Multiple spindle innervation and activity during contraction. J Physiol [Lond] 1951; 113:283–297.)

muscle length and allowing the monosynaptic reflex circuitry to regulate the extrafusal muscle tension. For example, stimulating γ-motor neurons alone raises tension on the intrafusal muscles. Although this tension is too weak to effect joint movement (Fig. 6.11), it does increase the tension on both the primary and secondary receptors. As a result, the frequency of action potentials on the $I_A$ and II axons increases. This increase in frequency exerts a powerful facilitation on the homonymous α-motor neuron pool that does effect muscle contraction and joint movement. As the muscle contracts under this reflex facilitation, the muscle spindle is unloaded, reducing the $I_A$

and II reflex facilitation until movement ceases. The muscle comes to rest, but at a new equilibrium length. In this way, *gamma activation determines the muscle length around which further motor regulation is established.*

Independent gamma activation is also necessary because the muscle spindles have a limited effective range; they cannot respond over the entire range of muscle length. To be maximally effective, the tension on the spindle must be maintained within a narrow range so that increases or decreases in muscle length cause appropriate changes in receptor activity. Activity on the γ-motor neuron adjusts the baseline tension on the muscle spindle receptor, matching it to the desired resting length of the muscle.

### Recruitment of Motor Neurons by Size

One of the important discoveries in physiology is that motor neurons are activated in a specific order during voluntary contraction of a muscle and deactivated in the opposite order as the contraction is voluntarily released. The significance of this observation is the discovery of two types of extrafusal muscle fibers. One type, the **slow, fatigue-resistant fibers,** develop tension slowly as frequency of action potential increases, and they can maintain this tension for long periods. These fibers have a broad dynamic range and can increase their tension 10- to 20-fold. The other type, the **fast, fatigable fibers,** develop tension rapidly but fatigue quickly. Speed is accomplished at the expense of dynamic range; the fast, fatigable fibers can produce only about a 2-fold increase in tension.

A relation exists between α-motor neuron size and muscle fiber type. Slow, fatigue-resistant fibers are generally innervated by small α-motor neurons, while the fast, fatigable muscle fibers are usually innervated by large α-motor neurons. This relation is important because neuron soma size determines the order in which motor units are recruited. Smaller neurons are brought to threshold first, since small neurons have a higher total membrane resistance than large neurons because of their smaller membrane surface area.

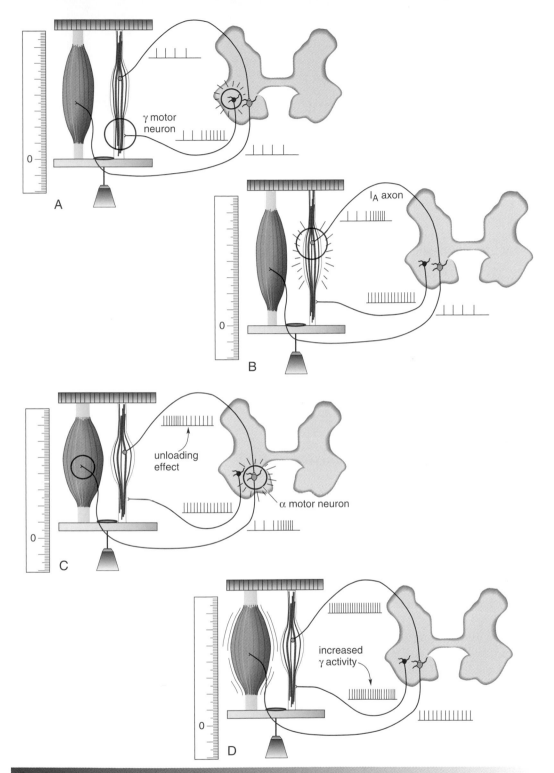

**Figure 6.11    Indirect action of γ-motor neuron activity**

The sequence of events necessary to establish a shorter set point for muscle length by increasing γ-motor neuron activity. The symbols over the axons represent action potential on that axon. **A.** Activity on the γ-motor neuron causes the contractile portion of the intrafusal muscle to contract. **B.** Contraction of the intrafusal muscle stretches the sensory portion of the fiber, depolarizing it and initiating action potential in the I_A axon. **C.** Activity in the I_A axon produces EPSPs in the α-motor neuron, causing it to fire and contracting the extrafusal muscle, which unloads the intrafusal fiber. **D.** The system reaches a new equilibrium at a shorter muscle length.

Consequently, all other variables being equal, the inward current flow initiated by an excitatory synapse generates a larger EPSP in a small neuron than in a large one.[6] Therefore, if a small supraspinal facilitation is distributed among all of the motor neurons in a pool, only the smallest neurons are brought to threshold. The middle-sized motor neurons are subliminally facilitated; they are brought to threshold only if the supraspinal facilitation is increased. This mechanism ensures that the steady, baseline muscle activity is borne by the least fatigable type of muscle fiber, leaving the fastest fibers in reserve for quick, short-lasting movements that are superimposed on the steady-state background tension.

## Development of Muscle Tension

The modulation of individual α-motor neuron firing rates regulates the tension produced by individual motor units. Under physiological conditions human α-motor neurons fire approximately 8 to 25 action potentials per second. At the lowest rate of discharge the motor unit produces approximately 10 to 25% of its maximum tension. As the firing rate of the α-motor neurons increases, muscle tension also increases.

Tension in a whole muscle is also regulated by the recruitment of motor units. The smooth application of tension during voluntary contraction is brought about both by increasing the force of contraction of individual motor units (modulated by α-motor neuron firing rate) and the recruitment of additional motor units (Fig. 6.12). The intrinsic organization of the spinal cord and the relation between the motor neurons and the muscle type ensures that the slow, fatigue-resistant motor units are recruited first and the fast, fatigable motor units are activated last. Therefore, descending motor commands need not be encoded for muscle fiber type. Only a general level of facilitation of the

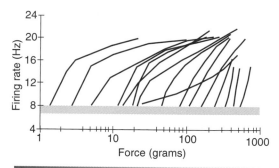

### Figure 6.12    Recruitment of motor units

This graph shows the recruitment of motor units during voluntary contraction of the extensor digitorum communis in the human. Each line represents the rate modulation of a single motor unit. The slope of the first units to be activated (slow, fatigue-resistant motor units) is much lower than that for the last units to be activated (fast, fatigable motor units). (Data from Monster AW, Chan H. Isometric force production by motor units of extensor digitorum communis muscle in man. J Neurophysiol 1977;40: 1432–1443.)

whole motor neuron pool must be incorporated in the motor command.

## INJURY AND REGENERATION OF THE PERIPHERAL NERVOUS SYSTEM

To appreciate the usefulness of MSR to neurological diagnoses, it is first necessary to have a fundamental understanding of how injury to the peripheral nervous system (PNS) can affect the MSR and muscle. The peripheral nerve may be injured in any of several ways. It can be cut cleanly in two; it can be constricted or crushed without severing the whole nerve; or it can be compromised by immunological or vascular disease. Although the neuronal response to injury in each of these cases is the same, the effectiveness of the regenerative process differs. Understanding these differences is important for determining the proper

---

[6] This phenomenon is a simple consequence of Ohm's law (E = IR). If the synaptic current (I) is constant, a larger voltage (E) is generated over a larger resistance (R). Of course this statement is an oversimplification because the electronic distance between the trigger zone and the synapse and a number of other factors must also be considered. However, these factors only modify the principle, which is that small neurons are more easily excitable than large ones.

treatment of nerve lesions and establishing a reasonable prognosis.

## Degeneration

When the axon is injured, neurons undergo specific degenerative changes. These changes are of two types: those proximal to the lesion and those distal to it.

### ORTHOGRADE DEGENERATION

When an axon is severed, the distal portion is removed from its source of metabolic nourishment. Without a continuous supply of trophic substances from the soma, the isolated axon soon dies. After the death of the axon, intraaxonal calcium is released from cisterns and sequestering molecules. The liberated calcium ions activate several enzymes that facilitate the disintegration of the axon. This process is called **orthograde** or **Wallerian degeneration.**

Secondary changes also occur after an axon dies. First, collagen and fibronectin production is stimulated in fibroblasts, causing hypertrophy of the endoneurium and perineurium. Second, because myelin cannot be maintained by the Schwann cell in the absence of an intact axon, the myelin becomes disorganized, disintegrates, and is phagocytized by Schwann cells and macrophages. Third, Schwann cells rapidly proliferate and organize themselves into columns of cells that take up the space vacated by the degenerated axon. Known as **Schwann tubes,** the columns play a critical role in the regenerative process (discussed later). Fourth, if the axon does not regenerate, eventually the Schwann cells cannot maintain themselves. Approximately a year after the injury, the Schwann tubes are replaced by connective tissue and the Schwann cells, by fibroblasts.

### RETROGRADE DEGENERATION

The neuronal cell body also undergoes characteristic changes after the amputation of its axon. The signal that apparently precipitates these changes is the loss of neurotrophic factors returned from the axon terminals to the soma by retrograde (from the periphery to the soma) axoplasmic flow. Instead, the soma receives materials released from degenerating

axons and Schwann cells at the site of the lesion. These materials may be enzymes released by Schwann cells or damaged axons. Although the precise nature of the signal is not known, the effect on the soma is apparent within hours of the amputation of an axon. The soma becomes swollen and the nucleus moves toward the periphery of the cell. The most conspicuous event is the reorganization of the rough endoplasmic reticulum and the mobilization of the ribosomes, after which the cell becomes less basophilic. Because the cell appears pale by light microscopy, light microscopists coined the term **chromatolysis** [G. *chroma*, color, and *lysis*, dissolution], which survives to this day.

### EFFECTS OF MUSCLE DENERVATION

Denervated muscle also undergoes conspicuous changes. These changes occur in three stages, signaled by fasciculations, fibrillations, and atrophy, in that order.

Following injury to the axon, **injury potentials** (potentials caused by depolarization of the membrane at the site of the lesion) evoke spontaneous action potentials that travel along the intact distal portions of the axon. For as long as the distal axon remains intact, these action potentials stimulate the muscle fibers of the still-complete motor unit to contract, eliciting a coordinated twitch among the muscle fibers. These contractions, which are visible to the careful observer, are known as **fasciculations** [L. *fascis*, bundle] (Fig. 6.13*A*). *Fasciculations are the earliest objective sign of muscle denervation.*

As the axon degenerates further, the terminal branches become isolated. Injury potentials are still generated and still cause muscular contractions. However, because the motor units are no longer joined by a functioning axon, the individual muscle cells no longer contract as a unit. These uncoordinated contractions, called **fibrillations** [L. *fibra*, fiber], are small and not visible on the body surface (Fig. 6.13*B*). They may be detected electrically by placing an electrode in the muscle and observing the muscle action potentials on an oscilloscope. This type of recording, an **electromyogram** [G. *electron*, amber; *mys*, muscle; and *gramma*, something writ-

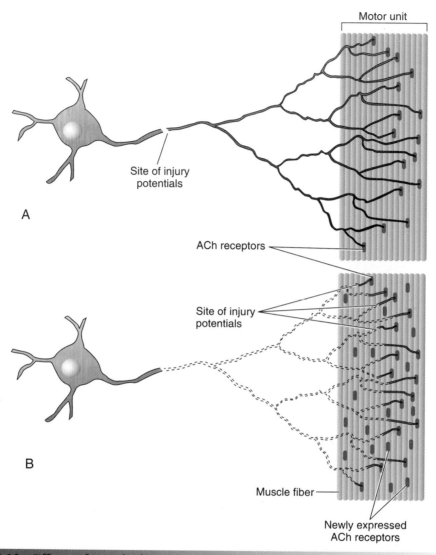

## Figure 6.13   Effects of muscle denervation

Fasciculations and fibrillations are caused by injury potentials generated at the site of injury to a motor neuron axon. **A.** Injury potentials cause all of the elements of the motor unit to contract simultaneously, producing a coordinated twitch (fibrillation) that is visible on the surface of the body. **B.** As the distal axon degenerates, the distal branches disconnect, and each has its own site where injury potentials are generated. Because the individual muscle fibers no longer contract as a unit, the twitches (fibrillations) are uncoordinated among the individual muscle fibers and not visible on the surface. In addition, as a consequence of denervation, the muscle fibers express numerous ACh receptors that make the muscle fibers hypersensitive to circulating ACh.

ten], or **EMG**, is used for objective documentation of muscle denervation.

After the distal axon has completely degenerated, the muscle becomes electrically silent. Degenerative changes in the muscle become apparent. Deprived of trophic substances delivered to the muscle by the neuron, the muscle undergoes **denervation atrophy.** This atrophy of denervation is not to be confused with the atrophy of disuse that occurs during immobilization. Denervation atrophy is much more profound and is an important clinical sign.

As a prelude to reinnervation, the denervated muscle develops a large number of acetylcholine receptor sites that serve as targets for regenerating axons. Denervated muscle can maintain these isolated receptors for about 2 years, after which, if no reinnervation occurs, they are lost. The presence of the uninnervated receptor sites also makes the muscle fibers hypersensitive to circulating acetylcholine, a condition that contributes to fibrillations.

## Regeneration

After a period of nuclear reorganization, injured neurons attempt to regenerate their original structure and to regain function. Since the embryonic conditions under which the neuron originally developed no longer exist, regeneration is not always successful. Success or failure depends on many factors, most of which are not completely understood. A few factors are discussed next.

### REGENERATION OF PERIPHERAL NERVE

In injured neurons, the production of proteins increases several-fold. Not only the amount of proteins but also the *types* of proteins change. The intact neuron produces materials necessary for synaptic transmission and general cell maintenance. The injured neuron produces materials necessary for the reconstruction of the distal axon and all of its terminals. Several growth-associated proteins that are essential for successful regeneration have been identified. Their transcription is triggered by axonal injury; they are not produced by intact neurons.

To accommodate this increase in protein synthesis, the *orthograde* (from the soma to the periphery) axoplasmic transport mechanisms are stimulated. The rate of slow axoplasmic transport is as much as doubled. Although the rate of fast axoplasmic transport is not altered, the amount of material transported increases by as much as 250%.

About 2 days after peripheral nerve injury, the proximal stump of the injured axon develops a specialized bulbous ending called the **growth cone.** Arising from the growth cone are about 10 to 50 sprouts called neurites that elongate and explore the interstitial space. If one of these neurites finds a favorable surface, its movement diminishes and the remaining sprouts shrink back into the body of the growth

cone. The remaining neurite enlarges and the growth cone redevelops at its distal terminus.

This regenerative process closely depends on the favorable interaction between the hydralike neurites and the interstitial environment. The Schwann cells are a critical part of this environment. **Laminin** and **fibronectin** are two glycoproteins found in the **basal lamina** [G. *basis*, base, and *lamina*, thin plate] of the Schwann cell. Both seem to stimulate the formation of growth cones. Laminin in particular is a favorable substrate for neurite attachment. Recall that a Schwann tube consists of a string of modified Schwann cells that occupy the space of a degenerated axon. Once it comes into contact with these cells, a growing neurite finds a laminin-rich basal lamina that provides a favorable environment for regeneration. By following the basal lamina provided by the continuous string of Schwann cells, the neurite can grow along the path of the degenerated axon to reach an appropriate target.

### REINNERVATION OF MUSCLE

When a regenerating motor neuron reaches a muscle, it is attracted to the acetylcholine receptors that have blossomed on its surface. Although the process is not completely understood, the acetylcholine receptor sites apparently secrete a chemotactic substance that attracts the regenerating axon. New myoneural junctions are established when a motor axon attaches to an acetylcholine receptor site. As myoneural junctions develop on the muscle, the unoccupied receptor sites are reabsorbed. Because the supplies of trophic substances from the axon are restored, the reinnervated muscle enlarges and the atrophy becomes much less prominent. However, since reinnervation of a muscle is rarely complete, it never regains its normal size.

### REGENERATION OF SENSORY RECEPTORS

Sensory receptors can also be regenerated, although the process is even less well understood than that for axons. The first sensation recovered is usually pain. The simplicity of the nociceptor terminals (free nerve endings) probably allows them to become functional at an early stage of regeneration. Other touch receptors can be renewed, but the full complement of sensory receptors is never fully restored. Therefore, natural sensory perceptions from a denervated area cannot be completely reestablished.

## Practical Considerations

This description makes it obvious that successful axonal regeneration is much more likely if the peripheral nerve is simply crushed and not severed (Fig. 6.14A). Following crush injuries, the regenerating axon is almost al-

ways directed into the Schwann tubes derived from its distal portion. The axon usually regenerates to its original target and good function can be restored. However, if the nerve is severed, new problems arise. For example, there may be a gap between the proximal and distal ends of the nerve. Growing axons can bridge gaps of several millimeters (Fig. 6.14B), but they may enter Schwann tubes that lead to inappropriate termination sites. A sensory axon may send a growth cone into a tube that

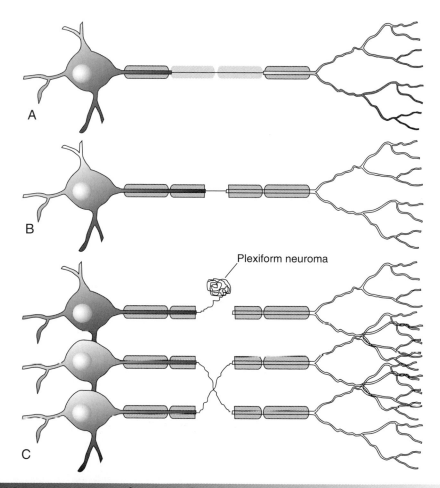

## Figure 6.14   Regeneration of peripheral axons

**A.** If the peripheral nerve is crushed, leaving the connective tissue intact, growth cones from the proximal segments of injured axons have little difficulty entering the Schwann tubes. Restoration of function is usually complete. **B.** If the nerve is severed but the stumps can be carefully anastomosed, growth cones have a good chance of entering appropriate Schwann tubes. Restoration of function is possible but rarely complete. **C.** If there is a large gap between the stumps of injured neurons, growth cones may not enter Schwann tubes. In such cases a plexiform neuroma is formed (*top*). In other cases motor axons may enter Schwann tubes that are derived from sensory nerves and vice versa. Little functional recovery occurs in such cases.

terminates on a muscle body and vice versa. Or motor axons may regenerate to muscles that are different from the ones they originally innervated. Functional recovery is less than complete in such cases.

If the gap is very large, neurites may not be able to cross it and find their way into a Schwann tube (Fig. 6.14C). Sensory neurons that wander beyond the protective field of the Schwann tubes may coil into a whorl of axons and connective tissue known as a **plexiform neuroma.** These neuromas can cause intense pain. More frequently, however, lost axons simply stop growing, and regeneration ceases. Eventually unconnected axons degenerate and ultimately the entire neuron dies.

Microsurgical techniques allow severed peripheral nerves to be sutured together, fascicle by fascicle, which is purported to improve functional recovery. This tedious process is not always practical. If the gap is large, the surgeon may have to insert a nerve graft between the stumps, and accurate fascicular realignment may be impossible. Yet, significant functional recovery is frequently attainable in such cases. Recent evidence suggests that exact fascicular alignment may not be necessary for good functional recovery, as was once believed. Under laboratory conditions severed nerves that are reapposed with a slight gap between the nerve ends regenerate with extraordinary precision. It appears that the regenerating axons have a remarkable ability to select a Schwann tube that will lead them to an appropriate target. Although a chemotactic signal is suspected, the process is not completely understood.

## CLINICAL EVALUATION OF MOTOR FUNCTION

Localizing a nervous system lesion is the essential first step in forming a correct neurological diagnosis. Many neurologists approach the problem of localization by mentally dividing the nervous system into several functionally distinct regions. Usually the patient's signs and symptoms allow the neurologist to exclude the lesion from one or more of these regions. Further analysis then allows refinement of the location.

Two functionally distinct regions of the nervous system are known as the **upper motor neuron** (UMN) and the **lower motor neuron** (LMN). This nomenclature is misleading, for neither of these so-called neurons exists as a discrete cell. Rather, each is a set of tracts or nerves and nuclei that form a *clinically recognizable functional system.* The concept of an upper and lower motor neuron is thus a generalization of the anatomical organization of the nervous system. Understanding the principles that define this concept is essential to neurologic diagnosis.

The ability to distinguish between lesions to the LMN and the UMN requires an understanding of how the physician uses the MSR to test the "lower motor neuron" and to evaluate neural dysfunction. *By definition, the "lower motor neuron" consists of the parts of the nervous system that when injured,* **decrease** *the strength of the MSR. Injuries to the "upper motor neuron"* **increase** *the strength of the MSR.* Understanding the basis of these definitions is essential to the neurological examination.

### Neurology of the MSR

Testing the MSR is fundamental to the neurological examination because *it allows the physician to distinguish between UMN and LMN injuries.* The physician uses a reflex hammer to sharply strike a tendon (Fig. 6.15). Striking a tendon places on the muscle a rapid stretch that *primarily stimulates the dynamic bag receptors,* causing a reflex contraction of the homonymous muscle. This reflex is commonly called the deep tendon reflex (DTR) because of the emphasis on striking the tendon with the reflex hammer.[7] This unfortunate term is so ingrained in medical parlance that it will probably never be replaced. The student is cautioned, however, to avoid associating the MSR with the GTO receptor. To avoid this confusion, this text uses the term MSR to designate this reflex, a usage that is gaining popularity among neurologists. Students are encouraged to adopt this terminology also.

The responsiveness of the MSR can be altered by trauma or disease. Only three findings

---

[7]This reflex is often called a muscle jerk because the muscle responds to the reflex hammer with a quick jerk.

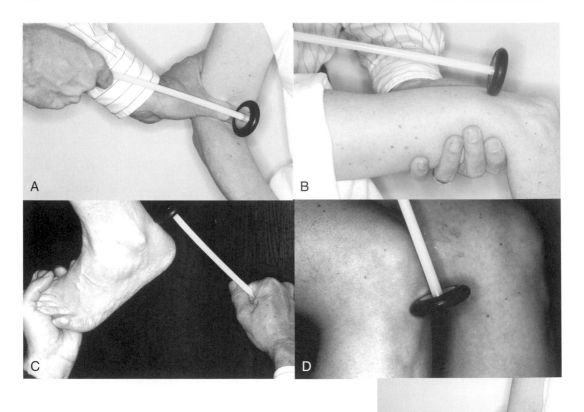

## Figure 6.15    Eliciting the MSR

Evocation of the five principal MSR reflexes: biceps (**A**), triceps (**B**), gastrocnemius (Achilles) (**C**), quadriceps (patellar) (**D**), and brachioradialis. The reflex hammer is used in three slightly different ways to stretch the muscle: by striking a tendon directly (**B, C,** and **D**); by striking the tendon indirectly, as when the examiner interposes a thumb between the hammer and the tendon (**A**); and by striking the muscle body directly (**E**).

can be observed: the reflex may be **hypoactive, normal,** or **hyperactive.** If the muscle does not contract with a quick, strong jerk in response to the reflex hammer, the reflex is said to be hypoactive, or reduced. It may be reduced to the point of absence. The reaction of the mus-

cle may be faster and stronger than normal, in which case the MSR is said to be hyperactive, elevated, or brisk (see Appendix 2). Many physicians use the plus nomenclature (Table 6.4) to describe the MSR response. It is not always easy to determine whether or not the

| Table 6.4 Clinical Notation Commonly Used to Describe MSR Responses | |
| --- | --- |
| Description | Interpretation |
| ++ | Very brisk, definitely abnormal |
| + | Brisk, probably abnormal |
| Normal | Within normal range |
| − | Weak, probably abnormal |
| − − | Very weak, definitely abnormal |
| Absent | Not perceptible |

MSR is elevated or reduced. Learning to make such judgments requires experience.

*Injury to any part of the PNS, including the muscle itself, reduces or eliminates the MSR.* Consider all of the elements of the nervous system that must perform correctly if this simple reflex is to function properly. The muscle sensory receptors (spindle apparatus), along with their primary afferent neurons (principally the $I_A$), must be intact. The axons of these neurons lie in the peripheral nerve and the dorsal roots. Thus, any injury to the peripheral nerve or the spinal roots that supply it adversely affects the reflex. The spinal cord, including the motor neurons, must also be intact where the root enters. The ventral root, peripheral nerve, myoneural junction, and muscle itself must be considered. *If any of these elements is damaged or destroyed, the MSR is either less responsive than normal* or, in extreme cases, absent altogether. The careful physician must consider all elements of the reflex path before forming conclusions about the motor system.

To illustrate, **peripheral neuropathies** are a class of diseases that affect the peripheral nerves. They are often associated with diminished reflexes because the disease process interferes with axonal transmission. A **compression injury** at the union of the dorsal and ventral root caused by a herniated intervertebral disk is a common cause of decreased reflexes in the extremities. **Tabes dorsalis** [L. *tabes*, wasting disease, and *dorsum*, the back], a

condition resulting from long-term infection by syphilis, destroys the large-diameter axons in the dorsal root, including the $I_A$ axons. This condition causes extreme paroxysmal pain (see Chapter 5) and because of the loss of the $I_A$ axons, decreased MSRs. **Polio myelitis**, a viral disease that frequently kills motor neurons in the spinal cord and brainstem, leads to paralysis and decreased or absent reflexes. **Myasthenia gravis**, which interferes with synaptic transmission between the motor end plate and the muscle, is manifested clinically by increasing fatigue and progressively diminished reflexes with exercise. Finally, the **muscular dystrophies** decrease or destroy reflexes by means of primary muscle disease that leads to eventual failure of the muscle.

This diverse group of neurological diseases have in common two elements: *all cause decreased or absent monosynaptic reflexes, and all affect the PNS or muscle.* This association between decreased MSRs and the aforementioned parts of the nervous system led to the clinical concept of the LMN, which is extraordinarily useful. With simple observations and a reflex hammer, the physician can quickly determine whether the neurological problem affects the CNS or PNS and localize it to a relatively small region. *Correctly using and interpreting the MSR is absolutely critical to the neurological examination.*

### Auxiliary LMN Signs

A reduction in the MSR is the only sign necessary to localize a lesion to the LMN. Under some circumstances, however, determining whether a reflex is depressed may be difficult. Therefore, ancillary signs are useful in corroborating the interpretation of the MSR and determining the presence of any LMN disease. Most prominent among these ancillary signs is **fasciculations**. Since damage to the α-motor neuron denervates the muscle, fasciculations are a useful indirect sign of nerve damage. At a later stage in the course of the disease, pronounced muscle **atrophy** serves the same purpose.

# C A S E   H I S T O R Y

## THE CASE OF THE EMBOTTLED MACHINIST

### HISTORY OF PRESENT ILLNESS, 7 JULY

Mr E. A. is a 55-year-old white man who is employed as a tool-and-dye maker for a large corporation. He was first seen by his physician on April 11, complaining of numbness in his feet. This numbness was of several months' duration. At that time it was determined that Mr. E. A. was an alcoholic, but he refused treatment for his alcoholism. Today, he is complaining of general weakness and numbness in his lower extremities, saying his symptoms have worsened since his last visit.

### MEDICAL HISTORY

Mr. E. A. has no history of other serious medical problems.

### PHYSICAL EXAMINATION

BP 155/95, otherwise unremarkable.

### NEUROLOGICAL EXAMINATION

#### Mental Status
Mr. E. A. gave a coherent and concise history. He was oriented to person, place, and time. He remembered the three items requested.

#### Cranial Nerves
No abnormalities in cranial nerve function were found.

#### Station and Gait
Mr. E. A.'s gait was safe but wide based and ataxic. He tended to slap his feet on the ground as he walked. He was unable to walk on his heels or toes.

#### Motor Systems
STRENGTH: His upper-extremity strength was bilaterally symmetrical and normal (5/5). There

was no drift as he held his arms out in front of his body. Lower-extremity strength was symmetrical but weak to direct strength testing (4/5). He could barely manage one deep knee bend.

TONE: There was no spasticity or rigidity (see Chapters 7 and 8).

BULK: Bulk was normal; there was no apparent atrophy.

ABNORMAL MOVEMENTS: There were no fasciculations or other abnormal movements.

#### Sensory Systems
Perception of pinprick was bilaterally dull, and vibration sense was absent from his knees down to and including his feet. Mr. E. A. could not determine the position of his toes or ankles when they were passively positioned by the examiner. When asked to stand on a narrow base, Mr. E. A. was fairly stable. When asked to close his eyes, he became unstable and would have fallen if not caught by the examiner (Romberg test). Sensations from the upper extremities were symmetrical and perceived as normal.

#### Reflexes
Both ankle MSRs (gastrocnemius-soleus muscle) were depressed (− −). Patellar (quadriceps muscle) and upper extremity MSR reflexes were normal. Plantar reflexes were flexor (normal; see Chapter 7).

#### Coordination and Control
Heel-to-shin, finger-to-nose, rapid alternating hand slapping, and rapid finger touching were easily accomplished.

#### Parietal Functions
There was no aphasia; optokinetic nystagmus was present in both directions. There were no atavistic signs.

### ANCILLARY STUDIES

None ordered.

## SUBSEQUENT COURSE

Mr. E. A. was again encouraged to seek treatment for alcoholism and he again refused. He was prescribed vitamin supplements and advised to improve his nutritional status.

## COMMENTARY

The first steps in analyzing a neurological case is to determine (a) the time course of the illness and (b) the distribution of the signs and symptoms. The time course helps to establish the cause of the disease, and the distribution of symptoms helps to establish the location of the lesion. Both factors are important to this case.

The history indicates that Mr. E. A.'s problems are localized to his lower extremities. The subjective impression gained from the history is confirmed by objective observation during the neurological examination. The decreased MSRs from the gastrocnemius-soleus muscles and the normal MSRs from the quadriceps muscles establish the peripheral nature of the disease process, the involvement of the LMN, and the localization to the distal portion of both lower extremities.

The loss of pinprick and vibration sensations from the lower extremities involves the entire distal portion. This stocking-and-glove pattern[8] is characteristic of diffuse peripheral nerve lesions and is in sharp contrast to the dermatome pattern associated with lesions of the roots or the patchy patterns associated with localized damage to a peripheral nerve (see Chapter 5). Mr. E. A. has difficulty walking because the sensory positional information from the skin and joints of his lower extremities is not being received in the spinal cord. The examination of joint position sense clarifies the reason for the gait disturbance: he has little proprioception from his ankles. The slapping of the feet is a common compensatory mechanism to increase sensory perception from the feet while walking. The importance of sensory feedback in motor control is discussed further in Chapter 7.

The history also reveals that Mr. E. A. has a long-term (several months), slowly progressing problem. It originally caused only sensory symptoms but has now progressed to involve both sensory and motor functions. Slowly progressive problems are not likely to be caused by strokes (intracranial thrombosis or hemorrhage) or traumatic injury. Expanding intracranial masses; metabolic, inflammatory, or immunological diseases, and toxins are more likely explanations.

Mr. E. A. presents a typical picture of peripheral neuropathy. Also known as **polyneuropathy,** peripheral neuropathy describes a clinical syndrome that includes both motor and sensory losses caused by diffuse lesions to peripheral nerves. The affected areas cannot be associated with the territory of a single nerve or spinal root. Frequently the pattern of loss is bilaterally symmetrical and has a stocking-and-glove distribution.

The lesions that can cause these losses are numerous and may be inherited or acquired. **Diabetes mellitus** is a common cause of peripheral neuropathy. In its later stages the microcirculation is disrupted. Many organs, including the peripheral nerves, undergo vascular damage. Peripheral neuropathies are also commonly associated with **toxins.** These include alcohol, heavy metals, metabolic toxins (associated with diseases such as diphtheria and with malignancies), and prescription drugs. **Nutritional and vitamin deficiencies,** particularly those involving the B group, are also associated with peripheral neuropathy. However, a large number of peripheral neuropathies are simply **idiopathic** [G. *idios,* self, and *pathos,* suffering], that is, disease of unknown cause.

Peripheral neuropathy is a common sequela to chronic alcohol abuse. The primary cause of the neuropathy is not known. Nutritional deficiency, particularly thiamine deficiency, is often a contributing factor for someone with a history of alcohol abuse like Mr. E. A.'s.

## FURTHER APPLICATIONS

6.1.   **Consider the history in this case. How does the distribution of the patient's symptoms help to determine which division(s) of the nervous system may be involved? How are the**

---

[8] Stocking-and-glove is generic and appropriate here even though Mr. E. A.'s hands are not yet involved in the peripheral neuropathy.

decreased MSRs consistent with this part of the history?

6.2. What makes the loss of position sense from the toes a significant finding? Is the preservation of position sense from the fingers also a significant finding? Explain.

6.3. What do you think causes the patient's ataxia? Does the Romberg test have any bearing on this observation?

6.4. No atrophy or fasciculations were noted, yet these are important signs of LMN pathology. Explain.

6.5. Consider the many causes of peripheral neuropathy. What mechanism might explain the stocking-and-glove pattern of sensory loss that is typical of these diseases?

# C A S E    H I S T O R Y

## THE CASE OF THE LIMPING LADY

### HISTORY OF PRESENT ILLNESS, 20 MAY

Mrs. N. B. is a 63-year-old white woman who went to her family physician complaining of pain in her lower back that extended down the side and back of her right leg. She walked with a noticeable limp. The pain began in April and has been getting worse. Mrs. N. B. reported that the pain was severe and after a week of complete bed rest said that the pain remained undiminished.

### MEDICAL HISTORY

Mrs. N. B. has no history of serious medical disease.

### PHYSICAL EXAMINATION

Mrs. N. B. is in good physical health. BP 135/80.

### NEUROLOGICAL EXAMINATION

#### Mental Status
Mrs. N. B. is oriented to person, place, and time. At the end of the examination she remembered the three items requested.

#### Cranial Nerves
No abnormalities in cranial nerve function were found.

#### Station and Gait
Mrs. N. B. walked with a limp, favoring her right leg. She could walk on her heels but had some difficulty toe walking, being unable to maintain the extension of her right foot.

#### Motor Systems

STRENGTH: Strength was 5/5 except at the right gastrocnemius-soleus muscle, which was 4/5.

TONE: There was no spasticity or rigidity (see Chapters 7 and 8).

BULK: Normal bulk for a woman of her age. There was no obvious atrophy.

ABNORMAL MOVEMENTS: There were no fasciculations or other abnormal movements.

SENSORY SYSTEMS: There was dullness to pinprick over the lateral border of her right lower extremity and foot. Mrs. N. B. was in great pain when she sat in a chair or stood. She was most comfortable while lying in bed with her knees flexed, although she was not free of pain even then. Passive straight leg raises were limited to 30° by pain on the right. The left leg could be raised to 90° nearly pain free.

### Reflexes

All MSRs were normal and symmetrical except for the right Achilles tendon, from which the MSR was absent. Plantar reflexes were bilaterally flexor (normal; see Chapter 7).

### Coordination and Control

All cerebellar tests were performed without difficulty.

### Parietal Functions

All parietal tests were normal.

### ANCILLARY STUDIES

MRI of the lumbosacral spine was ordered (Fig. 6.16).

### SUBSEQUENT COURSE

Mrs. N. B. underwent surgery the following day. The intervertebral disk was removed from between the L5 and S1 vertebrae without incident. She was prescribed a supervised program of physical therapy. Six months after her surgery she was pain free and had resumed her normal lifestyle.

### COMMENTARY

Low back pain is a common complaint that is often not successfully diagnosed and treated. Appropriate diagnosis for Mrs. N. B. was facilitated because her neurological examination provided objective, localized findings. When this is the case, treatment is very likely to be successful. We learn from the history that Mrs. N. B.'s pain is not associated with any notable injury. The pain is also highly localized to her right back and leg and is not relieved with bed rest. Also, the pain progressively worsened, reached a plateau, and remained undiminished.

Most notable among the objective findings of the neurological examination are weakness and absence of the MSR from the right gastrocnemius-soleus muscle. This finding establishes the peripheral nature of the problem. The facts that there is no other weakness and that all other reflexes are normal make the absent MSR more significant. The dull pinprick sensation from the lateral aspect of the right foot corresponds to the territory of the S1 dermatome (see Chapter 5). Particularly noteworthy is the fact that the gastrocnemius-soleus muscle receives its primary innervation from the S1 spinal root. Therefore, two independent lines of evidence, one sensory and one motor, help to localize the problem to a single spinal root.

Weakness, pain, and loss of somatosensory perceptions that can be attributed to one or two adjacent spinal nerves are the cardinal signs associated with **spinal disk syndrome.** This syndrome is caused by a displaced intervertebral disk that presses on one or two spinal nerves close to their egress from the spinal column (Fig. 6.17). Therefore, symptoms are the LMN type, involve both sensory and motor signs, and are highly localized. The present case is typical in these aspects.

Straight leg raises (placing the patient on the back, raising each fully extended leg independently, and noting the angle of the leg to the

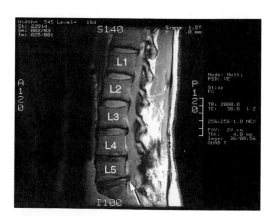

### Figure 6.16   Ms. N. B.

This proton density (2000/30) MRI illustrates the normal appearance of the intervertebral disks and one disk (*arrow*) that is protruding into the spinal canal, compressing the S1 spinal root. (MRI courtesy the Magnetic Imaging Center, South Bend, IN.)

## Figure 6.17 Relation of spinal nerves and the intervertebral disks

In this dorsal view of the lumbosacral spine, the dural sac and spinal nerves are shown in *black,* and the bony structures are shown in *outline.* In the L4-L5 and L5-S1 interspaces it is possible for a displaced intervertebral disk to compress either the nerve that exits at that level or the nerve that exits at the next most caudal level (the S1 entrapment by the L5-S1 disk). (Reprinted with permission from Curtis BA, Jacobson S, and Marcus EM. An Introduction to the Neurosciences. Philadelphia: WB Saunders, 1972.)

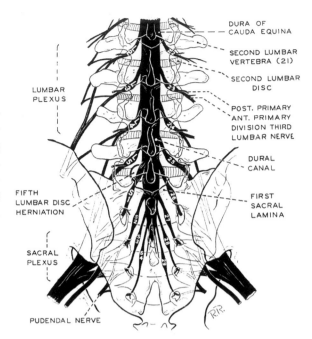

bed) are not diagnostic in these cases but are traditionally performed to quantify the severity of the symptoms. Raising the leg is said to stretch the sciatic nerve and can increase the pressure on the entrapped root. In many cases, however, raising the leg contralateral to the injured root causes increased pain but raising the ipsilateral leg does not.

At this point a diagnosis of right S1 spinal nerve entrapment at the L5-S1 vertebral interspace caused by a protruding intervertebral disk is reasonable. A disk in this position could place pressure either on the L5 or the S1 root (Fig. 6.17). It can be presumed that the S1 root is involved in this case because of the dermatome data and the loss of the MSR from the gastrocnemius-soleus muscle. The diagnosis should be verified by ancillary studies. In this case the MRI revealed a displaced intervertebral disk (Fig. 6.16).

## FURTHER APPLICATIONS

**6.6.** **The L5 spinal nerve exits at the interspace between the L5 and S1 verte-**brae, yet in this case it is the S1 nerve that is affected. Can you explain this apparent discrepancy?

**6.7.** **Suppose the L5 root was affected. Which disk would be the most likely cause of the problem? What symptoms would you expect to observe?**

**6.8.** **Most intervertebral disks rupture to one side, but occasionally one protrudes at the midline. What distribution of symptoms would you expect to observe for a midline rupture at the L5-S1 space?**

**6.9.** **In most cases the intervertebral disk is displaced in the lumbar region. However, displaced cervical disks are fairly common. What signs would you expect to observe if the disk between the C6-C7 interspace became displaced and pressed on the left spinal nerve?**

# S U M M A R Y

- **Striated muscles are endowed with a number of sensory receptors that convey to the CNS critical information about muscle dynamics.**

  The *muscle spindle apparatus* contains sensory receptors that furnish to the CNS information about muscle length and the velocity of length changes. The muscle spindle apparatus consists of specialized intrafusal muscle fibers enclosed in a capsule. There are two anatomically distinct intrafusal fibers, the nuclear bag and the nuclear chain. All of the chain fibers and some of the bag fibers are static receptors, responding primarily to muscle length. The bag fibers are dynamic, responding primarily to the velocity of length changes. The *GTO* is a sensory receptor that furnishes information about muscle tension.

- **Muscle receives both sensory and motor innervation.**

  Two types of sensory axons, group $I_A$ and group II, innervate the muscle spindle apparatus. $I_A$ axons originate in all bag and chain fibers and have both dynamic and static properties. Group II axons originate in static bag and chain fibers and have primarily static properties. A third type of fiber, the group $I_B$ axons, originate in GTOs.

- **The motor innervation of muscle falls into two classes, $\alpha$- and $\gamma$-motor neurons.**

  The $\alpha$-motor neurons innervate the main muscle mass, the extrafusal muscle, that provides the power necessary to move. The $\gamma$-motor neurons innervate the intrafusal muscle, the contractile portion of the muscle spindle apparatus. Although these spindle muscles are small and cannot directly cause movement of the entire muscle, they do regulate the sensitivity of the muscle spindle receptors.

- **The muscle sensory receptors make specific connections in the spinal cord that affect motor neuron activity.**

  The $I_A$ and II axons make excitatory monosynaptic synapses on homonymous $\alpha$-motor neurons. The $I_B$ axon synapses on interneurons that in turn make inhibitory synapses on homonymous $\alpha$-motor neurons. All of these axons also make numerous synapses on interneurons. The interneurons of laminae IV to VII are part of a synaptic network that coordinates synergistic neurons and provides for reciprocal innervation of antagonistic motor neuron pools.

- **The MSR is an important reflex that results from a rapid stretch of a muscle.**

  The rapid stretch almost exclusively stimulates the dynamic bag fibers. The signal enters the spinal cord over $I_A$ axons, which make excitatory synapses directly on $\alpha$-motor neurons. The motor neuron returns to the homonymous muscle, causing it to contract. The clasp knife reflex is not fully understood but probably originates in GTOs. The signals enter the spinal cord over $I_B$ axons, where they inhibit the homonymous $\alpha$-motor neurons through the action of an interneuron.

- **FRAs originate from cutaneous receptors.**

  The signal enters the spinal cord over group $A\beta$, $A\delta$, and C axons that make polysynaptic connections on interneurons in laminae IV to VII. Stimulation of FRAs typically elicits an ipsilateral flexion and a contralateral extension of the extremities.

- **Most supraspinal motor commands indirectly affect motor neurons, passing first through interneurons.**

  This strategy allows local spinal circuits to provide for reciprocal innervation and synergistic coordination automatically. Most motor commands also coactivate both $\alpha$- and $\gamma$-motor neurons so that the muscle spindle does not become unloaded during muscle contraction. Activation of $\gamma$-motor neurons alone causes a reflex contraction of the extrafusal muscle that establishes a new resting length for the muscle.

- **During voluntary contraction, tension is smoothly applied to a muscle.**

  Smooth application of tension is accomplished by modulating the frequency of action potentials on the $\alpha$-motor neurons as well as by recruiting more motor neurons. Motor neurons are recruited in a specific order, from the smallest to the largest. Small motor neurons innervate slow, fatigue-resistant muscle fibers, while the large motor neurons innervate fast, fatigable muscle fibers.

- **If an axon is severed, the axon undergoes both orthograde and retrograde degenerative changes.**

The neuron soma becomes chromolytic. The Schwann cells form Schwann tubes along the path of the degenerated distal axon. The distal end of a severed axon forms a growth cone that extends itself in an effort to regenerate the axon. Growth cones follow Schwann tubes and, under favorable conditions, form a new functional axon. Denervated muscle undergoes characteristic changes, first developing fasciculations that are followed by fibrillations. Eventually denervated muscle atrophies. If it is reinnervated by a motor axon, muscle function can be restored.

- **The LMN is a clinical concept.**

The LMN consists of all of the peripheral components of the MSR, including the muscle. Injury or disease can affect the MSR, making it either hyperactive or hypoactive. LMN pathology is characterized by hypoactive or absent muscle stretch reflexes. Diminished MSRs may also be accompanied by auxiliary signs, such as fasciculations, fibrillations, and atrophy.

## SUGGESTED READINGS

Brooks VB. The Neural Basis of Motor Control. New York: Oxford University, 1986.

Brown AG. Organization in the Spinal Cord: The Anatomy and Physiology of Identified Neurons. Berlin: Springer-Verlag, 1981.

Boulu P, Benoist M. Recent data on the pathophysiology of nerve root compression and pain. Rev Rhum Ed Engl 1996;63:358–363.

Kolb B. Brain Plasticity and Behavior. Mahwah, NJ: Lawrence Erlbaum, 1995.

Lundborg G. Nerve Injury and Repair. Philadelphia: Churchill Livingstone, 1988.

Partridge LD, Partridge LD. The Nervous System: Its Function and Its Interaction with the World. Cambridge, MA: MIT, 1993.

Ramon y Cajal S. Degeneration and regeneration of the nervous system. Raoul May RM, ed, trans. New York: Hafner, 1959.

# Motor Systems II: Descending Motor Systems

The motor circuits in the spinal cord are directly regulated by motor systems in the brainstem and cerebral cortex. These systems are composed of separate collections of neurons, each of which sends long tracts of axons into the brainstem and spinal cord, where they terminate. Consequently, these systems are called the **descending motor systems**. Like the ascending sensory systems (see Chapter 5), the descending motor systems are a parallel set of pathways with overlapping as well as complementary functions.

Four areas of the cerebral cortex generate motor commands. Although these areas are interconnected, each is concerned with different aspects of motor control. These areas are closely associated both functionally and anatomically with the basal ganglia and thalamus (see Chapter 8). Together the four cortical areas and the subcortical motor nuclei of the thalamus and basal ganglia produce the motor commands that descend to the brainstem and spinal motor areas. However, these motor commands reach the brainstem and spinal cord in a form that does not ensure precise motor performance. Therefore, control mechanisms in the spinal cord and cerebellum (see Chapter 9) fine-tune the motor commands, making supple, graceful, coordinated movement possible.

## ORGANIZATION OF THE DESCENDING MOTOR PATHWAYS

Motor neurons in the spinal cord are not randomly scattered in lamina IX but are precisely organized in a somatotopic arrangement that reflects the distribution of muscles in the extremities (Fig.7.1A). Imagine drawing a line that bisects the ventral horn. The motor neurons dorsolateral to that line innervate flexor muscles; those ventral medial to it innervate extensors. Furthermore, the most dorsomedial motor neurons supply the more proximal muscles, and the most ventral lateral ones supply the more distal muscles. This arrangement of motor neurons ensures that the descending motor tracts found in the lateral white column preferentially innervate flexor motor neurons and those in the ventral medial white column preferentially innervate extensor motor neurons (Fig.7.1B).

The descending motor pathways can be organized into four sets of tracts based on the origin of their cell bodies: the **corticobulbospinal tract**[1] (CBST), the **rubrospinal tract**,

---

[1]Many physicians call the CBST the pyramidal tract. Strictly speaking, the pyramidal tract refers only to the axons in the medullary pyramids. These axons are only a small subset of the CBST. The use of "pyramidal tract" as a synonym for the CBST is not only inaccurate but has led to even more unfortunate terms: pyramidal syndrome, extrapyramidal system, and extrapyramidal syndrome. Many authors advocate that these "pyramidal" terms be abandoned in favor of terms that more accurately express the anatomical and clinical situation.

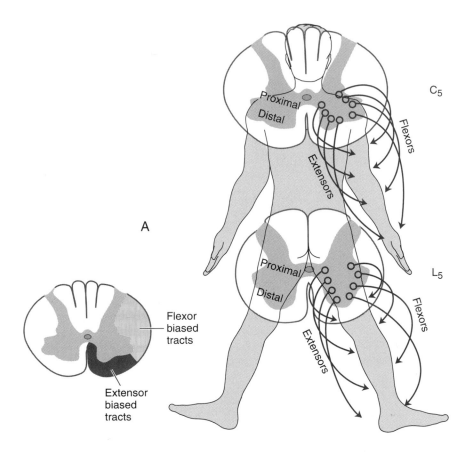

A

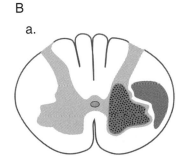

Flexor biased tracts

Extensor biased tracts

B

**Flexor Biased Tracts**

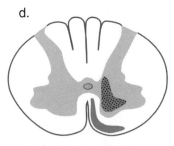

a.

Lateral corticospinal tract

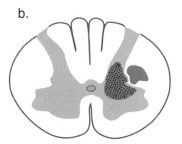

b.

Rubrospinal tract

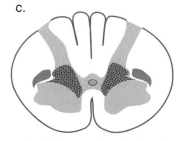

c.

Medullary reticulospinal tract

**Extensor Biased Tracts**

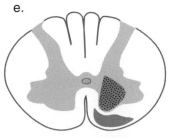

d.

Pontine reticulospinal tract

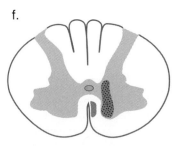

e.

Lateral vestibulospinal tract

f.

Medial vestibulospinal tract

the **reticulospinal tracts**, and the vestibu-lospinal tracts.

## The Corticobulbospinal Tract

The CBST originates in the cerebral cortex and descends into the brainstem and spinal cord motor systems. This tract consists of the **corticobulbar division** (fibers that terminate in the brainstem) and the **corticospinal division** (fibers that terminate in the spinal cord). Together the corticobulbar and corticospinal divisions of the CBST constitute the entire *voluntary cortical drive* to brainstem and spinal motor systems. These systems have many features in common, so it is logical to consider them as a single system with a single name.

### ORIGIN AND COURSE OF THE CBST

The CBST originates in three large areas of the cerebral cortex (Fig.7.2). Brodmann's **area 4** in the frontal lobe is the most specific cortical motor area and is usually designated the **primary motor cortex**, or **M-I**. About 31% of CBST axons originate in M-I. Another 29% originate in Brodmann's **area 6**, a motor region just anterior to M-I. Area 6 is divided into an inferolateral part, usually called the **premotor area** (PMA), and a superomedial part, usually called the **supplementary motor area** (SMA). The remaining 40% of the CBST arises from the parietal lobe. Specifically, **areas 3, 1, and 2, the somatosensory cortex (S-I)**, accounts for 31%, and **areas 5, 7, 39, and 40**, the **posterior parietal cortex**,[2] accounts for the remaining 9%. The axons from these cortical areas leave the cerebral cortex and collect in the posterior

portion of the posterior limb of the internal capsule. At the level of the mesencephalon the axons occupy a small region in the middle of the cerebral peduncle.[3] This tract becomes disorganized in the pons but is easily identifiable in the medulla as the medullary pyramid. In the spinal cord the CBST lies in the lateral white column (Fig.7.1*Ba*).

The primary motor area of the cerebral cortex, M-I, has a somatotopic organization that is essentially identical to the organization of the primary sensory cortex (Fig.7.3). The other motor areas, SMA and PMA, are also somatotopically organized. The motor areas are supplied by two cerebral arteries (see Chapter 1). The leg area of M-I and most of SMA is supplied by the anterior cerebral artery. The trunk, hand, and face area of M-I and the entire PMA are supplied by the middle cerebral artery.

The columnar organization in S-I, in which several columns serve slightly different functions for the same general somatotopically defined area, is also found in M-I. Some motor columns are organized so that they initiate activation of individual muscles. Other columns, when stimulated, cause contraction of several synergistic muscles simultaneously, producing movement in a preferred direction.

### TERMINATIONS OF THE CBST

Axons of the CBST terminate in the brainstem and spinal cord. Axons of the corticobulbar division synapse in the **red nucleus**, motor areas of the **reticular formation** (discussed later), and the various **motor nuclei of the cranial**

---

[2] A few authors include the frontal eye fields, Brodmann's area 8, in the CBST. Since the initiation and regulation of eye movements is considerably different from all other voluntary motor activity, it seems appropriate to keep area 8 separate from the CBST and consider it with the control of extraocular eye muscles.

[3] Many authors state that the CBST occupies the middle two-thirds of the cerebral peduncle. This is not possible. There are approximately 1 million corticospinal axons and probably an equal number of corticobulbar axons. Therefore, at most, the CBST at the level of the cerebral peduncle consists of 2 million axons. Because each cerebral peduncle contains at least 20 million axons, the CBST can occupy no more than 10% of its area.

---

**Figure 7.1   Descending motor tracts in the spinal cord**

**A.** The motor neurons in the spinal cord, distributed systematically within the gray matter of the ventral horn. **B.** The principal descending motor pathways in the spinal cord. Flexor biased tracts lie in the lateral white columns, between the dorsal and ventral horns. Extensor biased tracts lie in the ventral medial white columns. *Stippling,* terminus of the tract.

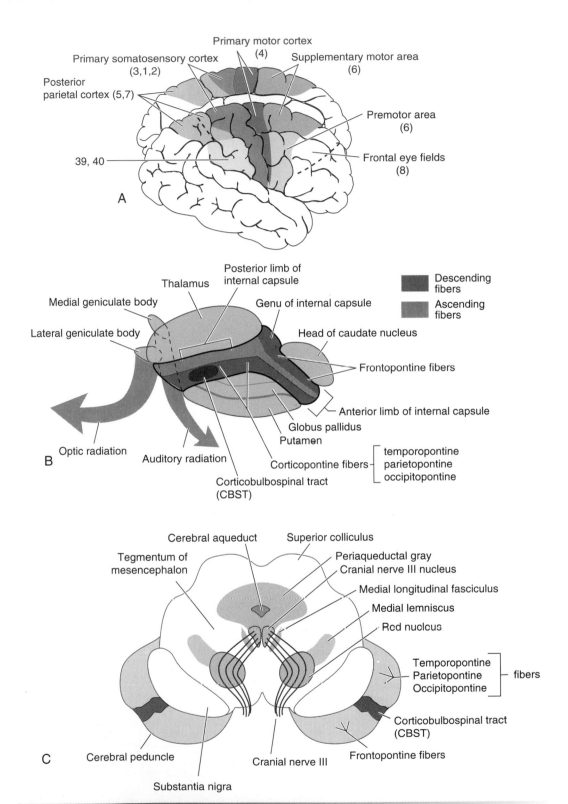

**Figure 7.2   Principal motor tracts rostral to the spinal cord**

**A.** The principal motor areas of the human cerebral cortex. The numbers refer to the Brodmann areas. SMA and PMA are both in area 6. **B.** A horizontal section through the brain showing the relations among the basal ganglia, thalamus, and internal capsule. The CBST axons are shown inside the internal capsule. **C.** CBST fibers in the cerebral peduncle at the level of the red nucleus.

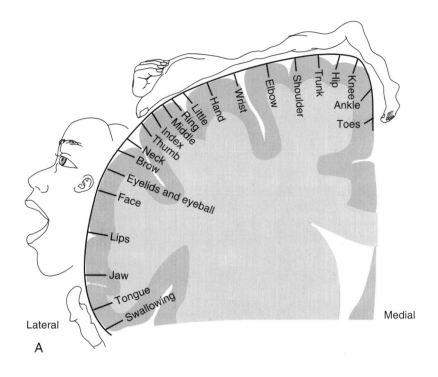

A

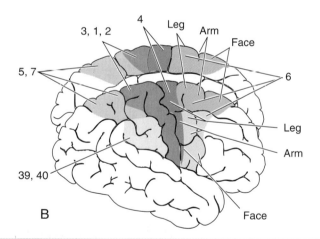

B

### Figure 7.3 Cortical motor areas

**A.** The somatotopic organization of the human M-I closely mirrors the organization of S-I. **B.** The somatotopic relations among M-I (*dark red*), PMA (*medium red*), and SMA (*light red*).

nerves[4] (Fig.7.4). The corticobulbar tract synapses are made ipsilateral or contralateral to the cells of origin, depending on the target. Corticobulbar axons destined for the red nucleus terminate exclusively in the ipsilateral nucleus, but axons synapsing in the reticular formation project bilaterally. Corticobulbar axons destined to terminate in the cranial nerve motor nuclei vary widely in their mode of distribution. Some nuclei receive strictly

---

[4] Some authors refer to the corticorubral or corticomedullary tract when discussing these specific connections.

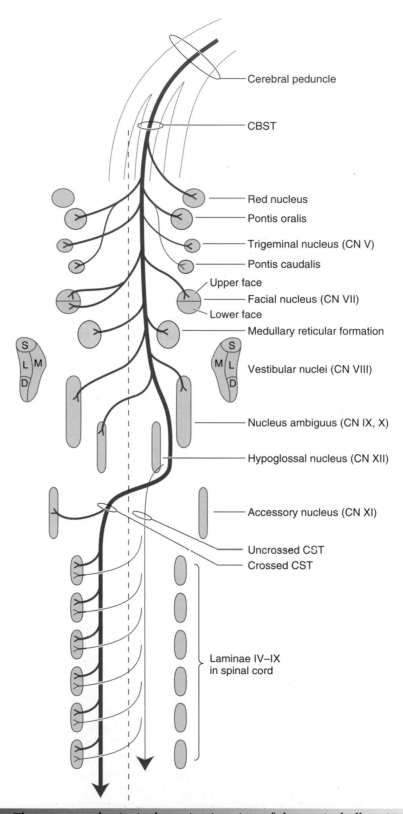

Cerebral peduncle

CBST

Red nucleus

Pontis oralis

Trigeminal nucleus (CN V)

Pontis caudalis

Upper face

Facial nucleus (CN VII)

Lower face

Medullary reticular formation

Vestibular nuclei (CN VIII)

Nucleus ambiguus (CN IX, X)

Hypoglossal nucleus (CN XII)

Accessory nucleus (CN XI)

Uncrossed CST

Crossed CST

Laminae IV–IX
in spinal cord

**Figure 7.4   The course and principal termination sites of the corticobulbospinal tract**

contralateral innervation; others receive bilateral innervation. These differences are discussed as each cranial nerve is presented (see Chapter 10).

In contrast to the corticobulbar division of the CBST, the vast majority of axons in the corticospinal tract [L. *cortex,* bark, and *tractus,* drawn out] cross the midline before terminating in spinal cord. Most corticospinal axons cross the midline at the pyramidal decussation in the lower medulla, becoming the **lateral corticospinal tract** in the spinal cord. A variable number of the corticospinal axons, probably not more than 10% of the total tract, continues uncrossed in the spinal cord as the **ventral corticospinal tract** (Fig.7.4). Most of these axons cross the midline at the level of their termination.

Corticospinal fibers terminate in laminae IV to IX of the spinal cord. Corticospinal axons originating from the parietal lobe terminate in the more dorsal regions of the spinal gray (laminae IV to VI); the terminations of axons from the frontal lobe are more broadly distributed (laminae V to IX) (Fig.7.1). It is clear from the location of corticospinal terminations that this tract synapses primarily on interneurons in the spinal cord. Consequently, excitation of α- and γ-motor neurons by the corticospinal tract is largely indirect, effected through polysynaptic pathways. Corticospinal axons make a few direct monosynaptic connections on α-motor neurons, particularly in primates. However, even in humans, who have the most monosynaptic connections, these direct connections constitute no more than a small percentage of the total contacts made by the corticospinal tract in the spinal cord.

In the spinal cord the corticospinal tract courses in the lateral white column. From this position one would expect the corticospinal tract primarily to facilitate flexor motor neurons. While that is generally true, the flexor dominance pertains mostly to the proximal muscles. Both flexor and extensor motor neurons supplying the distal muscles are facilitated by the corticospinal tract. Furthermore, the corticospinal neurons innervating distal muscles are more likely to make monosynaptic connections with motor neurons. Therefore, the corticospinal system has a definite functional bias toward fine control of the distal extremities and coarse regulation of the proximal flexors.

## The Rubrospinal Tract

The **rubrospinal tract** [L. *rubor,* red, and *spina,* thorn] (Fig.7.5) consists of axons originating from neurons in the red nucleus that terminate in the brainstem and spinal cord. The red nucleus is a nearly spherical body in the mesencephalon. In fresh cadaver sections the nucleus has a salmon color because of its high iron content. Immediately after leaving the nucleus, rubrospinal axons cross the midline, pass through the brainstem, and merge with the corticospinal tract in the cervical spinal cord. Within the spinal cord the rubrospinal tract and the corticospinal tract are completely intermingled. Rubrospinal axons terminate in approximately the same laminae as corticospinal axons (Fig.7.1*Bb*). Like corticospinal neurons, rubrospinal axons terminate primarily on interneurons that ultimately excite both α- and γ-flexor motor neurons. Efferent axons from the red nucleus also terminate in various nuclei of the brainstem, including the facial nucleus, the trigeminal nucleus, the vestibular nuclei, and the dorsal column nuclei.

The red nucleus receives most of its afferent connections from the cerebellum. (This pathway is discussed in Chapter 9.) It also receives a substantial number of afferents from the cerebral cortex. Monosynaptic corticorubral connections have been mapped in several species, and a somatotopic arrangement between the cerebral cortex and the red nucleus has been established. For example, pyramidal cells in the leg area of the motor cortex synapse on neurons in the leg area of the red nucleus, which in turn synapse on neurons in the lumbar spinal cord. Cortical afferents to the red nucleus arise from the ipsilateral M-I and SMA. Most of the cortical axons synapsing in the red nucleus appear to terminate there and are true corticorubral axons. However, a few corticospinal axons send collateral fibers into the red nucleus.

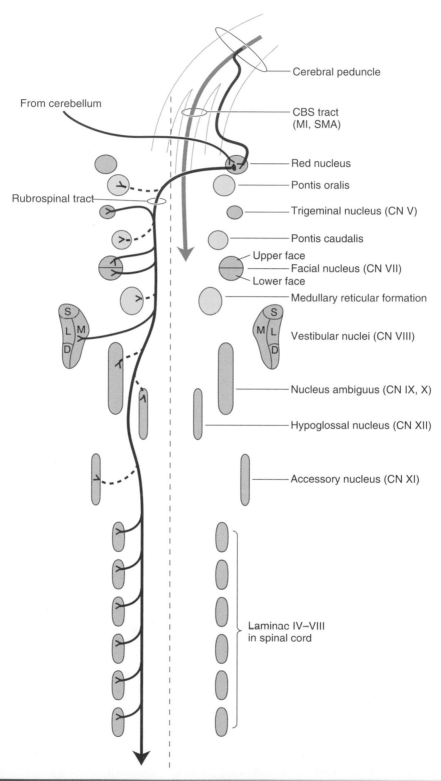

Cerebral peduncle

CBS tract
(MI, SMA)

From cerebellum

Red nucleus

Pontis oralis

Rubrospinal tract

Trigeminal nucleus (CN V)

Pontis caudalis

Upper face
Facial nucleus (CN VII)
Lower face

Medullary reticular formation

Vestibular nuclei (CN VIII)

Nucleus ambiguus (CN IX, X)

Hypoglossal nucleus (CN XII)

Accessory nucleus (CN XI)

Laminae IV–VIII
in spinal cord

**Figure 7.5   The course and principal termination sites of the rubrospinal tract**

*Broken lines* indicate probable connections.

## The Reticulospinal Tracts

The **reticulospinal tracts** originate in several nuclei of the brainstem reticular formation and descend to the spinal cord, where they terminate. The reticular formation consists of the brainstem tegmental gray matter that is not well organized into obvious nuclei. Areas of the reticular formation have been associated with specific functions, and neurons within these areas have been described and recognized as nuclei. Although the named nuclei in the reticular formation are not as discrete and prominent as the more typical nuclei associated with the cranial nerves, this does not diminish their importance. The motor nuclei of the reticular formation are discussed here, and other reticular nuclei are presented in subsequent sections.

The **medullary reticulospinal tract** arises from the **nucleus reticularis gigantocellularis** in the medulla (Fig.7.6). This tract descends *bilaterally* to all spinal levels, intermingled in the lateral white columns of the spinal cord with the rubrospinal and the corticospinal tracts (Fig.7.1*Bc*). Terminating primarily in laminae VII and VIII, it synapses on interneurons that facilitate α- and γ-flexor motor neurons.

The **pontine reticulospinal tract** arises from two pairs of nuclei, the more rostral **nucleus reticularis pontis oralis** and the **nucleus reticularis pontis caudalis** (Fig.7.5). Axons arising from these nuclei descend *ipsilaterally* to all spinal levels, coursing in the ventral medial funiculus (Fig.7.1*Bd*). They also terminate primarily in laminae VII and VIII and through interneurons facilitate extensor α- and γ-motor neurons.

The reticular motor neurons that give rise to the reticulospinal tracts receive afferents from the spinal cord, the cerebellum, and the cerebral cortex. The spinal connections of the **anterior lateral system** (ALS) that ascend to the reticular formation (called the spinoreticular division of the ALS) provide sensory input into the reticular motor nuclei, although the exact sensory modalities represented have not been worked out. Cerebellar afferents into the reticular formation are discussed in Chapter 9. Cortical afferents into the reticular motor nuclei arise from M-I and PMA. The cortical projections are distributed *bilaterally* in the reticular formation. Many monosynaptically excite the reticulospinal neurons that project into the spinal cord.

## The Vestibulospinal Tracts

The vestibular [L. *vestibulum,* small room] complex consists of four nuclei, the **superior, lateral, medial,** and **inferior vestibular nuclei,** all of which receive afferent connections from the vestibular nerve (part of cranial nerve VIII). Several long fiber tracts originate in the vestibular complex. Only two of them, the **medial** and **lateral vestibulospinal tracts,** are motor tracts that descend into the spinal cord (Fig.7.7).

The **lateral vestibulospinal tract** originates in the **lateral vestibular nucleus** (Deiter's nucleus). It descends to all levels of the spinal cord, coursing in the *ipsilateral* ventral medial funiculus (Fig.7.1*Be*). Its axons terminate in laminae VII and VIII. A few synapse on α-motor neurons in lamina IX, but these axons are clearly the minority. As one might expect from the ventral medial location of this tract, it primarily facilitates extensor α- and γ-motor neurons.

The **medial vestibulospinal tract**[5] originates in the **medial vestibular nucleus**. It descends to cervical and high thoracic levels only; there are no projections to the lumbar spinal cord (Fig.7.1*Bf*). Like the lateral vestibulospinal tract, it synapses on interneurons in the ipsilateral laminae VII and VIII, and it makes a few monosynaptic connections with α-motor neurons in lamina IX. The medial vestibulospinal tract primarily facilitates α- and γ-motor neurons, innervating muscles of the neck that stabilize the head. Its principal function is to provide a stable platform for the eyes, so this system is intimately connected with the pathways that regulate eye movement (see Chapter 10).

## THE CORTICAL MOTOR AREAS

Three principal areas of the cerebral cortex are directly concerned with motor control: the

---

[5] Formerly called the medial longitudinal fasciculus (MLF) of the spinal cord, this tract is now called the medial vestibulospinal tract by most authors.

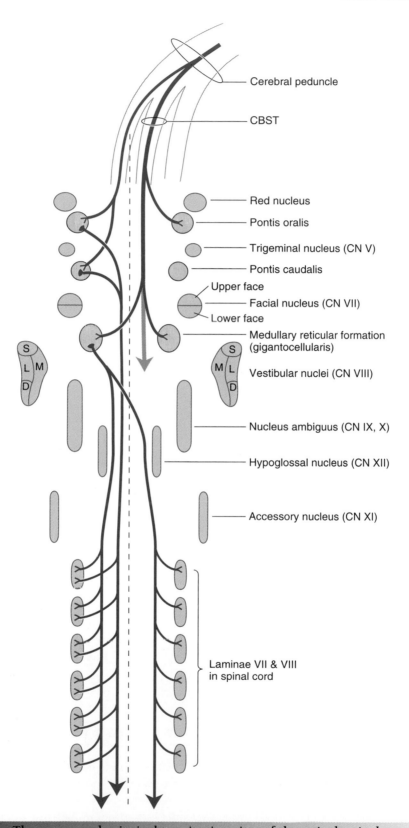

- Cerebral peduncle
- CBST
- Red nucleus
- Pontis oralis
- Trigeminal nucleus (CN V)
- Pontis caudalis
- Upper face
- Facial nucleus (CN VII)
- Lower face
- Medullary reticular formation (gigantocellularis)
- Vestibular nuclei (CN VIII)
- Nucleus ambiguus (CN IX, X)
- Hypoglossal nucleus (CN XII)
- Accessory nucleus (CN XI)
- Laminae VII & VIII in spinal cord

S
L  M
D

S
M  L
D

**Figure 7.6   The course and principal termination sites of the reticulospinal tract**

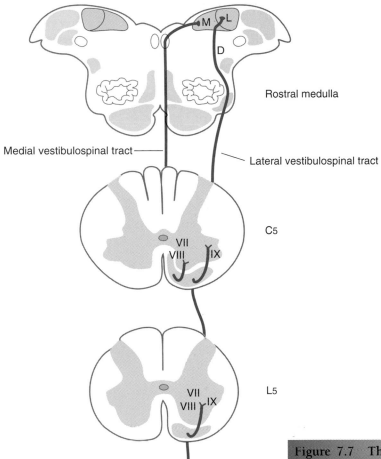

Rostral medulla

Medial vestibulospinal tract

Lateral vestibulospinal tract

C5

L5

**Figure 7.7 The course and principal termination sites of the vestibulospinal tracts**

primary motor area (M-I), SMA), and PMA (Fig.7.2). These regions are interconnected by intracortical short association fibers. Since the various motor regions serve different aspects of motor control, a brief review of these interconnections is a necessary basis for understanding the physiology of the region.

### Intracortical Connections

Somatotopically related areas of each of the three motor areas of the cerebral cortex are precisely interconnected (Fig.7.8). The short association axons that make these connections arise from pyramidal cells of cortical layer II.[6] The SMA and PMA are reciprocally interconnected, and both independently provide recip-

rocal connections to M-I, which receives afferents not only from these motor areas but also from sensory area 3a of S-I and areas 5 and 7 of the postcentral gyrus.

Pyramidal cells of cortical layer III in each of the motor areas also make somatotopically appropriate connections with the same motor areas in the contralateral hemisphere. These interhemispheric connections are most numerous between the areas corresponding to the trunk and proximal extremities. No interhemispheric connections are made between the areas representing the most distal part of the extremities, the hands and the feet. This relation apparently facilitates side-to-side coordination between the antigravity and pos-

---

[6] The pyramidal cell in the cerebral cortex is named for its shape, not for any relation to the so-called pyramidal tract (see Chapter 5).

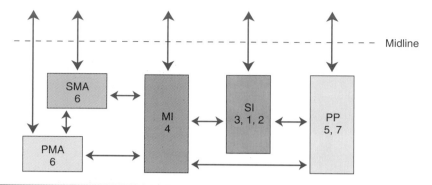

## Figure 7.8    Intracortical motor association pathways

Each of the three motor control regions of the cerebral cortex is somatotopically interconnected. Note the general convergence of signals onto M-I not only from traditional motor areas but also from parietal areas that are usually considered sensory. *Arrows* at the top depict callosal fibers crossing to the contralateral hemisphere. *SMA,* supplemental motor area; *PMA,* premotor area; *M-I,* primary motor cortex; *S-I,* primary sensory cortex; *PP,* posterior parietal cortex. The numbers refer to the Brodmann areas.

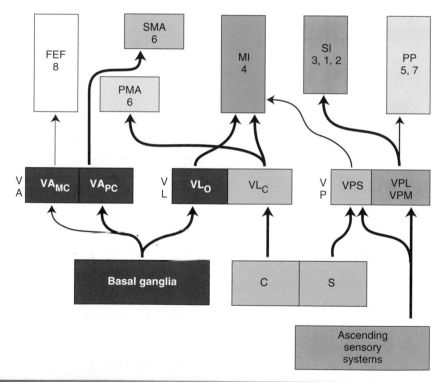

## Figure 7.9    Extracortical motor pathways

The principal connections between the thalamic nuclei and the sensorimotor areas of the cerebral cortex. The cerebellum is composed of cortical (*C*) and spinal (*S*) divisions. The numbers refer to the Brodmann areas. *FEF,* frontal eye fields; *SMA,* supplemental motor area; *PMA,* premotor area; *M-I,* primary motor cortex; *S-I,* primary sensory cortex; *PP,* posterior parietal cortex; *VA,* ventral anterior thalamic nucleus composed of VA$_{MC}$ and VA$_{PC}$; *VL,* ventral lateral thalamic nucleus composed of VL$_O$ and VL$_C$; *VP,* ventral posterior thalamic nucleus composed of VP$_L$, VP$_S$, and VP$_M$.

tural muscles while allowing for the relative independence of the prehensile hands and feet.

### Thalamic Connections

In addition to these intracortical connections, the motor areas of the cerebral cortex receive fibers from three noncortical areas: the *cerebellum, basal ganglia,* and *peripheral sensory systems.* All three of these systems are connected to the cerebral cortex through thalamic nuclei. Most of the details of these connections are discussed in Chapter 8. However, a few preliminary observations are appropriate here.

Specific nuclei in the thalamus make extensive reciprocal connections with the motor areas of the cerebral cortex (Fig.7.9). The **ventral lateral nucleus** (VL) and the **ventral anterior nucleus** (VA), which are both found in the ventral nuclear group of the thalamus, make the most extensive connections with the cortical motor areas. The ventral lateral nucleus consists of two subnuclei, the **pars oralis** ($VL_O$) and the **pars caudalis** ($VL_C$). The ventral anterior nucleus consists of the **magnocellular** ($VA_{MC}$) and the **parvicellular** ($VA_{PC}$) nuclei. While the nomenclature is confusing, the distinctions are based on cytological differences and the specific connections these nuclei make with functionally separate areas of the motor cortex. Two points regarding these connections are important. First, the three motor areas of the cerebral cortex (M-I, PMA, and SMA) each have their own thalamic connections. Second, pathways from the cerebellum and basal ganglia have separate feedback loops through the thalamus that converge on motor areas of the cerebral cortex.

### FUNCTIONAL RESPONSES OF CORTICAL MOTOR AREAS

Ablation experiments in animals trained to perform specific motor acts provide valuable information about cortical function. After the monkeys are trained, a region of the cerebral cortex is removed. By analyzing deficits in the animal's ability to perform the previously learned motor act, it is possible to gain insights into cortical function. Such experiments can have great clinical value when the lesions are made to mimic those that naturally follow cerebral injury in humans. A different approach is to measure the response of single cells while an intact animal is performing a volitional act. The analysis of the response properties of cortical neurons has provided unprecedented information about the functional organization of the cerebral cortex. Ultimately the results of animal studies must be correlated with evaluations of patients who have sustained accidental lesions and for whom good anatomical correlation with clinical findings is available. The following paragraphs summarize some of this information.

### The Primary Motor Area

The M-I cortical areas are called primary for many reasons. Stimulation of the M-I produces muscle movement at stimulus intensities far lower than those for any other part of the cerebral cortex. In addition, threshold stimulation of M-I produces highly localized motor responses that are often limited to a single motor unit within a specific muscle. Furthermore, physiological studies consistently show that activity in cortical neurons related to motor acts begins diffusely throughout the cerebral cortex and converges on M-I. The motor act occurs only after the activity in M-I reaches a peak.

Superficially, these observations suggest that an intact M-I is necessary for volitional motor activity—a common misperception. Voluntary motor functions are more complex than that. For example, recall that M-I, PMA, SMA, and large areas of the parietal lobe all contribute to the CBST. This arrangement implies that all of these areas influence brainstem and spinal motor centers. Also, experimental lesions in primates and lesions following stroke in humans consistently result in motor weakness and **apraxia** [G. *a,* negation, and *pratto,* to do] (inability to perform a learned motor skill in the absence of paralysis) but not total paralysis. Therefore, it is appropriate to ask whether the three motor areas of the cerebral cortex have separate functions, and if so, what are they?

Considerable evidence demonstrates that M-I neurons influence small groups of motor neurons in the brainstem and spinal cord, suggesting that this area exerts more direct control over motor activity than any other cortical region. Although it is tempting to assume a direct relation between a single cortical pyramidal cell and a single motor neuron in the brainstem or spinal cord, this is not the case. Small groups or *populations* of motor neurons are controlled by small populations of cortical neurons. The control is directed at the most distal muscles of an extremity and related to the most delicate and precise movements; as such, it is quite specific.

M-I neurons encode the *direction* of movement, which was demonstrated in one particularly interesting study. A monkey was trained to use its hand to push a lever in one of eight directions. During the movement action potentials were recorded from neurons in the M-I cortex. Individual neurons fired most during movement in one of the eight directions. However, their firing rates increased to some degree for about half of the directions and decreased for the other half (Fig.7.10). Hence individual cortical neurons in M-I are not like switches, each signifying a movement in one direction while all the other neurons remain silent. Rather, they are like a crowd in a football stadium. One group of spectators at one side of the stadium makes its presence known when one team scores, and another group at the other side becomes active when the opposing team makes a good play.

The mass action of M-I neurons can be visualized with a vector diagram in which each vector represents the relative activity of a single neuron and its preferred direction of movement. Summing all of the vectors produces a resultant vector for the entire population. The resultant vector closely matches the actual direction of movement (Fig.7.11).

M-I neurons also encode the *force* of muscle contraction. Force is encoded by the firing rate, which has been shown in many ways. For example, the rate of M-I firing is closely related to the *anticipated* load, before the motor act is initiated. How the nervous system computes the anticipated force required is an interesting but unanswered question. We all know, however, that the brain can be easily fooled. Each of us has experienced the disorientation associated with lifting a package that weighs substantially less than expected.

It has also been shown that the activity of cortical neurons increases if the load increases during a muscle contraction. This response is generated by sensory feedback. Part of the adjustment is accomplished by feedback through cerebellar circuits (see Chapter 9). However, part may also be derived from the parietal cortex, which may help explain its significant contribution to the CBST.

Neurons in M-I also encode the *velocity* with which a force is applied. The speed with which one moves an appendage is under voluntary control, so it seems appropriate that there are velocity-encoded neurons. They have in fact been observed in M-I, but they are less numerous than the force-encoding neurons. Many velocity-encoding neurons in M-I synapse in the red nucleus, and velocity-encoding rubrospinal neurons are far more numerous than velocity-encoding corticospinal neurons. In one study 10% of corticospinal neurons encoded velocity and 70% of the rubrospinal neurons did.

## The Premotor Area

The PMA in humans occupies about six times as much area as M-I. Despite its size the PMA contributes less to the CBST than M-I. Furthermore, electrical stimulation of PMA does not usually produce muscle movement unless the stimuli are much more intense than effective stimuli for the SMA or M-I. What then is the role of PMA in motor activity? A complete answer to that question is not known, but available data suggest that PMA is necessary to prepare M-I for the impending motor act.

Clever experiments using trained monkeys have provided some insight into PMA function. In one set of experiments a monkey was trained to rest its arm between trials in a specified location. Several targets were placed at various locations within reach. One of the targets would light, indicating a "ready" signal, but the mon-

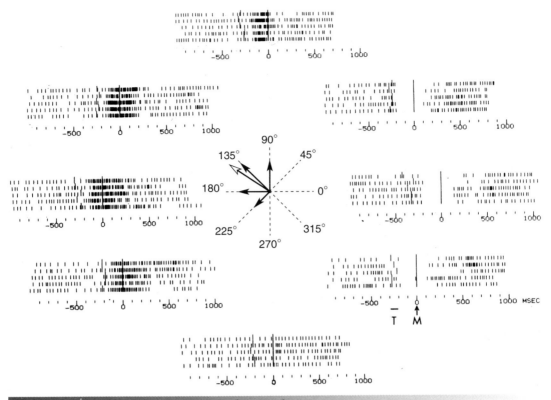

**Figure 7.10   Directional sensitivity of cortical neurons**

The firing patterns of one cell during arm movement in each of eight directions. Five trials are shown for each movement; each *horizontal line* represents one trial, and the *small vertical lines* within the *horizontal line* represent one action potential. The abscissa is in milliseconds relative to the beginning of movement at 0. This neuron increases its firing for about half of the directions (those to the left) and is inhibited for the other half (those to the right). The firing rate for this individual neuron increases most when movement is directed between 90 and 225°. The length of the vectors (*closed arrows*) in the center represenst the rate of neuron firing for each direction. The peak of the regression curve fitted to these data is the preferred direction for this neuron (vector with *open arrow* at 161°). (Adapted from Georgopoulos P, Kalaska JF, Caminiti R, Massey JT. On the relations between the direction of two-dimensional arm movements and cell discharge in primate motor cortex. J Neurosci 1982;2:1527–1537.)

key was not allowed to touch it until a second "go" light came on. At the go signal the monkey reached for the illuminated target to get a reward. The same paradigm was also established using an auditory ready signal instead of a visual signal. This experiment was designed to give the monkey time to anticipate and prepare for a precise motor act before the act was initiated.

Electrodes were placed in various parts of the motor cortex, and while the monkey was performing these tasks, the responses of individual cells were recorded. In the PMA many cells significantly increased their firing rate be-

tween the ready and go signals, but only if the anticipated movement was to be in a specific direction (Fig.7.12). Surprisingly, these PMA neurons usually decreased firing once the movement actually began.

These experiments suggest that many PMA neurons play a role in anticipating a specific complex motor act. Anticipation is based on multiple factors, since the behavior of these neurons is similar for both visual and auditory clues. PMA activity seems to facilitate multiple motor columns in M-I, preparing them for action. Prepared M-I neurons are close to thresh-

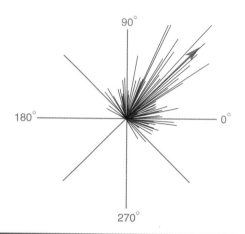

**Figure 7.11 Population vectors of M-I activity**

Each line in this diagram is a vector that indicates the preferred direction of a single neuron in M-I as determined by many experiments similar to the one illustrated in Figure 7.10. The length of the vectors indicates the discharge frequency of the neuron when the monkey moves its arm towards 45°. The sum of the vectors (*red arrow*) closely matches the direction of movement. (Modified from Ghez C. Voluntary movement. In: Kandel ER, Schwart JH, Jessell TM, eds. Principles of Neural Science. 3rd ed. Norwalk, CT: Appleton & Lange, 1991;617.)

old and more easily stimulated by other signals than unprepared neurons. As we have noted, lesions to the PMA in humans do not cause paralysis but slow complex limb movements. The slowing is apparently due to a lack of sufficient facilitation of the M-I neurons by the PMA. Because they are further from threshold when the go signal is received, the unprepared M-I neurons take longer to reach threshold.

## The Supplemental Motor Area

SMA lesions in humans, like M-I lesions, result in motor apraxia rather than paralysis. In animals, stimulation of neurons in the SMA elicits complex movements involving many muscle groups rather than the highly specific movements generated by M-I stimulation. For example, movements following SMA stimulation often involve the entire hand or arm and in some cases even postural movements of the whole body.

Controlled SMA lesions in trained monkeys have cast some light on the role of SMA. A unilateral ablation of SMA limits a monkey's ability to perform complex bimanual tasks. Following SMA ablation, both hands tend to mirror the other's movement, as if the remaining motor system is controlling both hands as a single unit. For example, in one classic experiment a monkey was presented with a raisin lodged in a hole in a transparent acrylic plate. To retrieve the raisin, a normal

**Figure 7.12 Cortical activity in PMA**

**A.** The functional role of PMA cortical cells was studied in monkeys. The animals were trained to rest their arm at a specific starting position (*1*) between trials. A target at one of the other stations would light (*2*), indicating the ready signal. Only when a second light at the same station, the go signal, appeared (*3*) would the monkey reach out (*4*) and touch the panel to extinguish the lights and receive a reward. The various periods were randomized as shown in the middle panel. **B.** Recordings of the activity of single PMA cells were made as the animals were performing this task. At the bottom of each of the four figures, each *line* represents one trial and each *dot* indicates an action potential. At the top of each figure is a composite histogram of all trials showing the number of action potentials versus time for all trials. All of the records are aligned on the left at the ready signal and on the right at the beginning of movement. (Because of the randomization of the trial lengths, some data in the center were deleted to keep all records the same physical length.) The PMA cells increased their firing rate after the ready signal only if the arm was to move to the right. The same cell was inhibited if the movement was to the left. The response was the same whether the ready signals were auditory or visual. These PMA cells did not participate in the actual motor act, since they were inhibited just before the arm began to move. (Reprinted with permission from Weinrich M, Wise SP. The premotor cortex of the monkey. J Neurosci 1982;2:1329-1345.)

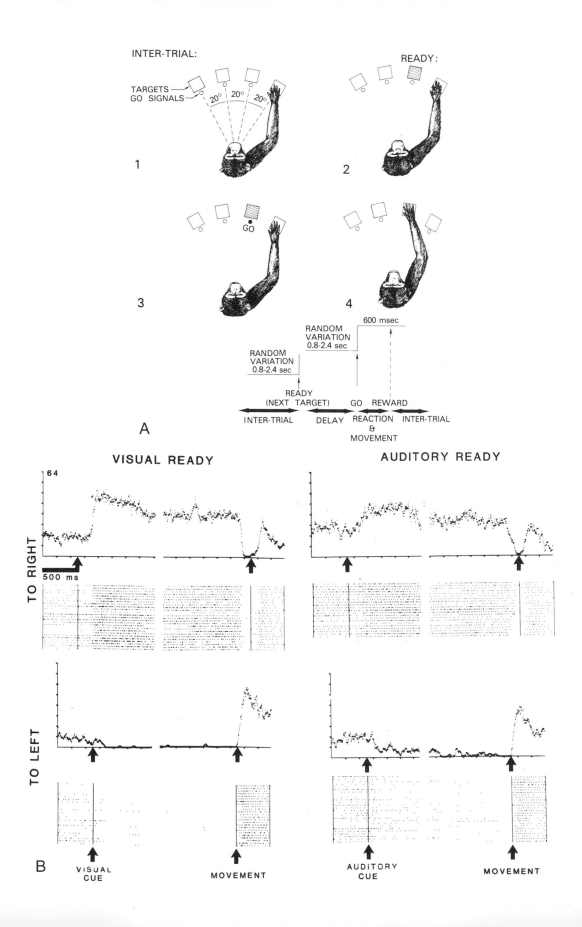

INTER-TRIAL:

TARGETS
GO SIGNALS

20° 20° 20°

1

READY:

2

GO

3

4

RANDOM
VARIATION
0.8-2.4 sec

600 msec

RANDOM
VARIATION
0.8-2.4 sec

READY
(NEXT TARGET)

GO    REWARD

INTER-TRIAL      DELAY    REACTION    INTER-TRIAL
                          &
                          MOVEMENT

A

**VISUAL READY**

**AUDITORY READY**

64

TO RIGHT

500 ms

TO LEFT

B

VISUAL
CUE

MOVEMENT

AUDITORY
CUE

MOVEMENT

monkey simply pushed it through the hole from the top with its finger, catching it beneath the plate in the palm of the other hand. After unilateral removal of the SMA, the monkey pushed the raisin from both sides simultaneously and was unable to retrieve the reward.

If the ipsilateral SMA and PMA are both removed, an entirely different apraxia occurs. For example, a monkey with such a lesion was presented with an apple slice behind a small acrylic barrier. The monkey could easily reach around the barrier to retrieve the apple with the hand ipsilateral to the lesion (recall that the motor cortex controls the contralateral body) but would also attempt to thrust its hand through the barrier with the arm contralateral to the lesion. If the lesion involved only M-I, the monkey could accomplish the task with either hand, although the hand contralateral to the lesion was weak and clumsy.

These experiments show that SMA and PMA are not necessary for *motivating* the monkey to perform the motor act, nor are they necessary for the monkey to *understand* how to accomplish the act, for the monkey would do just fine with the good arm. In addition, the monkey was not paralyzed. Somehow SMA and PMA are necessary to translate the knowledge of how to accomplish a motor act into a specific sequence of motor commands; in other words, *SMA and PMA are necessary for translating strategy into tactics.*

Experiments with humans have given some support to this interpretation of the monkey experiments. In humans, cerebral blood flow can be measured noninvasively with positron emission tomography (PET). Local cerebral blood flow increases as local neuronal activity increases. If a person is asked to contract the muscles controlling the index finger isometrically, blood flow in the M-I hand area increases. Tapping the same finger causes blood flow to increase over the hand area in both M-I and S-I, indicating that both the motor and sensory areas have become more active (Fig.7.13, *A* and *B*). If instead of simple finger tapping the subject is asked to perform a

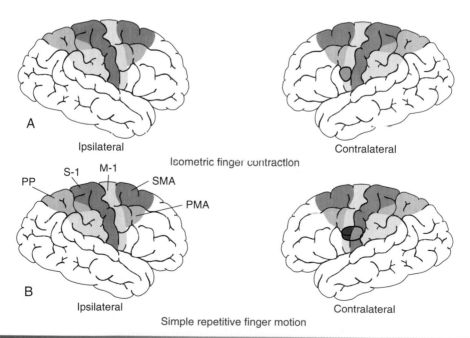

**Figure 7.13  Responses of cortical motor areas in the human**

Changes in regional blood flow, which can be measured by PET in the human, are presumed to reflect cortical activity. **A.** Isometric contraction of the fingers in the right hand is correlated with increased blood flow in the hand area of the left M-I (*pink area*). **B.** Repetitive finger tapping increases blood flow in the finger area of M-I and S-I.

complex sequence of movements with the fingers—a sequence that requires considerable concentration to perform accurately—blood flow increases in SMA as well as in S-I and M-I (Fig.7.13C). Finally, if the person is asked simply to think through the complex sequence without actually moving the fingers, blood flow increases only in SMA (Fig.7.13D). These experiments not only suggest a role for SMA in preparing for complex acts that require con-

scious effort but also show that SMA is not necessary for simple repetitive acts, such as finger tapping, that require little conscious thought or preparation.

## The Posterior Parietal Area

The posterior parietal [L. *posterus,* behind, and *paries,* wall] area is an enigmatic region of the cerebral cortex posterior to the S-I sensory cortex. Despite its distance from M-I and S-I

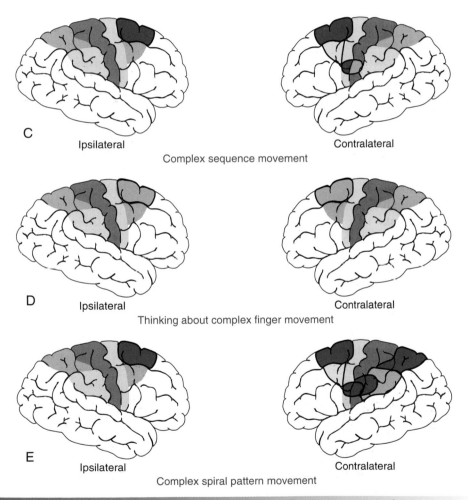

C  Ipsilateral                    Contralateral
Complex sequence movement

D  Ipsilateral                    Contralateral
Thinking about complex finger movement

E  Ipsilateral                    Contralateral
Complex spiral pattern movement

## Figure 7.13    Responses of cortical motor areas in the human—*continued*

**C.** A complex sequence of finger movements is correlated with a bilateral increase in blood flow to SMA and to the contralateral PMA in addition to the M-I and S-I increases associated with simple finger movements. **D.** When the subject thinks about the complex finger sequence that is performed in **C,** but no movement is generated, blood flow increases only in the SMA. **E.** When the subject is asked to draw an imaginary spiral in space, the posterior parietal area is activated in addition to the motor areas of the cortex. Amount of blood flow increase is indicated by density of coloration. (Data adapted from Roland PE, Larsen B, Skinhøf E. Supplementary motor area and other cortical areas in organization of voluntary movements in man. J Neurophysiol 1980;43: 1118–1136.)

and its location in what is usually considered sensory cortex, it contributes about 9% of the fibers found in the CBST. Stimulation of the posterior parietal cortex does not consistently result in motor activity. Its motor functions seem to be related to motivation or interest, qualities of behavior that are difficult to quantify and thus difficult to study.

Humans with lesions to the posterior parietal area display a behavior known as **neglect**. They seem *unaware* of the side of the body contralateral to the lesion. Although the sensory system has no demonstrable lesion, such patients ignore tactile or visual stimuli presented to the neglected side. This behavior is particularly evident if the lesion is to the nondominant hemisphere (see Chapter 15). Motor acts are similarly neglected, even though there is no demonstrable paralysis.

Single-unit recordings from trained monkeys performing specific tasks have provided some data that support the view that the posterior parietal cortex is an essential link between motivation and action. For example, some posterior parietal neurons in area 5 fire when the monkey reaches for something interesting, such as food, but do not fire during similar arm movements that are not associated with interesting objects. Similar neurons have been observed in area 7, but they are associated with eye movements that are directed toward interesting objects in the visual field. Humans with posterior parietal lesions, particularly those to the right hemisphere, often fail to move the contralateral limb on command. When the error is pointed out, however, the patient may move the affected extremity, thus proving that there is no paralysis and that the command was understood.

## Integration of Motor Commands

Having established that the descending motor tracts exert their control over final muscle contraction through multiple parallel pathways, we can now ferret out some of the differences in the ways these parallel tracts affect motor activity.

The corticobulbospinal tract primarily regulates the most discrete muscle contractions of the most distal muscles. This regulation is reflected in both the anatomy and physiology of

this tract. The monosynaptic corticospinal connections with motor neurons exist primarily on the distal motor neurons. Similarly, the cortical units with the lowest thresholds command the most distal muscles. Furthermore, corticospinal neurons are most active during the most delicate and precise finger movements. These same neurons may even decrease their firing rate if a strong, forceful gripping action is required. Rubrospinal neurons are similar to corticospinal neurons except that the rubrospinal tract preferentially innervates proximal muscles over distal muscles.

Stronger, sustained, forceful muscle contractions under cortical control are more closely associated with reticulospinal neurons that synapse more densely on the motor neurons supplying proximal muscles of the extremities and muscles of the trunk. The vestibulospinal tracts, especially the lateral vestibulospinal tract, also predominantly affect proximal muscles. The vestibulospinal tract is unique because it is not subject to direct cortical regulation. Because of its close association with the peripheral vestibular apparatus, vestibulospinal activity is most closely associated with orientation to gravity. Therefore, the reticulospinal and vestibulospinal systems may be collectively considered *postural*, since they establish a background level of activity that resists the effects of gravity and establishes the body's orientation in space.

## THE MOTOR SYSTEMS AS A CONTROL SYSTEM

The application of control system theory to physiological systems has provided important insights into their normal functions as well as a basis for understanding the ways in which these systems fail. Analysis of the motor systems in terms of control system theory is a useful exercise, as it establishes a framework against which clinical observations of patients with motor system lesions can be interpreted.

In the most general terms, control systems regulate an output variable in response to control signals. If the output variable does not affect the control signal, the system is said to be an **open-loop** system. However, if the control signal is modified in some way by the output variable, it is a **closed-loop** system (Fig.7.14A). Closed-loop control systems provide a *dynamic* mechanism through feedback regulation by which an output variable is regulated within certain limits around a desired value.

Control systems fall into two broad classes, **feed-forward** and **feedback** systems. Feedback systems measure the **controlled variable** (output) and compare it with the desired value, the **set point** (Fig.7.14B). If there is a discrepancy, an appropriate correction is applied by the controller to the input variable *after* the error has been detected. Feed-forward control systems anticipate the effect of environmental disturbances on a system and apply corrective action *in advance* of a measured error in the controlled variable (Fig.7.14C). Physiological motor systems have characteristics of both feed-forward

and feedback control systems. Feed-forward systems are considered in Chapter 9.

### Feedback Control Systems

The model of a feedback control system has six elements: the **sensor, set point** signal, **comparator, effector, controlled variable**, and **error signal**. For example, in one's home, *temperature,* the controlled variable, is regulated by a *heating and cooling system,* the effector. A *thermometer,* the sensor, monitors the temperature, which is compared by the *thermostat,* the comparator, with the *desired temperature,* or set point (Fig.7.15). The thermometer continuously monitors the house's temperature, and the thermostat continuously compares the temperature with the set point. If the temperature differs from the set point enough, the

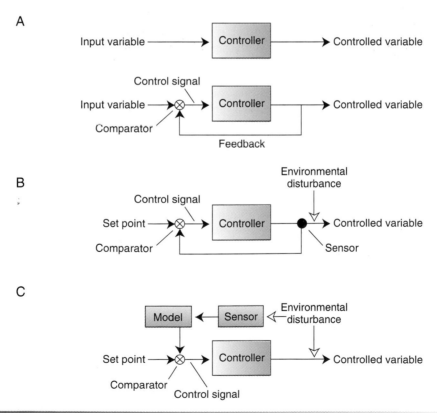

### Figure 7.14   Control systems

**A.** In an open-loop control system (*top*), the input variable to the controller drives the controller without modification by the output of the system. In a closed-loop control system (*bottom*), the output is used to modify the behavior of the controller. **B.** Feedback systems modify the control signal after an error in the controlled variable is detected. **C.** Feed-forward systems modify the control signal in response to events that are anticipated to affect the controlled variable.

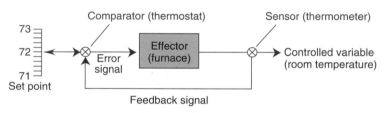

## Figure 7.15    Feedback control

A feedback control system modeled as a typical heating system that uses feedback regulation to control building temperature. In a typical home heating system, the thermostat contains the set point controller, the comparator, and the sensor (thermometer).

comparator sends an error signal to the heating or cooling system that turns it on. When the temperature matches the set point, the system goes off.

## SIMPLE CONTROLLERS

With a simple comparator like a thermostat, the error signal is either on or off. In other words, the thermostat can signal that the temperature is below the set point or above it. It cannot signal the amount of deviation (Fig.7.16). A simple on-off controller like a thermostat must not switch states the instant the temperature deviates from the set point because the effector needs time to function. Therefore, a delay, **hysteresis** [G. *hysteresis, a coming later*], is built into the comparator to allow the temperature to deviate a substantial amount from the set point before the effector is activated. Because of hysteresis, the controlled variable fluctuates within defined limits.

## PROPORTIONAL CONTROLLERS

In more sophisticated comparators the error signal is **proportional** to the degree of deviation from the set point. In these systems the response of the effector is also proportional. Using our furnace example, the *rate* at which heat is added to a building is a function of the magnitude of the error signal. Proportionally controlled systems can regulate a variable much more closely than a simple on-off system (Fig.7.17). Two concepts, gain and the damping factor, are used to describe the responsiveness of proportional controllers.

### Gain

The speed with which a proportional control system corrects a disturbance in the controlled variable is determined by the **gain** of the system. Gain is simply the amplification factor in the system that determines the magnitude of the applied correction relative to the magnitude of the error signal. In our heating system example, if the error signal is 10 arbitrary units and the furnace delivers 1000 Kcal/hour, the gain of the system is 100. If the furnace delivers 2000 Kcal/hour, the gain is 200. A system with a higher gain can respond more quickly to a disturbance.

At any given gain the response of the system is related to the magnitude of the error signal. Again, consider the furnace control system. If the gain is fixed at 100, the furnace delivers 1000 Kcal/hour when the error signal is 10. As the building warms up, the error signal diminishes. If the error signal drops to 2, the furnace delivers only 200 Kcal/hour. The key feature of a proportional control system is that the correction applied to the output variable is more refined as the variable approaches the set point. This element is similar to bringing an automobile to a stop. At 60 mph, one must step on the break hard to slow the vehicle rapidly. When approaching a stop sign, however, one gradually reduces the pressure to avoid an abrupt stop.

### Damping Factor

Another important characteristic of any proportional control system is the **damping factor**. The formal definition of the damping fac-

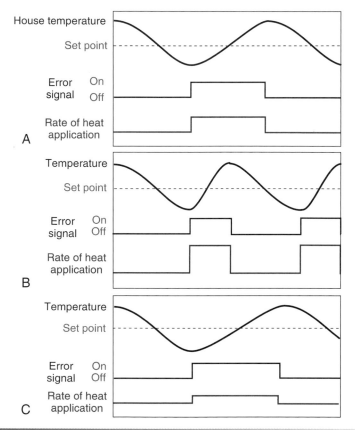

**Figure 7.16   Simple controllers**

**A.** With simple controllers such as is used with home heating systems, the controlled variable oscillates around the set point. Increasing (**B**) or decreasing (**C**) the furnace size does not affect the oscillations, but only affects the run time of the furnace.

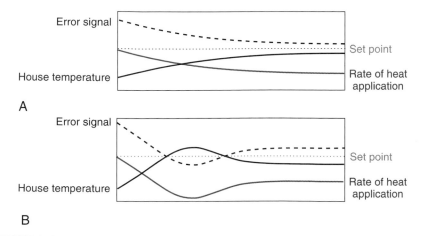

**Figure 7.17   Proportional controllers**

Proportional controlled heating systems can vary the amount of heat delivered by the furnace in proportion to the magnitude of the error signal. **A.** Critically damped systems smoothly approach the set point without oscillations. **B.** Slightly underdamped systems reach the set point sooner, but exhibit slight instability.

tor is mathematical and unnecessary for this discussion; the following description provides a broad overview of this concept. If the gain of a proportional control system is a little larger than optimal, the controlled variable follows a series of oscillations [L. *oscillare,* to swing back and forth] that get progressively smaller over time as the system returns to its set point (Fig.7.18). A system that responds with one or more oscillations is said to be **underdamped**. Underdamped systems quickly bring the controlled variable close to the set point but oscillate a bit before reaching a steady state.

If the gain of the system is optimal, the system approaches the set point as fast as possible without oscillating. The system is said to be **critically damped**. If the gain is reduced further, the system takes longer than the optimal time to achieve a steady state and is said to be **overdamped**. Most proportional control systems are slightly underdamped to maximize speed while minimizing the oscillations to acceptable levels.

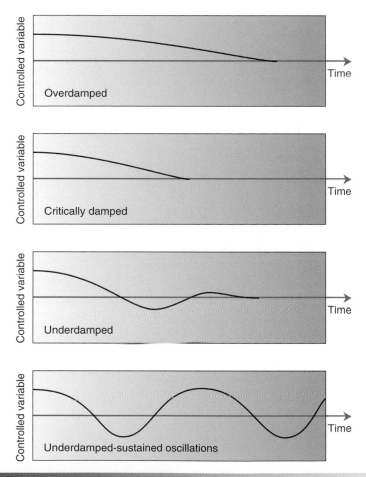

**Figure 7.18 Effect of gain on feedback systems**

Proportional control systems oscillate if the gain is too great. The tendency to oscillate is expressed as a damping factor. The gain of overdamped systems (*top*) is not optimal. Underdamped systems respond slowly to disturbances. The gain of a critically damped system is set just below the point where oscillations first appear, which brings the system to the set point in a minimal amount of time with no oscillations. In an underdamped system the gain is set so high that the system overshoots the set point, causing oscillations. The oscillations gradually diminish until the system becomes stable at the set point. Systems in which the gain is too high are unstable and oscillate indefinitely (*bottom*).

Proportional systems can become unstable if the gain is too large. As the gain of an underdamped system increases, each correction applied by the controller causes greater and greater swings in the output variable. Eventually the system enters a state of **sustained oscillations.** Everyone has experienced such oscillations in an auditorium equipped with an overamplified public address system. Sound from the loudspeakers is received by the microphone after a conduction delay across the auditorium. If the audio amplifier is properly adjusted, the system is stable and the audience hears the program. If the amplifier gain is at the critical point, one may hear a slight echo effect. If the gain is increased slightly, the audio system begins to oscillate, causing a high-pitched squeal irritating to audience and speaker alike.

## The Muscle Stretch Reflex As a Feedback Control System

*The muscle stretch reflex (MSR) operates as a feedback control system.* All of the elements of control systems can be identified. The controlled variable is muscle length. The nuclear bag receptors (sensors) detect changes in muscle length. Feedback signals from these receptors are transmitted to the spinal cord. The spinal cord contains circuitry (comparator) to compare the feedback signals with supraspinal command signals (set point) to control the muscle (effector). Lengthening the muscle causes the muscle spindle receptors to send an error signal to the spinal cord. The spinal cord then returns to the muscle a control signal that restores the original muscle length. The MSR acts as a proportional control system. The error signal from the receptors *varies in proportion to the change in length* of the muscle, and the control signal to the muscle also varies in proportion to the size of the error.

Under normal circumstances the gain of the MSR is set so that the system is *slightly underdamped.* If one elicits the MSR from the patellar tendon, the quadriceps muscle contracts moderately in response to the stretch and relaxes and contracts slightly again before returning to its resting length. Although only a single leg jerk is visible, the extra small contraction can be detected in the laboratory.

*Certain lesions to the central nervous system (CNS) change the gain of the MSR control system.* Under these pathological conditions the system *behaves as an unstable underdamped control system with excessive gain.* When the muscle is stretched, the leg swings more quickly and farther than normal. Instead of returning to its resting length after a single oscillation, the muscle contracts several times and the leg may visibly swing two or three times. MSRs that respond in this way are said to be **hyperactive.** Patients with hyperactive reflexes have jerky, **spastic** [G. *spastikos,* drawing in] movements (Fig.7.19).

If CNS damage is extensive, the gain of the MSR may be so great that the system becomes unstable. When instability occurs, numerous oscillations in the MSR can be evoked; this is **clonus** [G. *klonos,* tumult]. These rhythmic muscular contractions usually cease after several oscillations if the muscle is not otherwise stimulated. However, clonus may be **sustained** if the muscle is placed under a slight constant stretch. For example, the physician can sharply flex the patient's foot at the ankle and then hold the flexed position; a steady 5- to 7-Hz beating of the foot—sustained clonus—can be felt and often seen. Patients who have clonus can be considerably inconvenienced. Walking is very difficult, since each step can provoke a rhythmic beating of the affected limbs. Even propelling a wheelchair across rough pavement can cause enough passive limb movement to engage the MSR, which in turn evokes clonus.

Lesions to the CNS affect the dynamic properties of the MSR more dramatically than its static properties. Hyperactive reflexes are sensitive to the velocity of the muscle stretch, which is why the rapid stretch of the muscle caused by a sharp blow from a reflex hammer so effectively displays spasticity. The velocity sensitivity of spasticity can be shown in other ways as well. For example, if one slowly pronates and supinates a patient's arm, only a slight increase in resistance to passive movement is detected. However, if the limb is rapidly moved, a spastic muscle produces a sudden, brief catch in limb movement as the MSR is activated. This catch does not occur in normal subjects. The rapid increase in ten-

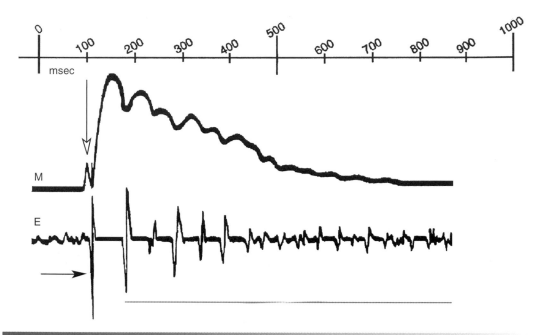

**Figure 7.19   MSR oscillations**

The electrical and mechanical responses from the quadriceps muscle demonstrate underdamping of the MSR. The muscle tension (*M*) and the EMG (*E*) are shown after a single tendon tap at the first small deflection in M (*open arrow*). The muscle stretch evokes a single large electrical discharge in the muscle (*closed arrow*) and an associated rapid increase in muscle tension. The initial electrical discharge is followed by a series of abnormal (*above pink line*) electrical discharges reflected in a series of waves of tension that diminish with time. (Reprinted with permission from Denny-Brown D. On the nature of postural reflexes. Proc Royal Soc 1929;B104:252–301.)

sion, or catch, in the muscle is momentary because the reflex increase in tension is great enough to invoke the **clasp knife reflex,** which causes massive inhibition of the α-motor neurons innervating the muscle (see Chapter 6).

The characteristic changes in the MSR following lesions to the CNS are caused primarily by alterations in the excitability of motor neurons. The exact source of the motor neuron facilitation is not known. It is known that motor neurons are innervated by inhibitory interneurons. Descending motor tracts, especially the rubrospinal tract, tonically facilitate these inhibitory interneurons, creating a resting background inhibition on both α- and γ-motor neurons. Consequently, removal of descending motor tracts that facilitate the inhibitory interneurons *disinhibits* the motor neurons, making them hyperexcitable (Fig.7.20).

## CLINICAL MANIFESTATIONS OF LESIONS TO THE DESCENDING MOTOR SYSTEMS

Differentiating between lesions to the peripheral nervous system (PNS) and to the CNS is an essential medical skill. It is most easily accomplished by differentiating between upper and lower motor neuron conditions. The concept of the lower motor neuron (LMN) is presented in Chapter 6; description of the upper motor neuron follows.

### The Upper Motor Neuron

Lesions to the descending motor systems cause a unique set of symptoms. This constellation of symptoms is so characteristic that the concept of the **upper motor neuron** (UMN) has evolved. This concept binds together several different but intimately interconnected anatom-

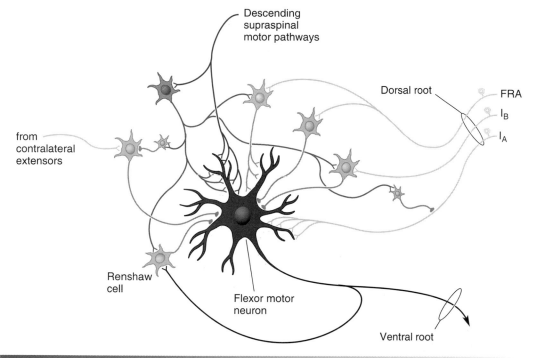

**Figure 7.20    UMN spasticity**

Hyperexcitability of the MSR following loss of the descending voluntary motor pathways is caused by loss of facilitation on inhibitory interneurons, which provides a net increase in excitation from IA primary afferent axons and a net decrease in facilitation from descending voluntary motor pathways. The net FRA influence is shifted from excitation to inhibition in this flexor motor neuron. FRA activity is the reverse for extensor motor neurons. *Closed circles,* inhibitory synapses.

ical entities, all of which are involved in motor control. Before presenting the salient features of the UMN, it is useful to recapitulate the clinical manifestations of LMN lesions (Table 7.1).

LMN lesions are characterized by a flaccid weakness or paralysis; decreased MSRs; and signs of muscle denervation (fasciculations, fibrillations, and atrophy). Frequently, muscles are involved individually rather than in groups. The distribution of weakness may be patchy. Patterns of sensory loss that accompany LMN symptoms follow the dermatomes or fragments of dermatomes according to the individual spinal or peripheral nerve involved. The LMN comprises a set of anatomical structures bound together by clinical observations. It is not a specific anatomical structure. Lesions to pe-

ripheral nerves, spinal roots, $\alpha$-motor neurons, and muscle can all cause LMN signs.

In contrast to LMN lesions, damage to the UMN produces *spastic weakness, hyperactive reflexes, and reversal of certain flexion reflex afferent (FRA)-driven reflexes but no signs of muscle denervation.* Muscles are affected in groups, an entire extremity or even half of the body. They are never affected individually. The patterns of sensory loss are similarly distributed, involving quadrants or halves of the body. Losses are never associated with specific dermatomes. Lesions that cause UMN symptoms invariably include damage to the corticobulbospinal tract, the rubrospinal tract, and the reticulospinal tracts. In human patients none of these tracts can be lesioned in isolation,[7] and therefore

---

[7] Isolated lesions to the corticospinal tract have been performed in various animal species. The results of these experiments have reinforced the general conclusion that UMN signs are not attributable to a single descending motor pathway.

**Table 7.1   Comparison of the Principle Features of the Upper and Lower Motor Neuron**

| Lower Motor Neuron | Upper Motor Neuron |
|---|---|
| Flaccid weakness or paralysis | Spastic weakness |
| Decreased or absent MSR | Increased MSR with or without clonus |
| Signs of muscle denervation; fasciculations, fibrillations, profound atrophy | No signs of muscle denervation |
| Muscles affected singly or in small groups innervated by a common nerve or spinal root | Muscles affected in large groups, organized by quadrants or halves of the body |
| FRA-driven reflexes normal | Some FRA-driven reflexes reversed (signs of Babinski and Bing), others absent (abdominal and cremasteric reflexes) |
| Sensory patterns: (a) stocking & glove; (b) follows dermatomes or fragments of dermatomes | Sensory patterns affect quadrants or halves of the body |

these three tracts can be considered an integrated UMN system. Damage to other parts of the motor system (see Chapters 5, 8, and 9) do not produce these symptoms.

WEAKNESS

The most prominent impairment that can be attributed to lesions involving the UMN is *weakness*. The usual term to describe voluntary muscle weakness is **paresis** [G. *paritemi*, let go], which is distinguished from a complete loss of voluntary motor control, or **plegia** [G. *plege*, a stroke]. Clumsiness and imprecise motor control accompany the weakness. Loss of precise motor control is most prominent in the distal extremities and is most closely correlated with damage to the corticospinal tract.

HYPERACTIVE REFLEXES

The increase in the MSR is the most characteristic sign of damage to the UMN. No other lesion to the nervous system causes this sign, so its importance cannot be overstated. As discussed earlier, the increase in the MSR is caused by depolarization of the motor neurons following the loss of descending motor tracts. Since this loss brings the motor neurons closer to threshold, less facilitation from any source is necessary to cause them to fire. Therefore, in the quiescent state there is little change in resting muscle tone. But once the muscle is stretched, even slightly, a rapid reflex contrac-

tion follows. During any simple voluntary movement the antagonist muscles reflexively contract as they are stretched. This reflex opposition to the desired movement makes the muscles seem stiff and **spastic**. The spasticity exacerbates the clumsiness and weakness.

REVERSAL OF CERTAIN FRA-DRIVEN REFLEXES

In addition to the MSR, several reflexes are commonly tested to verify suspected damage to the descending motor control systems. One such FRA-driven reflex is elicited by scratching the sole of the foot along its lateral margin, from the heel toward the toes. In normal persons the toes plantar flex. If the UMN is damaged, particularly the CBST, the toes extend and flare (Fig.7.21). The reversal of this FRA-driven reflex is called the **sign of Babinski**, named after the French physician of Polish heritage who first described it. This valuable sign is frequently masked in people who are very ticklish or who have unusually painful sensations from the bottoms of their feet. In such cases one can use a pin to stab the dorsum of the foot over the extensor hallucis longus tendon. The normal reaction is to extend the foot at the ankle away from the pin. The abnormal response indicating an UMN lesion, the **sign of Bing**, is to flex the toe and foot into the pin.

Two other FRA-driven reflexes, the **abdominal reflex** and the **cremasteric reflex** [I. *cremaster*, G. *kremaster*, suspender], are less commonly

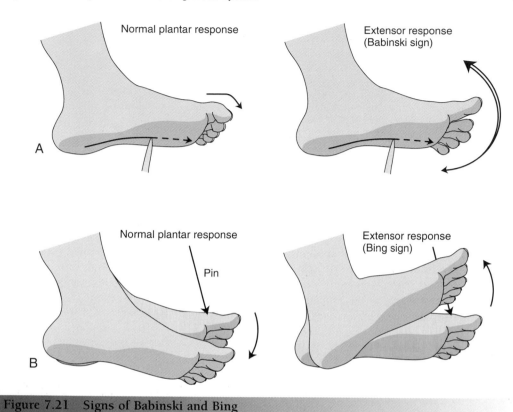

**Figure 7.21    Signs of Babinski and Bing**

**A.** The sign of Babinski indicates a lesion to the UMN. Scratching the lateral margin of the sole of the foot from the heel toward the small toe normally elicits a plantar (flexion) response. If the UMN has been damaged, the toes extend and flare. This reversal in the normal plantar FRA response is the sign of Babinski. **B.** A useful adjunct to the sign of Babinski is the sign of Bing. Sticking the dorsum of the foot with a pin normally makes one reflexively extend the foot at the ankle away from the pin. If the UMN has been lesioned, the foot is brought into the pin.

used to confirm an UMN lesion. Both reflexes are normally present but disappear if the descending motor systems are damaged. The abdominal reflexes are evoked by lightly scratching each quadrant of the abdomen with a pin. Normally the underlying muscles reflexively contract. The cremasteric reflex is invoked by gently stroking the medial surface of the thigh with a cotton swab. In the male patient one can see the ipsilateral testicle withdraw as the cremasteric muscle reflexively contracts. This response is not visible if the scrotum is cold and the testicles are already withdrawn, nor can it be seen in female patients.

## LACK OF MUSCLE SIGNS

By definition UMN lesions affect the CNS but spare the α-motor neurons of the brain-stem and spinal cord. Although the muscle may be spastic and paretic, it remains innervated. Consequently, fasciculations, fibrillations, and profound atrophy—all prominent signs of LMN lesions—do not follow UMN lesions.

## UMN Symptoms by Region of the CNS

Spastic weakness, hyperactive MSRs, reversed FRA-driven reflexes, and absence of the signs of muscle denervation are consistent signs of UMN lesions. Other important characteristic signs depend on the location of the lesion. The differences in the clinical picture of the various UMN lesions depend on the *different crossing patterns* of the motor and sensory tracts. Further distinctions can be drawn according to the *location of propinquitous CNS structures.*

These distinctions are illustrated in the following sections.

## SPINAL CORD LESIONS

Complete transection of the spinal cord produces three dramatic signs below the level of the lesion: (*a*) loss of voluntary movement, (*b*) total anesthesia, and (*c*) a temporary period of areflexia followed by permanent hyperreflexia. The loss of voluntary movement is due to the complete severance of motor commands descending from the brainstem and cerebral cortex. The level of transection determines the extent of motor loss. Cervical transections affect all four extremities, a condition known as **quadriplegia** [L. *quadri-*, four]. Lesions below the cervical enlargement produce **paraplegia** [G. *para*, beside]. If the lumbar cord is spared and only the sacral region or conus is involved, only partial paralysis of the lower extremities may be evident.

Anesthesia over the body below the site of spinal cord transection is due to the loss of the dorsal columns and the ALS. With all sensory tracts cut no sensory signals can reach cortical levels from the affected area. Eventually many patients do develop abnormal sensations called **paraesthesias** [G. *aisthesis,* sensation] from the affected areas. Paraesthesias are usually described as an unpleasant burning sensation. Although there is no satisfactory explanation for this phenomenon, it seems likely that a reorganization of synapses in the brainstem and spinal cord affects the thalamic targets of ALS transmission cells. This reorganization hypothesis is similar to the suggested reorganization following dorsal root avulsion (see Chapter 5) that produces similar painful paresthesias.

The areflexia, called **spinal shock**, following acute spinal injury is immediate and profound. Total flaccid paralysis below the site of the lesion includes both the voluntary and involuntary functions. The MSR is absent from all muscles. The bladder and bowels become atonic. Genital reflexes are absent, and autonomic functions (e.g., vasomotor tone, sweating) are lost. Spinal shock usually subsides after 1 to 6 weeks in humans. Spontaneous reflex emptying of bowels and bladder (see Chapter 13) and the vasomotor reflexes usually reappear first. Later muscle tone increases, especially in the flexor muscles and sphincters. Later still the exaggerated hyperactive MSRs associated with UMN lesions appear. Complex alterations in reflexes below the level of the lesion may continue for several months.

The mechanisms of spinal shock are not understood. Some evidence suggests that loss of the reticulospinal and vestibulospinal tracts is the most important factor. This hypothesis is supported by the observation that lesions more rostral than the pons do not produce a period of areflexia, but the essential explanation remains elusive.

Hemisection of the spinal cord, called **Brown-Séquard syndrome**, is an instructive lesion. For a hypothetical patient who has a perfect hemisection of the left spinal cord at T8[8], consider the findings of a neurological examination performed after the period of spinal shock (Fig.7.22). The patient is **monoplegic** [G. *monos*, single], having no voluntary motor functions of the left leg. Furthermore, he has **hyperactive reflexes** in the left leg and abnormal FRA-driven reflexes on the left (the signs of Bing and Babinski are present and the left abdominal and cremasteric reflexes are

---

[8] By convention, T8 refers to the eighth thoracic segment of the spinal cord, not to the vertebral column.

## Figure 7.22   The Brown-Séquard patterns of sensory and motor losses

*Bottom right,* distribution of signs in a patient with hemisection of the left spinal cord at T8. This harlequinlike distribution of sensory signs is an example of sensory dissociation. The sensory signs are the best indicators of the level of the lesion. *Arrows* at the feet are toe directions for the signs of Babinski and Bing. The schematic diagram of the CBST and the ascending sensory tracts illustrates how a spinal hemisection can produce these signs. For simplicity, only the CBST motor tract is shown. *Dark patch*, lesion.

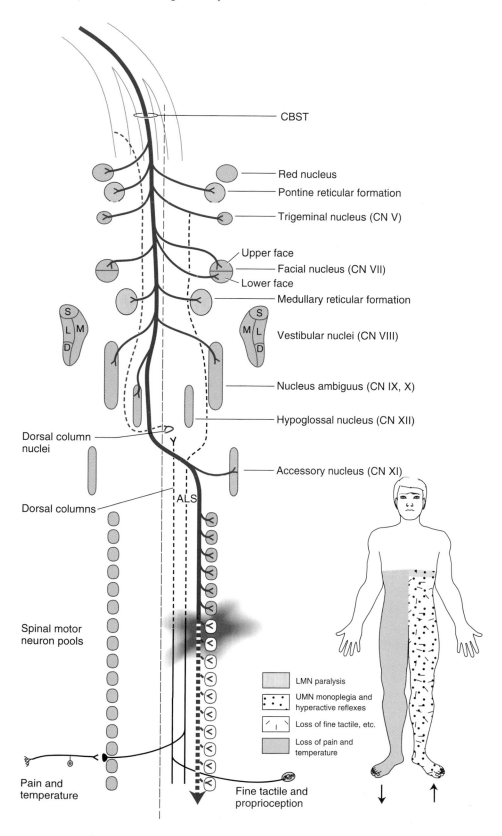

CBST

Red nucleus

Pontine reticular formation

Trigeminal nucleus (CN V)

Upper face
Facial nucleus (CN VII)
Lower face

Medullary reticular formation

S
L M
D
M L
D
S

Vestibular nuclei (CN VIII)

Nucleus ambiguus (CN IX, X)

Hypoglossal nucleus (CN XII)

Dorsal column
nuclei

Accessory nucleus (CN XI)

Dorsal columns

ALS

Spinal motor
neuron pools

LMN paralysis

UMN monoplegia and
hyperactive reflexes

Loss of fine tactile, etc.

Loss of pain and
temperature

Pain and
temperature

Fine tactile and
proprioception

absent). These motor disturbances are directly related to the loss of all of the descending motor tracts on the left; the lateral corticospinal tract, the rubrospinal tract, the medullary reticulospinal tract, the lateral vestibulospinal tract, the medial vestibulospinal tract, and the ventral corticospinal tract. Motor control and reflexes from the right leg are normal.[9]

The pattern of sensory losses allows one to locate the most rostral site of the lesion more precisely than the pattern of motor losses because sensations are absent below the last functional spinal segment. This level can be mapped to a dermatome. Our patient has lost pain and temperature sensations below approximately T8 on the right because the ALS axons on the left are severed. Since the ALS crosses at the level of origin, deficits associated with its loss are contralateral to and below the side of the lesion. In contrast, proprioception and fine tactile sensations are lost below the same level but ipsilateral to the side of the lesion because the dorsal columns remain ipsilateral throughout their course in the spinal cord. This dissociation of pain and temperature versus fine tactile perceptions is an important sign in spinal injuries.

As an exercise, write down the expected findings observed in a patient who suffered an infarct[10] [L. *infarcio*, pp. *infartus*, stuff into] in the territory of the anterior spinal artery.

## BRAINSTEM LESIONS

Brainstem lesions produce sensory and UMN deficits that are codistributed over the side of the body contralateral to the lesion. This con-

tralateral codistribution is seen because both sensory systems and the corticospinal tract cross the midline below the level of the middle medulla. Recall that the ALS crosses at the level of its origin in the spinal cord and that the medial lemniscus crosses at its origin at the most caudal regions of the medulla. Since the corticospinal tract crosses the midline at the transition between the medulla and the spinal cord, most of the principal sensory and motor tracts affected by brainstem lesions produce contralateral signs in the body.

The nuclei associated with the cranial nerves are in the brainstem; they are frequently affected by brainstem lesions (see Chapter 10). Several cranial nerves have motor nuclei that supply voluntary muscles. A brainstem lesion that involves one or more of these cranial nerve nuclei produces an ipsilateral LMN-type paralysis, since the α-motor neurons in the cranial nerve motor nucleus are lost. Because the brainstem is compact, lesions involving motor nuclei of the cranial nerves almost always involve the descending motor tracts as well. Therefore, brainstem lesions commonly present with an *ipsilateral LMN paralysis* of some motor function in the head, combined with a *contralateral UMN hemiparesis*. This **crossed paralysis** is characteristic of brainstem lesions.

Consider an idealized lesion in the left brainstem that affects the facial motor nucleus, the medial lemniscus, the ALS, and the CBST (Fig.7.23). Such a patient displays a complete paralysis of the mimetic muscles of the face on the left side due to the loss of the facial motor nucleus. The patient also has a

---

[9]In theory there ought to be some impairment of the right leg because of the loss of the medial corticospinal tract, since axons in that tract cross the midline at their level of termination. In practice no impairment is detectable by ordinary means.

[10]This word is so commonly misused that one should make special note of its meaning. Infarct means *death of tissue resulting from the arrest of circulation in the artery supplying the area*. This definition in no way suggests the process by which the circulation was arrested, and therefore the word lacks medical precision unless it includes either the artery involved or a description of the tissue killed. For example, *anterior myocardial infarct* is precise and informative; *cerebral infarct* is neither—unless one is describing the effects of decapitation.

## Figure 7.23   The crossed-palsy pattern of motor and sensory losses

The most diagnostic feature of brainstem lesions is the distribution of motor losses, which are characterized by cranial nerve paresis in the head and contralateral hemiparesis of the body. Sensory signs follow a similar pattern. This diagram illustrates how a brainstem lesion at the level of the facial nucleus can produce this pattern. *Dark patch*, lesion.

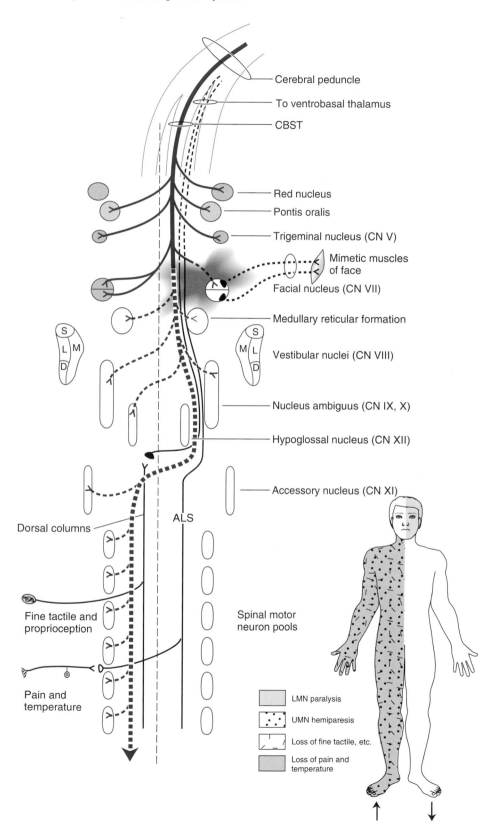

Cerebral peduncle

To ventrobasal thalamus

CBST

Red nucleus

Pontis oralis

Trigeminal nucleus (CN V)

Mimetic muscles of face

Facial nucleus (CN VII)

Medullary reticular formation

Vestibular nuclei (CN VIII)

Nucleus ambiguus (CN IX, X)

Hypoglossal nucleus (CN XII)

Accessory nucleus (CN XI)

Dorsal columns

ALS

Fine tactile and proprioception

Spinal motor neuron pools

Pain and temperature

LMN paralysis

UMN hemiparesis

Loss of fine tactile, etc.

Loss of pain and temperature

spastic (UMN) hemiparesis on the entire right side of the body due to the loss of the corticospinal fibers. This patient is not completely paralyzed on the right because the right rubrospinal and reticulospinal tracts, which have crossed the midline, can provide some motor control to the right side. Sensory losses include a loss of pain and temperature (ALS) and loss of proprioception and fine tactile sensations (medial lemniscus) from the right side of the body. Other specific abnormalities also affect cranial nerves below the level of the lesion. Details of these abnormalities are discussed in Chapter 10.

## LESIONS OF THE INTERNAL CAPSULE AND CEREBRAL CORTEX

Lesions to the internal capsule are commonly caused by strokes of the lateral striate arteries (see Chapter 1). These vessels are very narrow and they leave the parent artery at right angles, factors that make them susceptible to strokes. Because the CBST fibers are compressed in the posterior limb of the internal capsule and separated from the ascending sensory fibers, it is fairly common for capsular lesions to produce pure motor signs contralateral to the lesion. Therefore, a lesion producing a pure hemiparesis that spares the somatosensory system is almost certainly in the internal capsule contralateral to the side of the hemiparesis. However, since all tracts entering and leaving the cerebral cortex are found in the internal capsule, it is a mistake to assume that all capsular lesions produce a pure motor plegia. For example, the optic radiations (see Chapter 12), the fiber tracts that connect the lateral geniculate nucleus with the visual cortex, are particularly close to the CBST in the internal capsules. If these fibers are included in the internal capsule infarct, partial blindness[11] accompanies the hemiparesis.

Infarcts involving the motor areas of the cerebral cortex can occur in the territory of either the anterior or the middle cerebral artery. Infarcts in the middle cerebral artery produce motor and sensory losses that predominantly affect the contralateral face and arm while sparing somewhat the contralateral leg. Infarcts in the anterior cerebral artery do the opposite: they primarily affect the contralateral leg while sparing to some degree the contralateral arm and face. The explanation for these patterns lies in the distribution of the arteries (see Chapter 1).

Infarcts involving the motor regions of the cerebral cortex commonly affect areas other than those immediately adjacent to the central sulcus. Cortical areas with nonmotor functions are also frequently involved, and documentation of these nonmotor functional losses is frequently helpful in localizing the lesion to the cerebral cortex, even if motor losses may be minimal. These other functions are discussed in detail in Chapter 15.

### Stroke

Stroke is the consequence of cerebrovascular disease that interrupts blood flow to part of the brain, causing ischemia and infarction. Stroke is the third most common cause of death in the United States, and it accounts for about half of all neurological disease. It is the most common cause of UMN symptoms. Every physician has patients exhibiting the symptoms of cerebrovascular disease and therefore should be able to properly diagnose and evaluate this common condition.

The diagnosis of stroke depends on establishing the *time course* and *distribution of symptoms*. The symptoms of stroke rapidly develop over the course of a few seconds to a few hours. Few other neurological disease processes develop so rapidly. Therefore, determining the progression of the illness from the history is essential to diagnosing stroke. Furthermore, because stroke is primarily a vascular disease, the neurological deficits must be attributable to neuronal structures within the territory of a single artery. This information is gathered from the neurological examination.

There are three principal causes of strokes: **thrombosis** [G. *thrombosis*, curdling], **embolism** [G. *embolos*, wedge or stopper], and **hemorrhage** [G. *haima*, blood, and *rhegnynai*, burst forth]. Establishing the type of stroke is important both

---

[11] To be precise, a contralateral homonymous hemianopia results (see Chapter 12).

for the initial treatment of the patient and for follow-up care directed at reducing or eliminating the patient's risk factors for stroke. The following paragraphs briefly outline the major clinical features of the different types of stroke (Table 7.2).

## THROMBOSIS

Cerebral thrombosis, the development of a blood clot in a cerebral vessel, is caused by an atherosclerotic plaque in an artery. The plaque causes the vessel wall to degenerate and damages the endothelium. This damage attracts platelets and fibrin to the damaged site, and the thrombus slowly grows. Eventually, usually during a period of reduced blood pressure, the lumen closes and the distal circulation ceases. Decreased blood pressure may allow the vessel to narrow enough so that the lumen, compromised by the presence of the plaque, closes. This sequence of vascular events can be directly correlated with a sequence of neurological events characteristic of **atherothrombotic infarction**,[12] or **thrombotic stroke**.

About *60% of thrombotic strokes develop during sleep.* These patients awake paralyzed. They may be unaware of their condition and get out of bed, only to discover their impairment by falling to the floor. The probable cause of nocturnal onset is that blood pressure decreases during sleep.

About *20% of thrombotic strokes develop stepwise* over a several hours to a few days. In these situations initial neurological deficits appear, followed by a period without further deterioration. Another period of deterioration is heralded by expansion of the neurological signs.

This sequence of events is known clinically as a *stroke in evolution* and when the pathological process has stabilized, as a *completed stroke.*

**Transient ischemic attacks (TIAs)** [G. *ischein,* hold back] precede thrombotic stroke in about 40% of patients. TIAs are temporary neurological deficits caused by disturbed neural function that can be related to the territory of a single artery. The deficit usually clears within a few minutes and always within 24 hours. TIAs are presumed to be the result of the sloughing of small emboli from a thrombus that stick in a vessel and then quickly dissolve, allowing blood flow to resume. Or they may be caused by a temporary collapse of the arteriole at the plaque site. TIAs may herald an eventual thrombotic stroke by hours or months, or the stroke may never occur.

## EMBOLISM

An embolism is a foreign substance that occludes a blood vessel. Many embolisms are blood clots that broke free from a thrombus and lodged in a remote part of the circulation. Embolism can also be a mass of bacteria. Neurological signs develop rapidly with cerebral embolisms and usually do not progress. Only rarely are they preceded by a TIA. Cerebral embolism usually occurs during activity, and consciousness is usually preserved.

The source of the embolism is almost always the left side of the heart. Heart diseases that lead to the production of emboli include *atrial fibrillation, myocardial infarct,* and *defective* or *artificial heart valves,* particularly the mitral valve. Myocardial infarction frequently causes an akinetic region in the heart wall. A

---

[12]Unfortunately, it is common practice to call atherothrombotic infarction simply infarction. This usage is neither accurate nor precise (footnote 10).

## Table 7.2  Comparison of the Principal Types of Stroke

| Type | Place | When | Consciousness |
|---|---|---|---|
| Thrombosis | Occlusion at atherosclerotic plaque | Periods of decreased activity (sleep) | Preserved |
| Embolism | Displaced clot or bacterial mass occludes downstream artery | Periods of activity | Preserved |
| Hemorrhage | Rupture of vessel wall | Anytime | Stupor or coma |

thrombosis can develop within the immobile pocket of the ventricle. Pieces break off from the thrombosis, showering the vascular bed with emboli. Artificial or damaged heart valves are also common sites of embolus formation. Defective and artificial heart valves, because of their rough edges, attract platelets that precipitate clot formation. Atrial fibrillation can also cause emboli because the atrium does not completely empty.

## HEMORRHAGE

Intracerebral hemorrhage is associated with the sudden onset (minutes to hours) of neurological symptoms. It is frequently associated with severe headache. Unlike the occlusive strokes, in which consciousness is preserved, intracerebral hemorrhage may cause stupor or coma that may progress with time. These patients are usually hypertensive but not necessarily so, since **aneurysms** [G. *aneurysma,* a widening] and **arteriovenous malformations** may bleed spontaneously under normal pressure.

## RISK FACTORS

There are five important risk factors for stroke: **hypertension, hyperlipidemia, cigarette smoking, diabetes mellitus,** and **heart disease.** *Hypertension* damages the wall of small arterioles, making them susceptible to the development of atherosclerotic plaques, which in turn narrow the vessels, exacerbating the hypertension. The plaques become sites of thrombosis. Hypertension can also lead directly to arterial rupture, hence cerebral hemorrhage. The successful treatment of hypertension is the single most important factor in reducing the incidence of stroke (20% to 40%, depending on the study). *Hyperlipidemia, cigarette smoking,* and *diabetes mellitus* all accelerate the development of atherosclerosis. *Heart disease* is the most important risk factor for cerebral embolism. Since approximately 25% of the cardiac output reaches the brain, fragments from thrombi that develop in the left side of the heart have a high probability of becoming cerebral emboli.

# C A S E   H I S T O R Y

## THE CASE OF THE DROPPED DINNER FORK

### HISTORY OF PRESENT ILLNESS

Mr. R. B. is an 80-year-old white right-handed man who fell this morning on arising from bed at his usual waking time of 6:00 AM. His wife found him on the floor, awake and alert but unable to move his right arm and leg. She immediately called for an ambulance, which took him to the hospital. A few days before his fall, he dropped his fork during dinner and had some difficulty picking it up again. The clumsiness passed and neither he nor his wife thought much about it. He states that recently he has

had some minimal difficulty maintaining his balance.

### MEDICAL HISTORY

Mr. R. B. used to be hypertensive (220/110), but this condition is now well controlled with medication (150/90).

### NEUROLOGICAL EXAMINATION, 11 JAN, 7:30 AM

#### Mental Status
Mr. R. B. is able to converse and give a reasonable accounting of this morning's events. He knows the date and is aware of his surroundings and his physical condition. He is a little confused at times.

## Cranial Nerves

TRIGEMINAL: He reports that pinprick seems dull and cotton feels odd on the right side of the face but normal on the left side.

FACIAL: There is no movement from the lower right side of the face. The right nasolabial fold is quite flat in comparison with the left side. He can raise his eyebrows on both sides approximately equally.

There are other cranial nerve signs, all on the right side of the face. Specifics of cranial nerve examination are in Chapter 10.

## Station and Gait

Not tested.

## Motor Systems

STRENGTH: There is severe weakness of the right arm, with only a few flickers of motion noticed in the biceps and triceps (strength, 1/5). Mr. R. B. can raise his right leg off the bed by four fingers at the ankle, but it collapses quickly with the slightest pressure (strength, 4/5). Strength on the left side seems normal in all extremities (strength, 5/5).

TONE: There is a slight increase in muscle tone in the right arm; the right leg and left extremities display normal tone.

BULK: Symmetrical and apparently normal for a man of his age.

ABNORMAL MOVEMENTS: None were observed.

## Sensory Systems

Sensory testing (pin and cotton) on the right side of the body reveals an ill-defined area where there is a different feeling as compared with the left side, which the patient reports as feeling normal. The area of abnormal sensations clearly includes the right arm, shoulder, and chest. The patient's reporting of the right leg is unreliable. Sometimes he detects differences between the two sides and other times he does not. He cannot consistently delineate the boundaries on the right leg where sensory perceptions change.

## Reflexes

The MSRs are slightly brisk (+) from the right triceps, biceps, and brachioradialis; quadriceps and gastrocnemius are within normal limits. MSRs are normal on the left. The signs of Babinski and Bing are present on the right, absent on the left.

## Coordination and Control

The patient could not perform rapid finger touching with the right hand; he could with the left hand. Finger-to-nose and heel-to-shin were accomplished with the left arm and leg, but because of weakness, not with the right extremities.

## Parietal Functions

Mr. R. B. has mild expressive aphasia (see Chapter 15). Optokinetic nystagmus (OKN) was present both to the right and left. There were no atavistic signs.

## ANCILLARY STUDIES

Computed tomography (CT) of the head produced normal findings.

## SUBSEQUENT COURSE

Mr. R. B. was admitted to the rehabilitation unit of the hospital on 14 January. By this time there was some improvement in the strength of the right side of his body, but he could not stand without support, nor could he bring his right leg forward. A month later, on 14 February, Mr. R. B. was walking well with a cane and was beginning to negotiate steps. He still had considerable weakness and clumsiness in his right arm and hand. At the time of his discharge 2 weeks later, his right arm was clearly spastic with very brisk reflexes (++) and assumed a triple-flexion posture at rest. His walking had improved further and the MSR reflexes from the right leg were slightly brisk (+). The Bing and Babinski signs were still present on the right and absent on the left.

## COMMENTARY

At this point in your study of neurology, you have enough background to appreciate most of the neurological examination, so it is appropriate to introduce the basic concepts of neurological diagnosis. Correct diagnosis is essential, for it leads to proper treatment and appropriate management of risk factors. Also, especially in the case of untreatable disease, it is comforting to the patient and the patient's family.

Neurological diagnosis depends on establishing (a) an anatomical site of injury (the *anatomical diagnosis*), and (b) the process that led to the injury (*physiological diagnosis*). The physician begins the analysis of the case by listening to the patient's description of the course of the present illness. Having listened to the patient's history, the physician develops initial hypotheses about the illness. These hypotheses guide the physical examination, of which the neurological examination is a part. After the physical examination a list of differential diagnoses is developed. Ancillary diagnostic procedures further winnow this list and usually lead to a final diagnosis.

The history given by the patient (or a witness if the patient is unable to communicate) provides the physician with **symptoms** of the illness. Symptoms are felt; they are subjective impressions reported by the patient. The principal symptom, as defined by the patient, is the **chief complaint.** Mr. R. B.'s chief complaint is that he is weak on the entire right side of his body. One should also obtain from the history the **time course** of the illness. In this case the onset was rapid (he collapsed suddenly on arising) and there has been no notable progression of symptoms. Finally, one should elicit any observations that add significance to the chief complaint. In this case there is evidence of prodromal symptoms; Mr. R. B. dropped his fork at dinner, which was followed by temporary clumsiness of the right hand. It is also noteworthy that his neurological event apparently occurred while he was asleep. This history is consistent with a stroke in the left cerebral cortex affecting the descending motor systems—the initial hypothesis.

The neurological examination is designed to produce objective observations about the neurological state of the patient. Objective observations are **signs.** In this case it is significant that all of the neurological signs are on the right side of the body. Second, the sensory and motor losses coexist over the same parts of the body, which include the face, arm, and leg. Finally, Mr. R. B. has mild aphasia and is fully conscious, cooperative, and alert. The illness has left his mental faculties intact.

Having determined the clinical facts of the case, you are ready to interpret these facts in accordance with known anatomy and physiology. First determine whether the lesion is central or peripheral. The pattern of hemiparesis and sensory loss is consistent with a central lesion involving the descending motor system. The hyperactive MSRs and the signs of Babinski and Bing confirm the central origin of the problem.

Second, establish the approximate location of the lesion within the CNS. The lesion must be more rostral than the highest affected CNS structure, which in this case is the facial motor nucleus (brainstem). Since the facial nerve's weakness is ipsilateral to the arm and leg weakness, the lesion must affect the descending CBST fibers and not the facial nucleus; otherwise there would be a crossed palsy (Fig. 7.23). Furthermore, the face and arm are more affected than the leg. This dissociation suggests that the lesion must be in the left cerebral cortex because leg and arm areas of M-I are perfused by different arteries. If the lesion were in the internal capsule or cerebral peduncle, one would expect approximately equal involvement of the upper and lower extremities because in those structures the CBST is a compact structure (Fig. 7.2).

Finally, determine which side of the CNS is affected. Most of the corticobulbar fibers of the CBST cross the midline at the level of the motor nuclei they innervate. The corticospinal fibers cross at the junction of the spinal cord and medulla. Therefore, since the right side of the body is affected and the lesion is rostral to the facial nucleus, the lesion must be in the left hemisphere. Given this analysis, the anatomical diagnosis can be made: a lesion to the left cerebral cortex involving the arm and face area of M-I in the territory of the middle cerebral artery.

The anatomical diagnosis having been established, one must determine the cause of the illness. Neurological disease in adults is usually caused by metabolic, traumatic, neoplastic, or vascular abnormalities. The anatomical diagnosis in this case is highly focal, being limited to a specific area of one cerebral hemisphere. Therefore, disease processes that generally affect the entire nervous system, such as metabolic disease, are unlikely in this case. Trauma is also unlikely, given the history. Finally, symptoms associated with neoplastic disease usually develop slowly over weeks to months, not, as in the present case, over minutes to hours. Therefore, the cause of Mr. R. B.'s illness is probably vascular.

Having come to this conclusion, one must differentiate among cerebral hemorrhage, embolism, and thrombosis, because treatments are considerably different.[13] For that reason, CT of the head was ordered. *CT and MRI of nervous tissue within about 24 to 48 hours of an ischemic stroke (emboli or thrombosis) are normal,* whereas extravascular blood from an intracerebral hemorrhage is immediately visible. CT or MRI demonstrates an area of edema after about 48 hours after ischemic stroke. Mr. R. B.'s CT was normal, allowing the final diagnosis of thrombosis of the rolandic branch of the middle cerebral artery producing infarction of the inferior M-I area (Fig.7.24).

Once ischemic stroke is diagnosed, determining how much time has elapsed since the onset of symptoms is critical. Clot-dissolving agents, delivered within 3 to 4 hours of onset, can dramatically improve the prognosis of ischemic stroke. If such agents are given after 4 hours, the risk of intracerebral hemorrhage is greatly increased. In this case the CT was completed at 8:30 AM. Given the uncertainty of the exact time of onset, the administration of clot-dissolving agents was considered too risky.

## FURTHER APPLICATIONS

**7.1.** **Consider the neurological signs and symptoms one would expect to observe if Mr. R. B.'s thrombosis had occurred in the left anterior cerebral artery.**

**7.2.** **How would the history be different if Mr. R. B. had had a cerebral hemorrhage of the middle cerebral artery?**

**7.3.** **Could Mr. R. B. have an embolism rather than a thrombosis? What is the difference between these two types of stroke? How do their clinical pictures differ?**

---

[13]Discussion of treatment is beyond the scope of this text. Please refer to any of the clinical texts in the Suggested Readings at the end of this chapter.

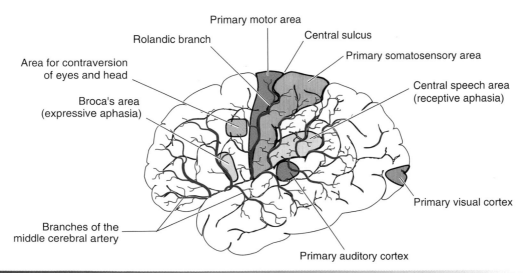

**Figure 7.24   Functional areas of the cerebral cortex correlated with the distribution of the middle cerebral artery**

The typical divisions of the middle cerebral artery and the principal functional regions served by its various branches.

# C A S E   H I S T O R Y

## THE CASE OF THE FALLING RUNNER

### HISTORY OF PRESENT ILLNESS

Ms. C. R., a 39-year-old woman and avid runner, was in good neurological health until January. At that time she fell while running and broke her left clavicle. Six weeks later, when the clavicle had healed, she resumed running. On her first day back she fell again, scraping both her hands and her knees. By September she had fallen frequently while running and on the stairs in her apartment building. She has reluctantly given up running. She says that at times her left leg feels like a piece of wood. Recently she has noticed that her left hand felt puffy and weak and performed somewhat clumsily. She has no family history of neurological disease.

### MEDICAL HISTORY

The patient has no history of serious medical disease.

### NEUROLOGICAL EXAMINATION, 2 SEPT

#### Mental Status
The patient gives a lucid history. She was able to remember all three items at the end of the examination.

#### Cranial Nerves
No abnormalities of cranial nerve function were found.

#### Station and Gait
Ms. C. R. walks with a limp, slightly dragging her left foot. She is not ataxic. She hops well on the right foot but not on the left. She can do three deep knee bends without difficulty.

### Motor Systems

STRENGTH: On direct strength testing her left arm and leg are weaker (4/5) than the corresponding right extremities (5/5). There is definite drift and supination of the left arm when she holds her arms outstretched.

TONE: There is increased tone in all extremities and definite spasticity in the left leg.

BULK: Muscle bulk is symmetrical and normal for a woman of her age.

ABNORMAL MOVEMENTS: No abnormal movements were observed.

### Sensory Systems
Appreciation of pinprick, light touch to cotton, vibration, and joint position are all within normal limits. The Romberg sign is not present.

### Reflexes
The MSRs from all extremities are brisk (+), with those from the left greater than those from the right. Two to four beats of unsustained clonus can be elicited from the left ankle. The sign of Babinski is present on the left, absent on the right.

### Coordination and Control
Rapid alternating movements of the left extremity are somewhat uncoordinated. Finger-to-toe and heel-to-shin maneuvers are performed reasonably well bilaterally (see Chapter 9).

### Parietal Functions
Not tested.

### ANCILLARY STUDIES

None ordered.

## COMMENTARY

Ms. C. R.'s chief complaint is weakness, which is making her unstable on her feet. The history indicates that her difficulties have been progressing slowly but relentlessly for several months. The neurological examination reveals that the weakness is greater on the left than the right. There are no sensory losses. The increased MSRs, clonus, and sign of Babinski prove the UMN nature of the disease. Hence the lesion is within the CNS and cannot be peripheral.

Given the patient's age and the general nature of her illness, a diagnosis of multiple sclerosis (MS) (see Chapters 2 and 12) is plausible. MS is an autoimmune disease directed against CNS myelin. This diagnosis depends on the absence of LMN signs, the presence of multiple CNS lesions that are anatomically distinct, and a history of exacerbation and remission of symptoms. No ancillary studies can provide a definitive diagnosis (see Chapter 12 for further discussion of MS). At this point Ms. C. R.'s difficulties can be explained by a single lesion, so the clinical picture of MS is incomplete. Multiple lesions cannot be proved and there is no history of exacerbations and remissions, so the diagnosis remains tentative.

## SUBSEQUENT COURSE

Ms. C. R. was examined again 11 months later. At that time her weakness had spread to all four extremities. By July her hands had become so weak that she had to quit her job.

## NEUROLOGICAL EXAMINATION, 19 AUG FOLLOWING YEAR

### Mental Status
Normal.

### Cranial Nerves
Normal.

### Station and Gait
Ms. C. R. is now in a wheelchair. She is very unsteady when standing and requires support. When she attempts to walk, she lurches and would fall without help.

### Motor Systems

STRENGTH: She is very weak in all four extremities (3/5).

TONE: Her upper extremities are very spastic, her lower extremities somewhat less so.

BULK: There is gross atrophy of the muscles in both hands and definite atrophy of the muscles in the shoulder girdle.

ABNORMAL MOVEMENTS: There are marked fasciculations in her tongue and occasional fasciculations in her right deltoid and over her lower ribs on the left.

### Sensory Systems
Ms. C. R. is able to perceive pinprick, cotton wisp, vibration, and joint position normally from all four extremities, trunk, and face.

### Reflexes
The MSRs from all four extremities are very hyperactive (++). There is sustained clonus from her left ankle. Unsustained clonus can be demonstrated from her jaw and right ankle. The signs of Babinski and Bell are present bilaterally.

### Coordination and Control
Not tested.

### Parietal Functions
The OKN is present in both directions. There is no aphasia or any atavistic signs.

### ANCILLARY STUDIES

None ordered.

### COMMENTARY

The passage of time often illuminates the neurological picture. Ms. C. R.'s condition has considerably worsened since her last examination. Her UMN signs have progressed to involve all four extremities. Most important, there are now definitive LMN signs—fasciculations and atrophy. Despite the progression of her motor difficulties to the point that she is bound to a wheelchair, Ms. C. R. has a normal sensorium. Her mental faculties remain undiminished.

The presence of LMN signs is incompatible with a diagnosis of MS. The symptoms of MS are limited to the CNS because only myelin produced by oligodendrocytes is damaged in that disease. The combination of UMN and LMN signs with normal somatosensory findings is characteristic of **ALS.**

Amyotrophic lateral sclerosis is a progressive degenerative disease of unknown etiology and is without effective treatment. Its diagnosis is based on the involvement of the voluntary motor systems with findings of simultaneous UMN and LMN signs. All other neurological systems remain intact. Patients remain fully sentient and mentally competent. The UMN signs are caused by the degeneration of the CBST, the rubrospinal tract, and the medullary reticulospinal tracts. These lesions are most evident in the spinal cord (Fig.7.25). The LMN symptoms are caused by the loss of the motor neurons in the ventral horn and the motor nuclei of the cranial nerves.

During the course of the disease the patient is eventually left with a total flaccid paralysis involving all voluntary motor systems except for the extraocular eye movements and the urinary sphincters. The relentless progress of the disease leaves the person intact in every other respect but imprisoned in a paralyzed body. Most persons with amyotrophic lateral sclerosis die within 5 years of the initial diagnosis. Patients can live a nearly normal life span with this disease if they are willing to endure continuous artificial ventilation and to be totally dependent on extensive nursing care. Such persons are rare.

## FURTHER APPLICATIONS

**7.4.** After the first examination Ms. C. R.'s symptoms can be explained by a single lesion. Where would you place that lesion?

**7.5.** Consider the value of the anatomical diagnosis in differentiating between MS and amyotrophic lateral sclerosis. Would alteration of epicritic sensory functions be helpful in differentiating these two diseases? Explain.

**7.6.** Explain how, after amyotrophic lateral sclerosis has run its course, the patient is left with a total flaccid paralysis. Why are there no UMN signs?

**7.7.** Consider the ethical questions this disease imposes on the physician. With respiratory assistance and proper nursing, patients can live for many years with amyotrophic lateral sclerosis, albeit totally helpless. Patients who choose not to take that course face death by aspiration or asphyxiation. Many choose suicide. Is physician-assisted suicide appropriate in such situations? What should be the obligation of society to provide, through state-supported insurance programs, long-term care for the amyotrophic lateral sclerosis patient who chooses ventilatory support? Later, if the patient chooses, is it appropriate to discontinue ventilatory support once it has been initiated? Should a health maintenance organization or other health care providers consider ventilatory support standard treatment and thus covered, or should it be extraordinary treatment and thus not covered?

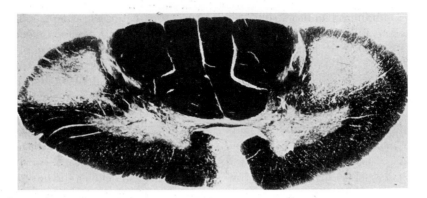

**Figure 7.25  Demyelination associated with amyotrophic lateral sclerosis**

This section of a cervical spinal cord, stained for myelin (*black*), was obtained from a patient who died of amyotrophic lateral sclerosis. Severe degeneration of the descending motor tracts is evident from the almost total loss of myelin from the lateral white columns (*white areas* in the lateral white columns). Not evident in this preparation is the loss of motor neurons from the ventral horns, because the section was not stained for cells. (Reprinted with permission from Rowland LP. Merritt's Textbook of Neurology. 8th ed. Philadelphia: Lea & Febiger, 1989;685.)

## SUMMARY

- **The CBST originates in a wide area of the cerebral cortex (Brodmann areas 4, 6, 3, 1, 2, 5, 7, 39, and 40).**

  CBST axons descend to the brainstem and spinal cord. Axons that terminate in the brainstem may be separately named the corticobulbar tract, and those that descend to the spinal cord may be called the corticospinal tract. CBST axons terminate in the red nucleus, the reticular formation, the voluntary motor nuclei of the cranial nerves (except the nuclei of ocular motion), and the spinal cord. Most of these connections cross the midline before terminating. Some structures in the brainstem are bilaterally innervated. CBST axons terminate primarily on interneurons, not motor neurons, and ultimately affect both α- and γ-motor neurons. In the spinal cord most axons facilitate flexor motor neuron pools. Some CBST axons terminate directly on α-motor neurons, primarily those innervating the most distal muscles.

- **The rubrospinal tract originates in the red nucleus.**

  Rubrospinal tract axons cross the midline immediately on leaving the red nucleus to descend through the brainstem and spinal cord. They terminate on interneurons and facilitate primarily flexor α- and γ-motor neuron pools of the proximal musculature. The red nucleus receives afferents from the motor areas of the cerebral cortex via corticobulbar axons and from the cerebellum.

- **The reticulospinal tracts originate in the pontine and medullary reticular formation.**

  Both tracts terminate on interneurons that affect the voluntary motor neuron pools. The medullary reticulospinal fibers primarily facilitate flexors, and the pontine reticulospinal fibers primarily affect extensors. Both systems receive afferents from the spinal cord, the cerebellum, and the motor regions of the cerebral cortex.

- The vestibulospinal tracts originate in the vestibular nuclei.

  The lateral vestibular nucleus gives rise to the lateral vestibulospinal tract, and the medial vestibular nucleus contains the cells of origin for the medial vestibulospinal tract. The medial tract descends only to cervical levels, innervating the muscles that stabilize the head. The lateral tract descends to all levels of the spinal cord, innervating extensor motor neurons. Both tracts terminate on interneurons, but the lateral tract also terminates extensively on α-motor neurons directly.

- The three named areas in the cerebral cortex that are closely associated with motor activity are the M-I, SMA, and PMA.

  All three areas are somatotopically organized and are reciprocally interconnected through short association axons.

- Cells in PMA facilitate specific sets of neurons in M-I required for a particular motor act.

  They fire before the evolving movement has been initiated.

- SMA is necessary for coordinated motor acts.

  SMA is necessary particularly for bimanual tasks, since unilateral lesions to the SMA produce mirror movements between the extremities. Neuronal activity in SMA and PMA converges on M-I neurons.

- M-I provides the most direct cortical control of the motor neurons.

  M-I pyramidal cells are connected quite precisely, mostly through interneurons, to individual motor units in the voluntary motor neuron pools. M-I neurons may be coded for the force, velocity, and direction of the motor task.

- The motor areas of the cortex receive ascending connections from the VA and VL thalamic nuclei.

  The thalamic nuclei are intermediate connections between the motor cortex and the cerebellum and basal ganglia.

- The concept of the UMN contrasts with that of the LMN.

  Certain CNS lesions produce a stereotyped constellation of symptoms that constitute a working definition of the UMN. They are (a) spastic paresis, (b) hyperactive MSRs, and (c) the reversal of certain FRA-driven reflexes (signs of Babinski and Bing). The CBST, the rubrospinal tract, and the medullary reticulospinal tract share many physiological functions associated with the UMN. Lesions of these tracts are closely correlated with UMN signs.

- The MSR exhibits properties of a proportional-control feedback system.

  The controlled variable is muscle length. Alterations in muscle length are fed back to the spinal cord, which generates an error signal that alters muscle tension to restore the original length. Damage to the UMN increases the gain of the MSR control system, underdamping it. This is manifested clinically as hyperactive MSR responses, muscle spasticity, and clonus.

- Strokes are the most common neurological problem and the third leading cause of death in the United States.

  Strokes are the result of cerebrovascular disease and fall into three classes. Atherothrombotic infarcts result from a thrombus within a cerebral vessel at the site of an atherosclerotic plaque. Cerebral embolisms occur when a clot breaks away from a remote thrombus and migrates into the cerebral vasculature. The most common site for the development of emboli is the left side of the heart. Cerebral hemorrhage occurs when a cerebral vessel, aneurysm, or arteriovenous malformation ruptures or leaks fresh blood into the tissue of the brain or its ventricles.

- MS is a degenerative disease of the CNS.

  It is probably an autoimmune disease; the antigen is CNS myelin. Clinically this disease is characterized by pure CNS lesions that are disseminated in both time and space. No ancillary studies are absolutely reliable in confirming the diagnosis of MS, although CSF protein studies and MRI are helpful. There is no cure for MS, but anti-inflammatory therapy may reduce the frequency of exacerbations.

- ALS affects both the UMN and the LMN.

  ALS is characterized by CNS lesions that are limited to the descending motor systems (CBST, rubrospinal, and reticulospinal tracts) and spare the sensory systems and higher cortical functions. Simultaneously, LMN symptoms also develop because of the loss of motor neurons in the brainstem and spinal cord. There is no effective treatment for this disease.

## SUGGESTED READINGS

Adams RD, Victor M, Ropper AH. Principles of Neurology, 6th ed. New York: McGraw-Hill, 1996.

Bradley WG, et al. Neurology in Clinical Practice, 2nd ed. Boston: Butterworth–Heinemann, 1996.

Brooks V. The Neural Basis of Motor Control. New York: Oxford University, 1986.

Haines DE. Neuroanatomy: An Atlas of Structures, Sections, and Systems. 5th ed. Baltimore: Williams & Wilkins, 1999.

Morrison BM, Morrison JH. Amyotrophic lateral sclerosis associated with mutations in superoxide dismutase: a putative mechanism of degeneration. Brain Res Brain Res Rev 1999;1:121–135.

Nieuwenhuys R, Voodg J, Van Huijzen C. The Human Central Nervous System. 3rd ed. Berlin: Springer-Verlag, 1988.

Rowland LP. Merritt's Textbook of Neurology, 9th ed. Baltimore: Williams & Wilkins, 1995.

Swash M. Early diagnosis of ALS/MND. J Neurol Sci 1998;160(suppl 1):S33–36.

Waddington M. Atlas of Cerebral Angiography With Anatomic Correlation. Boston: Little, Brown, 1974.

# Motor Systems III: The Basal Ganglia

The basal ganglia [G. *basis*, base, and *ganglion*, knot] provide the crucial physiological link between the *idea of movement* and the *motor expression of that idea*. Their influence on motor action is indirect, as they affect the motor regions of the cerebral cortex before motor commands are sent to the brainstem and spinal cord. Neuronal activity in the descending motor systems is closely correlated in time with the actual motor act. In contrast, most neuronal activity of the basal ganglia occurs before any movement begins. Disturbances in the function of the descending motor systems and the spinal cord result in paresis or paralysis. Lesions to the basal ganglia cause disturbances in the initiation or cessation of a motor event.

## NUCLEI OF THE BASAL GANGLIA

The basal ganglia are a set of nuclei that function as a bridge between the telencephalon and the diencephalon. Some of these nuclei are derived from the telencephalon, and others develop from the diencephalon. Information from the cerebral cortex enters telencephalic basal ganglion nuclei, passes into diencephalic regions of the basal ganglia, and proceeds to thalamic nuclei. From the thalamus the information returns to the cerebral cortex.

Our understanding of the functional role of the basal ganglia in motor control is changing rapidly. Originally thought to be a purely motor system, the basal ganglia are now recognized to participate in certain cognitive functions as well. The exact nature of this cognitive role is not understood. In part for this reason, there is legitimate disagreement about the structures that properly constitute the basal ganglia. For the purposes of this book, the basal ganglia consist of the following nuclei: the **caudate nucleus** [L. *caudatus*, having a tail], the **putamen** [L. *puto*, prune], the **nucleus accumbens** [L. *accumbens*, leaning], the **globus pallidus** [L. *globus*, sphere, and *pallidus*, pale], the **substantia nigra**, and the subthalamic nucleus.[1]

## The Striatum

The striatum [neuter of L. *striatus*, grooved], derived from the telencephalon, consists of the caudate nucleus, the putamen, and the nucleus accumbens (Figs. 8.1 and 8.2). Both cytoarchitectural and physiological studies confirm that these nuclei in fact constitute a single nucleus. Posteriorly the caudate and putamen are separated by the internal capsule. They merge at the most anterior portion; only a few threads of the anterior limb of the internal capsule pass between the caudate and the putamen.

The anterior portion of the caudate lies between the internal capsule and the lateral ventricle. It is larger than the remainder of the nucleus and is therefore called the **head**. Inferior to the head the caudate merges with the nucleus accumbens. The rest of the caudate

---

[1] Many authors include the claustrum in the basal ganglia. This enigmatic nucleus has major connections with the cerebral cortex, but because it does not have connections with specific thalamic nuclei, it seems prudent not to include the claustrum with the basal ganglia.

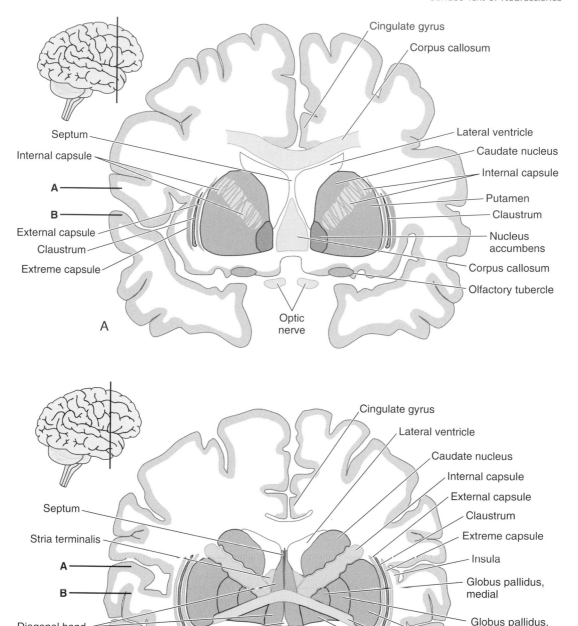

**Figure 8.1    Frontal sections through the frontal lobes**

**A.** Frontal section through the anterior portion of the basal ganglia. Threads of the caudate-putamen-accumbens pass through the anterior limb of the internal capsule, and the nucleus accumbens joins the caudate putamen at the ventral medial margin. **B.** Frontal section at the level of the anterior commissure. Note the relations among the septum, the diagonal band, and the nucleus basalis. Letters to the side correspond with the level of the sections in Figure 8.2.

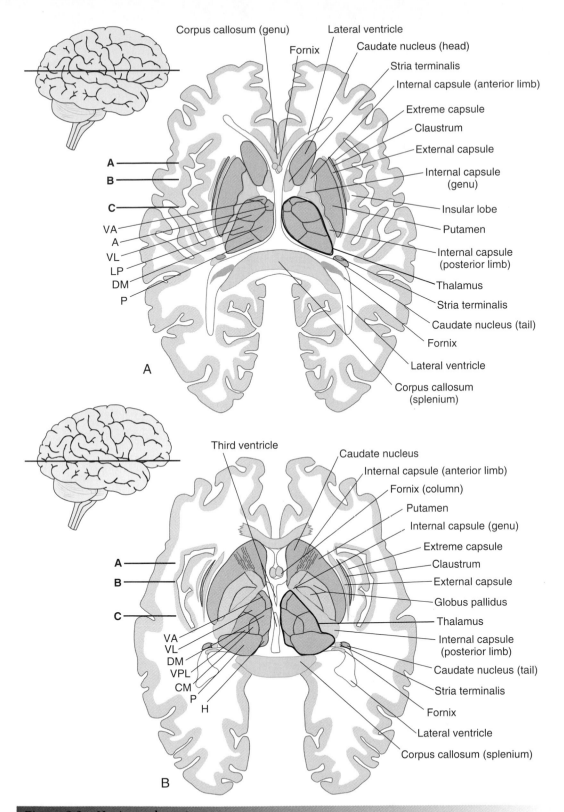

**Figure 8.2  Horizontal sections**

**A.** This horizontal section through the basal ganglia and the thalamus illustrates the relations of these structures to the internal capsule and the lateral ventricles. **B.** This horizontal section is at the level of the anterior commissure. Letters to the side correspond with the level of the frontal sections of Figures 8.1 and 8.4. Thalamic nuclei: *A,* anterior; *CM,* centromedian; *DM,* dorsal medial; *H,* habenula; *LP,* lateral posterior; *P,* pulvinar; *VA,* ventral anterior; *VL,* ventral lateral; *VPL,* ventral posterior lateral.

nucleus—the **body** and **tail**—wraps around the medial aspect of the internal capsule. The entire caudate nucleus forms part of the lateral wall of the lateral ventricle. It follows the wall into the temporal lobe, where it terminates at the **amygdaloid nuclei** [L. *amygdalum,* almond, and *eidos,* shape] just deep to the uncus. The putamen lies lateral to the internal capsule, between its anterior and posterior limbs.

Cells in the striatum are immunoreactive to several neurotransmitters and neuroactive peptides. More than 90% of striatal neurons are small and have spiny dendrites. They receive cortical afferents and are the principal source of efferent fibers from the striatum. **γ-Aminobutyric acid** (GABA) is the principal neurotransmitter released by all spiny neurons, and a neuroactive peptide is probably re-

leased with the neurotransmitter. The function of the neuroactive peptide is not known. Several classes of spiny neurons have been identified according to immunohistochemical data. The two most important groups are composed of cells immunoreactive to **substance P** (SP) and cells immunoreactive to **enkephalin** (ENK). Most of the other cells in the striatum are large, spiny, excitatory interneurons that release acetylcholine (ACh) as the neurotransmitter.

Neurons that stain for the various neuroactive peptides are unevenly distributed within the striatum. Immunohistochemically similar neurons are collected as isolated islands, or patches, within a continuous **matrix** (Fig. 8.3). The matrix stains heavily for acetylcholinesterase (AChE), which is much less prevalent within the patches.

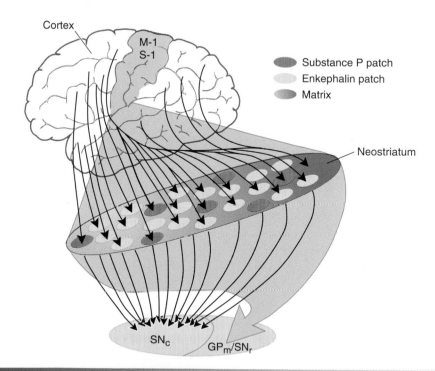

Substance P patch
Enkephalin patch
Matrix

Neostriatum

**Figure 8.3   Patch-matrix composition of the striatum**

The AChE-staining matrix (*pink area*), or background substance, of the striatum is punctuated with poorly staining patches. The patches (*black or gray areas*) contain neurons with different neurochemical properties. Some of the patches are immunoreactive for ENK; others are reactive for SP. The patches and matrix have discrete restricted connections both with the cerebral cortex from which they receive afferents and the globus pallidus and substantia nigra to which they project. *GP$_m$*, globus pallidus medialis; *SN$_c$*, substantia nigra pars compacta; *SN$_r$*, substantia nigra pars compacta.

The patch-matrix pattern seems to represent a basic division within the general organization of the basal ganglion system. The matrix receives afferents primarily from M-I and S-I and projects mainly to the medial globus pallidus/substantia nigra pars reticulata (GPm/SNr). In contrast, the patches are innervated primarily by the prefrontal lobe and certain limbic structures (see Chapter 14). Their principal projection is to the substantia nigra pars compacta (SNc).

The patches themselves are heterogeneous. Patches that stain for one neuroactive peptide do not necessarily overlap with patches that stain for another. This anatomical complexity suggests that within the striatum several physiological functions are served by parallel systems that are segregated both anatomically and neurochemically.

### The Pallidum

Derived from the diencephalon, the globus pallidus lies between the putamen and the internal capsule.[2] The globus pallidus consists of two nuclei, the **lateral** (GPl) and **medial** (GPm) divisions, which are separated by a thin layer of axons. Each nucleus has its own set of connections. The GPm is functionally identical to **the reticular division of the substantia nigra** (SNr). To acknowledge this functional similarity, they are designated **GPm/SNr** in this text. Most neurons within the pallidum are immunoreactive to GABA, which they probably use as a neurotransmitter.

### The Substantia Nigra

The substantia nigra, although a nucleus of the mesencephalon, is often considered to be a part of the basal ganglia because of its rich connections with the striatum (Fig. 8.4). It is composed of two subnuclei, the SNr and the **substantia nigra pars compacta** (SNc). Its name is derived from its black color in fresh cadaver brains. The black substance, **melanin**, is a byproduct of **dopamine** metabolism (Fig. 8.5).

Neurons in the SNc produce large amounts of dopamine and carry it by axoplasmic trans-

port to the striatum, where it is used as a neurotransmitter. Dopamine may also have other metabolic effects. Most of the dopamine-producing cells of the SNc also produce **cholecystokinin** (CCK), a neuroactive peptide. In addition to the striatum, these dual transmitter neurons project to the amygdaloid complex, the nucleus accumbens, and the prefrontal cortex. Neurons in the GPm/SNr project to the thalamus, the superior colliculus, and the brainstem reticular formation. These cells probably release GABA as a neurotransmitter.

### The Subthalamic Nucleus

Derived from the diencephalon, the subthalamic nucleus (STN) lies just medial to the internal capsule and ventral lateral to the thalamus proper (Fig. 8.4). Cells in this nucleus are immunoreactive to **glutamate** and may use it as a neurotransmitter.

## CONNECTIONS OF THE BASAL GANGLIA

The principal pathway by which the basal ganglia are interconnected with other parts of the nervous system (Fig. 8.6) originates in the entire cerebral cortex. Fibers project from the cerebral cortex to the striatum, which sends fibers to the pallidum. The pallidum sends axons to the ventral thalamus, which projects back to the principal motor areas of the cerebral cortex. While this general plan is quite simple, the details are somewhat more complex (Fig. 8.7).

### Afferent Connections

The striatum is the principal receptive area of the basal ganglia, as it receives afferent connections from nearly the entire cerebral cortex. These connections maintain the same spatial relations in the striatum as in the cortex; that is, the frontal lobe projects to the anterior caudate (the head of the caudate) and putamen; the parietal and occipital lobes project to the body of the caudate; and the tem-

---

[2] The term lentiform nucleus has historically been applied to the combined structures of the putamen and globus pallidus. This union cannot be defended on ontological, anatomical, or physiological grounds and therefore serves no function.

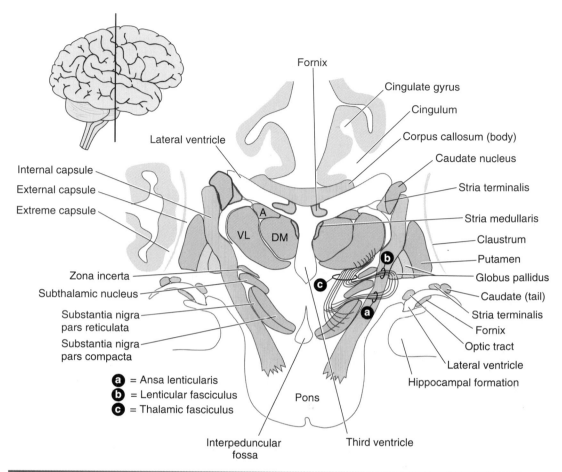

Fornix
Cingulate gyrus
Cingulum
Corpus callosum (body)
Caudate nucleus
Lateral ventricle
Internal capsule
External capsule
Extreme capsule
Stria terminalis
Stria medullaris
A
VL   DM
Claustrum
Putamen
Globus pallidus
Caudate (tail)
Stria terminalis
Fornix
Optic tract
Lateral ventricle
Hippocampal formation
Zona incerta
Subthalamic nucleus
Substantia nigra
pars reticulata
Substantia nigra
pars compacta

**a** = Ansa lenticularis
**b** = Lenticular fasciculus
**c** = Thalamic fasciculus

Pons

Interpeduncular
fossa

Third ventricle

### Figure 8.4 Frontal section through the diencephalon

Relations among the subthalamic nucleus, zona incerta, substantia nigra, and internal capsule. The internal capsule becomes the cerebral peduncle as it enters the pons. The globus pallidus and putamen lie lateral to the internal capsule, and the caudate lies medial to it and dorsal to the thalamus. Also note the position of the tail of the caudate nucleus and its relation to the stria terminalis and fornix. Fibers leaving the globus pallidus leave by two pathways, the ansa lenticularis (a) and the lenticular fasciculus (b), which merge to form the thalamic fasciculus (c). Thalamic nuclei: A, anterior; VL, ventral lateral; DM, dorsal medial.

poral lobe projects to the tail of the caudate. Not all areas of the cortex project equally to the striatum. For example, the head of the caudate is much larger than the body or tail, reflecting the caudate's more numerous connections with the frontal lobe than with the other lobes. Connections arising in the primary sensory and motor areas, S-I and M-I, project bilaterally from the frontal and parietal lobes to the putamen. Other areas of the neocortex project primarily to the ipsilateral caudate.

These cortical projections are well organized and maintain a topographic relation between the cerebral cortex and the striatum. Cortical afferent fibers terminate on the spiny neurons, making excitatory contacts with the heads of the spines. The striatum, particularly the putamen, also receives important projections from the SNc. Their actions are mediated by the transmitter dopamine, which has various actions depending on the nature of the dopamine receptor. To date, five receptors belonging to

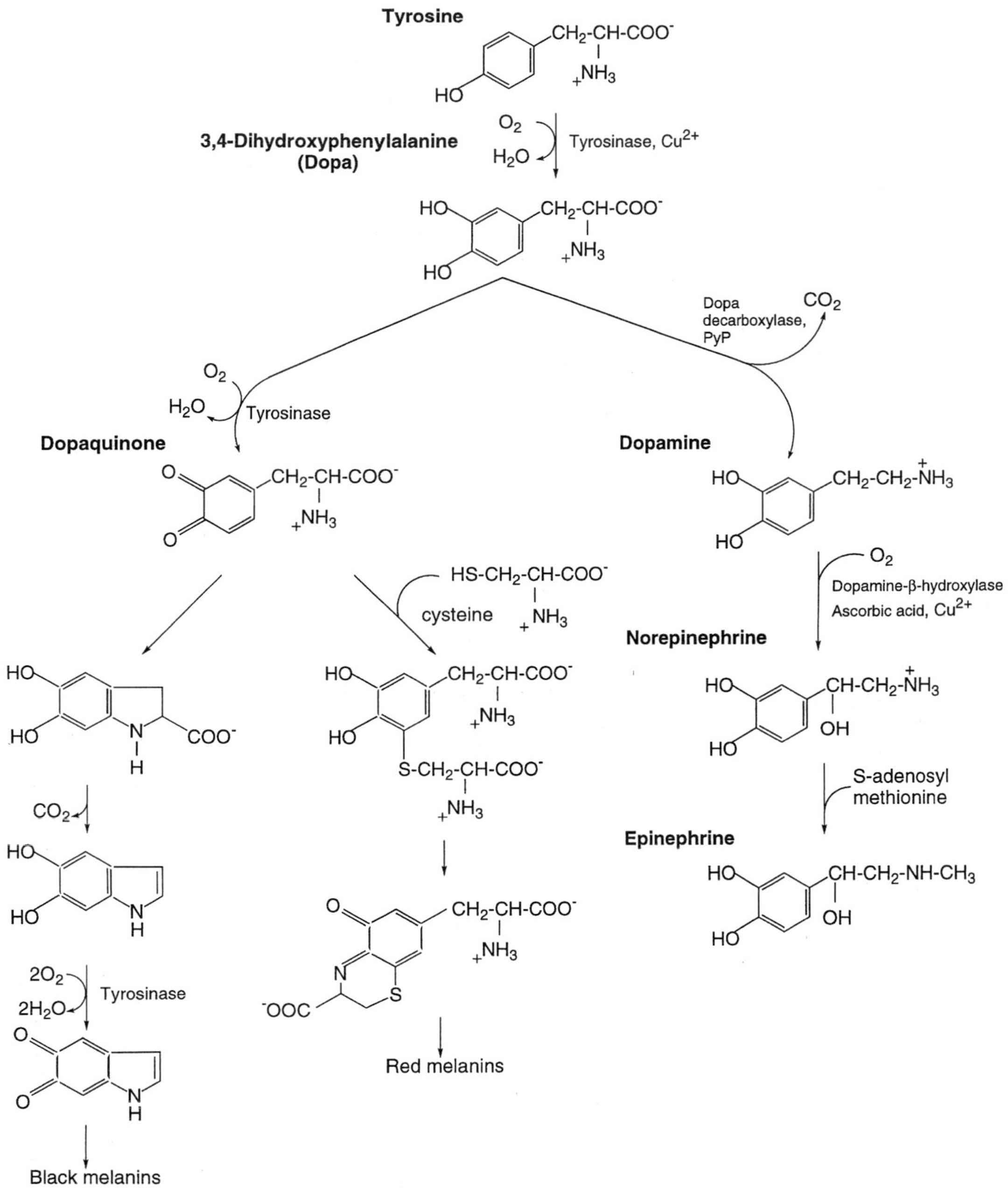

**Tyrosine**

**3,4-Dihydroxyphenylalanine
(Dopa)**

$O_2$

$H_2O$

Tyrosinase, $Cu^{2+}$

Dopa
decarboxylase,
PyP

$CO_2$

$O_2$

$H_2O$   Tyrosinase

**Dopaquinone**

**Dopamine**

HS-$CH_2$-CH-COO⁻

cysteine

**Norepinephrine**

$O_2$

Dopamine-β-hydroxylase
Ascorbic acid, $Cu^{2+}$

$CO_2$

S-adenosyl
methionine

**Epinephrine**

$2O_2$

$2H_2O$

Tyrosinase

Red melanins

Black melanins

**Figure 8.5    Metabolism of tyrosine**

two families of dopamine receptors have been identified; they are designated $D_1$ and $D_2$–like receptors.[3] Because receptors within the same family have similar actions, only

the families will be discussed in this book. The release of dopamine within the striatum reduces the release of GABA from ENK-containing neurons ($D_2$ receptor) and enhances

[3] The $D_1$ and $D_5$ receptors belong to the $D_1$ family; the $D_2$, $D_3$, and $D_4$ receptors belong to the $D_2$ family.

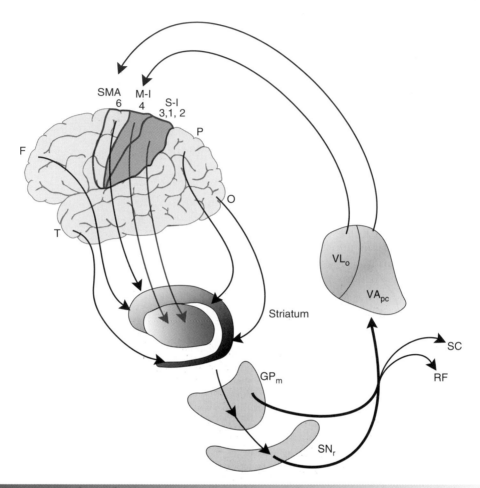

## Figure 8.6   Basal ganglia input-output connections

The principal pathway by which the basal ganglia are connected to other parts of the nervous system. The system forms a loop. Information originates from nearly the entire cerebral cortex and passes through the basal ganglia and thalamus before returning to the cortex. The modified information is returned primarily to the specific motor areas of the cerebral cortex, M-I and SMA. *F,* frontal lobe; *P,* parietal lobe; *O,* occipital lobe; *T,* temporal lobe; *SMA,* supplemental motor area; *M-I,* primary motor area; *S-I,* primary sensory area; *VA_{pc},* ventral anterior parvocellular; *VL_{o},* ventral lateral oralis; *SN_{r},* substantia nigra pars reticulata; *GP_{m},* globus pallidus medialis; *RF,* brainstem reticular formation; *SC,* superior colliculus. *Numbers* indicate Brodmann areas.

the release of GABA from SP-containing neurons ($D_1$ receptor). The location of the nigral inhibitory synapses on the necks of the spines suggests that these axons can selectively short-circuit excitatory postsynaptic potentials (EPSPs) originating on the heads in much the same way that inhibitory synapses on the base of dendrites can short-circuit EPSPs originating from more distal synapses (Fig. 8.8).

### Intrinsic Connections

The nuclei of the basal ganglia are connected by three principal pathways (Fig. 8.7). The first and largest pathway arises both from the matrix and from patches of SP-containing spiny neurons in the striatum. Most of these axons project to the GPm/SNr. The second set of intrinsic connections arises from patches of spiny neurons containing ENK. These axons project to the GPl. Neurons from GPl innervate the STN, which sends fibers to the GPm/SNr. The third pathway consists of axons that originate from patches of SP-containing spiny neurons in the striatum. This pathway terminates in the SNc. These axons are not collaterals of the axons that terminate in the GPm/SNr but are an anatomically and physio-

logically separate group. The dopaminergic SNc neurons project back to the striatum.

### Efferent Connections

The main source of axons leaving the basal ganglia is the GPm/SNr (Fig. 8.4). The efferent axons of the GPm/SNr terminate in the ventral

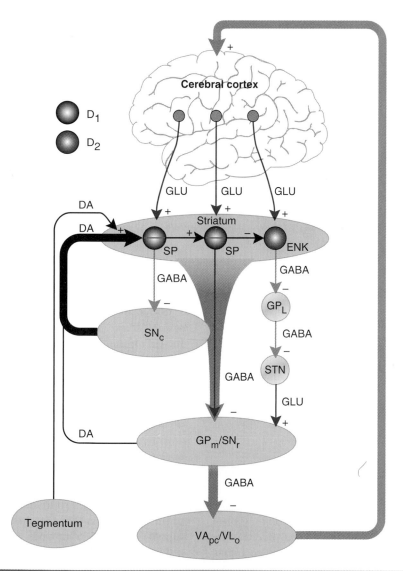

### Figure 8.7   Normal connections in the basal ganglia

The principal connections of the basal ganglia indicating the probable neurotransmitters and their apparent action (facilitation or inhibition). The *dark spheres* within the striatum are patches within the matrix. *GLU*, glutamate; *SP*, substance P; *ENK*, enkephalin; *GABA*, γ-aminobutyric acid; *DA*, dopamine; *SN*$_c$, substantia nigra pars compacta; *SN*$_r$, substantia nigra pars reticulata; *GP*$_L$, globus pallidus lateralis; *GP*$_m$, globus pallidus medialis; *VA*$_{pc}$, ventral anterior parvocellular; *VL*$_O$, ventral lateral oralis; *D*$_1$ and *D*$_2$ are two families of dopamine receptors. (Modified from Albin RL. The functional anatomy of basal ganglia disorders. Trends in Neurosci 1989;12:366–375.)

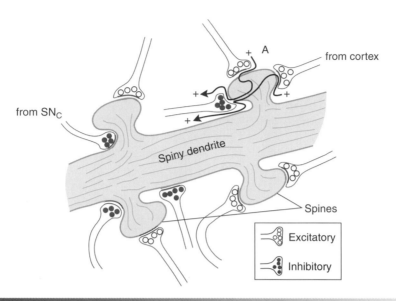

**Figure 8.8   Inhibition on dendritic spines**

The spines on dendrites not only greatly increase the surface area of the dendrite and thus the number of synapses it can receive but also can act as miniature dendrites themselves. Excitatory synapses, typically originating in the cortex, make contact on the heads of the spines of spiny neurons in the striatum. Inhibitory synapses (typically from SN$_c$) contact the necks of the spines. *Arrows* (spine A) indicate how the excitatory current is short-circuited. *SN$_C$*, substantia nigra pars compacta.

anterior parvocellular (VA$_{PC}$) and ventral lateral pars oralis (VL$_O$), specific thalamic nuclei that project primarily to the supplementary motor area (SMA) (area 6) and M-I (area 4) of the cerebral cortex (see Fig. 7.9). The GPm/SNr also sends efferent fibers to the superior colliculus and the brainstem reticular formation. These neurons are inhibitory (GABA). The neurotransmitters of the thalamocortical neurons are not known, but they are excitatory to the cerebral cortex.

## THE NEUROLOGY OF THE BASAL GANGLIA

The basal ganglia have great neurological importance because several common diseases have been correlated with specific lesions to this area. Damage to the basal ganglia produces movement disorders, or **dyskinesia** [G. *dys,* bad, and *kinesis,* movement]. Dyskinesia, a motor disorder that entails some loss of voluntary control and regulation, falls into two classes: those that result in spontaneous movements, or **hyperkinesia**, and those that result in

poverty of movement, or **hypokinesia.** Hyperkinesia is expressed as *involuntary spontaneous movements.* Hypokinesia causes the opposite effect, *the lack of spontaneous movements and a slowing of voluntary movement.* It is important to note that the motor system is otherwise intact, as are the knowledge and will to initiate and perform the motor act.

Dyskinesia differs from paralysis and paresis in two major respects. First, unlike paralysis or paresis, dyskinesia involves no dysfunction of the upper or lower motor neuron systems. Consequently, there is no weakness. Second, dyskinesia is not apraxia, the inability to plan or execute a complex motor act. Apraxia follows a lesion to the cerebral cortex and affects one's ability to conceptualize the task.

### Hyperkinetic Dyskinesia

Several clinical terms are used to describe involuntary spontaneous movements: **chorea, athetosis, dystonia, ballismus,** and **tic.** Although the terms imply discrete pathophysiological phenomena, recent research suggests that because all hyperkinesias arise from a common set of basal ganglia lesions, these terms actually signify variations of a single phenomenon.

Chorea [G. *choros,* dance] is a continuing series of rapid, jerky involuntary movements that are *fragments of purposeful movement.* For example, one's arm may suddenly abduct; this sudden abduction is actually a fragment of a more complex act of abduction and extension that occurs when reaching for an object. The motion is without conscious intention; it is spontaneous. People with chorea find the sudden spontaneous movement of an extremity extremely disconcerting. To cover the embarrassing moment, they may consciously incorporate the spontaneous movement into a purposeful act, such as adjusting their glasses. Although their constant activity may seem fairly normal to the casual observer, such people appear very restless. Chorea has been associated with atrophy of the striatum.

Athetosis [G. *athetos,* without position or place] is continual uncontrolled writhing. One spontaneous movement blends into the next, creating constant sinuous and purposeless motion. These spontaneous movements usually involve the hands and face, but all parts of the body can be affected. The movements are frequently combinations of alternating antagonistic motions, such as supination and pronation, flexion and extension, or inversion and eversion. Athetosis is an extension of chorea. Chorea consists of discrete, independent movements. As choreiform movements become more frequent, they may progress and take on the slower, more continual form of athetosis. This progression is common in Huntington's disease (discussed later in the chapter). In such cases, the term **choreoathetosis** is applied.

Dystonia [G. *tonos,* tension] is another type of involuntary movement. Its most extreme form, **idiopathic torsion dystonia** [G. *idios,* distinct, and *pathos,* disease; L. *torsio,* twist] (ITD) is a severe type of athetosis. Joints are forced into a locked position for a long period by extreme contraction of antagonist muscle groups. A fixed abnormal posture caused by continuous isometric muscle contraction may result. Al-

ternatively, various muscle groups may go into and out of spasms. The extreme tension with which the antagonistic groups work against each other forces the body into contorted positions. Because no gross central nervous system (CNS) lesions are detectable, most authorities assume that the lesion is a biochemical deficiency in the striatum.

The first signs of ITD begin to appear in childhood and relentlessly progress for 5 to 10 years, eventually leading to total disability for most patients. Most cases of ITD are inherited as an autosomal dominant gene (9q34) with a penetrance of about 0.3 to 0.4.

Adult-onset forms of dystonia present very differently. The most common form, **spasmodic torticollis**, is characterized by bizarre involuntary movements of the head and neck. Other forms involve involuntary movements of the orofacial musculature, which may be expressed as a forced closure of the eyelids, forced protrusion of the tongue, involuntary tooth grinding, or even spasms of the vocal cords.

Ballismus [G. *ballismos,* jumping about] is a violent involuntary movement of the proximal muscles that results in a flinging of the extremities. This dramatic but self-limiting condition evolves into a form of chorea or athetosis. Ballismus is caused by a discrete lesion to the STN contralateral to the affected side. The STN is excitatory to the GPm/SNr; therefore, its loss decreases the facilitation of GPm/SNr (Fig. 8.9). Since the GPm/SNr is inhibitory to the ventral lateral thalamus, loss of the subthalamic nucleus *disinhibits* the thalamus. Its facilitation of the motor cortex thus increases, resulting in the ballistic movements.

Tics [F. *tic,* convulsive] are a type of uncontrollable compulsive behavior. Like the movements of chorea, tics are quick fragments of a purposeful movement. They differ from chorea in that they are endlessly repeated in a stereotyped manner. Whereas chorea consists of many different randomly interspersed acts, tics are almost always repetitions of the same movement. Tics include sniffing, throat clearing, blinking, snorting, or even involuntary vocalizations. In Gilles de la Tourette syndrome, the spontaneous involuntary vocalizations can take the form of barking or swearing.

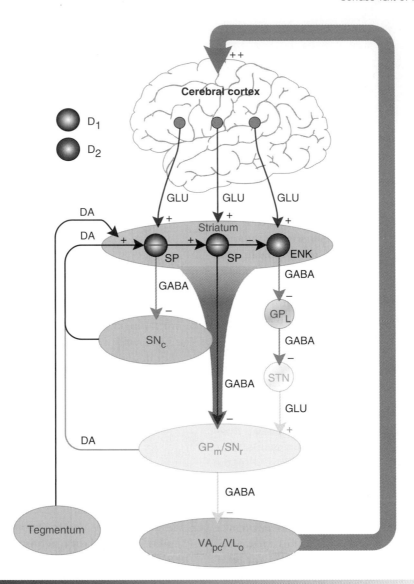

**Figure 8.9   Ballismus**

Hyperkinetic dyskinesia is thought to entail the functional removal of the STN from the basal ganglia circuitry. Removal of STN disfacilitates the GPm/SNr, which in turn disinhibits the $VA_{PC}$ and $VL_O$, freeing them to overstimulate the motor areas of the cortex. Abbreviations as in Figure 8.7. (Modified from Albin et al. Trends Neurosci 1989;12.)

## Hypokinetic Dyskinesia

Only one term, **bradykinesia** [G. *bradys,* slow], is used to describe the hypokinetic movement disorder. Bradykinesia is characterized by *poverty and slowness of movement.* Patients maintain a fixed posture for unusually long periods. The normal, restless shifting of one's posture and normal general fidgeting are reduced or absent. The facial expression is gaunt and fixed. The eyes seldom blink. When the patient walks, the arms do not swing. Patients with advanced disease have difficulty initiating even the most routine acts, such as rising from a chair. They have difficulty stopping when walking and often bump into furniture or walls. Even spontaneous swallowing is diminished, causing drooling, since the production of saliva remains undiminished. The principal hypokinetic disease is Parkinson's disease, discussed later in the chapter.

## DISEASES OF THE BASAL GANGLIA

Several specific diseases are associated with each of the involuntary movements. The most common are discussed next.

### Huntington's Disease

In 1872 George Huntington, a physician, reported on families living in eastern Long Island that he, his father, and his grandfather had treated. All of these families had members who shared the symptoms of **dementia**—the diminution of cognitive function due to organic brain disease—and chorea. The patients had no symptoms at birth. In middle age they developed peculiar personality changes and choreiform movements. Their symptoms progressed until they became incapacitated and died. All of these patients had a parent who displayed the same symptoms. Now known as **Huntington's disease** (HD), this condition is the most common of the hyperkinetic disorders known to originate from a defect in the basal ganglia.

In about half of patients with HD, dementia precedes the development of involuntary movements. The initial mental manifestations of the disease, when present, are alterations in personality. Patients may become irritable, impulsive, depressed, or violent. Later the patient may develop obvious dementia characterized by memory lapses and decreased attentiveness that progresses until the patient is incapacitated. Suicide is frequent, possibly because of the mental illness associated with the disease.

The choreiform movements associated with HD usually affect the hands and face first. Early in the course of the disease patients can mask the spontaneous movements by incorporating them into socially acceptable intentional acts. To the casual observer the patient may appear unusually fidgety or restless. As the disease progresses, more of the body becomes involved. Eventually the patient is in constant motion. At the terminal stages of HD, the chorea evolves into athetosis or dystonia.

### PATHOLOGY

The most consistent pathological finding in HD is a gross wasting of the caudate and putamen nuclei. This finding can be visualized with computed tomography (CT) or magnetic resonance imaging (MRI) (Fig. 8.10) as an enlargement of the lateral ventricles due to the atrophy of the caudate. The loss of striatal mass is

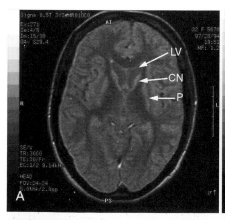 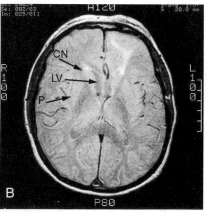

## Figure 8.10   MRI findings in HD

**A.** Proton density MRI of a patient with HD. Note the large lateral ventricles and the thin, atrophied head of the caudate nucleus and putamen. The putamen does not have its normal triangular shape. **B.** Proton density MRI from a normal patient. The head of the caudate is much fuller and the lateral ventricle is thinner and more wedge shaped than in **A.** The putamen is large and triangular. *LV,* lateral ventricle; *CN,* caudate nucleus; *P,* putamen. (MR images courtesy of the Magnetic Imaging Center, South Bend, IN.)

closely correlated with the development of involuntary movements. The ENK spiny neuron patches of the striatum are the most affected, at least in the early stages of the disease (Fig. 8.11). Their loss removes the striatal inhibition from the GPl, which increases the inhibition of the subthalamic nucleus. These changes effectively remove the STN from the circuitry of the basal ganglia, abolishing its facilitation of the

GPm/SNr. As with ballismus, these events disinhibit the ventral lateral thalamus (see discussion of ballismus, p. 295).

Also associated with HD is loss of neurons in the cerebral cortex, especially neurons from layer 3. Loss of these neurons results in some decrease in cortical mass and a widening of the gyri, which can usually be visualized with MRI. This cortical atrophy is much less strik-

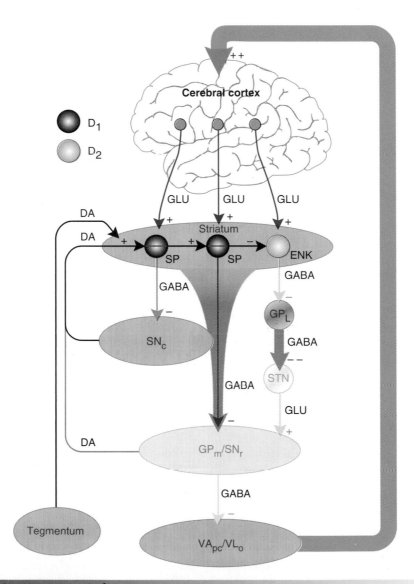

**Figure 8.11   Huntington's disease**

Degeneration of striatal enkephalinergic neurons. Their loss removes inhibition from the GP$_L$, which profoundly inhibits the STN, effectively removing it from the circuit, much as in ballismus (Fig. 8.9). Abbreviations as in Figure 8.7. (Modified from Albin RL. The functional anatomy of basal ganglia disorders. Trends in Neurosci 1989; 12.366–375.)

ing than the striatal atrophy seen in HD. In fact, it is so slight that it apparently cannot fully account for the mental changes associated with the disease.

Other types of dementia, such as Alzheimer's disease, are associated with profound cortical atrophy; they manifest certain mental disturbances not commonly associated with HD. For example, patients with Alzheimer's disease typically exhibit severe memory losses, a decrease in language and calculation skills, apraxia, and agnosia. HD patients are usually spared these difficulties. They are more likely to undergo personality changes, simple forgetfulness, apathy, depression, and generally slowed thought processes. These differences have led some researchers to suggest that HD produces subcortical dementia and Alzheimer's disease, cortical dementia. The concept of subcortical dementia implies sparing of the cerebral cortex, an implication that is not absolutely correct, since MRI and autopsy material consistently demonstrate cortical thinning in HD. Nevertheless, the term also implies that the basal ganglia play an important role in cognitive function. This implication correlates well with anatomy. The head of the caudate nucleus and the accumbens nucleus make numerous connections with the frontal lobes of the cerebral cortex. Therefore, atrophy of the head of the caudate can be expected to impair frontal lobe cortical function. For these reasons, distinctions between cortical and subcortical dementia are probably useful.

## ETIOLOGY

HD is caused by a mutation of the huntingtin gene on chromosome 4 (4p16.3). The mutation is expressed as an autosomal dominant disease. Approximately half of the children of an affected parent can be expected to be develop the disease (disease frequency 4 to 7 per 100,000). A study conducted in 1932 showed that nearly all affected people in the eastern United States were the progeny of 6 persons who emigrated to the New World in 1630 from a single village in Suffolk, England. Spontaneous mutations are apparently quite rare. A 1915 study of 962 patients with HD found that only 5 were thought to be de-

scended from unaffected parents and might be spontaneous mutations.

In most persons the disease is first recognized about age 35 to 40; however, various forms may manifest as early as age 4 and as late as age 70. The disease progresses until death occurs 10 to 15 years after the first symptoms appear. Because of the relatively late onset, most persons do not know that they are affected until after their reproductive years, which ensures the transmission of the gene to the next generation.

The huntingtin gene contains a repeating series of CAG nucleotide sequences. The number of repeats ranges between about 9 and 35 in normal individuals (mean, 19). A longer repetition of the sequence results in expression of HD (mean, 46 repeats). The age of onset of symptoms is inversely correlated with the length of the $(CAG)_n$ repeat, which explains the great variation in the age at which symptoms first appear.

The number of $(CAG)_n$ repeats is not passed on faithfully from one generation to the next. In normal persons (fewer than 35 repetitions), the $(CAG)_n$ length is quite stable. However, with increasing $(CAG)_n$ length, the gene becomes more unstable, and a greater number of repeats are passed on to the next generation. This instability is particularly evident when the gene is passed through the male gamete. Hence HD exhibits the phenomenon of **anticipation**, in which succeeding generations are affected at an earlier age than the parent, especially if the father is the affected parent. Thus the length of the $(CAG)_n$ sequence determines not only the age of disease expression but also the probability that the expansion will be increased in the next generation.

The huntingtin protein is expressed in normal persons, but its function is unknown. In animal models embryos fail to develop if the protein is absent. HD thus indicates a gain of function of the gene. The mechanism by which the defective huntingtin protein affects the nervous system is not known, but some speculation is appropriate. The CAG nucleotide sequence codes for glutamine, so the defective huntingtin protein contains a polyglutamine region. Polyglutamines can form cross-linkages with other proteins, a reaction that is catalyzed by transglutaminases (TGase). One of the proteins with which polyglutamines can cross-react is tubulin. Huntingtin has been shown to be closely associated with microtubules, suggesting that the defective protein may interfere with intracellular transport. Furthermore, TGase activity is greater than normal in people with HD, and its activity increases with age. This increase approximates the course of the disease. In normal persons TGase activity decreases with age. It has been postulated that long polyglutamate stretches are better substrates for TGase than short ones; if true, this finding would help to explain how the length of the $(CAG)_n$ sequence affects the age of onset of HD symptoms.

## Parkinsonism

Approximately 1% of the U.S. population over age 50 has parkinsonism, which James Parkinson described in 1817. The disease that now carries his name usually begins between ages 40 and 70. If untreated, Parkinson's disease (PD) progresses inexorably to death in about 10 to 15 years. PD is characterized by three signs: **bradykinesia, tremor,** and **rigidity.**

Perhaps the most prominent feature of PD is the 4- to 7-Hz tremor that almost always accompanies the disease. The tremor may begin in any extremity, and once begun, it tends to spread to the others. In the hand the tremor is quite characteristic, involving an alternating pattern of the thumb and fingers rubbing together. The more senior members of the neuroscience community say that it reminds them of ancient pharmacists making pills by rolling the ingredients between the thumb and fingers, so it is often called pill-rolling tremor. The tremor is seen only while the extremity is at rest; it disappears during intentional movement and sleep.

Although the tremor is the most noticeable and perhaps the most emotionally disturbing aspect of the disease for the patient and family members, bradykinesia is the most debilitating. The bradykinesia of PD is a true slowing of movement. All movement by the parkinsonism patient is reduced to the same slow velocity. When reaching for objects at various distances, normal persons increase the velocity of the movement as the distance increases. The parkinsonism patient, however, cannot increase the velocity of movement. The duration extends as the distance increases (Fig. 8.12). The parkinsonism patient is operating in slow motion.

Parkinsonism patients exhibit **rigidity,** a special type of resistance to passive movement of the limbs. Rigidity is a specific symptom that should not be confused with spasticity (see Chapter 7). To the physician, passively moving the patient's rigid limb feels like bending a lead pipe, which has led to the term **lead pipe rigidity.** The tremor can be felt superimposed on the rigidity, giving the sensation of two gears loosely meshing as each cog makes contact. The term **cogwheel rigidity** has evolved from this colorful description. Both

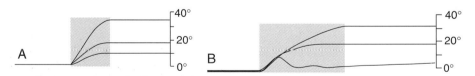

### Figure 8.12   Hypokinesia in Parkinson's disease

Parkinson's disease is hypokinetic dyskinesia. It results in overall slowing of muscle action. When moving an extremity, a normal person increases the velocity of muscle contraction as the distance moved increases, so that the total action takes place in approximately the same amount of time regardless of distance moved. In a person with PD, the contraction velocity remains constant. These graphs show elbow joint position following a flexion of 10, 20, and 40° in a normal person (**A**) and in a person with PD (**B**). The slope changes for each trial in the normal person but remains fairly constant in the PD patient, so that movement over the greatest distance takes much longer to complete than movement over a shorter distance. (Data from Hallett M, Khoshbin S. A physiological mechanism of bradykinesia. Brain 1980;103: 301–314.)

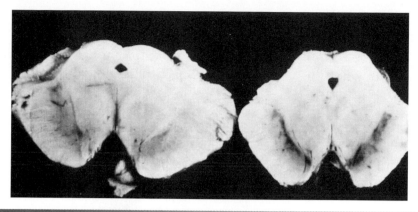

**Figure 8.13   Parkinson's disease pathology**

Loss of the pigmented cells of the substantia nigra in parkinsonism demonstrated at autopsy. Mesencephalon from PD patient (**left**) has very little color in the SN compared with the normal mesencephalon (**right**). (Reprinted with permission from Rowland LP. Merritt's Textbook of Neurology. 8th ed. Philadelphia: Lea & Febiger, 1989;659.)

terms are used to describe the rigidity of the parkinsonism patient.

Dementia is an inconsistent finding in parkinsonism. One study found that 32% of patients with PD had dementia; another, only 8%. Unquestionably, some parkinsonism patients have dementia, and MRI can demonstrate white matter lesions in most of these patients. It is not clear whether the dementia is caused by the same factors that cause PD or is an independent development. The number of patients exhibiting the characteristics of both PD and Alzheimer's disease (a specific type of dementia that is discussed in a later chapter) is higher than would be predicted by chance alone. However, no causal relation between PD and dementia has been established.

## PATHOLOGY

The most consistent pathological finding in patients with PD is the loss of the pigmented cells in the SNc (Fig. 8.13). Loss of these cells is accompanied by depletion of other pigmented cells of the CNS, the locus ceruleus, and the dorsal motor nucleus of the vagus. Because the SNc cells produce dopamine, SNc neurons facilitate the SP-containing spiny neurons of the striatum by acting through $D_1$ receptors. The loss of this facilitation reduces the inhibition of GPm/SNr neurons, increasing their firing rate. Since the

GPm/SNR neurons inhibit the ventral lateral thalamus, this nucleus is greatly inhibited (Fig. 8.14). As a result, the thalamic drive is removed from the motor cortex, producing hypokinesia.

In addition to facilitating the SP spiny neurons ($D_1$ receptors), the SNc dopamine pathway inhibits the ENK spiny neurons by acting through $D_2$ receptors. Removing this inhibition increases the inhibition of the GPL neurons, which decreases their firing rate. Decreasing the firing rate of the GPL neurons disinhibits the STN. Released in this way, the STN's facilitation of the GPm/SNr is increased. This inhibits the ventral lateral thalamus, hence removing thalamic drive to the motor cortex, which as discussed earlier, produces hypokinesia.

## ETIOLOGY

In 1817, when first described, PD appeared to be a single process with specific diagnostic criteria. Today, however, the picture is less clear. Many cases that resemble PD have a known cause. Nonidiopathic cases frequently respond differently to drug treatment and have a different clinical course from that of idiopathic PD. Other cases resemble PD and are idiopathic but have additional features that set them apart from true PD. For example, progressive supranuclear ophthalmoplegia is characterized by bradykinesia plus paralysis of the ex-

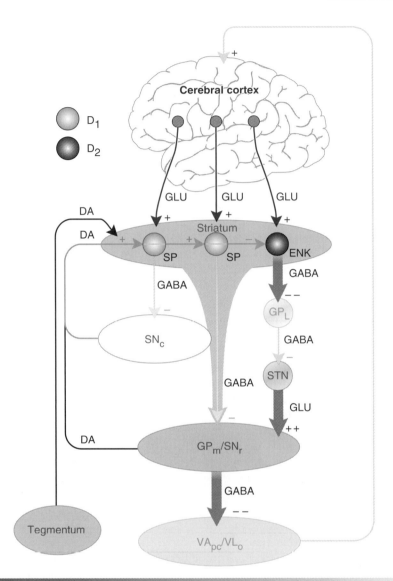

**Figure 8.14   Parkinson's disease**

Parkinsonism, a form of hypokinetic dyskinesia, is caused by loss of neurons in the SNc. Abbreviations as in Figure 8.7. (Modified from Albin RL. The functional anatomy of basal ganglia disorders. Trends in Neurosci 1989; 12:366–375.)

traocular eye muscles that is not related to the nuclei of ocular motion. This disease is often misdiagnosed as PD, but it is unresponsive to L-dopa treatment and has a much more malignant course. It appears that a number of disease processes include degeneration of the pigmented cells of the substantia nigra and the resulting clinical symptoms of bradykinesia and tremor. Since the prognosis and treatment of these variants is different from that of idio-

pathic PD, it is important to avoid labeling all of them as PD. The terms **parkinsonism** and **parkinsonian syndrome** with appropriate qualifications are gaining favor. The term PD, or **primary parkinsonism,** is reserved for the idiopathic form that has no complicating signs.

The cause of spontaneous SNc degeneration—PD, or primary parkinsonism—has yet to be identified. The parkinsonian syndrome can develop after various types of brain injury. **Head trauma**, particularly associated with prize fighting, is one of the preventable causes of parkinsonism. In one study 50% of professional boxers near the end of their career were diagnosed with punch-drunk encephalopathy, a syndrome that frequently includes parkinsonian symptoms.

**Encephalitis lethargica**, an influenza pandemic that enveloped the world between 1914 and 1930, has special importance in the history of PD. This deadly disease killed about 20% of those infected. Throughout the world more people died of this disease than in the hostilities of World War I. During the acute phase of the illness many patients exhibited symptoms now attributable to disease of the basal ganglia, including bradykinesia and chorea. A large number of survivors developed a form of parkinsonism a few months to 25 years after recovering from the infection. Encephalitis lethargica has not been seen in the United States since about 1930, but other forms of encephalitis and influenza are occasionally associated with parkinsonism. Although there is no evidence that ordinary influenza viruses cause parkinsonism, certainly it is possible that some viruses may selectively attack SNc neurons, much as the polio virus selectively attacks the α-motor neuron.

Certain toxins injure the brain in a way that produces parkinsonlike symptoms. Most notable are **carbon monoxide** and **manganese** poisoning. Recently a designer street drug, MPTP,[4] was accidentally produced in an illicit kitchen laboratory. Those who were exposed to the drug developed profound akinesia. It has been shown that this drug destroys nearly all the pigmented neurons in the SNc of primates and humans. The toxic agent is not MPTP itself, but a metabolite, MPP$^+$,[5] which specifically interferes with complex I of the electron transport chain in the mitochondria and thereby prevents the production of adenosine triphosphate (ATP). Without ATP the cell soon dies. MPTP is the first known neurotoxic agent that is specific to SNc neurons. Its conversion to MPP$^+$ apparently occurs only in the SN. This discovery supports the hypothesis that toxic agents can produce parkinsonism in humans.

Although no infectious or genetic cause has been consistently associated with primary parkinsonism, some researchers hypothesize that primary parkinsonism is an environmental disease caused by a number of possible toxins, particularly those that can be metabolized into reactive oxidative species (ROS). This hypothesis can be summarized as follows: (a) approximately 50% of the pigmented neurons in the SNc disappear in humans during the normal course of aging, but despite this loss, few people show signs of parkinsonism; (b) people who develop parkinsonism have lost approximately 66% of the pigmented neurons; (c) consequently, there is only a small safety factor in the number of neurons needed for normal function in the SNc throughout life; and (d) contact with a toxic agent, such as ROS, that kills as few as 15% of the SNc neurons during one's youth reduces the overall cell population enough that in later years too few neurons remain for normal function, resulting in parkinsonism.

As yet, no single toxic agent or group of toxins that can explain the high incidence of this disease has been identified. Furthermore, there are difficulties with the hypothesis. For example, it does not explain the higher incidence of the disease in whites (two to four times that of nonwhite races). Nor does it explain the relatively constant incidence of parkinsonism throughout the world. If environmental toxic agents were the cause of the disease, one would not expect a constant toxic exposure in all societies. Many important questions remain unanswered.

## TREATMENT

Once the connection between depletion of dopamine-producing cells and parkinsonian symptoms was made, replacement of the missing dopamine seemed a logical treatment. Since dopamine does not cross the blood-

---

[4] n-Methyl-4-phenyl-1,2,3,6-tetrahydropyridine.
[5] 1-Methyl-4-phenyl pyridine.

brain barrier, its precursor, L-dopa, is administered systemically. L-Dopa is converted to dopamine by cells in the SN. This treatment ameliorates symptoms in about 80% of patients (Fig. 8.15).

A second approach to treatment is to provide dopamine agonists rather than dopamine itself. A number of specific agonists of $D_2$ receptors are now being used clinically with good results. These dopamine agonists inhibit the ENK-containing striatal neurons and thereby facilitate the inhibitory striatonigral pathway (Fig. 8.14). They have the theoretical advantage over dopamine of not stimulating the $D_1$ receptors associated with the SP-containing striatal neurons. Traditional L-dopa treatment presumably stimulates both types of receptors.

A third form of treatment is reduction of the catabolism of dopamine. Dopamine is catabolized by monoamine oxidase-B (MAO-B).

Blockage of MAO-B maintains higher concentrations of dopamine in the synaptic cleft.

The catabolism of dopamine also produces the ROS hydrogen peroxide as a byproduct. ROSs damage cells by oxidizing proteins, membrane lipids, and DNA. Abnormally high concentrations of ROSs can also activate the permeability transition pore in the mitochondrial inner membrane, increasing the permeability of the inner mitochondrial membrane to water. As a result, water enters the matrix and causes the mitochondria to swell. The swelling disrupts the mitochondrial membranes, which increases the porosity of the outer mitochondrial membrane, allowing cytochrome $c$ to leave the mitochondria and enter the cytoplasm.

In the cytoplasm cytochrome $c$ initiates a biochemical cascade known as **apoptosis** [G. falloff, fr. *apo,* off, and *ptosis,* fall]. Apoptosis, or programed cell death, can be initiated by either intracellular or extracellular events. The induction of apoptosis by ROSs appears to be an important mechanism in a number of neurodegenerative diseases. Many investigators believe that apoptosis may be involved in Alzheimer's disease, PD, and perhaps HD and amyotrophic lateral sclerosis. It has been hypothesized that in PD peroxidases are deficient, which allows the concentration of hydrogen peroxide and possibly other ROSs to exceed normal levels, triggering apoptosis. If this hypothesis is correct, MAO-B inhibitors should slow the progression of the disease, and recent clinical trials have confirmed this prediction.

L-Dopa treatment and MAO inhibition do not curtail the relentless loss of nigral neurons. Despite treatment, the disease progresses. Eventually treatment becomes less effective and ultimately fails. The patients become immobilized to the point of confinement to bed, and they eventually succumb to *complications of the bedfast state.*[6] Before L-dopa therapy, primary parkinsonism caused death or severe disability in about 25% of patients within 5 years of the initial diagnosis.

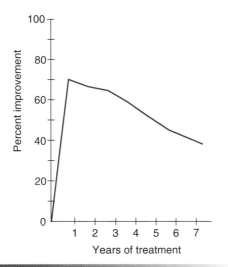

**Figure 8.15  Effectiveness of L-dopa therapy in parkinsonism**

The amount of improvement in parkinsonism symptoms with L-dopa treatment declines with duration of treatment. (Data from Rowland LP. Merritt's Textbook of Neurology. 8th ed. Philadelphia: Lea & Febiger, 1989;670.)

---

[6] Many neurological diseases such as parkinsonism are not fatal per se but immobilize the patient to the point that complications of immobility bring on death. These complications include pulmonary infections secondary to the aspiration of mucus or saliva, pulmonary congestion, urinary tract infections, and infections from decubitus sores.

About 80% died within 15 years. L-Dopa therapy reduces mortality by about 50%.

It is remarkable that L-dopa therapy is effective. It is still not known how flooding a system as complicated as the brain with L-dopa approximates the natural release of dopamine at synaptic boutons in the striatum. The answer may lie in the observation that the firing of SNc cells does not correlate with any of the dynamic parameters of muscle movement. Alterations in firing rate tend to be much slower than any motor act. This observation has led to the hypothesis that dopamine may act as a neurohumoral agent or modulator of overall striatal excitability. If this hypothesis is correct, systemic administration of L-Dopa could be expected to perform the same function, albeit crudely.

# C A S E    H I S T O R Y

## THE CASE OF THE GREAT STONE FACE

### HISTORY OF PRESENT ILLNESS

Mrs. A. R. is a 64-year-old woman who grew up in New Hampshire before moving to Indiana. She said the left side of her body felt weak and awkward. She has had a tremor for several years, but recently the tremor has been so bad that she went to her family doctor. He sought a neurology consultation because he thought she had had a stroke. She says she feels stiff all over and is having trouble initiating ambulation. She blinks rarely, and her granddaughter jokingly calls her the great stone face.

### MEDICAL HISTORY

Four years ago Mrs. A. R. developed a tremor in her left hand. Over a few months the tremor spread to her left leg. She said she did not have the flu during the great flu epidemic of the 1920s. She had no known occupational or social exposure to toxic levels of carbon monoxide, manganese, carbon disulfide, or MPTP. She had never been treated with phenothiazines, reserpine, haloperidol, or similar drugs. There is no history of neurological disease in her family.

## NEUROLOGICAL EXAMINATION, 1992

### Mental Status

She is alert, witty, and conversant. She is oriented to time and place. She can do serial subtractions by 7 and knows the U.S. presidents back to George Washington. There are no memory deficits.

### Cranial Nerves

All cranial nerve functions are within normal limits. Although her voice is very soft, there is no indication of hoarseness. The extraocular movements are full, symmetrical, and well coordinated.

### Station and Gait

Her countenance is expressionless, even when involved in animated conversation or telling a joke. She does not adjust her posture or make many subconscious movements when sitting in a chair. When standing, she is stooped and holds her arms slightly adducted and flexed. She has a shuffling gait and does not swing her arms while walking. On turning, she stands in one place and shuffles her feet, turning about on a single spot as if standing on a pedestal (**pedestal turning**). All of her movements are slow and deliberate.

### Motor Systems

STRENGTH: Strength is +5 everywhere.

TONE: There is a well-developed cogwheel rigidity in both arms and legs. She is somewhat more rigid on the left side than on the right; there is no sign of spasticity or clonus.

BULK: There is no atrophy.

ABNORMAL MOVEMENTS: There is an obvious 3- to 5-Hz resting tremor in all extremities. The left side is worse than the right side. During voluntary movements, the tremor decreases or even disappears. There are no fasciculations.

## Sensory Systems
Her perception of pinprick and cotton touches are symmetrical and within normal limits.

## Reflexes
MSRs are all within normal limits and symmetrical. Plantar signs are flexor.

## Coordination and Control
Not tested.

## Parietal Functions
The optokinetic reflex (OKN) is present to both the left and right. There is no aphasia or neglect.

## COMMENTARY

The history and physical appearance of this patient provide enough evidence for a diagnosis of parkinsonism. The patient's initial complaint is a tremor in the hands that progressed over several years. The neurological examination provides further corroborative evidence: cogwheel rigidity, shuffling gait, and slowing of spontaneous movements. The essential features of the parkinsonian state (bradykinesia, resting tremor, cogwheel rigidity, stooped posture with shuffling gait) are all well developed in this patient.

Once the initial diagnosis of parkinsonism is made, the patient should be questioned about possible causative factors, such as viral infections and exposure to carbon monoxide, manganese, or carbon disulfide. Eliminating causative and hereditary factors and observing the normal extraocular eye movements leads to the diagnosis of primary parkinsonism.

## SUBSEQUENT COURSE

Mrs. A. R. is taking a drug (Sinemet) that combines **carbidopa** and L-dopa in a single pill. Carbidopa is a decarboxylase inhibitor that does not cross the blood-brain barrier. It prevents the conversion of L-dopa to dopamine in the systemic circulation while allowing the conversion to take place in the cerebral circulation. This combination has greatly reduced the side effects associated with L-dopa alone. Mrs. A. R. is doing well. Her general motor performance is slower than normal, but she is able to walk unassisted and perform all of the activities of daily living. She is living independently and has an active social life.

## FURTHER APPLICATIONS

8.1.  Consider the criteria for the diagnosis of stroke. Are there any elements of this case that legitimately lead one to a diagnosis of stroke?

8.2.  Mrs. A. R. is not likely to have come into contact with MPTP, and inquiring about use of this drug in the history is mostly a matter of ritual on the part of the physician. However, the other chemicals may be significant to the history. Which of the substances mentioned in this case history would affect the diagnosis if the patient were exposed to them?

8.3.  L-Dopa treatment eventually fails to be effective in parkinsonism. Consider various hypotheses that may account for this failure. Would the mechanisms of L-dopa failure that you identify preclude the effectiveness of dopa agonists or MAO inhibitors?

8.4.  What side effects of L-dopa administration are alleviated by the coadministration of carbidopa?

# C A S E    H I S T O R Y

## THE CASE OF THE MEDICAL MERRY-GO-ROUND[7]

### HISTORY OF PRESENT ILLNESS

Ms. T. L. has a long history of rigidity that has recently kept her bedfast. Two days ago, after her family physician prescribed metoclopramide (Reglan) for a hiatal hernia, her condition immediately worsened. She became rigid to the point of nearly total immobility. She can no longer even turn the pages of a book. She is having great difficulty chewing, swallowing, talking, and breathing. The metoclopramide has been discontinued, but her condition has not improved. Recognizing the relation between metoclopramide and basal ganglia disease, her family physician, with great difficulty, persuaded her to see a neurologist at a major university medical center in another state. Having been through extensive neurological diagnoses twice before, she has entered the hospital very reluctantly, feeling that she will "end up in either a nursing home or a cemetery."

### MEDICAL HISTORY

Ms. T. L. is a 42-year-old woman who first began to have neurological problems when she was 4 years old. At that time she had trouble with her balance and fell down frequently. She was generally poorly coordinated. By age 5 her condition had worsened. Her left leg was quite rigid, and she held it almost constantly in a hyperextended position. Her other extremities were also somewhat rigid, but the left leg was worst. A spinal puncture was performed and analysis of the cerebral spinal fluid produced normal findings. She wore braces so she could walk in school.

By age 8 her rigidity had worsened and she was having more difficulty walking, and surgery was performed on her ankle to "stabilize" it. An electromyogram was read as normal. At age 13 she had such severe rigidity in both of her legs that she was walking only on her toes; she could not flex her feet at the ankle. Surgery to lengthen both Achilles tendons allowed her to walk somewhat better. Her condition progressed, however, so that by the time she entered high school, she was confined to a wheelchair.

She graduated from high school and entered college. Her condition continued to deteriorate, and she was forced to withdraw from school. She was referred to a specialty clinic, where she underwent a complete neurological examination. No diagnosis was made, and she was referred to a neurological team at a major university medical center. After another neurological evaluation the team concluded that her problem was a psychiatric illness and advised her to seek psychotherapy, which she did (1971).

The psychotherapy made her feel responsible for her problems. She was told that she "just wasn't trying hard enough." Her mother, her principal caregiver at the time, was told to "quit helping your daughter so much. She will never get better until she has to do things for herself." The psychotherapy brought on depression followed by feelings of anger, bitterness, and hostility toward the medical community. She removed herself from the "medical merry-go-round" and sought medical attention only for routine physical conditions. At that time (1971) she had no neurological diagnosis for her condition.

By 1991 she was essentially bedfast. For the past 4 years she has been attended by nurses from a local home care facility. She was very rigid. Her hands were continuously flexed and

[7] I am grateful to Dr. S. R. White for bringing this case to my attention.

her arms pronated and extended. Her legs were locked in extension. She could not tend to her personal hygiene or dress herself. She could read, watch television, and converse on the telephone. Her symptoms were somewhat milder in the mornings but progressed as the day wore on. By evening she was nonfunctional. During sleep her rigidity decreased significantly.

In accordance with this medical history, the attending neurologist immediately prescribed carbidopa/L-dopa. Within a few hours her rigidity waned slightly but noticeably. A week later she was mobile enough to enter physical therapy, and 6 weeks after entering the hospital and initiating L-dopa therapy, she went home. For the first time in her memory she was independent in her personal care. After 9 months she was walking normally, had obtained a driver's license, and had a job as an office manager at the home care facility that had provided her with nursing care for the previous 4 years.

## NEUROLOGICAL EXAMINATION, MARCH 1993

### Mental Status
Ms. T. L. is an animated, articulate, and very pleasant person who is able to give a full and detailed history. She is oriented to person, place, and time.

### Cranial Nerves
All tested within normal limits.

### Station and Gait
She walks with an awkward but safe gait. She lifts her feet very high as she walks. She has a substantial foot drop. She gestures quite noticeably with her hands and arms as she talks.

### Motor Systems
All four of her extremities seem loose and a little floppy as she walks or gestures. There are no dystonic movements.

### Sensory Systems
Perception to pinprick and cotton is symmetrical and everywhere intact.

### Reflexes
All MSRs are normal. Plantar signs are flexor.

### Coordination and Control
Not tested.

### Parietal Functions
Not tested.

## ANCILLARY STUDIES

MRI revealed no abnormalities. Ms. T. L. agreed to participate in a research program and submitted to positron emission tomography (PET), which revealed a normal density of active dopamine receptors in the striatum.

## COMMENTARY

Ms. T. L. has a relentlessly progressing disease that affects her motor systems. The description that she provides in her history is that of dystonia, a basal ganglia disease of unknown etiology, pathology, and until recently, treatment. It is common for people with dystonia, as in the case of Ms. T. L., to submit to numerous orthopaedic procedures that are directed at restoring mobility. These measures usually offer only temporary benefit because of the progression of the disease. What is remarkable in this case is that despite two extensive neurological evaluations, Ms. T. L.'s dystonia remained undiagnosed.

Her family physician would probably not have prescribed metoclopramide if her condition had been properly diagnosed, because this drug is contraindicated in patients with basal ganglia disease. The exact mode of action of metoclopramide is not known, but it seems to act like a dopamine antagonist. Acute dystonic reactions and parkinsonism are well-recognized side effects of this drug. In the case of Ms. T. L., the exacerbations of her underlying dystonia were so severe that despite her reluctance to become involved with the medical system again, she was persuaded to submit to reevaluation. Fortunately, the attending neurologist recognized her symptoms and instituted appropriate therapy.

**Dopa-responsive dystonia (DRD)**[8] is a variant of dystonia. It is characterized by early onset,

---

[8] Called L-dopa-responsive dystonia (LRD) by some authors.

toe walking in childhood, diurnal variation in the severity of its symptoms, and immediate and dramatic response to L-dopa. DRD is an autosomal dominant hereditary disease. The gene, on chromosome 14q, shows incomplete penetrance. The prevalence of DRD is unknown, but it is estimated that it accounts for as many as 10% of all cases of dystonia. It is hypothesized that DRD is caused by a defect in the release of dopamine from the terminals of the SNc neurons, for there is no pronounced atrophy of the substantia nigra, and PET reveals functional dopamine receptors in the striatum. Patients treated with L-dopa have shown little decrease in effectiveness of the drug, in contrast to response by patients with parkinsonism.

## FURTHER APPLICATIONS

**8.5.   DRD is frequently misdiagnosed as juvenile parkinsonism, in part because DRD is sometimes associated with a tremor. Consider the similarities and differences between dystonia and parkinsonism and develop your own criteria for differentiating between these two diseases. Are there causes of tremor other than parkinsonism?**

**8.6.   Consider the role of the family physician in this case. Had he not been alert to the connection between metoclopramide and the manifestations of basal ganglia disease, Ms. T. L.'s condition would still be improperly diagnosed. On the other hand, should he have recognized dystonia before he prescribed the metoclopramide?**

**8.7.   Speculate about possible mechanisms of DRD. Account for the continued responsiveness to L-dopa therapy with DRD and the failure of long term L-dopa therapy with PD.**

## S U M M A R Y

- **The basal ganglia are a set of nuclei at the base of the cerebral hemispheres.**

  They serve as a bridge between the cerebral cortex and the thalamus. Signals originating from all parts of the cerebral cortex pass through the striatum into the thalamus. From the thalamus they are returned primarily to the motor areas of the cortex. Several shorter loops also exist. The subthalamic nucleus, for example, receives fibers from the globus pallidus and sends fibers to it and to the substantia nigra. The substantia nigra receives axons from the caudate and putamen, to which it also projects.

- **The basal ganglia are essential in translating the conception of motor acts into action.**

  Therefore, disturbances of basal ganglia function cause spontaneous movements or the opposite, a poverty of movement. These two extremes of basal ganglia disorders are exemplified by HD and PD, respectively.

- **HD is a genetic disorder that results in the early death of neurons of the striatum.**

  Clinically it is characterized by dementia and chorea. Because it is caused by an autosomal dominant gene, 50% of the progeny of an affected person may be expected to develop the disease. There is no effective treatment.

- **Parkinsonism is a biochemical disease of the basal ganglia that is characterized by the loss of the dopaminergic neurons of the SNc.**

  It produces bradykinesia, tremor, and cogwheel rigidity. Dementia is inconsistently associated with parkinsonism. Most parkinsonism is idiopathic (primary parkinsonism), but it may be caused by head trauma, viral infection, or exposure to neurotoxins, most notably carbon monoxide, manganese, and antipsychotic drugs. The symptoms of parkinsonism can usually be at least partially alleviated by the administration of L-dopa. Dopamine agonists and MAO-B inhibitors are also helpful.

- **Dystonia is a disease of the basal ganglia of unknown causation.**

    It is characterized by nearly continuous contractions of various muscle groups. These contractions can lock joints into abnormal postures. These patients may be rigid in various extremities, the trunk, or the whole body. Unlike the rigidity associated with PD, the rigidity of dystonia is due to active contraction of antagonistic muscle groups. Some forms of dystonia respond to the administration of L-dopa.

## SUGGESTED READINGS

Green RD, Reed JC. Mitochondria and apoptosis. Science 1998;281:1309–312.

Mello Luiz EA, Villares J. Neuroanatomy of the basal ganglia. Psychiatr Clin North Am 1997; 20:691–703.

Nygaard TG, Marsden CD, Duvoisin RC. Dopa-responsive dystonia. Adv Neurol 1988;50:377–383.

Online Mendelian Inheritance in Man (OMIM).[9] Baltimore: Johns Hopkins University. MIM 128230. Dystonia, progressive with diurnal variation.

Online Mendelian Inheritance in Man (OMIM). Baltimore: Johns Hopkins University. MIM 128100. Dystonia 1, Torson.

Online Mendelian Inheritance in Man (OMIM). Baltimore: Johns Hopkins University. MIM 143100. Huntington disease; HD.

Online Mendelian Inheritance in Man (OMIM). Baltimore: Johns Hopkins University. MIM 168600. Parkinsonism.

Online Mendelian Inheritance in Man (OMIM). Baltimore: Johns Hopkins University. MIM 601104. Supranuclear palsy, progressive.

Palermo-Neto J. Dopaminergic systems: dopamine receptors. Psychiatr Clin North Am 1997;20: 691–703.

Wexler NS. The Tiresias complex: Huntington's disease as a paradigm of testing for late-onset disorders. FASEB J 1992;6: 2820–2825.

---

[9] OMIM can be reached at http://www3.ncbi.nlm.nih.gov/omim/.

# Motor Systems IV: The Cerebellum

The cerebellum regulates posture and coordinates motor acts. Disturbances of cerebellar function produce disturbances of gait, balance, and stability and diminish the accuracy of reaching motions. Cerebellar lesions also affect the ability to improve motor skills. Loss of cerebellar function does not produce paralysis, paresis, apraxia, or deficits in the initiation or termination of voluntary motor acts.

## ANATOMY OF THE CEREBELLUM

The cerebellum (see Fig. 1.19) is a large, compact structure attached to the pons by three pairs of tracts, the **cerebellar peduncles** [ML. *pedunculus,* a little foot, stalk, or stem, dim of L. *pedum,* shepherd's staff, fr. L. *pes,* foot]: the **superior** (brachium conjunctivum), **middle** (brachium pontis), and **inferior** (restiform body) peduncles.[1] The body of the cerebellum is divided into two hemispheres that are continuous with the **vermis** [L. *vermis,* worm] at the midline. An intermediate zone that is not visible on gross inspection lies between the vermis and the hemispheres. Like the cerebral cortex, the cerebellar cortex is deeply folded into **folia** [L. *folium,* pl. *folia,* leaf] that increase its surface area. Some of the folds are deeper than others, and the deep folds separate the cerebellum into lobes. The **flocculus** [L. *flocculus,* small wool tuft] and **nodulus** [L. *nodulus,* little knot], together known as the **flocculonodular lobe,** are noteworthy because specific clinical signs are attributable to lesions of this lobe (discussed later in the chapter). The main body of the cerebellum is divided into an **anterior lobe** and a **posterior lobe** by the **primary fissure.** Lesser folds further divide the cerebellum into smaller lobes. These anterior posterior divisions do not correspond to the functional divisions of the cerebellum, and little is to be gained by learning their names.

### Microanatomy of the Cerebellar Cortex

The cerebellar cortex is the superficial cell-containing region of the cerebellum. It consists of three layers. The deepest cortical layer is the **granule cell layer;** the most superficial is the **molecular layer.** A single layer of cells, the **Purkinje cell layer,** lies between them (Fig. 9.1). Five principal neuronal cell types are found in the cerebellar cortex. The cells and their probable neurotransmitters are summarized in Table 9.1. The synaptic relations among these cells are summarized in Figure 9.2.

**Purkinje cells** have a large goblet-shaped cell body and an immense fan-shaped dendritic tree that extends toward the cerebellar surface into the molecular layer and perpendicular to the long axis of the folium. In addition to their extensive branching, Purkinje cell dendrites have numerous spines that greatly increase the synaptic surface area. Axons from Purkinje cells are the only fibers that leave the cerebellar cortex. Most of these axons synapse in the deep nuclei; a few leave the cerebellum to synapse in brainstem nuclei. All make inhibitory synapses on their targets. The neuro-

---

[1] The names in parentheses are the traditional names of the cerebellar peduncles.

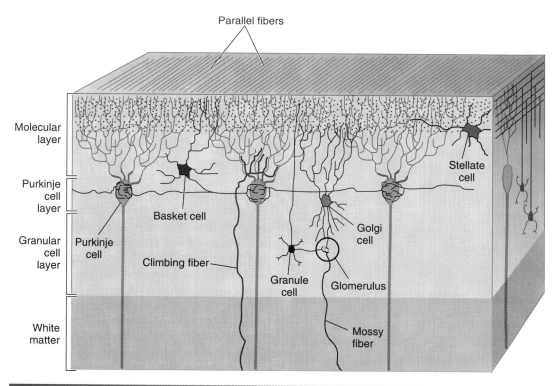

**Figure 9.1    The three-dimensional arrangement of the cerebellar cortex**

The parallel fibers run perpendicular to the fan-shaped dendritic tree of the Purkinje cell. Basket cell axons run perpendicular to the parallel fibers. Granule cells, Golgi cells, and mossy fibers synapse together in the glomerulus.

**Table 9.1    Transmitters in the Cerebellum**

| Synaptic Source | Target | Transmitter |
| --- | --- | --- |
| Purkinje cell | Deep cerebellar nuclei | GABA (−) |
| Granule cell | Purkinje cell dendrites (via parallel fiber) | Glutamate (+) |
| Basket cell | Purkinje cell | GABA (−) |
| Golgi cell | Granular cell glomerulus | GABA (−) |
| Stellate cell | Purkinje cell dendrites | Taurine (−) ? |
| Mossy fiber | Granular cell glomerulus | ACh (+) ?? |
| Climbing fiber | Purkinje cell | Aspartate |

transmitter is probably γ-aminobutyric acid (GABA).

**Granule cells**, the most numerous type of neuron in the brain, are found in the cerebellar granule cell layer. Axons from these cells project directly to the surface of the folia. Here they bifurcate, sending the two branches about 6 to 10 mm along the folia. Because the axons of granule cells lie parallel to one another, they are known as **parallel fibers**. About 400,000 parallel fibers run through the branches of the dendrites of a single Purkinje cell. Each parallel fiber traverses the dendritic fields of about 1,000 Purkinje cells that are lined up in an orderly row along the length of the folia, much like the wires that run through the arms of roadside telephone poles. Parallel fibers make excitatory synaptic contacts with Purkinje cells.

**Basket cells** lie in the deepest part of the molecular layer. Their dendrites extend into the superficial region of the molecular layer and receive excitatory synaptic input from parallel fibers. The axons of basket cells extend across the folia at the junction of the molecular and Purkinje cell layers and perpendicular to the parallel fibers. As they traverse this interface, each axon extends a collateral branch to a Purkinje cell that envelops its soma like a basket. Basket cells make powerful inhibitory synapses on Purkinje cells that can temporarily silence it. The inhibition is so powerful because the synapses are on the Purkinje cell soma, very close to the trigger zone.

**Stellate cells** [L. *stellatus,* starry, star-shaped, fr. *stella,* star], which lie in the molecular layer, receive excitatory contacts from parallel fibers.

The stellate cell makes inhibitory synapses on the dendrites of Purkinje cells. Like basket cells, stellate cells send their axons across the folia perpendicular to parallel fibers. In contrast to the inhibition produced by basket cells, the inhibition produced by stellate cells is discrete because it is directed at individual branches of dendrites. In effect, stellate cells electrically prune the dendritic tree by temporarily removing dendritic limbs from the Purkinje cell, negating their influence.

**Golgi cells** lie slightly deep to the Purkinje cell layer. Their dendritic fields extend into the molecular layer, where parallel fibers make excitatory synaptic contacts with them. Golgi cell axons enter the granule cell layer and make inhibitory synapses with the dendritic extensions of the granule cells. Together the Golgi cell axons, granular cell dendrites, and mossy fibers (discussed later in the chapter)

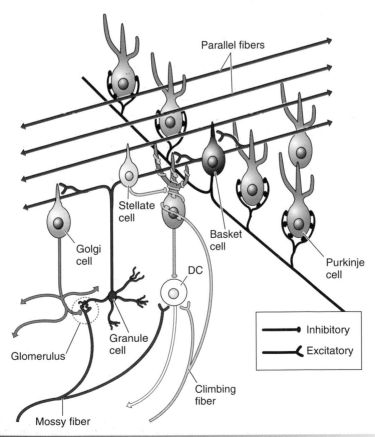

Parallel fibers

Stellate cell

Golgi cell

Basket cell

DC

Purkinje cell

Granule cell

Glomerulus

Climbing fiber

Mossy fiber

● Inhibitory

< Excitatory

**Figure 9.2   Synaptic relations among cerebellar cortical cells**

*DC,* deep nuclear cell.

constitute a structure known as the **cerebellar glomerulus** [L. *glomerulus,* little ball, cluster, fr. *glomus,* a ball-shaped mass]. The cerebellar glomerulus is a complex synaptic structure contained within a glial capsule (Fig. 9.3). The three cell types make numerous synaptic contacts within the confines of the glomerulus.

It is reasonable to expect a somatotopic map of the body represented in the cerebellar cortex, analogous to the somatotopic maps in the primary sensory cortices and thalamic nuclei. Although recent evidence confirms that the deep cerebellar nuclei are mapped to the body, no convincing somatotopic maps of the cerebellar cortex have been discovered.[2] The significance of the lack of cortical mapping is discussed later in the chapter.

### Afferent Connections

Although the cerebellum receives information from all parts of the nervous system, the axons

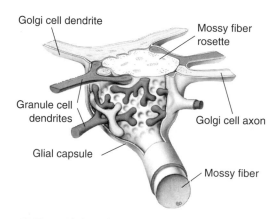

Golgi cell dendrite
Mossy fiber rosette
Granule cell dendrites
Golgi cell axon
Glial capsule
Mossy fiber

**Figure 9.3   The glomerulus of the cerebellum**

The mossy fiber terminal, called a rosette, synapses on the granule cell and Golgi cell dendrites and receives synaptic contact from Golgi cell axons. The granule cell dendrite also synapses with Golgi cell dendrites. (Reprinted with permission from Carpenter MB, Sutin J. Human neuroanatomy. 8th ed. Baltimore: Williams & Wilkins, 1983.)

that enter the cerebellum make only three types of synaptic contacts in the cerebellar cortex. Most of the afferent fibers are classified by the morphology of their synaptic endings as either **mossy fibers** or **climbing fibers**. The third type of axon entering the cerebellum contains monoamines, which presumably are used as neurotransmitters.

### MOSSY FIBERS

Mossy fibers are the most numerous type of axon entering the cerebellum. They arise from four principal parts of the central nervous system (CNS): (*a*) the spinal cord, (*b*) the vestibular nuclei, (*c*) the brainstem reticular formation, and (*d*) the deep pontine nuclei. After entering the cerebellum, mossy fibers divide into two branches: one branch terminates in a deep cerebellar nucleus, and the other ascends to the cerebellar cortex. The cortical branches make excitatory contacts with granule cells and Golgi cells in cerebellar glomeruli. These endings look like tufts of moss, giving these fibers their name.

Mossy fibers excite granule cells that in turn excite Purkinje cells via parallel fibers. The extent of this excitation is remarkable. A single mossy fiber innervates approximately 600 granule cells. Each granule cell, through its parallel fiber, synapses with about 1,000 Purkinje cells. Therefore, assuming no overlap (not a reasonable assumption), a single mossy fiber may excite approximately 600,000 Purkinje cells. Even if there is considerable overlap, the amount of synaptic divergence in this system is impressive.

The synaptic convergence on Purkinje cells is just as remarkable. Each granule cell receives synapses from about four mossy fibers, and each Purkinje cell receives about 80,000 synapses from parallel fibers. Again, assuming no overlap, each Purkinje cell potentially receives information from approximately 320,000 mossy fibers.[3]

Parallel fiber synapses on Purkinje cells produce small-amplitude excitatory postsy-

[2] Many textbooks offer illustrations of homuncular maps drawn on the surface of the cerebellum. These maps are based on recordings of evoked potentials from the cortical surface. There are many difficulties with this technique, and several authors question the validity of the maps. Although the issue remains unsettled, direct topographic mapping of the body onto the cerebellar surface now seems unlikely.

[3] These numbers are based on observations from the cat. It is not possible to make such estimates from human material.

naptic potentials (EPSPs) (0.02 to 4 mV when recorded at the Purkinje cell soma). These EPSPs are caused by the opening of sodium ion selective channels in response to the granule cell neurotransmitter (probably **glutamate**). The amplitude of the EPSP is increased when many parallel fiber synapses are simultaneously active. If the spatial and temporal summation of EPSPs is sufficient, threshold is reached and an action potential is produced in the Purkinje cell. Since the synaptic activity from parallel fibers is very high, Purkinje cells have a high background firing rate, about 70 spikes per second.

## CLIMBING FIBERS

The inferior olivary nuclei are the source of all climbing fiber input into the cerebellum. Axons leave the inferior olive, cross the midline, and enter the cerebellum through the inferior cerebellar peduncle. From the inferior peduncle the axons divide extensively to innervate wide areas of the cerebellar hemisphere.

The projections from the inferior olive to the cerebellum are quite orderly and reciprocal. For the purposes of clinical medicine it is not necessary to learn the details of all of the afferent connections to the inferior olive. It is sufficient to know that all parts of the sensory and motor systems project into the inferior olive in an organized way. From the spinal cord, direct connections to the inferior olive are transmitted by the **spino-olivary tract**, which courses in the ventral funiculus of the spinal cord. Fibers from the dorsal column nuclei reach the inferior olive after crossing the midline. The inferior olive also receives afferent fibers from the vestibular nuclei, red nucleus, superior colliculus, and mesencephalic reticular formation. Finally, axons from the sensory and motor areas of the cerebral cortex project widely into the inferior olive. It is apparent from these widespread and diverse inputs that the inferior olivary nuclei are a major staging area through which sensory and motor information is transmitted to the cerebellar cortex.

Similar to mossy fibers, climbing fibers divide into a deep branch and a cortical branch after entering the cerebellum. The cortical branch further divides, sending collaterals into several lobes. Each collateral branch makes approximately 300 synapses on a single Purkinje cell. Each Purkinje cell receives only one climbing fiber. The climbing fiber is so named because it contacts only the soma and basal dendritic branches of the Purkinje cell, ascending the dendrite as if it were climbing a tree. The synapses are intensely excitatory.

The climbing fiber neurotransmitter **aspartate** opens calcium ion channels in the soma of Purkinje cells, which produces EPSPs. The calcium-dependent spikes initiated by climbing fiber input are much less frequent (only about 1 per second) than the sodium-dependent spikes initiated by the mossy fiber–parallel fiber input. Yet the EPSPs are so intense that a single climbing fiber calcium spike triggers an action potential. The synapse between a climbing fiber and a Purkinje cell is one of the few obligatory synapses in the mammalian CNS.

The significance of the calcium spike, however, probably has nothing to do with the action potential it initiates in the Purkinje cell. Calcium spikes generated by climbing fibers are outnumbered by parallel fiber–generated sodium spikes by about 70:1. Therefore, the effect on the stream of action potentials leaving the Purkinje cell is negligible. The real significance of the calcium spike is that it represents the inward flow of calcium ions, which have the potential to affect the metabolism of the Purkinje cell. Calcium ions are important intracellular messengers that can exert a variety of long-lasting effects (see Chapter 3). Some evidence suggests that the calcium-dependent spikes in Purkinje cells are a critical component of the cerebellar mechanism responsible for motor learning (motor plasticity, discussed later in the chapter).

## MONOAMINERGIC FIBERS

The monoaminergic fibers that supply the cerebellum originate in the raphe nuclei (serotonin-containing axons) and locus ceruleus (norepinephrine-containing axons). Because their terminals have no special morphology, these fibers carry no special name. The monoaminergic axons branch extensively and terminate in all layers of the cerebellar cortex. The physiological role of the mono-aminergic systems is unknown.

## Efferent Connections

All axons leaving the cerebellar cortex originate in Purkinje cells. Almost all terminate in the deep cerebellar nuclei, which as their name implies, lie deep in the white matter of the cerebellum. Some of the Purkinje cells in the flocculonodular lobe terminate in the vestibular nuclei. Except for a few Purkinje cell axons from the flocculonodular lobe, all fibers leaving the body of the cerebellum originate in the deep cerebellar nuclei. There are three pairs of deep nuclei, the **fastigial** [L. *fastigium,* ridge, summit], **interpositus**[4] [L. *inter,* between, and *positus,* positioned], and **dentate** [L. *dentatus,* toothed, notched]. The axons from the cells in the deep nuclei leave the cerebellum through the cerebellar peduncles and synapse in the thalamus, the brainstem motor centers, or the vestibular nuclei.

The cells of the deep cerebellar nuclei are somatotopically arranged and independently mapped; each map represents one complete body half (Fig. 9.4). This independent multiple representation of the body is particularly significant, since each nucleus, along with the corresponding portion of the cerebellar cortex that projects to it, serves a different aspect of motor coordination. This arrangement divides the cerebellum into three independent motor control systems.

## FUNCTIONAL DIVISIONS OF THE CEREBELLUM

The cerebellum can be classified into three divisions based on the connections with the nervous system that each division makes. These divisions are called the **vestibulocerebellum,** the **spinocerebellum,** and the **cerebrocerebellum** (Fig. 9.5). These functional divisions do not correspond to the prominent fissures that divide the cerebellum into lobes, with one exception: the vestibulocerebellum is congruent with the flocculonodular lobe. The functional divisions, however, are much more useful than the gross anatomical divisions in understanding the physiology of the cerebellum and interpreting its neurology.

## The Vestibulocerebellum

The vestibulocerebellum is composed of the flocculus and the nodulus. This flocculonodular lobe receives most of its afferent fibers from the vestibular nuclei; a few come from the vestibular nerve (cranial nerve [CN] VIII) directly (Fig. 9.6). They terminate as mossy fibers. Most of the axons from the Purkinje cells leave the vestibulocerebellum via the inferior cerebellar peduncle to synapse in the ipsilateral vestibular nuclei.

The few primary afferent fibers from the vestibular nerve that innervate the vestibulocerebellum originate in the labyrinthine receptors of the inner ear (see Chapter 10). Signals from these receptors are critical for two important physiologic functions: (*a*) to coordinate head movements with eye movements, and (*b*) to regulate gait and posture.

Clear vision depends on the coordination of head and eye movements so that an image can be maintained on the retina of the eye. For example, if while reading this page, you move your head from side to side, your eyes scan in a direction opposite the motion of your head to keep the printed word fixed upon the retina. The vestibular system provides information about the dynamics of head movement. The cerebellum, with its associated vestibular nuclei, and the nuclei of ocular motion integrate this information and provide the necessary motor commands to the neck muscles and the extraocular eye muscles to effect this coordination. The details of this system are discussed in Chapter 10.

Through its extensive connections with the lateral vestibular nucleus, the vestibulo-

---

[4] In humans, the **globose** and the **emboliform** nuclei correspond to two regions in the interpositus nucleus in other primates. The emboliform nucleus is homologous to the anterior region of the interpositus, and the globose nucleus corresponds to the posterior region. Most efferent axons from the interpositus nucleus arise in the anterior region, the analogue of the larger emboliform nucleus, which is many times larger than the globose nucleus. Nothing is lost but much is gained in simplicity by learning the connections of both nuclei under the single name interpositus.

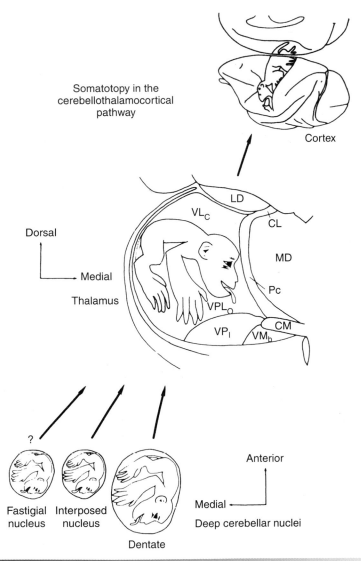

Somatotopy in the
cerebellothalamocortical
pathway

**Figure 9.4    Somatotopic relations in the deep cerebellar nuclei**

The somatotopic organization of the dentate, interpositus, and fastigial nuclei compared with the same organization in the thalamus and M-I cortex. The data are based on experiments with monkeys. Major thalamic nuclei that correspond with the human are the *CM*, centromedian; *LD*, lateral dorsal; *MD*, medial dorsal; *VL$_C$*, ventral lateral compacta; and *VP$_{LO}$*, ventral posterolateral oralis. (Reprinted with permission from Thach WT, Goodkin HP, Keating JG. The cerebellum and the adaptive coordination of movement. Annu Rev Neurosci 1992;15:403–442.)

cerebellum also regulates gait and posture. Recall that the lateral vestibulospinal tract originates in the lateral vestibular nucleus and facilitates the motor neurons innervating the antigravity muscles (see Chapter 7). These connections are fast and direct, as many of them make monosynaptic connections with α-motor neurons. The inner ear senses alterations in the body's orientation to gravity and sends appropriate corrective signals to the spinal cord to modify the activity of these motor neurons.

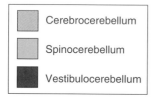

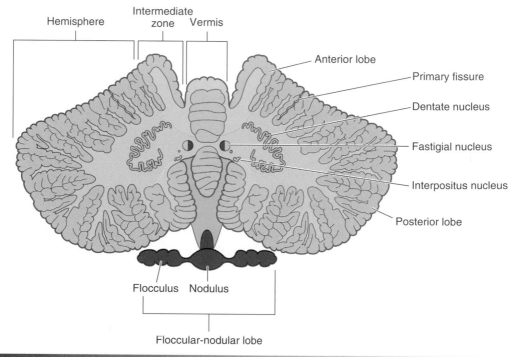

**Figure 9.5  Functional divisions of the cerebellum**

## The Spinocerebellum

The spinocerebellum corresponds to the vermis and the intermediate zone, a small strip of the cerebellar hemispheres immediately adjacent to the vermis (Fig. 9.5). Most of the information reaching the spinocerebellum arrives from the spinal cord. Sensory information from the muscles and the lower half of the body surface travel to the spinocerebellum over two principal fiber tracts, the **dorsal spinocerebellar tract** (DSCT) and the **ventral spinocerebellar tract** (VSCT) (Fig. 9.7).

The DSCT carries specific proprioceptive information to the spinocerebellum. Cutaneous information from touch and pressure receptors and proprioceptive information

from muscle spindle receptors, Golgi tendon organs, and joint receptors enter the spinal cord over IA, IB, and group II primary afferent axons. The receptors associated with these axons have restricted sensory fields and thus supply discrete information to the CNS. In addition to the synaptic connections discussed in Chapter 6, these primary afferent axons send collateral branches that synapse in the ipsilateral **nucleus dorsalis (Clarke's column)**, a collection of large cells in lamina VII at the base of the dorsal horn (Fig. 9.7). Axons leaving this nucleus collect in the dorsal lateral funiculus just inferior to the dorsal root entry zone without crossing the midline. The axons ascend the spinal cord as the DSCT and enter

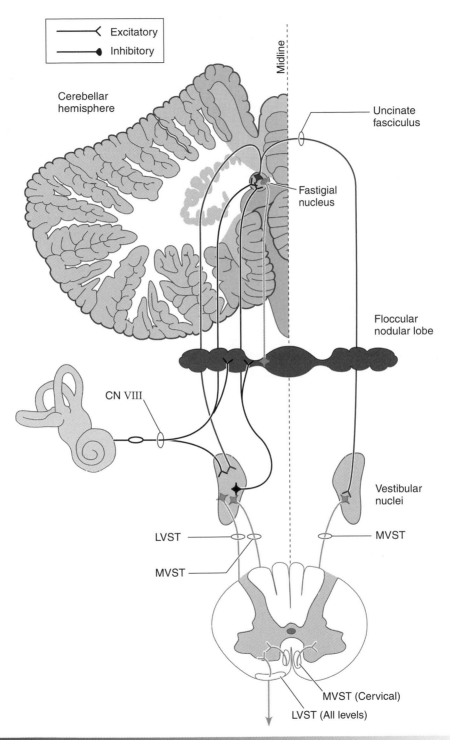

**Figure 9.6  Connections of the vestibulocerebellum.**

*MVST,* medial vestibulospinal tract; *LVST,* lateral vestibulospinal tract.

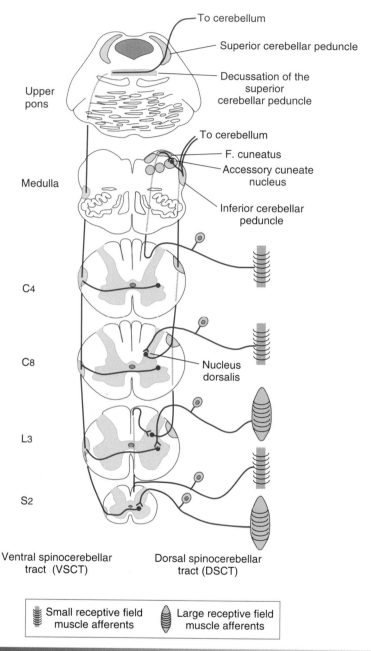

**Figure 9.7   The spinocerebellar tracts**

The major features of the dorsal spinocerebellar tract (*right*) and the ventral spinocerebellar tract (*left*). These tracts transmit qualitatively different information to the spinocerebellum. Note the various crossing patterns that ultimately keep the information ipsilateral to the origin.

the cerebellum through the inferior peduncle, where they terminate as mossy fibers. Since the nucleus dorsalis exists only from about C8 to L3, the DSCT carries information only from

the trunk and lower extremities. An analogous system for the upper extremity consists of a few fibers from the fasciculus cuneatus that break away from the medial lemniscus and synapse in the **accessory cuneate nucleus** [L. *cuneus,* wedge]. Axons from this nucleus form the **cuneocerebellar tract** and join the DSCT to enter the cerebellum through the inferior cerebellar peduncle.

The VSCT originates in large cells in lamina VII that border the dorsolateral boundary of the ventral horn. Axons from these "border cells" cross the midline in the ventral white commissure of the spinal cord and collect in the ventral lateral funiculus (Fig. 9.7). From this location they ascend the spinal cord, pass through the brainstem, and enter the spinocerebellum through the superior peduncle. Because the superior cerebellar peduncle is a crossed tract, axons of the VSCT ultimately terminate ipsilateral to the cells of origin. The border cells that give rise to the VSCT are polysynaptically innervated by flexion reflex afferents (FRAs), as well as by a few afferent fibers from muscle spindles and Golgi tendon organs. They also receive monosynaptic contacts from collateral branches of all of the descending motor tracts (corticospinal, reticulospinal, vestibulospinal, and rubrospinal).

The information that the VSCT conveys to the spinocerebellum is qualitatively different from that conveyed by the DSCT. For the most part VSCT sensory information arises from sensory receptors with large receptive fields. They are also innervated by the CBST and can therefore return to the cerebellum copies of the motor commands that are arriving at the motor neuron pools. In contrast, the DSCT carries direct information from the muscle and joint receptors that indicates the actual effect of the motor commands on limb placement.

Purkinje cells of the spinocerebellum send axons into the **ipsilateral fastigial** and **interpositus nuclei** (Fig. 9.8). Cells in the vermis project to the fastigial nucleus; those in the intermediate zone terminate in the interpositus. Most of the efferent fibers from the fastigial nucleus cross the midline within the cerebellum as an arch of fibers, the **uncinate fasciculus** [L. *uncinatus,* hooked, fr. *uncus,* hook, barb], and then leave the cerebellum through the contralateral inferior peduncle. Most of these crossed fibers terminate in the lateral and infe-

rior vestibular nuclei and the motor portions of the reticular formation. A smaller number of fastigial axons have ipsilateral connections, terminating in the lateral and inferior vestibular nuclei. A few fastigial axons find their way to the thalamus (ventral lateral pars oralis [$VL_O$]), the superior colliculus, and the cervical spinal cord (lamina IX).

Purkinje cells in the intermediate zone project to the interpositus nucleus. Axons from the interpositus nucleus leave the cerebellum through the superior peduncle. Because this tract is crossed, all interpositus axons terminate on the side contralateral to their origin. Most of the axons terminate in the red nucleus, but about one-third pass through the nucleus and terminate in the $VL_C$ of the thalamus.

### The Cerebrocerebellum

The cerebrocerebellum, which consists of most of the cerebellar hemispheres, receives afferent connections from the **deep pontine nuclei** (Fig. 9.9). About 20 million axons from these nuclei are sent into the contralateral cerebellum through each middle cerebellar peduncle. Within the cerebellum they are distributed to the cerebellar hemispheres, where they terminate as mossy fibers. The cerebrocerebellum receives afferent connections indirectly from the cerebral cortex because the deep pontine nuclei receive most of their afferent fibers from all four cortical lobes (Fig. 9.10). The most massive projections come from the precentral and postcentral gyri. The most widely represented cortical regions are areas 6, 4, 3, 1, 2, and 5, which correspond with the principal motor and sensory areas. There are important projections from the primary visual cortex (area 17) as well. The corticopontine axons leave the cerebral cortex, descend through the internal capsule, and collect in the cerebral peduncle. Those from the frontal lobe lie in the ventral medial part, and those from the remaining lobes lie in the dorsolateral part. The two groups of axons are separated by the corticobulbospinal tract (CBST). These cortical projections onto the deep pontine nuclei are topographically precise and well organized.

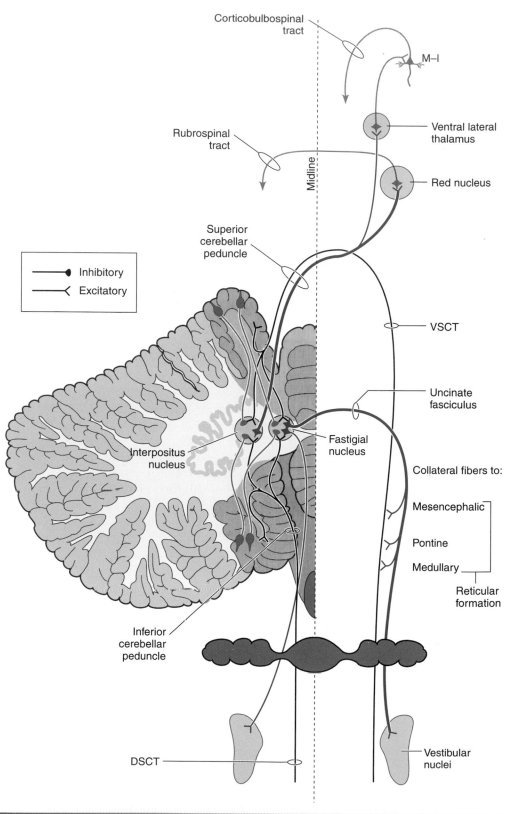

**Figure 9.8   Connections of the spinocerebellum**

The fastigial nucleus receives Purkinje cell axons from the vermis, the interpositus from the intermediate zone. *DSCT*, dorsal spinocerebellar tract; *VSCT*, ventral spinocerebellar tract; *M-I*, primary motor cortex.

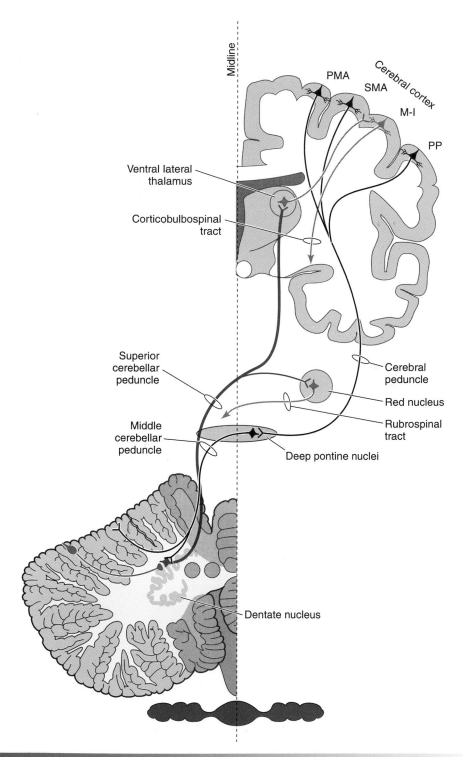

**Figure 9.9 Connections of the cerebrocerebellum**

*PMA,* premotor area; *SMA,* supplementary motor area; *PP,* posterior parietal cortex; *M-I,* primary motor cortex.

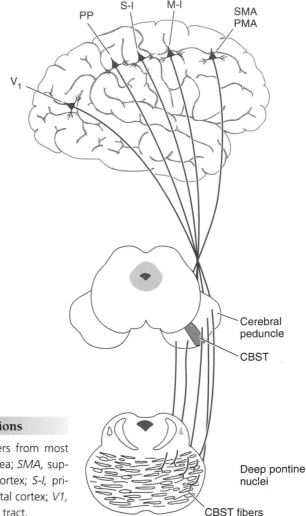

**Figure 9.10   Cerebropontine connections**

The deep pontine nuclei receive afferent fibers from most parts of the cerebral cortex. *PMA,* premotor area; *SMA,* supplementary motor area; *M-I,* primary motor cortex; *S-I,* primary somatosensory cortex; *PP,* posterior parietal cortex; *V1,* primary visual cortex; *CBST,* corticobulbospinal tract.

Purkinje cells of the cerebrocerebellum project to the dentate nucleus. Axons leaving the dentate nucleus pass through the superior cerebellar peduncle and terminate in the contralateral $VL_C$ of the thalamus. A smaller number of axons terminate in the red nucleus contralateral to the hemisphere of origin. In this respect, dentate projections mirror those from the interpositus nucleus.

## The Cerebellum As a Control System

Lesions to the cerebellum do not produce paralysis. Cerebellar lesions do not cause weakness, nor do they affect the ability to initiate or terminate voluntary movement. With- out the cerebellum, however, precise, coordinated movements are impossible. These observations suggest that the cerebellum acts as a regulatory system that modifies motor acts initiated by other regions of the CNS. The anatomy of the connections of the motor systems supports this view. For example, the arrangement of the vestibular and spinal divisions of the cerebellum suggests that they operate as a typical feedback control system (Fig. 9.11A). Both divisions receive sensory information about either body position or muscle action. The output affects the descending motor systems at the brainstem level (red nucleus, motor nuclei of the reticular formation,

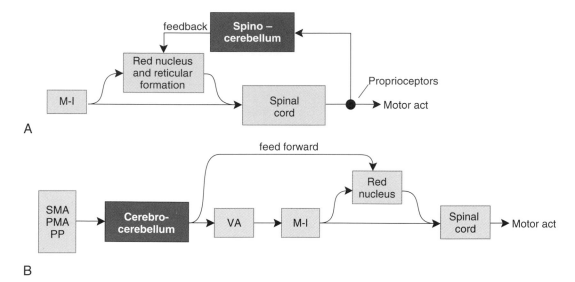

A. The spinocerebellum acts as a feedback control system, taking information from the motor act as it is evolving in time, computing corrections, and applying the corrections to the integrating motor centers in the brainstem. **B.** The cerebrocerebellum lies between the sensorimotor-motor cortex and the primary motor cortex (*M-I*) and can act as a feed-forward controller. It receives information about the impending motor act, computes corrections, and applies the corrections to the nuclei where the final motor commands are assembled (thalamus and primary motor cortex).

and vestibular nuclei). This information is used to affect the motor act *while it is in progress.* In other words, the state of the output variable—motor activity—is used to alter the motor command input.

The cerebrocerebellum is arranged differently (Fig. 9.11*B*). It receives most of its information from the motor, premotor, and sensory areas of the cerebral cortex. The sensory areas of the parietal lobe convey sensory information about the postural state of the body, and the motor areas of the frontal lobes, especially from the supplementary motor area (SMA) and premotor area (PMA), convey the motor command that *is about to be executed.* The output from the cerebrocerebellum feeds back to the red nucleus and the primary motor cortex (M-I), where it can affect the motor command *before the execution of the command.* In other words, the cerebrocerebellum is arranged to act like a feed-forward control system. Feed-forward control systems modify the action of control systems before an action takes place by measuring environmental variables that may

affect how the control system as a whole operates. To measure these variables, they must have some internal representation or model of the control system and how the environmental variables affect it. Developing and retaining this model may be one function of the cerebellar cortex.

## CLINICAL ASPECTS OF CEREBELLAR FUNCTION

The function of the cerebellum is best appreciated by observation of patients with cerebellar lesions. The motor disturbances are unique and clearly distinguishable from disturbances associated with lesions to the basal ganglia or the upper or lower motor neuron systems.

The cerebellum is functionally uncrossed with respect to the midline; hence, lesions to it affect the ipsilateral side of the body. This characteristic can be appreciated by considering the various crossing patterns of the afferent and efferent fiber tracts to the cerebellum. The DSCT carries ipsilateral information and enters the cerebellum over the inferior peduncle, an un-crossed tract. The VSCT, however, which carries information from the contralateral side of the body, enters the cerebellum over the superior peduncle, a crossed tract. Similarly, the dentate efferent fibers leave through the superior peduncle and cross the midline to innervate the red nucleus and the thalamus. Axons leaving the red nucleus immediately cross the midline before projecting to the spinal cord. Information from the thalamus is sent to the ipsilateral (to the thalamus) cerebral cortex, but motor commands leaving the cerebral cortex cross before innervating the motor nuclei of the brainstem and spinal cord.

The principal signs of cerebellar dysfunction are (*a*) an **ataxic gait** [G. *a*, without, and *taxis*, order], (*b*) **nystagmus** [G. *nystagmos*, nod (n.), fr. *nystazo*, to drowse], (*c*) **dysmetria** [G. *dys*, bad, and *metron*, measure], (*d*) **dysdiadochokinesia** [G. *diadochos*, working in turn, and *kinesis*, movement], and (*e*) **decomposition of movement**. Nystagmus and ataxia are most closely associated with damage to the vestibulocerebellum; the remaining signs are closely associated with damage to the spinocerebellum and cerebrocerebellum.

### Signs of Vestibulocerebellar Injury

Because the flocculonodular lobe of the cerebellum is so closely coupled to the vestibular system, it is difficult to distinguish between injury to the vestibulocerebellum and to the vestibular nuclei or the peripheral vestibular apparatus. Ataxic gait and nystagmus, the two principal symptoms associated with lesions to the vestibulocerebellum, are also the principal symptoms associated with vestibular end-organ disease. These signs are associated with highly automated (i.e., walking and eye coordination) motor tasks.

The most obvious sign associated with vestibulocerebellar lesions is a staggering, ataxic gait with a tendency to fall *toward the side of the lesion* (Fig. 9.12). This ataxia is closely related to the inability to coordinate body position (proprioceptive information) with gravity-associated changes in body motion (vestibular information). As one starts to fall, the changing body position must be assessed relative to gravity to compute the ap-

propriate corrective action. Without a functioning vestibulocerebellum and/or peripheral vestibular system, corrections are too slow to be effective.

Injury to the vestibulocerebellum also produces a characteristic spontaneous eye movement called nystagmus. This term describes an oscillating eye movement in which the eyes move slowly in one direction and rapidly in the other. A lesion to the flocculonodular lobe, the vestibular nuclei, or the vestibular end organ can cause nystagmus. These lesions are also frequently associated with **vertigo** [L. *vertigo*, dizziness, fr. *vertere*, to turn], the sensation of the world spinning around. Some students may be familiar with these symptoms, having experienced nystagmus and vertigo upon lying in bed after an intemperate evening of entertainment. Purkinje cells and possibly the labyrinth itself are unusually sensitive to the toxic effects of ethanol, which produces a temporary flocculonodular lesion. Nystagmus and the vestibular apparatus are discussed in detail in Chapter 10.

### Signs of Spinocerebellar and Cerebrocerebellar Injury

Lesions to the spinocerebellum and cerebrocerebellum produce somewhat different signs from those of lesions to the vestibulocerebellum. Recall that cerebrocerebellar output is directed primarily to the M-I motor cortex via the ventral lateral thalamus and that spinocerebellar output is directed to brainstem motor nuclei. Therefore, spinocerebellar and cerebrocerebellar lesions produce defects that affect the most precise movements of the extremities. A number of clinical terms succinctly describe these effects.

#### DYSDIADOCHOKINESIA

Cerebellar lesions result in a disruption of the *timing* of muscle contractions, which causes a *delay* in the initiation and termination of motor commands. Therefore, the *sequence* of individual muscle contractions is disrupted. The velocity of motor acts is normal, in contrast to the situation caused by basal ganglia lesions, which slow velocity (see Chapter 8).

The disruption in timing leads to a number of specific motor deficiencies. Perhaps the eas-

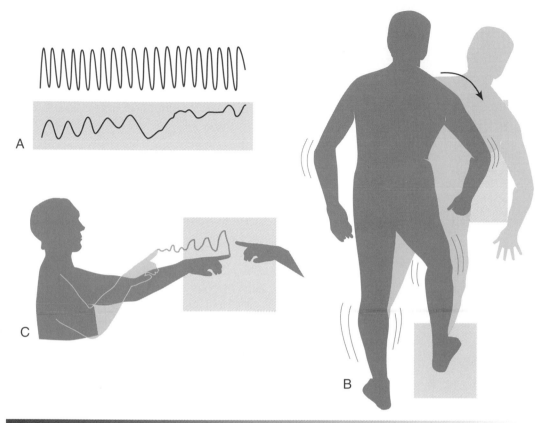

**Figure 9.12    Typical effects of cerebrocerebellar dysfunction**

**A.** Position of a hand during rapid alternating pronation and supination. The *upper record* is from a normal person, the *bottom* from one with a cerebellar lesion. **B.** The lack of coordination caused by cerebellar lesions may be revealed by a wide-based staggering gait with a tendency to fall toward the side of the lesion. **C.** People who have cerebellar lesions have great difficulty accurately reaching toward a target. The deviations become greater as the motor act progresses.

iest to observe is the *inability to perform repetitive tasks.* Performing such tasks requires precise timing between antagonistic muscle groups. For example, a normal subject has no trouble rapidly pronating and supinating the hands. If the cerebellum is not functioning, this simple act becomes impossible, as the coordinated timing between the various muscle groups is disrupted (Fig. 9.12). The inability to perform rapid alternating movements is called dysdiadochokinesia.

## DYSMETRIA

Timing derangements can also be demonstrated by having a patient touch the examiner's finger and then touch his own nose. The normal patient can make the finger travel a di-

rect, straight course from one target to the other, even with the eyes closed. If the cerebellum is dysfunctional, the finger travels a wandering course that deviates more and more from the straight line as the finger approaches the target (Fig. 9.12C). *Performance deteriorates as the motor act progresses.* This condition is properly described as dysmetria.

The unsteadiness seen in target-directed movements is sometimes called intention tremor. Superficially dysmetria resembles a tremor that is expressed only during a voluntary act, in contrast to the tremor of rest associated with parkinsonism. However, dysmetria is not rhythmic or constant in frequency or amplitude. True tremor has all of these characteristics and seems to be the result of continuous oscillatory behavior in central motor areas that is independent of external events. Thus, the term tremor is best reserved for the latter situation, while the term dysmetria most aptly describes a form of incoordination that results from cerebellar dysfunction.

## DECOMPOSITION

The poor timing of motor acts that occurs with cerebellar lesions can be seen as a decomposition of movement. To complete a motor act, the patient divides the synergistic components into separate acts in an effort to remove the necessity of precise timing between the components. For example, in reaching for an object, the patient may first move the shoulder joint, then the elbow, followed by the wrist and fingers. This strategy fails, of course, since each joint has antagonist muscles that must be coordinated. Nevertheless, decomposing the movement does improve performance somewhat. The disruption of the precision of motor acts that is associated with spinocerebellar and cerebrocerebellar lesions can manifest as ataxia. Dysmetric ataxia, however, is not associated with vertigo, the cardinal sign of vestibulocerebellar or vestibular end-organ disease.

## REFLEXES

The most objective signs of cerebellar dysfunction are **pendular muscle stretch reflexes** (MSRs) and **hypotonia**. To demonstrate pendular reflexes, a limb must be allowed to swing freely. For example, to test the quadriceps MSR, the patient should sit on the edge of an examining table. The MSR contraction occurs after the tendon is struck, but the distal extremity swings back and forth several times like a pendulum instead of damping quickly after one or two swings.

Pendular reflexes and hypotonia are related signs. Animal studies show that removal of the cerebellum or its deep nuclei reduces the facilitation of $\gamma$-motor neurons. This loss of gamma drive in effect reduces the gain of the negative-feedback MSR control system and lessens the reflex's effect in regulating muscle length. Muscle tone is reduced because the decreased facil-

itation of the $\gamma$-motor neurons is reflected in a decreased facilitation of the $\alpha$-motor neurons (see Chapter 6). With less resting muscle tone, there is less resistance to passive movement after the initial MSR contraction. Therefore, a limb such as the lower leg swings back and forth like a pendulum because of its own mass, not because of active muscle contractions.

## MOTOR PLASTICITY

Abundant evidence suggests that the cerebellum is capable of modifying its function in relation to experience. This feature is called **motor plasticity** or **motor learning**. Motor plasticity is not a new observation. Anyone who has learned to ride a bicycle or play a musical instrument has experienced motor plasticity. When learning to ride a bicycle, for example, one must consciously think about every aspect of riding: balance, pedaling, braking, steering, and so on. The overall act is consciously decomposed into its parts. As long as it is necessary to think about the process, corrections are too slow, and one falls off a lot. But with practice, the motor skills necessary to ride a bicycle become more automatic. Eventually it is not necessary to think about the specific *tactical* motor acts required to ride. Conscious efforts are directed instead toward the overall *strategy,* such as the best route. The execution of the motor tactics becomes unconscious. In fact, the transfer of motor tactics from the realm of the conscious to the unconscious is absolutely necessary if motor proficiency is ever to be achieved. Patients with cerebellar lesions cannot perform motor tasks unconsciously; they revert to conscious direction. For this reason, everything they do is decomposed and resembles a youngster learning to ride a bicycle.

Although the evidence is not complete, there is a growing consensus that the cerebellum is the part of the nervous system largely responsible for motor plasticity. If that is true, the cerebellum must have a mechanism that can alter synaptic efficiency in response to experience. The climbing fiber synapse is believed to be that mechanism. Two lines of evidence support this view.

First, activation of the climbing fiber synapse causes calcium ions to enter the Purkinje cell. Calcium is a potent intracellular messenger. It can modulate the phosphorylation of proteins by activating protein kinase C or calmodulin. Once activated, these proteins have the potential to increase the production of neurotransmitter receptors or signal the production of different receptors. Finally, some receptors can be directly phosphorylated, which can modulate their sensitivity to neurotransmitters. Although the exact effects on the intracellular metabolism of the Purkinje cell is not known, the climbing fiber synapse may exert profound changes in the Purkinje cell's long-term electrical behavior.

Second, climbing fiber activity is altered during a period of motor learning. In a classic experiment, monkeys were trained to move a lever into a target zone using only wrist flexion or extension. Once the monkeys had learned the task, climbing fiber spikes in Purkinje cells occurred randomly and infrequently (about 1 to 2 Hz). But when the load on the lever was changed so that a slightly different coordination between flexors and extensors was required to place the lever in the target zone, climbing fiber activity increased to about 4 to 6 Hz. In addition, the activity was no longer random, but became correlated with the lever displacement. After the new task was learned, climbing fiber activity once again declined and became random and infrequent. Furthermore, spike activity from parallel fibers decreased during the learning period and remained at the lower level after the new task was learned and the climbing fiber activity had returned to prelearning levels.

## THEORY OF CEREBELLAR FUNCTION

Despite our fairly detailed knowledge of the anatomy and physiology of the cerebellar circuits, there is no comprehensive and coherent model of overall cerebellar function. However, some promising ideas have been presented that are described in the following sections. One theory of cerebellar function follows from the observation that the principal function of the cerebellum seems to be the *coordination of muscle contractions across synergistic groups*. This coordination is achieved by *regulating the timing* of individual muscle contractions.

### Role of Parallel Fiber Excitation

Although the parallel fibers in the molecular layer of the cerebellum synapse with hundreds of Purkinje cells, these parallel fiber synapses are not all active simultaneously. Because of the small diameter of parallel fibers, action potentials travel relatively slowly[5] across the folia, exciting one Purkinje cell after another in series. Thus a wave of Purkinje cell excitation spreads down a folium, following the action potentials along the parallel fibers. The inhibitory basket cells and stellate cells are also excited by this wave. However, because their axons run perpendicular to the parallel fibers, the wave of basket cell–Purkinje cell inhibition spreads across the folia perpendicular to the parallel fiber–Purkinje cell excitatory wave (Fig. 9.13) that occurs simultaneously.

The Purkinje cells that are lined up along a beam of parallel fibers send axons into one of the deep cerebellar nuclei. Here they synapse in an orderly manner across the nucleus that is somatotopically mapped to the body. Therefore, as the Purkinje cells fire sequentially along the folia, the cells in the deep cerebellar nuclei are also affected sequentially. Thus the timing of the cerebellum's motor regulatory activity is predetermined by the relation of the Purkinje cells to the parallel fibers and the sequence of muscles affected by the relation of the Purkinje cells to the deep nuclear cells (Fig. 9.14).

A single row of Purkinje cells receives hundreds of thousands of synapses with parallel fibers. Each of those synapses has the potential to produce EPSPs with different amplitudes and time courses. Since each parallel fiber may

---

[5] Parallel fibers are unmyelinated and average about 0.2 $\mu$m in diameter. Such fibers conduct at about 0.5 M/sec/$\mu$m. Therefore, an action potential takes about 50 msec to travel from the center to the end of a 10-mm parallel fiber.

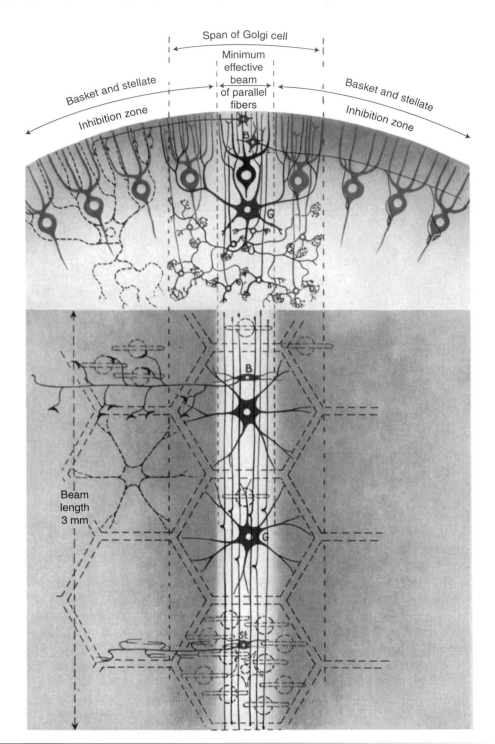

## Figure 9.13  Excitation and inhibition patterns in the cerebellar cortex

The spreading wave of excitation by parallel fibers and inhibition by basket cells and stellate cells. **Top.** The cerebellar cortex in cross-section. *Arrows* across the top of the figure, inhibition zone of the basket and stellate cells. **Bottom.** The cerebellar cortex viewed from the surface. *White path* in the center, the zone of parallel fiber excitation that intersects Purkinje cells (*dashed cells,* not labeled), basket cells (*B*), Golgi cells (*G*), and stellate cells (*St*). The intensity of the purple shading indicates the wave of inhibition spreading laterally across the folium. This inhibitory wave decreases the excitability of Purkinje cells that are not in the beam of parallel fiber excitation. Basket cell inhibition may act to deselect alternate sets of Purkinje cells that affect the same synergistic set of muscles as the selected beam (Fig. 9.14). (Reprinted with permission from Eccles JC, Szentagothai J. The Cerebellum As a Neuronal Machine. New York: Springer-Verlag, 1967.)

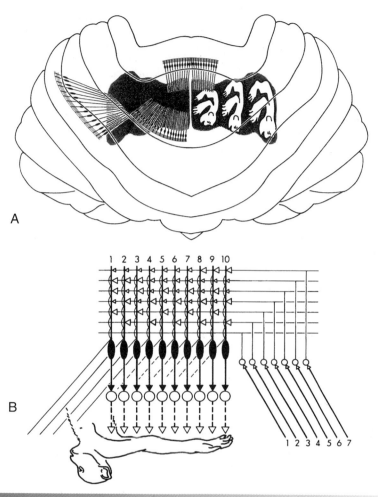

### Figure 9.14 Hypothesis of cerebellar function

**A.** A beam of parallel fibers selects a set of Purkinje cells that project across one of the deep cerebellar nuclei. This projection automatically affects synergistic muscle groups because the nucleus is somatotopically organized. The timing is determined by the slow progression of excitation along the parallel fibers. **B.** The same beam of Purkinje cells may be selected by numerous parallel fiber pathways, each of which represents different sensory stimuli projected through the granule cell synapse. The various parallel fiber pathways do not all necessarily activate the Purkinje cells to the same degree. The effectiveness of the parallel fiber–Purkinje cell synapse is depicted by the size of the triangular synapse. Each of the seven parallel fibers may represent a slightly different coordination of the same set of synergistic muscles. (Reprinted with permission from Thach WT, Goodkin HP, Keating JG. The cerebellum and the adaptive coordination of movement. Annu Rev Neurosci 1992; 15:403–442.)

have a different effect on a Purkinje cell, the selection of parallel fibers is crucial to the function of the cerebellum. In effect, each parallel fiber represents a differently computed program of precisely timed motor sequences. Therefore, different sequence adjustments can

be imposed on a motor act by Purkinje cell activity triggered by different sets of granule cell–parallel fiber selection (Fig. 9.14).

Parallel rows of Purkinje cells in the cerebellar cortex control different but closely related sequences of muscle coordination.

Slight differences in sequencing can be established by the slightly different connections that the Purkinje cells make in the deep nuclei. The radiating pattern of basket cell and stellate cell inhibition that spreads across the folia perpendicular to parallel fiber excitation suppresses the competing parallel representations of coordination sequences (Fig. 9.13). Therefore, as one Purkinje cell beam is excited, its immediate neighboring beams are inhibited.

## Clinical Corroboration

These ideas of cerebellar function correlate well with two clinical observations. First, small lesions to the cerebellum produce few symptoms. Lesions must be quite large, involving most of a lobe, for example, before obvious cerebellar

symptoms appear. This observation is consistent with the hypothesis that the cerebellar circuitry includes a lot of functional redundancy. As described earlier, if multiple repetitions of Purkinje cell sets represent only variations on essentially the same motor sequence, then moderate lesions can be absorbed with only very subtle changes in motor function observable. Second, clinical experience and recent experimental evidence in animals have demonstrated that unlike the cerebral cortex, the cerebellar cortex has no well-defined somatotopic organization. This observation is also consistent with the stated hypothesis because it is the cerebellar *output* that is somatotopically mapped through the deep nuclei. The input is redundantly reproduced on the cortical surface by the granule cell–parallel fiber path.

# C A S E   H I S T O R Y

## THE CASE OF MUSHROOMS AND COCAINE[6]

### HISTORY OF PRESENT ILLNESS

Mr. T. H. is a 34-year-old man who collapsed one morning while dressing. He was unable to move any extremity, had double vision, and had difficulty speaking. He was fully conscious and remained so during the ambulance ride to the emergency department, where he arrived within an hour of the initial onset of symptoms.

### MEDICAL HISTORY

He had an inguinal herniorrhaphy 3 years earlier. There is no recent history of head or neck trauma. He does not use alcoholic beverages, but he did admit to the occasional use of hallu-

cinogenic mushrooms and cocaine. The most recent use of cocaine was 3 days before the present illness. His grandmother died of a stroke at age 60; his grandfather died of a heart attack at the age of 73.

### PHYSICAL EXAMINATION

On admission his vital signs were blood pressure, 150/100; heart rate, 120; respirations, 12.

### NEUROLOGICAL EXAMINATION

**Mental Status**
Mr T. H. is awake and oriented to person, place, and time. He can give a good history, although there is a severe dysarthria.

**Cranial Nerves**

OLFACTION: Not tested.

---

[6] This case was brought to my attention by Dr. Rahman Pourmand of the Indiana University School of Medicine.

VISION: Visual fields were full to confrontation. The patient reported horizontal diplopia and "blurry vision"; fundi were normal in appearance (no papilledema).

OCULOMOTION: Mr. T. H. is unable to adduct the right eye on left lateral gaze or adduct the left eye on right lateral gaze. Both eyes adduct on convergence (bilateral internuclear ophthalmoplegia; see Chapter 10). Left and right abduction and vertical eye movements were full. There was right ptosis.

PUPILS: The right pupil was 7 mm; the left, 3 mm (anisocoria).

TRIGEMINAL: Light touch and cold were poorly perceived over the right side of the face. Masseter strength was not noted.

FACIAL: There was mild weakness of the lower right face.

AUDITION: Mr. T. H. could hear light finger rubbing bilaterally. Air conduction was more sensitive than bone conduction bilaterally (Rinne test), and the Weber test was perceived in the midline. The patient reported that there was no tinnitus (see Chapter 11).

VAGOGLOSSOPHARYNGEAL: Palatal elevation was symmetrical and full. Gag reflex was present bilaterally. Phonation was normal.

ACCESSORY: Trapezius and sternocleidomastoid strength was 4/5 bilaterally.

HYPOGLOSSAL: The tongue protruded in the midline. There was no atrophy or fasciculations.

STATION AND GAIT: Mr. T. H. was unable to walk.

## Motor Systems

STRENGTH: There was slight weakness in all groups (4/5).

TONE: Slight spasticity was observed in all muscle groups in all extremities.

BULK: Mr. T. H. is well muscled. The extremities were symmetrical.

ABNORMAL MOVEMENTS: There were no involuntary movements or fasciculations.

## Sensory Systems

Mr. T. H. perceived light touch and pinprick equally from all extremities, both proximal and distal.

## Reflexes

The MSRs were symmetric and slightly elevated (+) from all muscle groups in all extremities. The Babinski sign was present bilaterally.

## Coordination and control

There was severe bilateral dysmetria and dysdiadochokinesia in the upper and lower extremities. This was so severe that Mr. T. H. could not walk. There was pronounced dysarthria with scanning speech.

## Parietal Functions

There is no aphasia or atavistic signs. Optokinetic reflex (OKN) was present bilaterally.

## ANCILLARY STUDIES

Computed tomography (CT) of the head taken in the emergency department was read as normal. Magnetic resonance imaging (MRI) 3 days after admission revealed bilateral paramedian midbrain infarctions (Fig. 9.15). Magnetic resonance arteriogram (MRA) demonstrated a thrombus in the distal 7 mm of the basilar artery. Transesophageal echocardiography (TEE) demonstrated a patent foramen ovale with a right-to-left shunt demonstrated with microtubules. There was also an atrial septal aneurysm. Venous Doppler sonography did not demonstrate any deep vein thrombi.

## SUBSEQUENT COURSE

After a period of recovery and rehabilitation, Mr. T. H. returned to his home and lives independently. He has residual bilateral intranuclear ophthalmoplegia, dysarthria, dysmetria, ataxia, and occasional diplopia. He can walk only with assistance and uses a wheelchair for mobility. He is unable to work. He is taking fluoxetine (Prozac), warfarin (Coumadin), and propranolol (Inderal).

## COMMENTARY

The history of rapid onset of symptoms and the retention of consciousness suggest that Mr. T. H. has had a stroke. CT at the time did not demonstrate intracranial bleeding, so the stroke was probably caused by a thrombus or an embolus (see Chapter 7).

Having hypothesized a stroke, the next step is to determine the location of the lesion. The most striking feature of this case is the dysarthria, ataxia, and scanning speech. The ataxia is so severe that the patient cannot walk. These are the cardinal signs of cerebellar injury, but they do not localize the lesion more specifically than to the cerebellum and its connections (peduncles).

Fortunately for purposes of diagnosis, there are more signs and symptoms in this case than dysarthria and ataxia. Mr. T. H. has facial weakness, facial hypoesthesia [G. hypo, under, and

aisthesis, feeling], ptosis, and anisocoria [G. aniso, unequal, and kor, pupil], all on the right side. These signs point to CN III, V, and VII.

In the case of CN signs, it is necessary to decide whether the nerve itself or its central connections are involved in the lesion. In the case of the facial nerve, only the lower right part of the face is weak; the upper face is spared. This is a sign of upper motor neuron facial paresis; therefore, the nucleus itself is spared (see Chapter 10 for a discussion of facial palsy) and the corticobulbar fibers rostral to the facial nucleus and contralateral to the facial weakness must be involved.

Similarly, the oculomotor nerve, which controls the lifting of the eyelid and the pupillary diameter as well as all but two of the extraocular muscles, is not affected because there is no weakness of the extraocular muscles. This lack of

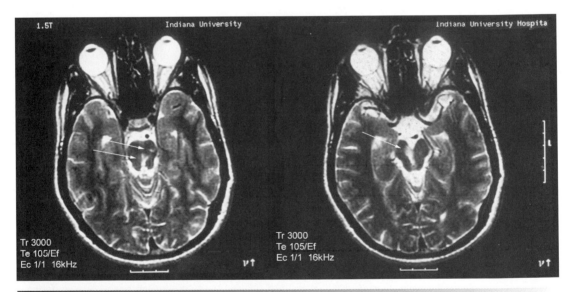

**Figure 9.15    MRI of Mr. T. H.**

**Left.** Two areas of high signal in the pons (*arrows*). The central enhancement involves the decussation of the superior cerebellar peduncles and part of the central tectum, including the MLF. The smaller enhancement is in the basis of the pons and may involve some CBST fibers. **Right.** The large enhancement in the central pons. It involves a small portion of the right cerebral peduncle, the decussation of the superior cerebellar peduncle, and the MLF. (MRI courtesy of Dr. Raymond Pourmand, Indiana University Hospitals.)

weakness is a subtle point because the patient cannot adduct either eye on contralateral gaze. However, since the patient can adduct both eyes on convergence (looking at a close object, which causes both eyes to adduct), the medial recti muscles and their innervation must be intact. This **internuclear ophthalmoplegia** is caused by a lesion to the medial longitudinal fasciculus (MLF). The central pathways that control eyelid elevation and pupillary diameter are in the tectum of the midbrain (see Chapter 10 for a discussion of eye movements).

This analysis indicates two lesions, one on the left rostral to the facial nucleus but caudal to the internal capsule. The second lesion is in the midbrain, probably on the right. Multiple lesions are anathema to neurologists because most neurological disease produces a single lesion. In this case, however, the increased MSRs, weakness, and Babinski signs are bilateral, which supports bilateral lesions. The most prominent neurological signs in this case are dysarthria and ataxia. These can be explained by midbrain lesions if the superior cerebellar peduncles are involved.

The analysis of all these data suggests that there are two lesions in the midbrain, one on the right, the other on the left. Both lesions involve the superior cerebellar peduncles, the CBST, and the pretectal area. The superior cerebellar peduncles are probably most severely affected because the cerebellar signs are so pronounced. The CBST is only minimally involved because the weakness and increased MSRs are slight. The pretectal lesion is probably on the right, affecting the fibers leading from it to the oculomotor nucleus but not the nucleus itself. This hypothesis was confirmed by MRI (Fig. 9.15).

The next step is to determine whether the stroke was caused by a thrombus or an embolus (see Chapter 7). The MRA, which was ordered to differentiate between these possibilities, revealed an occlusion of the rostral portion of the basilar artery. Most of the remaining ancillary studies were directed at locating the source of any emboli. Investigation with TEE unexpectedly revealed a patent foramen ovale and atrial septal

aneurysm in the heart with right-to-left shunting. Sonography of the large deep veins did not reveal any thrombi, so it is presumed that blood collected in the pocket of the aneurysm and coagulated. The clot or pieces of it broke off and entered the left circulation through the foramen ovale. Mr. T. H. remains at risk for developing further emboli.

## FURTHER APPLICATIONS

9.1. When analyzing a case of neurological deficit, it is often useful to ask yourself if the lesion could be located in (a) the cerebral cortex or internal capsule, (b) the basal ganglion or thalamus, (c) the brainstem, (d) the cerebellum, (e) the spinal cord, or (f) the peripheral nervous system. What signs or symptoms point to or eliminate each of these general areas as the site of the lesion in this case?

9.2. Justify the use of MRI 3 days after a CT revealed no lesions in the brain.

9.3. Explain why deep vein thrombi present more than ordinary concern in this case.

9.4. Explain the diminution of light touch sensations from the right face while light touch is preserved throughout the rest of the body.

9.5. Mr. H. T. is taking fluoxetine, warfarin, and propranolol. What is the specific usefulness of each drug in this case?

9.6. Is the use of hallucinogenic mushrooms and cocaine medically significant?

9.7. What major neurological disease is characterized by multiple CNS lesions? Why is that diagnosis not likely in this case?

## S U M M A R Y

- The cerebellum is composed of a pair of hemispheres joined in the midline by the vermis and the flocculonodular lobe.

  The cerebellum is attached to the brainstem by three pairs of peduncles, the superior, middle, and inferior. The cerebellum has a superficial cortex that contains most of the cerebellar cells and a central core that contains three pairs of nuclei. The Purkinje cell is the only cortical cell that projects out of the cortex; the remainder of the cells—the basket, Golgi, granule, and stellate cells—are interneurons in the cerebellar cortex.

- There are three types of fibers entering the cerebellum: mossy fibers, climbing fibers, and monoaminergic fibers.

  Climbing fibers arise only from the inferior olive. They synapse with the soma and basal dendrites of Purkinje cells, activating calcium ion channels. Mossy fibers excite granule cells. The granule cell axon becomes the parallel fibers of the cerebellar cortex and are the principal excitatory input to Purkinje cells. The monoaminergic fibers originate in the raphe nuclei and the locus ceruleus (norepinephrine-containing axons). Their physiological function is unknown.

- The cerebellum is functionally divided into three parts: the vestibular, spinal, and cerebral regions.

  Each division of the cerebellum has its principal input and output connections with the division of the CNS for which it is named. The vestibular and spinal divisions of the cerebellum are arranged as a feedback loop. These divisions use proprioceptive information to modify the activity of the descending motor systems after the commencement of the motor act. Output from the vestibular and spinal cerebellum synapses in the red nucleus,

the motor areas of the reticular formation, and the vestibular nuclei. The cerebrocerebellum is arranged as a feed-forward loop. It receives sensory information from the cerebral cortex about current limb position as well as information about impending motor commands. Its efferent fibers project back to the thalamus and from the thalamus to the primary motor areas of the cerebral cortex. At the cerebral cortex these fibers can affect the final development of the motor command before it is initiated.

- Motor learning occurs in the cerebellum.

  The improvement in motor skills that occurs with practice is due to alterations in cerebellar function. This neuronal plasticity is believed to be accomplished by the calcium ion current induced by the climbing fibers. It is thought that the increased calcium concentration activates appropriate protein kinases that eventually modify the efficiency of the simultaneously active parallel fiber synapses.

- Disturbances of cerebellar function desynchronize activity among synergistic muscles.

  The clinical manifestations of cerebellar dysfunction are nystagmus and ataxia arising from the vestibulocerebellum and dysmetria, dysdiadochokinesia, hypotonic MSRs, and decomposition of movement arising from the spinocerebellum and cerebrocerebellum.

### SUGGESTED READINGS

Eccles JC, Szentagothai J. The Cerebellum As a Neuronal Machine. New York: Springer-Verlag, 1967.

Thach WT, Goodkin HP, Keating JG. The cerebellum and the adaptive coordination of movement. Annu Rev Neurosci 1992;15:403–442.

# The Cranial Nerves

A thorough understanding of the anatomy and physiology of the cranial nerves is essential for diagnosing many neurological conditions. Because the cranial nerve nuclei reside at all levels of the brainstem, deficits in cranial nerve function provide essential clues to the integrity of brainstem functions, such as the regulation of respiration, cardiovascular reflexes, and even consciousness. Furthermore, analysis of abnormal cranial nerve function often leads to the precise localization of intracranial lesions, an essential step in developing a neurological diagnosis. Three cranial nerves innervate the intrinsic and extraocular muscles of the eyes, and these nerves are in turn affected by the tectum and the vestibular system. Therefore, eye movements and ocular reflexes are an important part of the neurological examination, making the eyes an important window to the brain. Most of the cranial nerves, beginning with the hypoglossal, are discussed in this chapter. Because cranial nerves are composed of more than one functional element or modality, each modality will be discussed separately.

The concept of **neural modalities** and the associated nomenclature are presented in Appendix 1, Box A.1. This nomenclature arises from the developmental segregation of the neuroblasts into a series of columns (Fig. 10.1; see Appendix 1, Figs. A.9 and A.10). Each column represents a different neural function. Traditionally, the functional divisions of the cranial nerves are described in terms of these embryologically derived modalities. However, many of the distinctions between the various modalities blur during development. Further-

more, no one cranial nerve expresses all of the modalities. Therefore, the organizational description of the functional components of the cranial nerves can be simplified to include only **afferent, efferent, somatic,** and **visceral modalities,** a useful approach that is employed in this chapter. Table 10.1 summarizes the traditional classification scheme.

The afferent and efferent components of the cranial nerves are associated with nuclei that lie in the **alar** and **basal** plate regions of the brainstem, respectively (see Appendix 1). The division between these two embryonic regions is marked in the brainstem, most prominently in the medulla, by a shallow groove, the **sulcus limitans** (Fig. 10.2). In the medulla, the basal-alar division is marked by an imaginary line that extends from the sulcus limitans ventral laterally to the margin of the brainstem. This imaginary line becomes more horizontal as it ascends the brainstem. Ventral and medial to the sulcus lie the basal plate derivatives, the motor nuclei. Dorsal and lateral to the sulcus lie the alar plate derivatives, the sensory nuclei. The nuclei of the **visceral** cranial nerve components generally lie close to this imaginary line; the nuclei of the **somatic** components lie more medially (motor) or laterally (sensory). This chapter discusses all of the cranial nerves except the olfactory, optic, and acoustic nerves, which are addressed in later chapters.

## THE HYPOGLOSSAL NERVE (XII)

The hypoglossal nerve is purely motor and is served by a single nucleus in the medulla. The

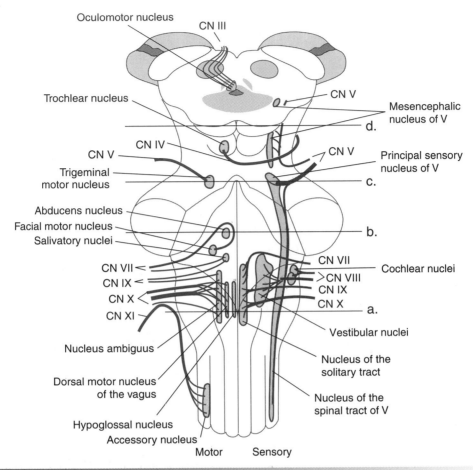

**Figure 10.1   Location of cranial nerves and associated nuclei**

This transparent view from the dorsal surface of the brainstem illustrates the location and extent of the cranial nerve nuclei and the internal course of their axons. The motor nuclei and nerves are shown on the *left;* the sensory nerves and nuclei are shown on the *right*. Not shown: the cranial nerve ganglia associated with each of the sensory nerves (except the mesencephalic division of V). The lines marked *a, b, c,* and *d* indicate the level of the corresponding cross-sections in Figure 10.2.

motor neuron cell bodies of the hypoglossal nerve lie in the **hypoglossal nucleus.** This small, compact tubular nucleus lies close to the midline in the caudal medulla, immediately ventral to the fourth ventricle (Fig. 10.3). It receives afferent connections from the *contralateral* corticobulbar tract. As they leave the nucleus, hypoglossal axons take a ventral and slightly lateral course and emerge from the brainstem between the medullary pyramid and the inferior olive. The hypoglossal nerve leaves the skull through the **hypoglossal canal.** Its axons innervate the *ipsilateral* tongue, supplying

the **intrinsic muscles** of the tongue and the **styloglossus, hyoglossus, genioglossus,** and **geniohyoid** muscles.

Damage to the hypoglossal nucleus or nerve at any point along its course causes typical lower motor neuron (LMN) signs in the ipsilateral half of the tongue. These signs include paresis or paralysis, depending on the severity of the lesion. Fasciculations in the tongue are easily seen, followed in a few days by obvious atrophy. On palpation, the affected side of the denervated tongue feels soft and flaccid. When the patient is asked to stick the tongue straight

## Table 10.1  Summary of Cranial Nerves

| Nerve | Component[a] | Function | CNS Nuclei |
|---|---|---|---|
| I Olfactory | SSA[b] | Olfaction | Periamygdala and entorhinal cortex |
| II Optic | SSA[c] | Vision | Lateral geniculate nucleus |
| III Oculomotor | GSE | Oculomotion and elevation of eyelid | Oculomotor nucleus |
| | GVE | Pupillary constriction and lens accommodation | Edinger-Westphal nucleus |
| IV Trochlear | GSE | Superior oblique muscle | Trochlear nucleus |
| V Trigeminal | SVE | Muscles of mastication | Motor nucleus of V |
| | GSA | Sensory, light touch | Principal sensory nucleus of V |
| | GSA | Sensory, pain, and temperature | Nucleus of the spinal tract of V |
| | GSA | Sensory, proprioception | Mesencephalic nucleus of V |
| VI Abducens | GSE | Lateral rectus muscle | Abducens nucleus |
| VII Facial | SVE | Mimetic muscles | Facial motor nucleus |
| | GVE | Lacrimation and salivation | Superior salivatory nucleus |
| | SVA | Taste, anterior two-thirds of tongue | Nucleus of the solitary tract of V |
| | GSA | Sensory, pain, and temperature | Nucleus of the spinal tract of V |
| VIII Acoustic and vestibular | SSA | Balance | Vestibular nuclei |
| | SSA | Hearing | Cochlear nuclei |
| | SSE[d] | Regulate vestibular hair cell function | Periabducens nuclei |
| | SSE | Regulate cochlear hair cell function | Periolivary nuclei |
| IX and X Glossopharyngeal vagus | SVE | Muscles of soft palate, pharynx, and larynx | Nucleus ambiguus |
| | GVE | Salivation (IX) | Inferior salivatory nucleus |
| | GVE | Regulation of digestive organs | Dorsal motor nucleus of the vagus |
| | GVE | Regulation of the heart | Nucleus ambiguus |
| | SVA | Taste, posterior third of tongue (IX) | Nucleus of the solitary tract |
| | GVA | Sensory from viscera, baroreception, and chemoreception | Nucleus of the solitary tract |
| | GSA | Sensory, pain, and temperature | Nucleus of the spinal tract of V |

[a] See Box AI.1 for explanation of classification schema.

[b] The true olfactory nerve consists only of the axons of the bipolar receptor cells. It is appropriately classified as SSA based on its origin from a placode.

[c] The classification scheme does not apply to the optic nerve because the so-called nerve consists of second-order axons that are myelinated by oligodendrocytes, characteristics that classify it as a CNS tract. The true cranial nerve of vision consists of axons of the retinal bipolar cells derived from the optic cup, a placode.

[d] The efferent vestibulocochlear fibers are not usually included in this classification scheme; the SSE designation is appropriate.

**Table 10.1　Summary of Cranial Nerves—*continued***

| Nerve | Component[a] | Function | CNS Nuclei |
|---|---|---|---|
| XI Accessory | SVE[e] | Trapezius and sterno-cleidomastoid muscles | Accessory nucleus in spinal cord C2-C5 |
| XII Hypoglossal | GSE | Intrinsic muscles of the tongue | Hypoglossal nucleus |

[e] The SVE classification is based on data that show the accessory nucleus of the spinal cord to be a displaced fragment of the nucleus ambiguus. This nerve has been classified as GSE by some authors and left unclassified by others.

out, the tongue deviates *toward the side of weakness.* This deviation is a result of the way each genioglossus muscle extends and adducts [L. *adduco,* bring to] the tongue. When both muscles are active, the adductor forces from each side balance, and the tongue extends in the midline. If one genioglossus is paralyzed, its opposite member adducts the tongue across the midline upon extension. Damage to the corticobulbar tract above the level of the nucleus of cranial nerve (CN) XII causes an upper motor neuron (UMN) type of paresis of the tongue contralateral to the lesion. Since it is impractical to test the muscle stretch reflex of the tongue, the UMN nature of the lesion can be ascertained only by the absence of LMN signs in the tongue.

Deviation of the tongue indicates a neurological problem affecting the motor control of the tongue, but deviation per se does not localize the side of the lesion. If the lesion is in the nerve or nucleus, tongue deviation is toward the side with the lesion. If the lesion is the UMN type, the tongue deviates away from the side of the lesion. In both cases, *deviation is toward the side of weakness.* Observing the presence or absence of fasciculations and atrophy and noting tongue muscle tone are essential in evaluating hypoglossal function.

**THE ACCESSORY NERVE (XI)**

The accessory nerve, which is also purely motor, is supplied by a single nucleus. The motor

neurons are in the **accessory nucleus,** a column of motor neurons that reside in the dorsolateral portion of the spinal cord.[1] Axons from the accessory motor neurons do not leave the spinal cord in the ventral root but exit the cord just dorsal to the dentate ligament, between the dorsal and ventral roots (Fig. 10.4). Accessory rootlets join one another as they ascend in the subdural space along the side of the spinal cord. Entering the cranium through the **foramen magnum,** they briefly join the vagus nerve rootlets before leaving the cranium through the **jugular foramen.** Just outside the skull the accessory nerve separates from the vagus nerve and innervates the ipsilateral **sternocleidomastoid** and **trapezius** muscles.

Isolated lesions to the accessory nerve are not common. Loss of accessory nerve function causes a LMN paralysis of the muscles it innervates. Contraction of the sternocleidomastoid muscle causes the head to rotate from side to side on the atlas and thrusts the chin down and laterally toward the side opposite the muscle. Weakness of the sternocleidomastoid can be easily tested by asking the patient to turn the head to one side while the examiner resists the movement by holding the chin. The chin moves *away from the muscle being tested.* The trapezius is a major muscle of the back and shoulder. If it is paralyzed, shrugging the shoulder and elevation and outward rotation of the arm are all compromised on the ipsilateral side.

[1] The accessory nucleus is a fragment of the nucleus ambiguus. The accessory nucleus fragment separates from the main nucleus during development and migrates into the spinal cord, drawing the peripheral nerve fibers with it. This developmental peculiarity explains the unusual peripheral course of the accessory nerve. Because it originates in the nucleus ambiguus, the cranial division of the accessory nerve is described as part of the vagus nerve.

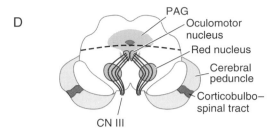

D

PAG
Oculomotor
nucleus
Red nucleus
Cerebral
peduncle
Corticobulbo–
spinal tract
CN III

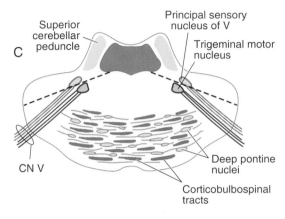

Superior
cerebellar
peduncle

C

Principal sensory
nucleus of V
Trigeminal motor
nucleus

CN V

Deep pontine
nuclei

Corticobulbospinal
tracts

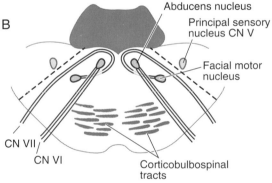

B

Abducens nucleus
Principal sensory
nucleus CN V

Facial motor
nucleus

CN VII
CN VI

Corticobulbospinal
tracts

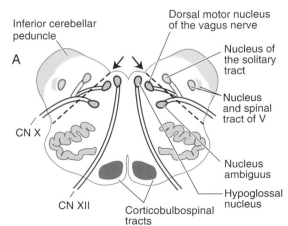

Inferior cerebellar
peduncle

A

Dorsal motor nucleus
of the vagus nerve

Nucleus of
the solitary
tract

Nucleus
and spinal
tract of V

CN X

Nucleus
ambiguus

Hypoglossal
nucleus

CN XII
Corticobulbospinal
tracts

**Figure 10.2   Alar–basal plate divisions in the brainstem**

Cross-sections of the brainstem at the level of the medulla (**A**), the pontomedullary junction (**B**), the pons (**C**), and the mesencephalon (**D**). The junction between the alar and basal plate is indicated by the broken line. Sensory components are shown in *gray;* motor, in *pink.*

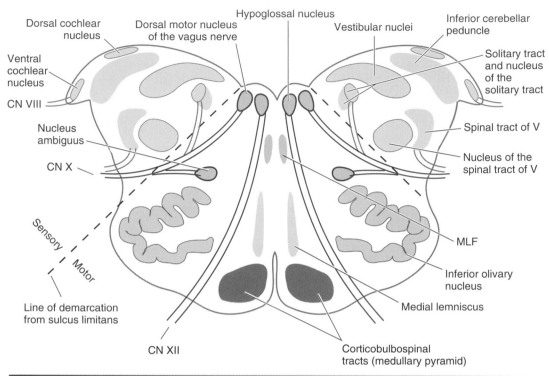

Dorsal cochlear nucleus

Ventral cochlear nucleus

CN VIII

Nucleus ambiguus

CN X

Sensory / Motor

Line of demarcation from sulcus limitans

CN XII

Dorsal motor nucleus of the vagus nerve

Hypoglossal nucleus

Vestibular nuclei

Inferior cerebellar peduncle

Solitary tract and nucleus of the solitary tract

Spinal tract of V

Nucleus of the spinal tract of V

MLF

Inferior olivary nucleus

Medial lemniscus

Corticobulbospinal tracts (medullary pyramid)

**Figure 10.3   Cranial nerves of the medulla**

The accessory nucleus is innervated by axons in the corticospinal tract. Since the nucleus lies caudal to the pyramidal decussation, almost all UMN types of lesions involving the accessory nucleus occur contralateral to the side of paralysis. However, as lesions to the corticospinal tract generally produce a hemiparesis, the sternocleidomastoid and trapezius muscles are not affected in isolation. Therefore, noting their involvement in UMN types of lesions is generally not diagnostically significant.

## THE VAGUS (X) AND GLOSSOPHARYNGEAL (IX) NERVE COMPLEX

The vagus and glossopharyngeal nerves are separate structures in the periphery, but centrally they share the same anatomy and functions. All of the axons belonging to these nerves penetrate the brainstem dorsal to the

inferior olive as a series of rootlets that extend along the medulla throughout the length of the inferior olive. Unlike the hypoglossal and accessory nerves, the vagus and glossopharyngeal nerves have several afferent and efferent components. Within the medulla, axons belonging to the various functional components are associated with five nuclei (Figs. 10.3 and 10.5).

### Efferent Components

Efferent axons of the vagus and glossopharyngeal nerves arise from three nuclei: the **nucleus ambiguus**, the **dorsal motor nucleus of the vagus**, and the **inferior salivatory nucleus.**

THE NUCLEUS AMBIGUUS

The nucleus ambiguus is a large motor nucleus in the ventral lateral portion of the medullary reticular formation just dorsal to the inferior olive. It receives *bilateral innerva-*

*tion* from the corticobulbar tract. Axons destined to join the glossopharyngeal nerve arise from the most rostral portions of the nucleus; those joining the vagus arise from the caudal region. Axons leaving the nucleus ambiguus innervate the intrinsic voluntary muscles of the larynx (laryngeal nerve, a branch of the vagus); the constrictor muscles of the pharynx (the **palatoglossus** and **levator palati**, the pharyngeal branch of the vagus); and from the glossopharyngeal nerve, the **stylopharyngeus muscle** (an elevator of the pharynx). The nu-

cleus ambiguus also innervates the heart. Neurons in the nucleus ambiguus slow the heart rate and decrease atrioventricular conduction within the heart.

## THE DORSAL MOTOR NUCLEUS OF THE VAGUS

The parasympathetic preganglionic axons of the vagus nerve arise from the **dorsal motor nucleus of the vagus** (DMN). The DMN receives afferent fibers primarily from the hypothalamus and the nucleus of the solitary tract (discussed

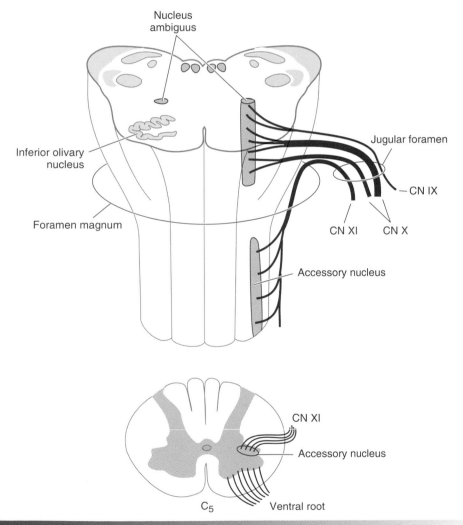

**Figure 10.4   The accessory nucleus and nerve**

**Top.** The peripheral course of the accessory nerve showing how it briefly joins the most caudal rootlets of the vagus nerve intracranially before separating from it. **Bottom.** Location of the accessory nucleus in the spinal cord and the separate egress of its axons from the ventral root when leaving the cord.

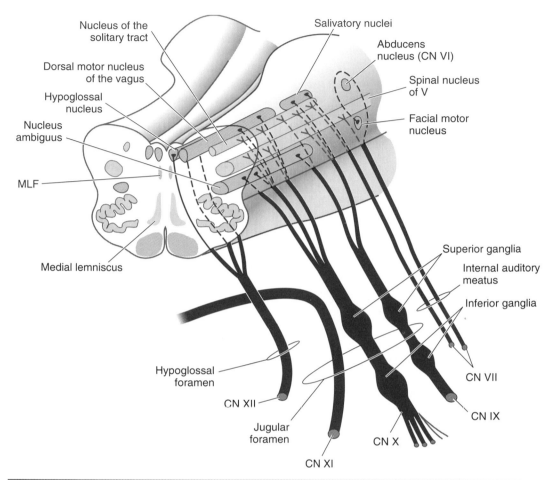

**Figure 10.5   The cranial nerves of the medulla and their nuclei**

later in the chapter). Axons leaving the DMN are widely distributed throughout the viscera. In addition to the heart, they innervate all of the alimentary canal and the digestive organs, including the pharynx, esophagus, trachea, bronchi, stomach, liver, pancreas, small intestine, and most of the colon. Short postganglionic axons synapse with glands or smooth muscle within these various target tissues.

## THE INFERIOR SALIVATORY NUCLEUS

Preganglionic parasympathetic fibers innervating the parotid gland arise from the inferior salivatory nucleus. This small nucleus contributes axons only to the glossopharyngeal nerve. The axons separate from the main nerve almost immediately after passing

through the jugular foramen, forming the tympanic nerve. The tympanic nerve enters the temporal bone through the tympanic canaliculus and forms a plexus in the middle ear that innervates its mucous membranes. From the middle ear the nerve continues as the lesser petrosal nerve, passing once again through the temporal bone and reentering the cranium. It leaves the cranium for the last time through the foramen ovale and synapses in the **otic ganglion**. Postganglionic axons leave the otic ganglion to supply the parotid gland.

## Afferent Components

The cell bodies of the primary afferent axons of the vagus and glossopharyngeal nerves reside in peripheral ganglia. Each nerve is associated with two ganglia, the superior and the inferior. Like the neurons in the dorsal root ganglia of the spinal nerves, the sensory neurons in the cranial nerve ganglia are pseudo-unipolar. In the ninth and tenth nerves the peripheral sensory axons arise from a variety of locations but synapse in the central nervous system (CNS) in one of only two nuclei, the **nucleus of the solitary tract** (NST) or the **nucleus of the spinal tract of V** (NSTV).

## THE NUCLEUS OF THE SOLITARY TRACT

Most sensations from the viscera are not consciously felt.[2] However, these sensations are important for the regulation of many cardiovascular, respiratory, and gastrointestinal functions. Primary afferent axons of the glossopharyngeal and vagus nerves carrying visceral sensations arise from the same areas that are innervated by the efferent fibers of these nerves: the pharynx, larynx, trachea, bronchi, lungs, heart, and digestive organs. The cell bodies for these axons lie in the inferior ganglion of the two nerves. As they enter the brainstem, the sensory axons destined for the NST form a prominent bundle called the **solitary tract**. Axons entering this tract bend caudally and descend in the medulla before terminating. Along its course fibers leave the solitary tract and synapse in cells that line its lateral border. These cells form the NST (Figs. 10.3 and 10.5).

Axons that originate in specialized visceral receptors are particularly important in cardiovascular reflex regulation. Sensory axons in the glossopharyngeal nerve innervate the chemoreceptors of the **carotid body** and the baroreceptors of the **carotid sinus**. The sensory components of the vagus nerve innervate similar receptors in the **aortic arch**. The chemoreceptors detect oxygen tension in the blood; the baroreceptors measure blood pressure.

In humans, the glossopharyngeal is the principal nerve that conveys the sensation of taste. It innervates the taste buds in the posterior third of the tongue; the facial nerve innervates the taste buds from the anterior two-thirds of the tongue. The few taste buds on the epiglottis are innervated by the vagus nerve,

but these degenerate in infancy. The various taste buds contain cells specialized for chemoreception. Sensory axons that innervate the taste buds enter the brainstem over their respective nerves and synapse in the most rostral portion of the NST.

Neurons in the NST make extensive central connections. Local projections to the nucleus ambiguus, the DMN, the **dorsal raphe**, and the **medullary reticular formation** have been described, as have remote projections to the **hypothalamus** and the **amygdaloid complex**. These latter connections are undoubtedly important in the regulation of many autonomic functions. The reticular formation in particular participates in several reflex functions, including swallowing, vomiting, respiration, and cardiovascular regulation (see Chapter 15).

Rostral solitary neurons project directly to the ventral posterior medial (VPM) nucleus of the thalamus and to the hypothalamus. The VPM nucleus projects to the primary sensory cortex, where a gustatory area near the tongue representation in the primary sensory cortex has been identified in humans. This pathway is presumably responsible for the conscious sensations of taste. Projections to the hypothalamus probably are the afferent path for the feeding reflexes and perhaps some of the emotional affect associated with feeding.

## THE NUCLEUS OF THE SPINAL TRACT OF V

The glossopharyngeal and vagus nerves have axons that carry somatic sensations (i.e., from the body surface) to the CNS. The cell bodies of these axons are in the superior ganglion of each nerve. The **auricular nerve** innervates a small portion of the concha, the external auditory meatus, and the external surface of the tympanic membrane; it joins the vagus before entering the brainstem (Fig. 10.5). Sensory information from the posterior third of the tongue and the surface of the pharynx travel in the glossopharyngeal nerve. The central axons of the glossopharyngeal and vagus nerves become incorporated in the **spinal tract of V**. These axons terminate in the nucleus that lines the medial side of the tract, the nucleus

---

[2] Visceral pain is brought to consciousness over axons of the sympathetic nervous system that enter the spinal cord (see Chapter 5).

of the spinal tract of V (NSTV), which carries primary afferent axons from four cranial nerves: the trigeminal, facial, glossopharyngeal, and vagus (Fig. 10.5). The central connections of the NSTV are described in the discussion of the trigeminal nerve.

## Clinical Considerations

Peripheral lesions to the glossopharyngeal and vagus nerves are not common. Unilateral loss of the glossopharyngeal nerve results in paralysis of the *elevator muscle of the pharynx* and a loss of the *gag reflex* from the affected side. When the patient is asked to phonate, the paralyzed side of the pharynx droops in comparison with the intact side, where the elevator muscles draw the raphe into an arch.

Loss of the vagus nerve results in paralysis of the soft palate that frequently causes the *uvula to tilt toward the intact side*. Swallowing is impaired by the loss of the constrictors of the pharynx and the palatoglossus, a muscle at the base of the tongue that helps to initiate swallowing. During swallowing, food and fluids tend to be regurgitated into the nasopharynx because of the general loss of tone in the pharynx and soft pallet. More serious effects can occur as a result of *paralysis of the vocal cord* on the affected side. The paralyzed cord collapses and partially occludes the air passage, causing hoarseness. In the case of unilateral lesions, the hoarseness subsides with time. Bilateral lesions, however, can be life threatening because the collapse of both vocal cords can severely impair air flow. The most common lesion affects the left recurrent laryngeal nerve. Its involvement can signal disease in the thorax or mediastinum, since this nerve hooks under the aortic arch. Aortic aneurysms, enlargement of the tracheobronchial lymph nodes, and mediastinal tumors can all cause hoarseness by involvement of the left recurrent laryngeal nerve. Thyroidectomy and thymectomy are frequently complicated by injury to the laryngeal nerve.

Central lesions in the brainstem that involve the corticobulbar tracts do not produce dramatic vagal or glossopharyngeal symptoms because *the nucleus ambiguus is innervated bilaterally*. Consequently, lesions above the brainstem that affect corticobulbar fibers cause minimal symptoms. Brainstem lesions that directly affect the nuclei, however, produce the same LMN symptoms as direct lesions to peripheral nerves. For example, poliomyelitis is an infectious disease that kills motor neurons. Although it usually affects the lumbar spinal cord, it occasionally affects the brainstem, where it can cause weakness in swallowing, hoarseness, and tongue paralysis. Severe cases cause death. Vascular lesions may also directly affect the nuclei. The most common of these lesions is *occlusion of the posterior inferior cerebellar artery* (**Wallenberg's syndrome**). Another lesion directly affecting the brainstem nuclei is *chronic bulbar palsy*. This disease is caused by degeneration of the voluntary motor nuclei of the lower cranial nerves (V, VII, IX, X, and XII).

## THE VESTIBULOCOCHLEAR NERVE (VIII)

The vestibulocochlear nerve is mixed. Almost all of its axons are afferent, innervating the cochlea and the vestibular apparatus. However, a small efferent component innervates both the cochlea and vestibular apparatus, regulates the sensitivity of the receptors, and modulates the afferent synapses. In the following section only the vestibular apparatus and the vestibular division of CN VIII are described. The cochlea and the central auditory pathways are described in Chapter 11.

## The Labyrinth

The vestibulocochlear sensory organ evolved from the lateral line organ of bony fish. The lateral line organ consists of specialized sensory cells, called hair cells, that contain "hairs" extending from the apex of the cell into the slime on the surface of the fish. Bending of the hairs, which occurs whenever the slime in which the hairs are embedded is moved, excites the hair cells. Hair cells can therefore detect any movement of the water around the fish that disturbs the slime. Derivatives of the lateral line organ in mammals, the cochlea and the vestibular apparatus, detect sound pressure waves in air (hearing) and head movement (vestibular apparatus) by a mechanism that is essentially unchanged from that found in the fish—the bending of the cilia of hair cells in response to fluid movement.

In mammals, the vestibulocochlear system consists of a **bony labyrinth** and a **membranous labyrinth** (Fig. 10.6). The bony labyrinth consists of a series of interconnected cavities within the temporal bone that are filled with **perilymph,** a fluid similar in composition to cerebrospinal fluid. Suspended within the bony labyrinth is the membranous labyrinth, which consists of a series of ducts and sacs that enclose the sen-

sory epithelia of the auditory and vestibular systems. It is filled with **endolymph,** a fluid unique to the vestibulocochlear system and similar in composition to intracellular cytoplasm but without the inclusions and cytoskeletal elements. Endolymph has a high potassium ion concentration, about 140 mM, and a low sodium ion concentration, about 26 mM (Table 10.2).

Four distinct regions are found in the membranous labyrinth (Fig. 10.6). The **cochlea** is the organ of hearing. The **utricle** is a large, bulbous structure that lies at the base of three **semicircular ducts.**[3] The **saccule** lies between

---

[3] In the vernacular one usually sees the term semicircular canal. Strictly speaking, the canal is the cavity within the temporal bone; the duct is the space enclosed by the membranes.

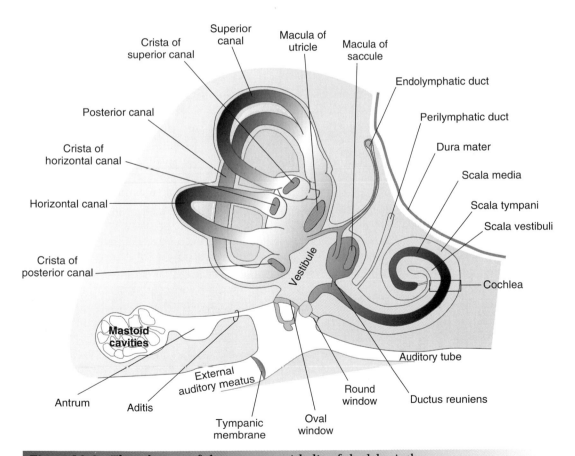

**Figure 10.6   The relations of the sensory epithelia of the labyrinth**

The membranous labyrinth (*gray*), which is filled with endolymph, is surrounded by the perilymphatic space (*pink*). The membranous labyrinth is a continuous structure. The small ductus reuniens maintains communication between the cochlear division and the vestibular division. The cochlear and mastoid structures are discussed in Chapter 11.

**Table 10.2   Ionic Composition of Body Fluids (mEq/L)**

|          | Plasma    | CSF   | Perilymph | Endolymph |
|----------|-----------|-------|-----------|-----------|
| Protein  | 6000–8000 | 10–38 | 75–100    | 10.0      |
| $K^+$    | 20        | 12–17 | 15        | 140.0     |
| $Na^+$   | 140       | 150   | 148       | 26.0      |
| $Cl^-$   | 600       | 750   | 120       | 14–0      |
| $Mg^{++}$| 1–3       | 2     | 2         | 0.9       |
| $Ca^{++}$| 7         | 3     | 3         | 3.0       |

the utricle and the cochlea. The *endolymphatic space of all four structures is continuous but closed*; it does not communicate with any other fluid space. The endolymphatic system is surrounded by a perilymphatic space that generally follows its contours except in the region of the utricle and saccule. There the perilymphatic space bulges to form a large cavity, the **vestibule**. An oval hole called the **oval window** lies in the wall separating the vestibule from the middle ear cavity. It is normally filled by the footplate of the stapes (see Chapter 11).

### The Vestibular Sensory Epithelia

The utricle and the saccule each contain a neuroepithelial sensory receptor called a **macula**. The base of each semicircular duct is enlarged, forming the **ampulla** that contains another neuroepithelial sensory receptor, the **crista ampullaris**. The three cristae and the two maculae contain the hair cells, which are the sensory transducers.

## THE VESTIBULAR HAIR CELLS

The hair cell is the sensory transducer throughout the vestibulocochlear system. This highly specialized cell is named for the hairlike processes that extend from its apical surface (Fig. 10.7). Vestibular hair cells have two types of hairs: a single **kinocilium** and between 50 and 110 **stereocilia**. The kinocilia are complex organelles containing the 9 + 2 internal structure common to motile cilia. The stereocilia are much simpler. Their external limiting membrane is a continuation of the hair cell membrane. The stereocilia contain a dense network of actin filaments. A spikelike structure, the rootlet, extends from the base into the cuticular plate at the apex of the hair cell. The stereocilia are arranged in rows of varying heights. The longest, about 100 μm, is the row adjacent to the kinocilia. Each subsequent row is shorter until the stereocilia are only about 1 μm long. This arrangement polarizes the hair cell anatomically, with the kinocilium at one edge of the

### Figure 10.7   The vestibular hair cells

**A.** The type I hair cell axon terminal is shaped like a chalice and envelopes the entire cell; the axon terminals on the type II hair cell are simpler, resembling typical CNS synapses. The afferent synapses are not highly vesiculated. Specialized densities in the hair cell, the synaptic ribbons, mark the active site of the afferent synapse. The efferent axons form highly vesiculated endings that have active sites on both the type II hair cell and on the afferent endings. Not shown: the efferent synapses on the afferent chalice. (Reprinted with permission from Fawcett D, Raviola E. A Textbook of Histology. 12th ed. New York: Chapman and Hall, 1994.) **B.** Electron micrograph cross-sections taken near the bases of several cilia. The kinocilium (*k*) is recognizable because of its characteristic 9 + 2 internal structure. The stereocilia have a much simpler internal structure of actin filaments. The rootlet (*r*) is visible in one stereocilia. Not shown: the fine bridges that connect adjacent stereocilia, ensuring that shearing forces will be distributed to all the stereocilia and that they will bend as a unit. (Reprinted with permission from Friedmann I, Ballantyne J. Ultrastructural Atlas of the Inner Ear. London: Butterworth, 1984.)

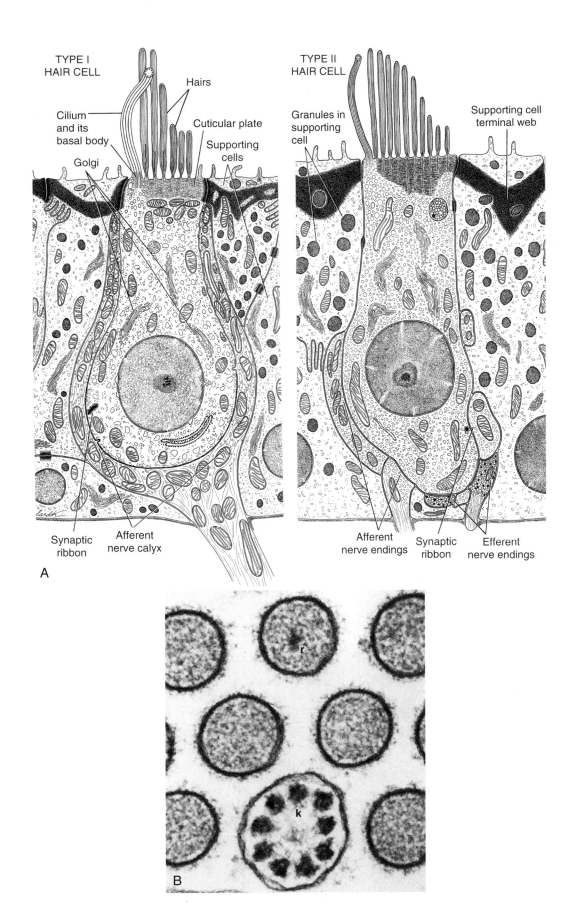

TYPE I HAIR CELL

Hairs

Cilium and its basal body

Cuticular plate

Golgi

Supporting cells

Synaptic ribbon

Afferent nerve calyx

TYPE II HAIR CELL

Granules in supporting cell

Supporting cell terminal web

Afferent nerve endings

Synaptic ribbon

Efferent nerve endings

A

B

r

k

hair cell and the stereocilia distributed across the top of it.

The hair cells are also polarized physiologically. The stereocilia are stiff. A force directed perpendicular to the shaft causes the hairs to bend at the base, where the stereocilia extends into the cuticular plate. This bending causes changes in the ionic flux across the hair cell membrane. Bending the stereocilia toward the kinocilium depolarizes the entire hair cell and produces action potentials on the afferent axons. Bending the stereocilia in the opposite direction hyperpolarizes the cell. The ionic details of hair cell stimulation and synaptic activation are discussed in Chapter 11.

There are two types of vestibular hair cells, type I and type II (Fig. 10.7). The differences between the two types are based on the type of innervation they receive. The afferent fiber innervating the type I hair cell terminates as a calyx [G. *kalyx,* the cup of a flower], which envelops nearly the entire hair cell. Multiple active zones lie between the hair cell and the nerve terminal. The type II hair cells are innervated by the more familiar nerve terminal boutons. The vestibular hair cells appear to release aspartate or glutamate as the neurotransmitter.

## THE MACULAE

The maculae are the neurosensory epithelia of the saccule and utricle. Each macula consists of numerous hair cells surrounded by supporting cells resting on a base of connective tissue (Fig. 10.8). The surface of the macula extends into the cavity of the membranous labyrinth and is bathed by endolymph. The macula is covered by the **otoconial membrane**, which is composed of three layers. The first layer is a loose veil that lies close to the apical surface of the hair cells. Immediately above this veil is the second layer, a thick gelatinous substance on which is piled the third layer, a mass of calcium carbonate crystals called **otoconia**. These otoconia greatly increase the mass of the entire structure (Fig. 10.9).

The stimulus for the macula is the relative movement between the otoconial membrane and the surface of the hair cells, which causes the hairs to bend. Such relative movement is possible because of the inertia of the otoconial membrane. When the head moves in the plane of the macula (**linear acceleration**), the macula moves with it because its base is firmly attached to the temporal bone. Inertia retards the movement of the otoconial membrane with its otoconia, resulting in the generation of shearing force across the apex of the hair cells. This shearing force bends the hairs, causing an ionic current flow in the hair cells that initiates the release of neurotransmitter at the base of the cells. The terminal boutons of the afferent axons have receptors for the neurotransmitter that when activated, produce action potentials that are carried to the CNS. *Linear acceleration is the adequate stimulus for the maculae.*

Not all of the hair cells of the maculae are arranged in the same direction of anatomical polarization. There are two levels of organization. First, the hair cells are lined up back to back along a dividing line, the **striola**, that runs approximately down the middle of the macula, so that the direction of polarizations are 180° apart (Fig. 10.10). Second, the striola bends about 90° across the surface of the macula. This arrangement ensures that movement

## Figure 10.8  Structure of the vestibular maculae

**A.** The macula of the saccule and the macula of the utricle are sensory epithelia containing both type I and type II hair cells. The cilia of the hair cells are embedded in the otoconial membrane, which has a gelatinous layer where the calcium carbonate crystals (otoconia) lie. (Reprinted with permission from Iurato S. Submicroscopic structure of the inner ear. New York: Pergamon Press, 1967.) **B.** The size and shape of the otoconia vary across the surface of the saccule (*a*) and utricle (*b*). The size variation corresponds with the striola, the line that marks the interface between the hair cells of opposite orientations. A typical macula is shown in oblique view (*c*). (Reprinted with permission from Paparella M, Shumrick D, eds. Textbook of Otolaryngology, vol 11. Philadelphia: Saunders, 1991.)

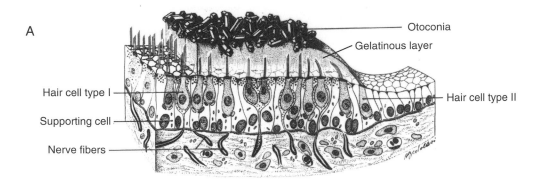

A

Otoconia

Gelatinous layer

Hair cell type I

Supporting cell

Nerve fibers

Hair cell type II

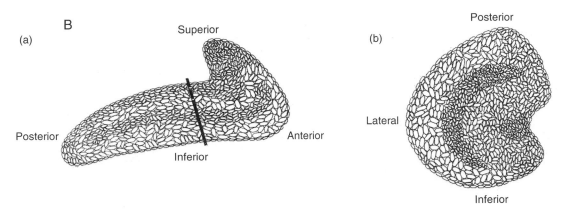

B

(a)

Superior

Posterior

Anterior

Inferior

(b)

Posterior

Lateral

Inferior

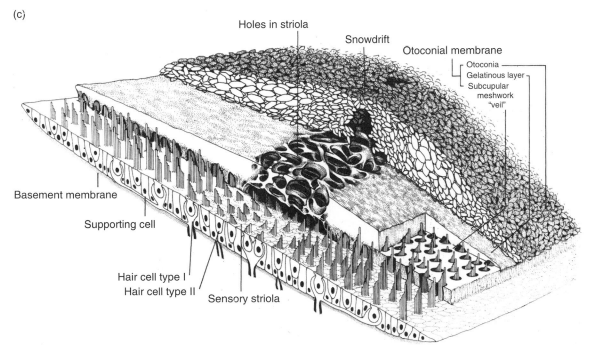

(c)

Holes in striola

Snowdrift

Otoconial membrane
- Otoconia
- Gelatinous layer
- Subcupular meshwork "veil"

Basement membrane

Supporting cell

Hair cell type I

Hair cell type II

Sensory striola

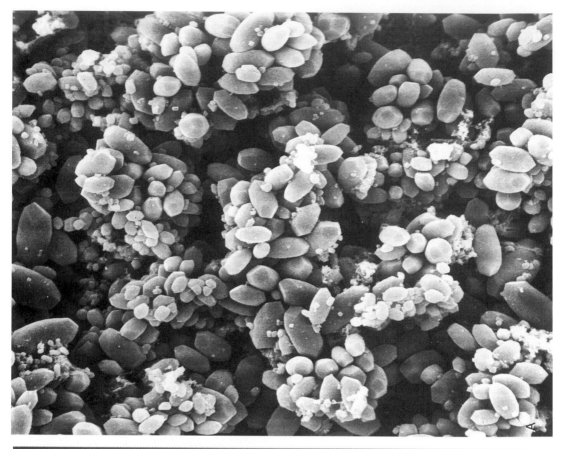

**Figure 10.9    SEM of the otoconia**

(Original micrograph courtesy of Dr. C. Gary Wright, University of Texas, Dallas, Tx.)

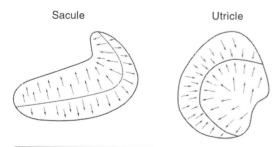

Sacule                          Utricle

**Figure 10.10    Polarity of macular hair cells**

*Arrows* show the direction of movement (toward the kinocilium) that stimulates the hair cells in that region. The *arrowheads* are aligned in two groups, which shows how the hair cells in each group point 180° apart. The imaginary line that separates the two groups is the striola. (Modified from Lindeman HH. Studies on the morphology of the sensory regions of the vestibular apparatus. Adv Anat Embryol Cell Biol Vol. 42. New York: Springer-Verlag, 1969 vol. 42.)

of the otoconial membrane in any direction in the plane of the macular surface excites some hair cells and inhibits others.

To ensure that hair cells will be stimulated by any linear movement of the head, the two maculae lie perpendicular to each other. In the upright human the saccule lies approximately in the sagittal plane; the utricle lies nearly in the horizontal plane. Because of its vertical position, the constant linear acceleration of gravity constantly affects the otoconia of the saccule. When the head is tilted, the utricle is also affected by gravity. Consequently, the maculae are very sensitive to static head position.

### THE CRISTAE

The crista ampullaris is the sensory epithelium of the semicircular ducts. The crista is housed in the ampulla, a small swelling of tissue at the base of each semicircular duct. Each crista contains hair cells and supporting cells that rest on a connective tissue base (Fig. 10.11). The hairs are embedded in a gelatinous mass, the **cupula**, that extends into the endolymphatic space across the full diameter of the semicircular duct.

The semicircular ducts are receptors for **angular acceleration**. The hair cells are sheared by the differential movement of the endolymph and the crista (Fig. 10.12). To see how this differential movement affects the hair cells, imagine your head rotating in the plane of a semicircular duct. During the initial acceleration the endolymph lags behind the movement of the crista because of its inertia. This relative movement between the endolymph and the crista places pressure on the cupula, deflecting it and bending the hairs of the hair cells. The crista therefore *is stimulated by angular acceleration of the head in the plane of the semicircular duct.*

Note that a constant angular *velocity* is not an appropriate stimulus for the semicircular ducts, because there is friction between the endolymph and the wall of the duct. As the head rotates at a constant angular velocity, the angular force gradually is transferred to the endolymph. Eventually the fluid and the crista rotate at the same velocity and the shear across the cupula ceases. However, if the head is brought to rest (negative angular acceleration), the endolymph tends to continue to flow through the semicircular duct. This movement of endolymph again shears the hairs of the crista, but in the direction opposite to the original stimulus.

The three semicircular ducts are oriented in approximately orthogonal planes (Fig. 10.13). The **horizontal** duct is inclined toward the anatomical horizontal plane at about −25°. The **anterior** duct[4] meets the sagittal plane anterior laterally at about 41° , and the **posterior**

---

[4] Formerly called the **superior** canal.

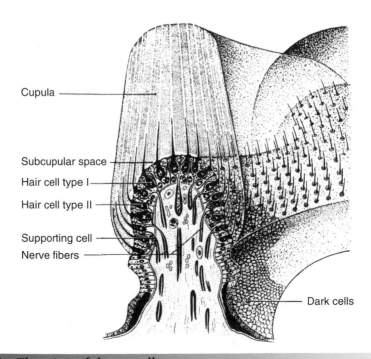

**Figure 10.11  The crista of the ampulla**

Like the maculae, the cristae contain both type I and type II hair cells. The cilia are embedded in a gelatinous membrane, the cupula. The cristae have no otoconia. (Reprinted with permission from Iurato S. Submicroscopic structure of the inner ear. New York: Pergamon Press, 1967.)

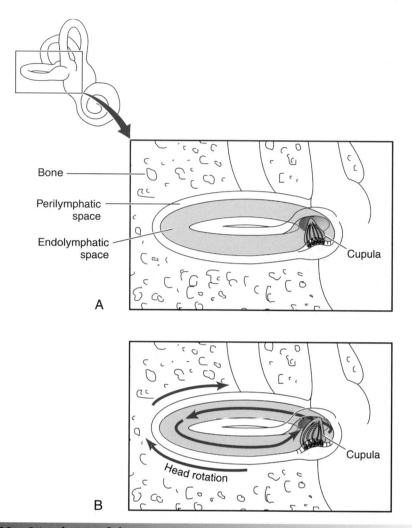

Bone

Perilymphatic
space

Endolymphatic
space

Cupula

A

Cupula

Head rotation

B

**Figure 10.12    Stimulation of the cristae**

In the absence of head rotation the cupula of the crista lies approximately perpendicular in the lumen of the
semicircular duct (**A**). During head angular acceleration the inertial drag of the endolymph tilts the cupula and
its embedded hair cells in the direction opposite to that of the head rotation (**B**).

duct intersects it at about 56°. This arrangement places the posterior duct on one side in
nearly the same plane as the anterior duct on
the other side; the two horizontal ducts lie approximately in the same plane.

Unlike hair cells in the maculae, the hair
cells of the cristae are all oriented in the same
direction. For the horizontal cristae deflection
of the hairs toward the utricle results in depolarization of all the hair cells. Deflection in the
opposite direction hyperpolarizes them. The
anterior and posterior cristae are oriented in

the opposite direction; deflection toward the
utricle hyperpolarizes them. In either case angular acceleration that stimulates the hair cells
in one duct simultaneously inhibits the hair
cells in the complementary duct on the contralateral side. Thus, just as in the maculae, for
any given movement some hair cells are stimulated as others are inhibited (Fig. 10.14).

THE VESTIBULAR NEURONS

The primary afferent vestibular neurons are
true bipolar neurons. Their cell bodies are in

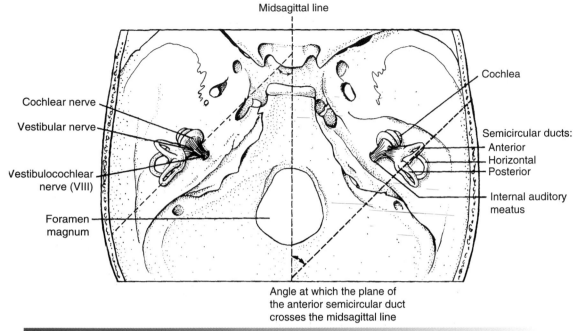

Midsagittal line

Cochlear nerve

Vestibular nerve

Vestibulocochlear nerve (VIII)

Foramen magnum

Cochlea

Semicircular ducts:
Anterior
Horizontal
Posterior

Internal auditory meatus

Angle at which the plane of the anterior semicircular duct crosses the midsagittal line

**Figure 10.13 Orientation of the semicircular ducts in the skull**

The arrangement of the semicircular ducts pairs the anterior duct of one side with the posterior duct of the contralateral side because they lie in the same plane (two parallel broken lines). The two horizontal ducts lie in approximately the same plane, hence pair each other. The two members of each pair are polarized in opposite directions. Therefore, stimulation of one duct inhibits its contralateral mate. (Reprinted with permission from Kelly JP. The sense of balance. In: Kandel ER, Schwartz JH, Jessell TM, eds. Principles of Neural Science. 3rd ed. Norwalk, CT: Appleton & Lange, 1991;506.)

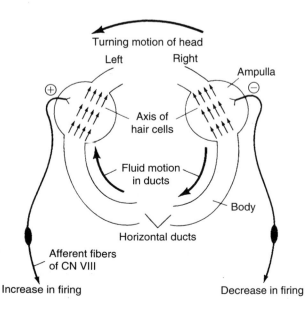

Turning motion of head

Left    Right

Ampulla

Axis of hair cells

Fluid motion in ducts

Body

Horizontal ducts

Afferent fibers of CN VIII

Increase in firing

Decrease in firing

**Figure 10.14 Paired stimulation of the semicircular ducts**

Head rotation stimulates the semicircular duct toward which the head is turning and inhibits the contralateral duct in the same plane. (Reprinted with permission from Kelly JP. The sense of balance. In: Kandel ER, Schwartz JH, Jessell TM, eds. Principles of Neural Science. 3rd ed. Norwalk, CT: Appleton & Lange, 1991;507.)

two peripheral ganglia, Scarpa's ganglia, in the **internal auditory meatus** (Fig. 10.6). The peripheral axons of vestibular neurons contact the vestibular hair cells and are the postsynaptic elements of the afferent synapse (Fig. 10.7). When stimulated, hair cells probably release a neurotransmitter that depolarizes the afferent synaptic bouton of the vestibular neuron. The central axons of vestibular neurons enter the brainstem at the pontomedullary junction. Nearly all vestibular afferent fibers bifurcate immediately after entering the CNS. The ascending branches synapse in the superior, medial, and lateral vestibular nuclei; the descending branches synapse in the inferior and medial nuclei. A few axons enter the flocculus, nodulus, and uvula of the cerebellum, where they terminate as mossy fibers.

Vestibular efferent axons arise bilaterally from a small collection of cells just lateral to the abducens nucleus. These axons travel with the vestibulocochlear nerve and terminate with highly vesiculated endings on the vestibular hair cells (Fig. 10.7). They terminate directly on type II hair cells but synapse with the calyx on type I hair cells, forming an axoaxonic synapse. The efferent terminals contain acetylcholine, which is probably the neurotransmitter.

## The Central Vestibular Connections

The vestibular nuclei make connections with three functional areas of the nervous system, the **spinal cord**, the **cerebellum**, and the **nuclei of ocular motion**. The connections of the vestibular nuclei with the spinal cord are discussed in detail in Chapter 7. To recapitulate, the **lateral vestibular nucleus** contains large neurons that project to all levels of the ipsilateral spinal cord as the **lateral vestibulospinal tract**. These axons are excitatory on extensor motor neuron pools. The **medial vestibular nucleus** gives rise to the **medial vestibulospinal tract**. These axons descend only to cervical levels, innervating motor neurons that primarily stabilize the head. This action provides a stable platform for the eyes.

The connections of the vestibular nuclei with the cerebellum are discussed in Chapter 9. These contacts originate primarily from the **lateral vestibular nucleus**, which makes extensive contacts with the **flocculonodular lobe**. The connections with the nuclei of ocular motion are discussed later in this chapter, after the external connections of these nuclei.

## Clinical Considerations

One's sense of place in space is computed from information garnered from three principal senses: vision, proprioception, and the vestibular sense. By itself, the vestibular sense does not provide adequate information to provide stability with reference to gravity and one's three-dimensional orientation in space. Vestibular information must be supplemented by either vision or proprioception. The inadequacy of the vestibular sense alone is the basis of the Romberg test (see Chapter 5). However, inappropriate signals from the vestibular system can disrupt one's sense of stability even when visual and proprioceptive signals are normal.

The principal symptoms associated with vestibular dysfunction are **nystagmus** and **vertigo**. Nystagmus is a particular type of eye movement characterized by a slow conjugate gaze in one direction followed by a rapid return of the eyes in the opposite direction. Nystagmus is discussed later in relation to all types of eye movements. Vertigo has a specific medical meaning that is often misrepresented in everyday speech. Clinically, vertigo *is the sense that the world is spinning around or that one's head or body is whirling.* It is an illusion of motion. Patients usually describe vertigo as "dizziness," a common term that includes not only vertigo but also **syncope**, a feeling of light-headedness, and **fainting**, which is associated with hypotension, weakness, and numerous other nonspecific conditions. In response to the perceived motion of vertigo, an affected person often leans against the perceived motion, as if being drawn by a magnet. Falling is common. In severe cases patients involuntarily fling themselves to the ground. Vertigo is commonly accompanied by nausea, vomiting, tinnitus (a ringing in the ears), and deafness.

**Positional vertigo** is produced when the head assumes certain positions. The cause of positional vertigo appears to be the detachment of part of an otoconium from the otoconial membrane of the utricle, which becomes lodged in or near the posterior ampulla, rendering it sensitive to the force of gravity. In certain critical positions the otoconial crystals can stimulate the cupula in the posterior duct, giving rise to abnormal vestibular sensations. The patient is seized with vertigo that rarely lasts for more than 40 seconds. The episodes recur, however, until the crystals relocate or disperse, which usually occurs in a few days or weeks. About 17% of the cases of positional vertigo are precipitated by head trauma that presumably dislodges the otoconia. Another 15% of cases are associated with viral labyrinthitis. Positional vertigo is not associated with hearing loss.

Vertigo is also the most prominent symptom of **Ménière's syndrome**. Unlike positional vertigo, Ménière's vertigo is almost invariably accompanied by tinnitus and hearing loss as well as nausea and vomiting. Furthermore, the attacks last a few minutes to several hours, much longer than those of positional vertigo. Ménière's syndrome is probably caused by an imbalance between the production and reabsorption of endolymph. If the production of endolymph exceeds its reabsorption, the endolymphatic space expands (**endolymphatic**

hydrops) and eventually ruptures, allowing the sodium-rich perilymph to contaminate the endolymph. The contamination of the endolymph with sodium ions causes depolarization of the afferent axons. This depolarization is sustained until the appropriate ionic milieu is reestablished. The contamination also kills hair cells. Each attack, therefore, causes progressive damage to the labyrinth and the cochlea with which it communicates (see Chapter 11). Eventually, in cases of long duration involving multiple episodes, the affected side goes completely deaf and loses all labyrinthine function. However, most people with Ménière's syndrome recover spontaneously, and recurrences cease after a few years. The disease can be treated with some success by the introduction of a shunt that drains perilymph into the cerebrospinal fluid through a pressure-sensitive valve. Other surgical approaches entail destruction of the labyrinth or section of the vestibular nerve.

## THE FACIAL NERVE (VII)

The facial nerve is a mixed nerve associated with four brainstem nuclei. Its axons leave the brainstem at the pontomedullary junction just medial to the vestibulocochlear nerve (Fig. 10.15). Both the facial and vestibulocochlear

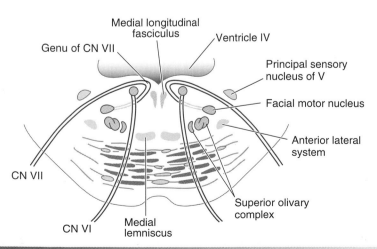

Figure 10.15   The facial and abducens nerves

nerves enter the temporal bone through the **internal auditory meatus**. Within the temporal bone the facial nerve divides into three branches, the **chorda tympani**, the **greater petrosal nerve**, and the **facial nerve** (motor component) (Fig. 10.16).

## Efferent Components

There are two efferent components to the facial nerve. The visceral motor axons originate in the facial motor nucleus and innervate the mimetic muscles of the face. The visceral preganglionic parasympathetic axons arise from the superior salivatory nucleus and mediate lacrimation and salivation.

## THE FACIAL MOTOR NUCLEUS

The main branch of the facial nerve innervates the voluntary **mimetic muscles** of the face, or-

bicularis oculi, **stapedius, stylohyoid, posterior belly of the digastric**, and **platysma**. The motor neurons are in the **facial motor nucleus**, a collection of cells in the caudal pons that lie within a triangle formed by the NSTV, the superior olivary complex, and the abducens nucleus. Axons leaving the facial motor nucleus take an unusual course, being directed dorsomedially toward the roof of the pontine tegmentum. They reach the vicinity of the abducens nucleus and wrap around it to form the **internal genu** of the facial nerve. The axons briefly course rostrally, proceed ventral laterally between the facial motor nucleus and the NSTV, and leave the brainstem at the cerebellopontine angle (Fig. 10.15). The facial nerve leaves the cranium by passing through the internal auditory meatus of the temporal bone. Within the temporal bone it makes a sharp bend (**external genu**) before finally leav-

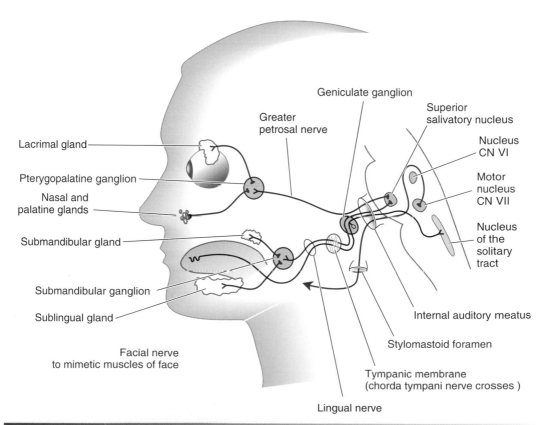

**Figure 10.16   Peripheral distribution of the facial nerve components**

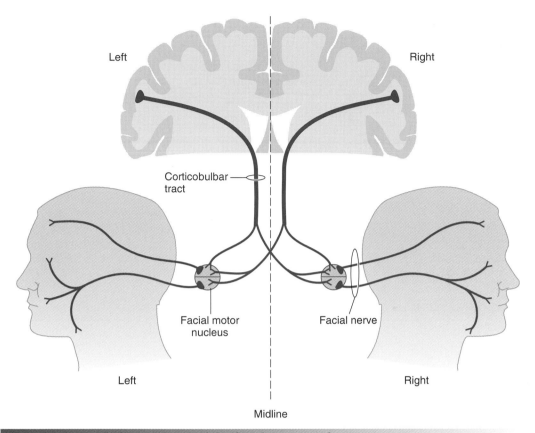

Left

Right

Corticobulbar
tract

Facial motor
nucleus

Facial nerve

Left

Right

Midline

**Figure 10.17    Dual innervation of the facial motor nucleus**

The motor neurons innervating the mimetic muscles of the lower face receive only contralateral corticobulbar fibers; the motor neurons innervating the mimetic muscles of the upper face receive bilateral innervation.

ing the skull through the **stylomastoid foramen** (Fig. 10.16).

The facial motor nucleus receives cortical motor commands via the corticobulbar tract. The termination of this tract within the nucleus is divided so that motor neurons innervating the upper portion of the face (eyebrows and forehead) receive *bilateral innervation;* the motor neurons innervating the *lower face receive only contralateral innervation* (Fig. 10.17). This arrangement allows the examiner to differentiate lesions to the nucleus from those affecting only the corticobulbar tract. Lesions to the facial motor nucleus cause an ipsilateral paresis of the entire face; lesions to the corticobulbar tract affect only the lower face.

The facial motor nucleus also receives afferent fibers from several other sources. One source of particular importance is the reticular formation. Tactile and pain stimuli from the cornea are transmitted via the trigeminal nerve to the reticular formation from the NSTV. Both facial motor nuclei receive signals from the reticular formation that initiate *bilateral* contraction of the *orbicularis oculi,* the muscles that *close the eyelids* (Fig. 10.18). This contraction is known as the **corneal reflex.** Although slow (latency more than 40 msec), this reflex protects and cleanses the eye of debris that could injure the cornea. Since reflex closure of the eye is mediated by the reticular formation, other stimuli, particularly those that are novel and startling, like flashes of light or loud noises, can also initiate blinking. The unconscious continual blinking of the eye, important for maintaining proper corneal hydration, is probably also mediated by the reticular formation.

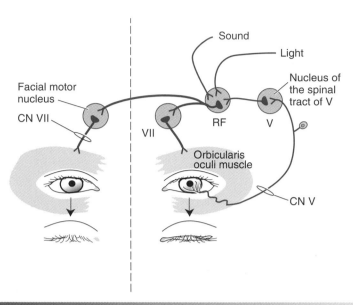

**Figure 10.18   The corneal reflex**

The corneal reflex involves two nerves. Pain afferent fibers from the cornea enter the CNS over the trigeminal nerve (CN V) and synapse in the NSTV. Within the brainstem secondary axons from the NSTV synapse in the reticular formation (RF), which in turn makes bilateral contact with the facial motor nuclei. From the facial motor nuclei, motor axons in the facial nerve (CN VII) innervate the orbicularis oculi muscles, closing the eyelid. The reticular formation also receives afferents from other sensory modalities that can also initiate lid closure.

## THE SUPERIOR SALIVATORY NUCLEUS

The facial nerve contains parasympathetic axons that arise from the **superior salivatory nucleus** (SSN). The preganglionic parasympathetic axons innervate the **pterygopalatine** and the **submandibular ganglia**. The pterygopalatine ganglion sends postganglionic fibers to the **lacrimal glands** and the mucous membranes of the nose and oral cavity; postganglionic fibers from the submandibular ganglion innervate the **sublingual** and **submandibular salivary glands** (Fig. 10.16).

The SSN, like the inferior salivatory nucleus (ISN), is not a well-organized collection of neurons. Both nuclei consist of a few scattered cells in the dorsal lateral area of the reticular formation. Their axons progress directly ventral laterally to join the main body of the facial (SSN) or glossopharyngeal (ISN) nerve. In the facial nerve the parasympathetic fibers remain separated from the voluntary motor axons that form the main part of the facial nerve, and they follow the motor root into the internal auditory meatus of the temporal bone. Since these fibers lie between the acoustic nerve and the main fa-

cial nerve and can be isolated during gross dissection, they are frequently called the **intermediate nerve**. The peripheral course of the intermediate nerve is complex and not described in detail here. It is sufficient to note that at the external genu of the motor root of CN VII the intermediate nerve divides into the greater petrosal nerve and the chorda tympani. The greater petrosal nerve terminates in the pterygopalatine ganglion. The chorda tympani follows the motor nerve for a short distance before separating from it. The parasympathetic fibers of the chorda tympani terminate in the submandibular ganglion.

### Afferent Components

There are two afferent components of the facial nerve, neither of which has great clinical significance.

### THE NUCLEUS OF THE SOLITARY TRACT

Axons that terminate in the NST convey the sensations of taste from the anterior two-thirds of the tongue. These axons leave the tongue in the lingual nerve and later join the chorda tympani (Fig. 10.16). As previously described, the corda tympani joins the main motor root of the facial nerve and follows it into the brainstem. The cell bodies of the sensory fibers lie in the **geniculate ganglion**, a collection of cell bodies found at the external genu of the facial nerve. The central connections of the nucleus of the solitary tract are described earlier in the chapter, in the section on the glossopharyngeal nerve.

## THE NUCLEUS OF THE SPINAL TRACT OF V

The second sensory component of the facial nerve carries somatic sensations from a small area within the pinna (Fig. 10.5). These sensory axons join the motor root of the facial nerve and follow its course through the temporal bone to the brainstem. Their cell bodies are also in the **geniculate ganglion**, and they synapse in the NSTV.

### Clinical Considerations

The importance of recognizing the differences between paralysis of an entire half of the face and paralysis of only the lower quadrant is discussed earlier in the chapter (see page 359). To recapitulate, the motor neurons serving the upper quadrant of the face are supplied bilaterally by axons of the corticobulbar tract. This dual innervation makes these neurons somewhat refractory to unilateral supranuclear (above the level of the facial motor nucleus) corticobulbar lesions. Motor neurons supplying the lower quadrant of the facial muscles have no dual innervation. They are supplied only by contralateral corticobulbar fibers. Thus supranuclear lesions result in a marked weakness of the lower facial muscles contralateral to the lesion; the upper face is spared. For example, cerebral infarction in the territory of the middle cerebral artery or infarction of the cerebral peduncle causes marked weakness of the contralateral lower facial muscles. This weakness is readily seen as a flattening of the nasolabial fold and drooping of the corner of the mouth. A voluntary grimace is obviously asymmetrical. Wrinkling of the forehead or raising of the eyebrows is essen-

tially normal. In contrast to this pattern, paresis or frank paralysis of the entire half of the face results from lesions that affect the facial motor nucleus directly or the peripheral facial nerve.

**Bell's palsy** affects the peripheral portion of CN VII and causes complete paralysis of the mimetic muscles of the involved side. The eye cannot be closed, the brow wrinkled, or a smile produced on the side ipsilateral to the lesion. The corner of the mouth droops and the nasolabial fold is flattened. This disfigurement is very traumatic to the patient. The loss of the blink reflex is also a great concern, since the patient cannot close the eye. Drying, clouding, and ulceration of the cornea can result from the lack of corneal hydration normally supplied by lacrimation. Steps must be taken to protect and artificially hydrate the cornea.

Although its exact cause is unknown, Bell's palsy is most likely the result of compression of CN VII within the facial canal in the temporal bone. Compression is probably caused by inflammation secondary to a viral infection. The inflammation changes the water content of the nerve, making it visible on magnetic resonance imaging (MRI) (Fig. 10.19). Although the condition is dramatic, the rate of spontaneous recovery is high. Approximately 80% of patients recover within 3 months. If the nerve is severely damaged, complete regeneration of the nerve is required, which may take as long as 2 years, and in that case recovery is usually not complete. Occasionally during regeneration axons originating from mimetic motor neurons cross over into the distal Schwann tubes of the parasympathetic motor fibers. Thereafter, the patient upon smiling may shed a few tears due to this inappropriate innervation, the so-called crocodile tears of Bell's palsy.

## THE TRIGEMINAL NERVE (V)

The trigeminal nerve is associated with four nuclei in the brainstem; one is motor and the remaining three are sensory. The motor axons innervate the muscles of mastication. The sensory fibers innervate the face and most of the internal surface of the nasal and oral cavities, including the tongue and teeth.

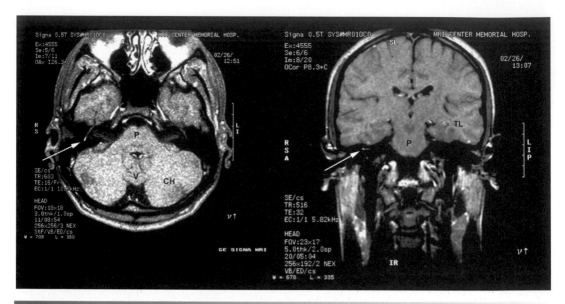

Figure 10.19    MRI of a patient with Bell's palsy

The horizontal section (**left**) shows signal enhancement of the facial nerve on the right (*arrow*). The coronal section (**right**) of the same patient shows signal enhancement of the nerve near the genu (*arrow*). The normal facial nerve is not visible on the contralateral side. (Courtesy of the Magnetic Resonance Imaging Center, South Bend, IN.)

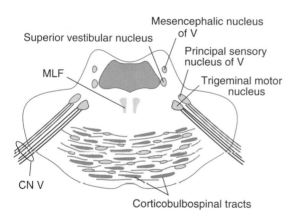

Figure 10.20    The trigeminal nerve in the pons

## Efferent Component

The **trigeminal motor nucleus** lies in the pons at the level where the trigeminal nerve leaves the brainstem. The nucleus lies in the lateral portion of the tegmentum but medial to the **principal sensory nucleus of V (PSNV)** (Fig. 10.20). Motor axons from the nucleus leave the brainstem in the trigeminal nerve and are incorporated into the mandibular ($V_3$) division. Leaving the skull through the foramen ovale, $V_3$ innervates the **muscles of mastication**, the **tensor palatini**, the **tensor tympani**, the **mylohyoid**, and the **anterior belly of the digastric muscle**. The motor nucleus receives bilateral connections from the corticobulbar tract. Consequently, supranuclear lesions do not produce dramatic signs of weakness in mastication.

## Afferent Components

Three nuclei are associated with the sensory functions of the trigeminal nerve: the **mesencephalic nucleus of V**, the NSTV, and the PSNV (Figs. 10.20 and 10.21).

### THE MESENCEPHALIC NUCLEUS OF V

The mesencephalic nucleus consists of a thin line of pseudounipolar neurons that lie in the mesencephalon along the lateral margin of the fourth ventricle as it begins to narrow before becoming the aqueduct. These neurons are

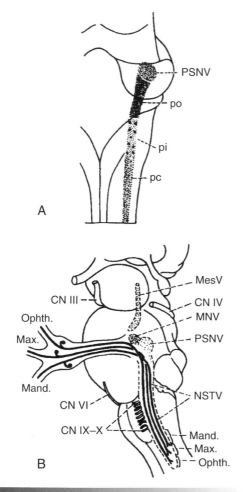

**Figure 10.21    The nuclei of the trigeminal nerve**

**A.** Dorsal view of the brainstem showing the relation between the principal sensory nucleus of V (*PSNV*) and the nucleus of the spinal tract of V (*NSTV*). The NSTV is divided into three regions, pars oralis (*po*), pars intermedialis (*pi*), and pars caudalis (*pc*). **B.** Lateral view of the brainstem showing the relation between the mesencephalic nucleus of V (*MesV*), the motor nucleus of V (*MNV*), and PSNV. The three divisions of the trigeminal nerve do not all terminate at the same level in the NSTV. (Reprinted with permission from Brodal. Neurological Anatomy. New York: Oxford University, 1981.)

pseudounipolar and receive no synaptic connections. They constitute a displaced peripheral ganglion. Their peripheral axons innervate the spindles and proprioceptors of the muscles innervated by the trigeminal motor

root. Some evidence suggests that they also innervate the muscle receptors of the extraocular eye muscles. The central axons form synapses in the motor nucleus and PSNV.

### THE TRIGEMINAL SOMATOSENSORY CONNECTIONS

The cell bodies of the sensory axons of the trigeminal nerve are in the trigeminal (semilunar) ganglion. The peripheral axons are distributed over all three divisions of the nerve, the **ophthalmic** ($V_1$), **maxillary** ($V_2$), and **mandibular** ($V_3$). They innervate the skin of the face and the mucous membranes of the oral and nasal cavities as well as the most inferior portion of the meninges. There is essentially no overlap in the peripheral distribution of the three divisions. Thus the dermatome pattern of the facial innervation is clinically important (Fig. 10.22).

On entering the pons, sensory axons in the central branch of the trigeminal nerve segregate. The largest axons leave the main branch of the nerve and terminate in the **principal sensory nucleus**; the smaller axons enter the spinal tract of V to synapse in the NSTV. The larger axons convey fine tactile sensations and proprioception. They have small receptive fields and adapt rapidly. The smaller axons carry pain and temperature sensations, have large receptive fields and adapt slowly. Many primary afferent trigeminal axons bifurcate on entering the pons, sending one branch to the principal nucleus and the other to the spinal nucleus. The bifurcation of these axons may account for the fact that electrical potentials related to tactile stimuli can be recorded from both nuclei.

The NSTV is a large structure at the lateral margin of the brainstem. Extending from the mid pons to the cervical spinal cord, it is accompanied on its lateral aspect by the spinal tract of V, a collection of primary afferent axons that synapse in the nucleus. At its caudal pole it merges with the dorsal horn of the spinal cord. In the pons it merges with the principal sensory nucleus at the level where the trigeminal nerve enters the pons. Although axons from four cranial nerves (V, VII, IX, and X) synapse in this nucleus, axons from the trigeminal nerve are by far the most numerous.

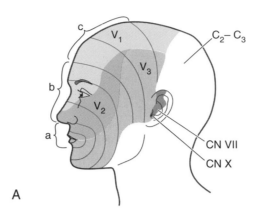

A

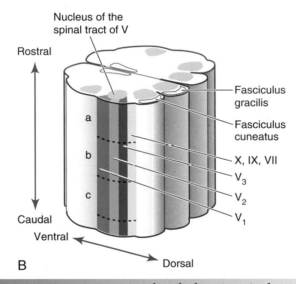

B

## Figure 10.22   Dermatome patterns associated with the trigeminal nerve

**A.** In the head, the sensory receptors of the skin are supplied by the trigeminal nerve and the C2 and C3 dorsal roots; this shows the pattern of distribution. Note the boundaries of the three divisions of the trigeminal nerve ($V_1$, $V_2$, and $V_3$) and the division between the trigeminal and the cervical roots. The angle of the jaw is supplied by C2 and the anterior aspect of the pinna is supplied by CN VII. The external auditory meatus is supplied by CN X, and the lining of the middle ear cavity, by CN IX (not shown). A second dermatome pattern is based on the termination of trigeminal primary afferent axons in the nucleus of the spinal tract of V. This pattern makes an onion skin–like pattern on the face surrounding the lips. **B.** This oblique view of the lower medulla shows how the axons of the spinal tract of CN V are organized. The three divisions of the trigeminal nerve are segregated, with the ophthalmic division lying most lateral. The fibers originating from the somatosensory divisions of the vagus, glossopharyngeal, and facial nerves lie most medially within the tract. The axons supplying the area around the lips terminate in the NSTV most rostrally (*a*); those serving more peripheral areas of the face terminate more caudally (*b* and *c*). Because the trigeminal axons enter the brainstem in the pons and descend toward the spinal cord, severing the spinal tract of V near the rostral pole of the nucleus (*arrow* between *a* and *b*) cuts nearly all the fibers but spares the most rostral fibers serving the central part of the face, preserving sensation around the lips. Sections at a lower level (*b* and *c*) spare an increasingly wide area.

Axons that terminate in the NSTV enter the pons and descend as the spinal tract of V (Fig. 10.21). The axons from the three divisions of the trigeminal nerve remain segregated along the length of the tract; $V_1$ axons are most lateral; $V_3$ axons are most medial. The few axons from CN VII, IX, and X that terminate in the NSTV are also in the spinal tract of V. They lie between the $V_3$ axons and the fasciculus cuneatus (Fig. 10.22).

In addition to the principal dermatome pattern associated with the three divisions of the trigeminal nerve, a second dermatome pattern is associated with the spinal tract of V. Axons innervating the region of the lips terminate in the most rostral part of the NSTV. A pattern of ever-widening circles radiates from the lips; axons innervating these circles descend more caudally in the spinal tract of V before terminating in the nucleus.

Most neurons in the NSTV send axons across the midline to synapse in the reticular formation of the medulla and pons. Very few of these axons appear to ascend to the thalamus. Nociceptive sensory information from the face presumably travels over reticulothalamic fibers of the anterior lateral system (ALS) to the thalamus.

The PSNV is a relatively small globular structure in the dorsolateral pons at the most rostral pole of the NSTV and lateral to the trigeminal motor nucleus. The neurons in the PSNV send axons to the contralateral VPM nucleus of the thalamus. Most of the axons leaving the PSNV cross the midline and join the contralateral medial lemniscus. About a third of the axons ascend in the ipsilateral medial lemniscus and terminate in the ipsilateral VPM.

The PSNV is functionally analogous to the dorsal column nuclei. Fine tactile and proprioceptive information passes through it to the ventrobasal thalamus via a fast and direct pathway. The NSTV, by contrast, is analogous to the laminae in the dorsal horn of the spinal cord that receive pain and temperature information. Both the spinal and the trigeminal nociceptive systems project to the ventrobasal thalamus by polysynaptic pathways. Although a few nociceptive fibers proceed directly to the thalamus, most synapse in the reticular forma-

tion from which the final thalamic projections arise. Thus the separation of fast versus slow and tactile versus nociceptive pathways also applies to sensations from the face.

Secondary fibers from the trigeminal sensory nuclei are also distributed locally to other brainstem structures. These connections are important for local reflexes. The corneal reflex, discussed in association with the facial nerve (see page 359), is particularly important. The afferent limb of this reflex traverses the ophthalmic division of the trigeminal nerve and synapses in the NSTV. From there secondary fibers innervate the facial motor nucleus indirectly through the reticular formation. Efferent axons from the facial motor nucleus arise and innervate the orbicularis oculi muscle, closing the reflex path. The reflex relaxation of the masseter muscles and withdrawal of the tongue after biting one's tongue or cheek is presumably effected by analogous connections involving motor nuclei V and XII.

### Clinical Considerations

The most conspicuous neurologic problem associated with the trigeminal nerve is **trigeminal neuralgia,** or **tic douloureux** [Fr., *tic,* spasmodic movement, and *douloureux,* painful]. This condition is characterized by paroxysms [G. *paroxysmos,* sharpen, irritate] of severe pain in the territory of the trigeminal nerve, usually the maxillary or mandibular division. The pain is intense, often described as burning, tearing, cutting, stabbing, or electric shock–like. The pain lasts for several seconds. Several episodes may run together and last for hours. An attack can be triggered by the slightest tactile (not painful) stimulus in specific areas within the territory of the trigeminal nerve (called trigger zones). Fear of eliciting an attack may cause the patient to restrict eating, shaving, brushing the teeth, or even talking.

Trigeminal neuralgia is generally considered to be idiopathic. However, one study found an association between trigeminal neuralgia and vascular anomalies that irritate the nerve root (84% of 411 patients). A small percentage of cases may be caused by tumors or multiple sclerosis. Although the disorder is not caused by seizures, it is often successfully

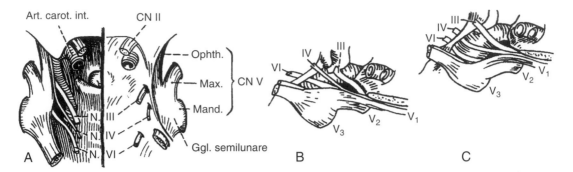

**Figure 10.23    Cranial nerves in the cavernous sinus**

**A.** The region of the cavernous sinus showing the relations among the carotid artery, the three nerves of ocular motion, and the three divisions of the trigeminal nerve. The dura has been removed on the left and retained on the right. **B.** A lateral view of the cavernous sinus shows the normal relations of the structures. **C.** An aneurysm of the carotid artery displaces cranial nerves VI and IV. This displacement also exerts pressure on the trigeminal nerve, resulting in the ominous combination of facial pain and ophthalmoplegia. (Reprinted with permission from Brodal A. Neurological Anatomy. New York: Oxford University, 1981.)

treated with anticonvulsive drugs. Temporary relief can be provided by injecting the affected peripheral branch of the trigeminal nerve with absolute alcohol, which blocks nerve conduction for several months. Permanent relief can often be obtained by means of surgery. Decompression of the microvessels at the nerve root is frequently successful (about 80% of patients), as is section of the sensory nerve root. However, these procedures have their risks. Severe keratitis [G. *keras,* horn, and *itis,* inflammation] and ulceration of the cornea usually follow section of the ophthalmic division, eventually leading to loss of vision in the affected eye. A less risky and equally effective surgical approach is to stereotaxically direct a probe into the ganglion and carefully heat it with radiofrequency current. This procedure probably destroys only the A and C fibers, which preserves some elements of touch and the corneal reflex.

The trigeminal nerve can also be affected by aneurysms of the internal carotid artery. Because of its location in the region of the cavernous sinus, the expanded artery can exert pressure on the nerve roots (Fig. 10.23). Since the nerves of ocular motion (III, IV, and VI) also travel in the same area, frequently one or more of them are also affected by pressure. Therefore, facial pain, diminished corneal re-

flex, and ocular palsy (see next section) in any combination is an ominous constellation of symptoms that demands immediate investigation. Similar combinations of symptoms may also arise from hypophyseal tumors that have expanded into the cavernous sinus.

## THE NERVES OF OCULAR MOTION (III, IV, AND VI)

Three cranial nerves, the **abducens** (VI), **trochlear** (IV), and **oculomotor** (III), innervate the extrinsic muscles of the eye, which move the eye in its orbit. In addition, the oculomotor nerve innervates the **levator palpebrae**, the muscle that lifts the eyelid. Also, parasympathetic fibers that regulate the size of the pupil and the shape of the lens are associated with the oculomotor nerve.

### The Extrinsic Muscles of the Eye

Six muscles, the **medial** and **lateral rectus**, the **superior rectus** and **inferior oblique**, and the **inferior rectus** and **superior oblique**, control the position of the eye in the orbit (Fig. 10.24). The *medial* and *lateral rectus* muscles rotate the eye around an imaginary **vertical axis.** Contraction of the medial rectus causes **adduction** of the eye; contraction of the lateral rectus causes **abduction** [L. *abduco,* draw away]. The other eye movements are more complex because the remaining muscles do not pull perpendicular to any single axis during forward gaze. Since they lie medial to the sagittal axis of the eye, their force is exerted obliquely to all three axes. If the patient's gaze is directed straight ahead, contraction of the *superior rectus* muscle causes *elevation, medial rotation,* and *adduction* of the eye. Similarly, contraction of the *superior oblique* causes *depression, medial rotation,* and *abduction* of the eye. Contraction of the *inferior rectus* causes *depression, lateral rotation,* and *adduction;* the *inferior oblique* produces *elevation, lateral rotation,* and *abduction* of the eye (Table 10.3).

When evaluating eye movements, ideally each muscle should be tested in isolation. The medial and lateral rectus muscles may be tested in isolation by adduction and abduction from direct forward gaze. The remaining muscles can be isolated by noting that the superior and inferior rectus muscles act as pure elevators or depressors if the eye is abducted about

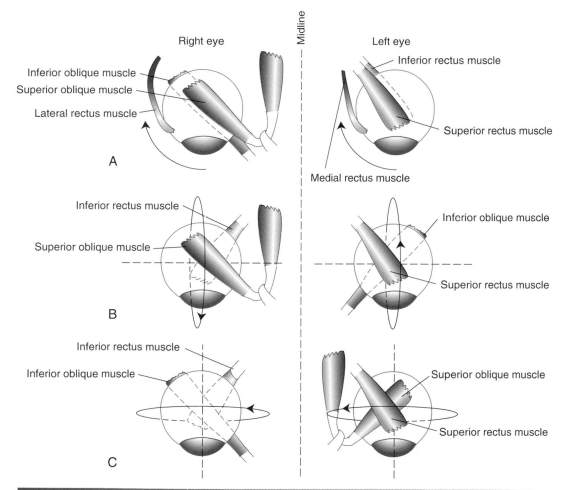

**Figure 10.24   The action of the extrinsic muscles of the eye in each of the three imaginary axes of rotation**

The view from above as the patient faces the examiner. Movement in any of the anatomical planes requires the coordination of several muscles. **Top.** Horizontal plane. **Middle.** Sagittal plane. **Bottom.** Coronal plane (rotation of the eye).

**Table 10.3   Action of Extrinsic Eye Muscles**

|  | Elevate | Depress | Medial Rotation | Lateral Rotation | Abduct | Adduct |
|---|---|---|---|---|---|---|
| Superior rectus | ✔ |  | ✔ |  |  | ✔ |
| Inferior oblique | ✔ |  |  | ✔ | ✔ |  |
| Inferior rectus |  | ✔ |  | ✔ |  | ✔ |
| Superior oblique |  | ✔ | ✔ |  | ✔ |  |
| Medial rectus |  |  |  |  |  | ✔ |
| Lateral rectus |  |  |  |  | ✔ |  |

23°, which corresponds to the angle of insertion of these muscles into the globe. The oblique muscles become pure elevator-depressors when the eye is adducted approximately 39°. Therefore, when testing the extrinsic eye muscles, elevation and depression of the eyes during right lateral gaze isolates the two rectus muscles on the right and the two obliques on the left and conversely on left lateral gaze (Fig. 10.25).

### The Abducens Nucleus

Motor neurons in the abducens nucleus, near the midline of the pons at the internal genu of the facial nerve (Fig. 10.15), send axons to the ipsilateral lateral rectus muscle over the abducens nerve (VI). This nerve exits the basis of the pons near the midline at the pontomedullary junction. It courses in the posterior fossa until it enters the area of the cavernous sinus. It leaves the cranium through the superior orbital fissure before innervating the lateral rectus muscle.

### The Trochlear Nucleus

Motor neurons in the **trochlear nucleus** innervate only the superior oblique muscle. The trochlear nucleus lies in the mesencephalic

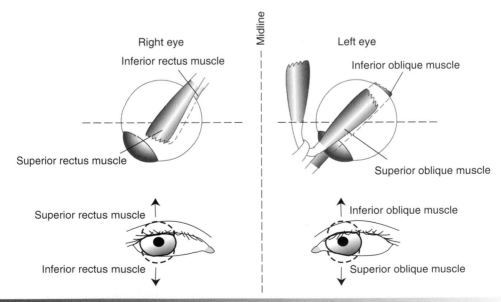

**Figure 10.25   Isolating the extraocular muscles for testing**

Elevation and depression of the eye can be accomplished by single pairs of antagonistic muscles if the gaze is shifted about 23° from center. On lateral gaze the superior and inferior rectus muscles are tested in the abducted eye; the inferior and superior oblique muscles are tested in the adducted eye.

tegmentum at the level of the inferior colliculus (Fig. 10.26A). The trochlear nerve (IV) crosses the midline before leaving the roof of the brainstem. It wraps around the lateral aspect of the cerebral peduncle before entering the region of the cavernous sinus. Like the abducens nerve, it leaves the cranium through the superior orbital fissure.

### The Oculomotor Nucleus

All of the other extrinsic muscles of the eye are innervated by motor neurons that reside in the **oculomotor nucleus**. This nucleus lies in the mesencephalon just rostral to the trochlear nucleus, at the level of the superior colliculus (Fig. 10.26B). The oculomotor nerve (III) leaves the nucleus and travels ventrally through the red nucleus and the medial portion of the cerebral peduncle before leaving the brainstem. Like CN VI and IV, it enters the area of the cavernous sinus and leaves the cranium through the superior orbital fissure. Once in the orbit, the oculomotor nerve divides into branches that innervate the superior, inferior, and medial rectus muscles; the inferior oblique; and the levator palpebrae.

## EYE MOVEMENTS

Clear vision requires stable congruence of the retinal images in the two eyes; otherwise **diplopia** (double vision) results. To prevent diplopia, movements of the two eyes must be coordinated so that an image falls on complementary portions of the retina in each eye. If an object moves in space, the two eyes must track it to keep its image appropriately fixed on the two retinas. Tracking a moving object usually requires at the very least the adduction of one eye, abduction of the other, and compensation in the vertical and horizontal planes. Since the eyes are in the head, an unstable platform, the computation of eye movements must take head motion into account. Therefore, the coordination of eye movements involves the vestibular system as well as the visuomotor nuclei, and their interconnections.

This section concludes with a brief description of the function of the gaze centers.

### Types of Eye Movements

The control of eye movements is quite different from the control of skeletal movements. Most skeletal movements are initiated and closely directed by neurons in the cerebral cortex, specifically those in the premotor area (PMA), supplementary motor area (SMA), and primary motor cortex (M-I). The regulation of skeletal movements by the muscle stretch reflex and cerebellar regulation enhances the precision of the consciously directed motor act. Although the range of skeletal movements runs from the subtle stroke of the artist's fingers drawing a brush across a canvas to the boxer's knockout punch, all skeletal muscle activity is basically the same: a smooth, coordinated contraction among many muscle groups. The velocity of skeletal motor activity is continuously variable and smoothly regulated.

Eye movements are quite different. The most striking difference between skeletal and eye movements is the two mutually exclusive types of eye movements, **smooth pursuit** and **saccades** [Fr. *saccade*, sudden check of a horse]. Smooth pursuit movements are also called **eye tracking** because they are employed only when the eye is following a moving object.

Acute vision depends on the ability to maintain the image of an object on the **fovea**, the central 1° of the retina[5] (see Chapter 12). Any movement of the target's image on the fovea causes the smooth-pursuit system to move the eyes *reflexively* to restore the image to its original foveal position. Smooth-pursuit eye movements maintain the image of a target of interest on the fovea. Once the target has been acquired, the smooth-pursuit motor system fixes on it and causes the eyes to track it. As long as the target is moving between about 5 and 100° /second and it remains within the visual field, this system allows the eyes to track it and maintain its image on the fovea. Fixation can be initiated voluntarily (as when we decide to follow a soccer player dribbling around the field) or involuntarily (as when

---

[5] The fovea is specialized for high-resolution imaging (see Chapter 12).

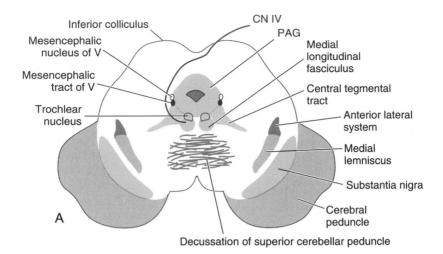

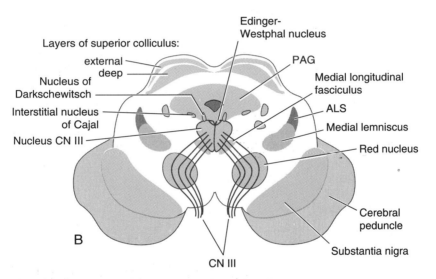

**Figure 10.26   Cranial nerves of the mesencephalon**

Cross-section of the mesencephalon at the level of the trochlear nuclei (**A**) and of the oculomotor nuclei (**B**).

our eyes follow the cars of a train when we are stopped at a railroad crossing). Fixation can also be terminated by voluntary action. However, the actual smooth, variable-velocity contraction of the extraocular muscles cannot be accomplished voluntarily; there must be a moving target to follow. For this reason, smooth-pursuit eye movements are often called *involuntary eye movements*.

Saccades direct the gaze from one target to another. Saccades can be divided into several classes. One class, **intentional saccades**, are voluntarily initiated, as when one decides to look from the base runner to the pitcher while watching a baseball game. Consequently, saccades are often called *voluntary eye movements*. Despite this term, another class of saccades, **reflexive saccades**, are initiated involuntarily, as when the phone rings and one reflexively looks at it. Motion in the peripheral visual field can also reflexively initiate a saccade, which places the image of the moving object on the fovea. In contrast to smooth-pursuit eye movements, the velocity of the saccade is constant, about 800°/second. There is no voluntary control over the velocity of saccades.

All types of saccades can quickly direct the gaze toward an object of interest. Smooth-pursuit eye movements are subsequently employed to keep the eyes on the object as it moves. It is easy to demonstrate these two types of eye movement to yourself. First try to shift your gaze slowly between two objects in the room. It cannot be done. Your eye movements between the objects are broken into a series of short saccades. If, however, you focus on your finger and slowly move it about, you can follow it at very slow velocities with no interrupting saccades.

### Eye Movement Reflexes

Two important reflexes combine saccades and tracking eye movements. The **vestibulo-ocular reflex** (VOR) moves the eyes in response to head movement; the **optokinetic reflex (OKN)** captures an image for subsequent fixation and tracking. Both reflexes have important clinical applications.

#### THE VESTIBULO-OCULAR REFLEX

During visual tracking or scanning of an object, the specific muscle contractions required to keep the object centered on the fovea are affected by both the static position of the head and by any head movements that may occur. Head movements that occur during eye movements necessitate modification of the signals sent to the eye muscles. The vestibular apparatus detects both static head position and dynamic head movements and uses its central connections with the nuclei of ocular motion to adjust the eye movements to compensate. This reflex movement of the eyes in response to vestibular stimulation is the VOR.

You can readily appreciate the sophistication of the VOR by tilting your head while reading these lines. What had previously required a simple adduction and abduction movement of the eyes now requires that the eyes move in all axes. Information about head position, detected and measured by the saccule and utricle, is used to adjust the action of all six of the nuclei of ocular motion.

The VOR can compensate for dynamic movement as well as static head position. For example, when you are sitting in a barber's chair[6] and the barber turns you to the left, your eyes automatically move toward the right. Rotation of the head to the left stimulates the crista of the left horizontal duct and inhibits the right horizontal crista (Fig. 10.13). The excitatory signals are passed from the left vestibular nuclei to the contralateral abducens nucleus, causing abduction of the right eye. The left oculomotor nucleus is also excited, causing adduction of the left eye. Conversely, inhibitory signals are sent to the motor neurons of the right medial rectus muscle and the left lateral rectus.

Consider what happens when the slow rotation to the left continues: the eyes slowly track an imaginary object to the extreme right. At this point they do not lock in place as you might first suspect, but a saccade moves the eyes back to the forward gaze position. They then slowly track to the right again. This slow tracking movement followed by a fast centering saccade in the opposite direction is called **rotatory nystagmus.** It is named for the *fast* component, so in our example rotating someone to the left will produce a *left lateral nystagmus* and vice versa.

If the barber notices your nauseated state and stops rotating the chair, inertia causes the endolymph to continue to flow through the horizontal duct. Since the head is now stationary, the cristae are stimulated in the opposite direction and a *right lateral postrotatory nystagmus* occurs. Postrotatory nystagmus is a disorienting phenomenon familiar to pilots, astronauts, and devotees of merry-go-round rides.

The VOR is an important tool for evaluating brainstem injury in unconscious patients. When the patient is lying face upward, the horizontal ducts lie nearly in the vertical plane. After determining that there is no injury to the cervical spine, the examiner simply rotates the head left and right for maximum stimulation of the horizontal cristae. Normally the VOR conjugately moves the eyes in the direction opposite to movement of the head. The action re-

---

[6] The proper medical term is the Bárány chair, named for the man who first studied vestibular nystagmus with such an apparatus.

sembles that of a china doll with eyeballs that look forward no matter how the head is tilted. This procedure is therefore often called the **doll's eye maneuver**. If the eyes do not track together and react appropriately to head movement, a brainstem lesion is almost certain.[7] This procedure takes advantage of the scattered location of the structures necessary for the reflex—the vestibular system, the nerves and nuclei of ocular motion, and the pathway interconnecting them—from the medulla to the mesencephalon. Brainstem injury almost certainly affects one or more of these structures and consequently disrupts the VOR.

## OPTOKINETIC NYSTAGMUS

Brainstem and cortical visuomotor centers can also initiate oculomotor reflexes. For example, if an object is moving across the visual space, the visuomotor centers initiate a saccade to bring its image onto the fovea and track the image, keeping it on the fovea as the object moves.

This **fixation reflex** is highly developed in humans. The fixation reflex is responsible for a phenomenon sometimes called **railroad nystagmus**. A person sitting in a moving train often fixes the eyes on a passing object, for example the utility poles that line the tracks. Once fixed on the object, the eyes track it until it passes from view. Then the eyes saccade back to the forward gaze position and fix on the next pole. The slow tracking eye movements in one direction followed by a fast saccade in the opposite direction has the exact same appearance to an observer as rotatory nystagmus. The clinical name for railroad nystagmus is optokinetic nystagmus (OKN). OKN can be elicited by any repetitive visual stimulus. It is conveniently elicited during the neurological examination by pulling a ribbon with a simple pattern across the visual field of the patient.

## SPONTANEOUS NYSTAGMUS

In contrast to rotational and optokinetic nystagmus, both of which are normal reflex responses to specific stimuli, **spontaneous nystagmus almost always indicates an underlying pathological condition.** Lesion to the labyrinth, vestibular nerve, brainstem, or cerebellum can cause spontaneous nystagmus. Lesions that involve the labyrinth or the CN VIII directly (*unilateral peripheral lesions*) cause nystagmus, vertigo, nausea, and unsteadiness with a tendency to fall. These symptoms result from an imbalance in vestibular stimulation between the two ears. This imbalance mimics natural stimulation. Hence, if the lesion affects the right vestibular nerve, the left vestibular signal is greater than the right. This signal is similar to the stimulus (considering only the horizontal duct) of the head turning toward the left. Therefore, the nystagmus fast phase is to the left (away from the lesion) and the patient has a tendency to fall to the right (into the perceived motion and toward the side with the lesion).

If the vestibular nerve is affected directly, as happens with **acoustic neuromas**[8] (see Chapter 11), these symptoms are accompanied by a diminished or total loss of hearing on the affected side because the acoustic and vestibular branches of the nerve share the confined space of the internal auditory meatus. With end-organ or nerve damage, the vestibular symptoms are usually transitory, an observation that can be explained by the ability of the CNS to compensate for the loss of the sensory signals from one labyrinth if the contralateral labyrinth is intact. Certain ototoxic drugs, particularly **aminoglycoside antibiotics,**[9] may destroy the vestibular hair cells bilaterally. In these cases the patient may completely lose vestibular function, hence permanently lose the VOR. Spontaneous nystagmus does not occur, because vestibular signals from both sides are absent and consequently there is no imbalance. However, without the VOR, clear vision is impossible because the retinal image can no longer be stabilized in reaction to slight movements of the head.

*Central lesions of the brainstem* produce many of the same vestibular symptoms as pe-

---

[7] Beware of patients with glass eyes!

[8] Tumors of the VIII nerve.

[9] Three aminoglycosides commonly in use today are anikacin, gentamycin, and tobramycin.

ripheral lesions, but vertigo is usually absent. Nystagmus may be caused by any disease affecting the brainstem. Nystagmus derived from brainstem lesions is usually permanent, since no compensation is possible if the brainstem nuclei are destroyed. Nystagmus caused by lesions to the *cerebellum* commonly depends on head position and is usually prominent in only one static head position. Otherwise it may be indistinguishable from labyrinthine nystagmus. The most common cause of nystagmus is alcohol intoxication, a condition that renders the cerebellum dysfunctional because of its particular sensitivity to this drug. Experienced Saturday night bed pilots are quite familiar with the positional sensitivity of cerebellar nystagmus.

## The Motor Centers Controlling Eye Movements

Perhaps the most remarkable fact about the control of eye movements is that unlike most voluntary motor systems, the motor neurons controlling the extraocular eye muscles are not directly regulated by motor areas in the cerebral cortex. Rather, cortical control of voluntary eye movements is indirect, acting through brainstem visuomotor centers. The **vestibular nuclear complex** plays a critical role in adjusting eye movements in response to head movement. The **superior colliculus** is a unique structure that receives a variety of sensory inputs and initiates motor commands to direct head and eye movements toward the stimulus. The **paramedian pontine reticular nucleus (PPRN)**, the **rostral interstitial nucleus of the medial longitudinal fasciculus (riMLF)**, the **interstitial nucleus of Cajal (INC)**, and the **pretectal region** are integrating centers that direct horizontal and vertical gaze. These four nuclei constitute the **accessory oculomotor nuclei**. It is necessary to understand these structures and their interconnections to appreciate how eye movements are initiated and regulated.

### THE VESTIBULAR NUCLEI

The vestibular nuclear complex consists of four nuclei that receive sensory information about the movement of the head and its rela-

tion to gravity from the vestibular receptors. This information is used to stabilize the body relative to gravity by regulating postural reflexes, to control eye movements in response to changes in head position, and to stabilize the head to provide a more stable platform for the eyes. As discussed in Chapter 7, the lateral vestibular nucleus regulates the antigravity muscles via the lateral vestibulospinal tract that emanates from it. The medial vestibular nucleus stabilizes the head via the medial vestibulospinal tract. Eye movements are controlled by vestibular neurons originating in the medial and superior vestibular nuclei. Axons from the medial and superior vestibular nuclei project to the nuclei of ocular motion, the tectal nuclei, and the accessory oculomotor nuclei (see gaze centers, later in the chapter) over a fiber tract called the **medial longitudinal fasciculus** (MLF). The MLF is a paired structure that lies very close to the midline in the tegmentum just ventral to the fourth ventricle and courses the entire length of the brainstem (Figs. 10.3, 10.15, and 10.26).

### THE SUPERIOR COLLICULUS

The superior colliculus is part of the tectum of the mesencephalon. It is a complex structure composed of several strata of cells and fibers. For simplicity these strata can be divided into a **superficial** and a **deep** layer (Fig. 10.27). The superficial layer receives information about the visual space from two sources. Afferent fibers originating in the *retina* constitute one source, and afferent fibers from the *visual cortex* (areas 17, 18, and 19) are the other source. Certain cells in the superficial layer of the superior colliculus receive information about the same visual space from both sources.

The most prominent efferent projections from the superficial layer are to the pulvinar, a thalamic nucleus that projects in turn to the cerebral cortex. This circular organization (visual cortex → superior colliculus → thalamus → cerebral cortex) is reminiscent of the organization of the basal ganglia. The superficial layer also projects to the pretectal nuclei (described later in the chapter). There are probably no projections into the deep layer.

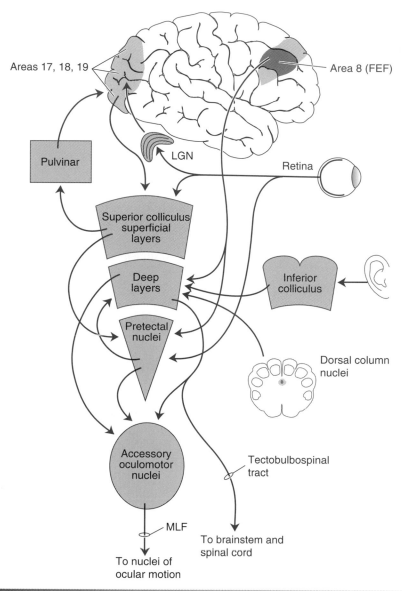

**Figure 10.27   Role of the superior colliculus in tracking eye movements**

The deep layer of the superior colliculus receives information from nonvisual cortical areas. *Somatosensory signals* reach the deep layer from several sources. Although a few fibers arise from lamina IV of the spinal cord, the majority come from the dorsal column nuclei and the nucleus of the spinal tract of V. The inferior colliculus supplies auditory information to the deep layers. Information about voluntary saccades is supplied by a region in the frontal lobes of the cerebral cortex known as the **frontal eye fields**, part of area 8 (Fig. 10.27).

The deep layer of the superior colliculus projects to several structures. The small **tectospinal** tract leaves the deep layer, crosses the midline, and descends near the surface of the tegmentum. At the lower medulla it becomes incorporated into the medial vestibulospinal tract and terminates in the cervical spinal cord. These fibers are important in directing head movements toward novel visual and auditory stimuli. **Tectobulbar fibers** terminate primarily in the PPRN. *There are no direct connections from the superior colliculus to the nuclei of ocular motion* (Fig. 10.27).

## THE GAZE CENTERS

Eye movements are characterized as either horizontal or vertical gaze because they can be dissociated by specific CNS lesions. The following sections describe the clinical gaze conditions associated with lesions to specific anatomical structures.

### Horizontal Gaze

Horizontal and vertical eye movements are coordinated by different parts of the PPRN, a collection of cells that lies lateral to the MLF between the abducens and the trochlear nuclei. This nuclear complex receives afferent fibers from the deep layer of the superior colliculus and from the vestibular nuclei.

Horizontal eye movements are regulated by neurons in the caudal part of the PPRN and interneurons in the abducens nucleus (Fig. 10.28). Signals received from the superior colliculus activate excitatory burst neurons (EBNs) in the PPRN. As their name implies,

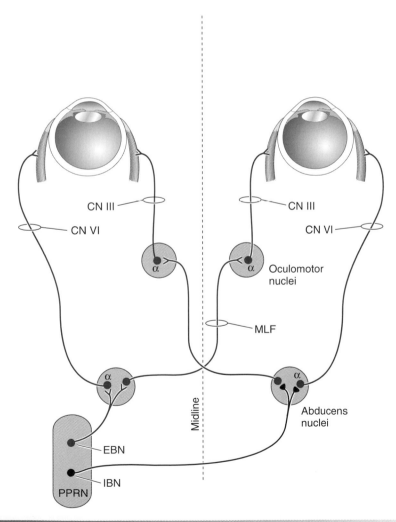

**Figure 10.28  Simplified circuit for the regulation of horizontal gaze**

EBN, excitatory burst neuron; IBN, inhibitory burst neuron; PPRN, paramedian pontine reticular nucleus.

these neurons send a burst of action potentials into the abducens nucleus, exciting the lateral rectus motor neurons and causing a horizontal saccade. Similarly activated inhibitory burst neurons (IBNs) send axons to the contralateral abducens nucleus, inhibiting the contralateral lateral rectus muscle. Interneurons in the abducens nucleus cross the midline and ascend in the MLF to innervate the contralateral oculomotor nucleus and control the medial rectus muscles.

Saccade signals must be followed by a hold signal if the eye is to remain in place following the saccade. Otherwise the eye drifts back to center gaze, which is the relaxed position of the extraocular muscles. The hold signal (position) is produced by the mathematical integration of the saccade signal, a velocity signal (Fig. 10.29). The location of the neural integrator for horizontal gaze is thought to be in the medial vestibular nucleus and the flocculus of the cerebellum. If the integrator fails, no hold signal is generated, and the eye drifts back to center gaze. A new saccade must then occur to place the eye back on the target. This process repeats, producing a nystagmus known as **gaze-evoked nystagmus**. This type of nystagmus is present only when the gaze is off center. It disappears on forward gaze because no hold signal is required to maintain forward gaze.

### Vertical Gaze

The control of vertical eye movements is similar to that of horizontal eye movements. EBNs for vertical saccades have been identified in the riMLF, a small collection of cells just ventral to the nucleus of Darkschewitsch. The riMLF receives direct afferent fibers from the rostral PPRN and the vestibular nuclei and projects directly to the oculomotor nucleus. Neural integrator cells for vertical gaze have been identified in the INC. All of these structures lie in the mesencephalon, so pressure on the rostral brainstem or small lesions to this area disrupt vertical eye movements, leaving horizontal eye movements intact.

### OPHTHALMOPLEGIA

Disturbances of extraocular eye movements, ophthalmoplegia [G. *ophthalmikos,* relating to the eye, and *plege,* stroke], can be caused by lesions to any of three parts of the nervous system. They are classified as **nuclear** if they involve the

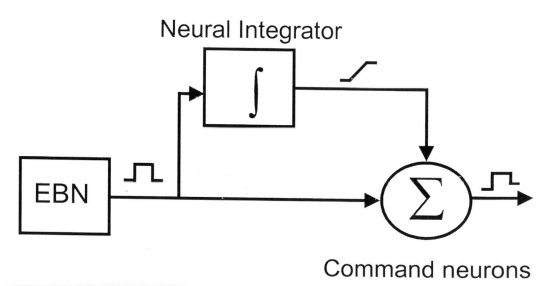

**Figure 10.29   Circuit for the neural integrator**

Neural signals that initiate saccades are velocity signals initiated by EBNs. A neural integrator, probably in the cerebellum, generates a position (static hold) signal by integrating the velocity signal. The velocity saccade command and the position command are summed by the command motor neurons.

nuclei of oculomotion or the associated cranial nerves, *internuclear* if the lesion involves the MLF, and **supranuclear** if the lesion involves the cerebral cortex, the descending corticomesencephalic fibers, or the brainstem gaze centers. Each type of lesion produces distinctive disturbances in ocular motion.

## Nuclear Ophthalmoplegia

Lesions to CN III, IV, or VI or their associate nuclei produce weakness of the muscles innervated by the nerve. For example, a lesion to the abducens nerve or nucleus produces loss of lateral gaze to the ipsilateral side due to the paralysis of the lateral rectus muscle. On forward gaze the eye is diverted medially because of the lack of normal resting tone in the lateral rectus muscle, which the patient experiences as diplopia. A lesion to CN III or its nucleus produces a downward and outward gaze in the eye ipsilateral to the lesion. Muscle tone is retained only in the superior oblique and lateral rectus muscles because the oculomotor nerve supplies all of the extraocular eye muscles except for these two. The combined action of these muscles draws the eye laterally (lateral rectus) and downward (superior oblique).

## Internuclear Ophthalmoplegia

Unilateral lesions to the MLF produce characteristic derangements in eye movements. These lesions are described as internuclear because the source of the oculomotor paralysis originates between the nuclei of ocular motion. Internuclear lesions are not only clinically important but also instructive. Therefore, a brief discussion of two common internuclear lesions is appropriate.

A unilateral lesion to the MLF between nuclei III and VI disrupts the adducting saccades on the ipsilateral side because of the loss of the fibers originating in the contralateral abducens nucleus that innervate the oculomotor nucleus (Fig. 10.30). Convergence is preserved, since coordination between the two oculomotor nuclei does not require that fibers pass through the MLF. The adduction of both eyes during convergence proves that both oculomotor nu-

clei and nerves are intact. This syndrome is called **internuclear ophthalmoplegia** (INO).

If the lesion involves one MLF and the ipsilateral abducens nucleus, saccades for both adduction and abduction are lost in the ipsilateral eye and adducting saccades are lost in the contralateral eye (Fig. 10.30). Only contralateral abduction remains. Because all horizontal saccades are lost from one eye and half of the horizontal movements are lost from the other, this finding is called the **one-and-a-half syndrome**. Both INO and one-and-a-half syndrome are commonly caused by multiple sclerosis or pontine stroke.

## Supranuclear Ophthalmoplegia

Lesions above the brainstem gaze centers interrupt voluntary saccades, but reflex eye movements remain intact. These lesions disrupt the descending corticomesencephalic fibers that carry the signals for voluntary saccades and separate the burst neurons in the brainstem from cortical control. The connections with the vestibular nuclei remain intact. Therefore, voluntary saccades are absent but reflexive saccades, such as those associated with the VOR, are preserved. Progressive supranuclear palsy (see The Case of the Frozen Eyes, later in the chapter) is probably the most common form of this disorder.

Lesions to the pons involving the posterior commissure, pretectal area, or riMLF disrupt vertical gaze. Axons from the riMLF innervate the third and fourth nuclei bilaterally, with many of the axons crossing in the posterior commissure. Since upward and downward saccades are driven by burst neurons in the riMLF, disruption of this nucleus or any of its efferent axons affects vertical saccades. Vertical gaze is often affected this way when a process such as a pineal tumor presses on the rostral mesencephalon.

The *frontal eye fields* (FEF) *of the frontal lobes* (approximately area 8) project to the deep layer of the superior colliculus and to the PPRN and riMLF. The FEFs seem to be most important in inhibiting fixation, hence lesions to the FEFs produce a form of supranuclear palsy that is usually described as **enhanced fixation**. Persons with this disorder also cannot

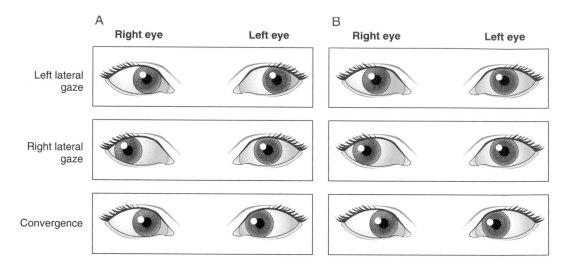

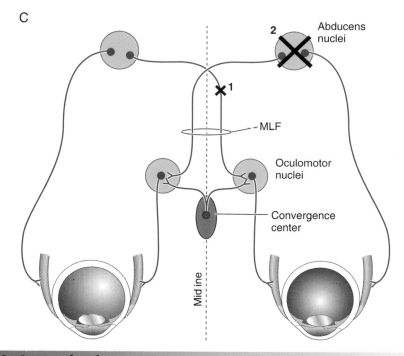

**A.** Internuclear ophthalmoplegia: a lesion in one MLF (patient's left in illustration; lesion 1, below) between the abducens and the oculomotor nuclei. The patient is unable to adduct the left eye on the affected side during contralateral gaze. Because the convergence does not depend on signals traversing the MLF, the patient is able to adduct on convergence. **B.** One-and-a-half syndrome: lesions involving both the MLF and abducens nucleus on one side (lesions 1 and 2, below). The only horizontal movement possible is abduction of the contralateral eye and convergence. **C.** Pathways involved in the lesions.

initiate saccades toward the side opposite the lesion. A small area of the *prefrontal cortex* (approximately area 46) inhibits the generation of unwanted reflexive saccades, such as saccades directed toward a moving object in the peripheral visual field. Lesions involving this area, which commonly occur in Huntington's disease, lead to innumerable saccades directed at every distracting movement in the environment. A small area in the posterior parietal cortex (PPC), approximately the angular gyrus, areas 39 and 40, functions by directing attention toward visual objects. The PPC projects to the FEF, which apparently sends the signal that releases the eyes' fixation on one object and thus allows a saccade toward an object of greater interest. Lesions to the FEF or the PPC severely disrupt the VOR, which is why the VOR is an important part of the neurological examination.

### The Ocular Reflexes

Clear vision also requires compensation of the lens and the pupil to adjust the eye for subject distance and brightness. These adjustments occur automatically through certain ocular reflexes.

## CONSTRICTION OF THE PUPILS

When light shines into the eye, the constrictor muscle in the iris contracts, narrowing the pupil. Although it is the iris that contracts, by convention this reaction is known as **pupillary constriction.** The constriction of the pupil is usually tested by shining the light from a small flashlight into each of the patient's eyes in turn and observing the pupils.[10] Normally, both pupils constrict when the light shines into one eye, which is called the **consensual light reflex.**

The pathways for the light reflex are not known with certainty (Fig. 10.31). It is generally agreed, however, that direct retinal afferent fibers synapse in the pretectal area. Axons from the pretectal area innervate both **Edinger-Westphal nuclei;** the contralateral connections pass through the posterior commissure before synapsing on the contralateral nucleus. From these nuclei arise preganglionic parasympathetic axons that leave the brainstem over the **oculomotor nerves** and innervate the **ciliary ganglia,** on the globes. Postganglionic fibers innervate the **constrictor muscle of the iris.** Therefore, the light reflex depends on two cranial nerves, the optic (II) and the oculomotor (III).

## ACCOMMODATION AND CONVERGENCE

In addition to adjusting the iris to changes in ambient light, the shape of the lens must be altered to focus on both near and distant objects (see Chapter 12). At rest the lens is thin, allowing the eye to focus on distant objects. When viewing nearby objects, the eyes must converge to avoid diplopia; to improve visual acuity by reducing the effect of spherical aberrations in the lens, the pupils constrict. To focus on nearby objects the lens must thicken, a process known as **accommodation.** All three actions—*accommodation, convergence, and constriction*—which occur together when a person views close objects, are collectively known as the **accommodation reflex.**

The mechanisms of the accommodation reflex are only partly understood. The test of this reflex requires that the patient be able to see and to cooperate with the examination. Therefore, the occipital visual cortex must be functional. Signals from the occipital cortex are probably transmitted to the pretectal area, which bilaterally innervates the Edinger-Westphal nuclei (Fig. 10.31). As mentioned earlier, these nuclei supply the parasympathetic preganglionic neurons that innervate the **ciliary ganglion** by way of the oculomotor nerve. Postganglionic axons from the ciliary ganglion innervate not only the pupillary constrictor muscle but also the **ciliary muscles** in the eye. The ciliary muscles are arranged so that their contraction shortens the suspensory ligament of the lens. This ligament normally places tension on the lens, lessening its curvature; when this tension is relieved by ciliary contraction, the lens passively thickens.

---

[10] Of course, if the patient is in a brightly lit room, shining a light into the eyes does not make the pupils constrict; they are already constricted because of the ambient light.

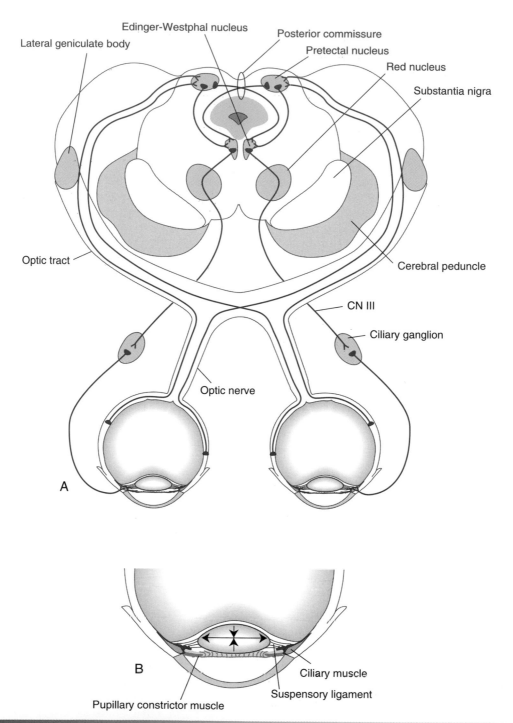

**Figure 10.31    The light reflex pathways**

**A.** The probable pathways that mediate the pupillary light reflex. The afferent path is the optic nerve (CN II), and the efferent path is the oculomotor nerve (CN III). Visual information from the eye reaches the contralateral pretectal nuclear complex via fibers in the posterior commissure. (Adapted from Crosby E. Correlative Anatomy of the Nervous System. New York: Macmillan, 1962.) **B.** The suspensory ligament places tension on the lens while the ciliary muscle is relaxed, thinning the lens and allowing it to bring distant objects into sharp focus on the retina. Contraction of the ciliary muscle relieves tension on the suspensory ligament and consequently the lens thickens.

# C A S E    H I S T O R Y

## THE CASE OF THE RETIREMENT PARTY[11]

### HISTORY OF PRESENT ILLNESS

Mr. A. M., a 44-year-old factory worker, was building shelves in his garage late one Sunday evening when he noticed that his left arm and left leg felt a little weak. He decided to stop working for the evening, concluding that he was probably overtired and that it was time to turn in for the night. By the following morning, his left-sided weakness was much worse. In addition, his right hand and leg felt numb and tingly. Despite these difficulties, he resolved to go to work that morning because he did not want to miss a friend's retirement party at lunchtime. He vowed to call his family doctor immediately on his arrival to see if she could see him that afternoon.

Over the next several hours Mr. A. M.'s weakness worsened. At approximately 10:00, during his morning coffee break, he began to have difficulty speaking. As he took a sip of his soda, he had trouble swallowing and began to cough. Embarrassed and visibly shaken, he explained to his colleagues that his mouth "wasn't working right." He nervously recounted the nature of the other difficulties that he had been having over the past 2 days. Disturbed by his noticeably slurred speech, a coworker volunteered to take him to the emergency department of a nearby hospital. Mr. A. M. is a heavy, long-time smoker (3 packs of cigarettes a day for 25 years) and a former heavy drinker (2 cases of beer per week). He states that he no longer drinks alcoholic beverages but continues to smoke.

### PHYSICAL EXAMINATION

Mr. A. M. weighs 253 pounds and is 5 feet 11 inches tall. His blood pressure is 180/110 with a resting heart rate of 93. The physical examination is otherwise unremarkable.

### NEUROLOGICAL EXAMINATION

#### Mental Status

Mr. A. M. was alert, cooperative, and oriented to person, place, and time. Memory test was not reported.

#### Cranial Nerves

OLFACTION: Not tested

VISION: Fields were full to confrontation (see Chapter 12).

OCULOMOTION: Not tested.

PUPILS: Pupils were equal and reactive to direct and consensual light reflex. Accommodation was not tested.

TRIGEMINAL: There was decreased sensation to pinprick on the right side of the face. Responses to cotton and the corneal reflex were not tested.

FACIAL: The right nasolabial fold was somewhat flattened and the mouth was slightly drooped on the right. The motility of the eyebrows was not tested.

AUDITION: Patient could hear the rubbing of fingers held close to the pinna. Hearing was grossly normal from each ear.

VAGOGLOSSOPHARYNGEAL: Voice was normal. The gag reflex, and the appearance of the pharyngeal arches and uvula, were not tested.

ACCESSORY: Not tested.

HYPOGLOSSAL: The tongue deviated to the right on protrusion.

#### Station and Gait

His gait was slightly ataxic and broad based. He was unable to perform a tandem walk. He could

---

[11] This case was given to me by Dr. Carl Marfurt of the Northwest Center for Medical Education, Indiana University School of Medicine.

walk on his heels and toes with difficulty and required support.

## Motor Systems

STRENGTH: Muscle strength was moderately
weak (3/5) in all four extremities.

TONE: Not tested.

BULK: Not tested

ABNORMAL MOVEMENTS: No abnormal movements were noted.

## Sensory Systems

There was decreased sensation to pinprick on
the entire left side of the body. Perceptions of vibration and joint position were intact bilaterally.

## Reflexes

All muscle stretch reflexes were 2+. There were
bilateral Babinski and Bing signs (see Chapter 7).

## Coordination and Control

There was some dysmetria on finger-to-nose and
heel-to-shin bilaterally and dysdiadochokinesia
bilaterally. The right side was worse than the left.

## Parietal Functions

Not tested.

## ANCILLARY STUDIES

MRI of the head revealed that the basilar and
right vertebral arteries were tortuous and dilated. A fusiform aneurysm of the mid to upper
basilar artery with an intraluminal thrombosis
was noted. No extravascular blood was demonstrated.

## SUBSEQUENT COURSE

Early the next morning Mr. A. M. had sudden onset of vertigo, nausea, and vomiting. He could
no longer hear out of his right ear. Neurological
examination revealed a spontaneous left-sided
nystagmus. The next day audiometry confirmed
a total loss of hearing on the right. Another MRI
was ordered (Fig. 10.32A). In addition to the vascular abnormalities seen in the first MRI, it
showed two areas of decreased signal in the
pons at the level of the middle cerebellar peduncle. One area of low signal was in the midline;
the other was to the right.

A cerebral angiogram was performed 2 days
later (Fig. 10.32B). It demonstrated a marked
enlargement of the basilar and right vertebral
arteries. There was also evidence of a fusiform
basilar artery aneurysm with intraluminal
thrombosis.

The aneurysm was considered inoperable.
The patient was prescribed anticoagulative drugs
and given physical and occupational therapy. He
was advised to stop smoking. On follow-up 2
months after discharge (3 months after his initial
symptoms), he was much improved. He no
longer smoked and had lost 30 pounds. His
blood pressure was 130/90 with a resting heart
rate of 81. He still had a total hearing loss in the
right ear, but his cerebellar deficits were greatly
improved. He had a residual mild loss of pinprick
sensation on the left side of his body. All muscle
stretch reflexes (MSRs) were 2+, and he had bilateral signs of Babinski.

## COMMENTARY

Defining the physical extent of a lesion is a de-
ductive process. First the parts of the nervous
system that are not functioning properly are determined by observing the capabilities of the patient. Second the lesion is localized by analysis of
the anatomical relations of the neurological
structures at various levels of the nervous system
so as to determine the site or sites where the involved structures are in proximity. A step-by-step
analysis of this case follows to show how to approach a neurological diagnosis.

1. First determine the approximate rostrocaudal
   level of the lesion. In general *cerebral lesions*
   produce symptoms on the entire contralateral
   half of the body. *Brainstem lesions* produce
   crossed symptoms—one side of the head and
   the opposite side of the body. *Spinal lesions*
   spare the cranial nerves and commonly produce paraparesis, quadriparesis, or sensory
   dissociation (pinprick preserved while light
   touch is lost over the same area or vice versa).
   By the time Mr. A. M. reached the emergency
   department, crossed symptoms were apparent. The right side of his face drooped, the
   labionasal fold was flattened, and his tongue
   deviated to the right. There was decreased
   perception of pinprick to the right side of his

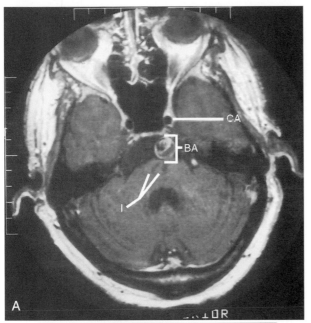

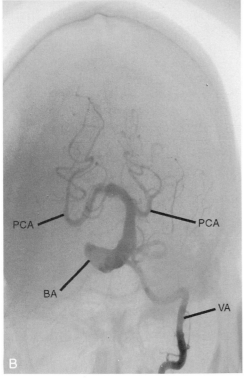

**Figure 10.32   Ancillary studies for Mr. A.M.**

**A.** Mr. A. M.'s second MRI shows an enlarged basilar artery indicative of an aneurysm and two areas of decreased signal (dark areas) in the middle and right pons, which indicates two infarcts (I). The basilar artery is abnormally large (compare with the carotid arteries) and appears to have a dissected wall and intraluminal material. *CA,* carotid artery; *BA,* basilar artery. **B.** Mr. A. M.'s arteriogram reveals a tortuous and greatly enlarged basilar artery with intraluminal material, suggesting a thrombus. *PCA,* posterior cerebral artery; *BA,* basilar artery; *VA,* vertebral artery.

face and the entire left half of his body. The *loss of pain and temperature* points to the ALS. Because the entire left half of the body is involved, the lesion must be above the neck and on the right, since the tract crosses at the level of origin in the spinal cord. The loss of pain and temperature on the *right side of the face* points to the right spinal tract of V. The right facial weakness suggests involvement of the right facial motor nucleus.

2. Once the approximate level of the lesion has been determined, attempt to identify a small, specific structure that is dysfunctional. In this case the spinal tract of V and the facial motor nucleus are implicated. The former runs the entire length of the medulla and pons. Its size limits its usefulness in localizing the lesion. However, because the facial motor nucleus is small and compact, you should concentrate on proving or disproving its involvement. If the lesion is in the right facial motor nucleus, you expect to observe facial paralysis involving both the upper and lower face. Since the abducens nerve and nucleus are very close to the facial motor nucleus, you might also expect to observe a weakness of abduction in the right eye. If the paralysis involves only the lower part of the face, look above the level of the nucleus for a corticobulbar lesion. Unfortunately, in the case of Mr. A. M., the physician not only failed to observe the extent of facial weakness but also did not report Mr. A. M.'s eye movements. These are serious omissions. We can surmise with some certainty that the facial motor nucleus has a lesion. If the left corticobulbar tract had a lesion above the facial motor nucleus, the facial weakness and body numbness would be on the same side, because both tracts (ALS and corticobulbospinal tract [CBST]) cross the midline before innervating the affected structures. Since facial weakness and body numbness occur on opposite sides, this hypothesis must be false. Therefore, we have two possibilities: the lesion involves the facial motor nucleus or there are two lesions widely separated in space. The latter possibility is less likely than the former.

3. Having determined that the lesion is in the right brainstem involving the facial motor nucleus, you must now study the patient's disabilities to determine what other structures may be involved. Do these other structures lie close enough to the facial motor nucleus to be involved in the lesion? Mr. A. M. has *increased MSRs* in all four extremities and bilateral signs of Babinski and Bing. These classic UMN signs point to a lesion that affects the CBST bilaterally. However, Mr. A. M. is not to-

tally paralyzed. He can walk, although not well. He has voluntary but not normal control over all four extremities. Therefore, the CBST lesion is undoubtedly incomplete. At the level of the pons the CBST is not a small, compact bundle as it is in the medulla. Its fibers are widely separated in the basis of the pons. A small vascular lesion near the midline in the pons may easily damage some CBS fibers bilaterally, resulting in the type of minimal UMN signs in all four extremities that are observed in this patient. The patient clearly has *signs of cerebellar involvement.* There is bilateral dysdiadochokinesia and dysmetria, which are somewhat worse on the right than on the left. Such signs may be produced by a lesion of the cerebellum itself, but given the other findings, such a lesion seems unlikely. The basis of the pons, however, contains both the deep pontine nuclei and their axons, which form the middle cerebellar peduncle. A midline lesion would be expected to injure these fibers, producing bilateral cerebellar signs. The fact that the signs are somewhat more pronounced on the right suggests that the lesion may be asymmetrical, perhaps involving the left deep pontine nuclei or the right peduncle (remember that cerebellar signs are ipsilateral to the lesion, but the middle cerebellar peduncle is a crossed tract). The pattern of *decreased sensation to pinprick* and the *dissociation between intact proprioception and vibration along with diminished pain and temperature perception* have paramount diagnostic value. The loss of pain and temperature from the left side of the body can be explained by the selective loss of the ALS in the brainstem on the right. In the pons the ALS is very close to the facial motor nucleus, and the loss of one of these structures would very likely be accompanied by the loss of the other. Since the ALS contains secondary fibers at this point, the information carried by these fibers originates from the contralateral side of the body. At this level the ALS has not yet joined the medial lemniscus, so preservation of proprioception, vibratory perceptions, and fine tactile sensations would be expected.

The spinal tract of V also lies very close to the facial motor nucleus. It consists of primary axons, so its loss would produce decreased perception of pain and temperature on the ipsilateral side of the face. The problems that Mr. A. M. has with *swallowing* are probably caused by the loss of corticobulbar fibers to the nucleus ambiguus. Since this nucleus receives bilateral supranuclear innervation, these losses are not expected to be dramatic. Examination of the pharynx and evaluation of the gag reflex would have been helpful in analyzing this case. Given the analysis so far, *tongue deviation* to the left as a result of the loss of the corticobulbar axons on the right can be expected. The observed right-sided deviation of the tongue may be due to left corticobulbar involvement with selective sparing of the corresponding fibers on the right. Given the other lapses in observation that the reporting physician made in this case, it seems more likely that the deviation was recorded in error and that the tongue actually moved toward the left on protrusion. The physical boundaries of the lesion determined by this analysis are illustrated in Figure 10.33.

4. Having localized the lesion as accurately as possible, you must now determine its cause.

Developing a full differential diagnosis for Mr. A. M.'s difficulties is beyond the scope of this book, but a few points are worth mentioning. Mr. A. M. is an overweight heavy smoker with high blood pressure. These facts place him at high risk for stroke. Given the relatively slow stepwise development of his symptoms, an evolving thrombotic stroke (see Chapter 7) should be considered. If the diagnosis of stroke is correct, the lesion must be placed within the territory of a single artery. In the present case occlusion of a **paramedian** and **short right circumferential branch of the basilar artery** may account for all of Mr. A. M.'s initial symptoms. The second episode of vertigo, nausea, and deafness can be explained by a second thrombus that occluded the **right labyrinthine** artery. Occlusion of this artery causes loss of the cochlea, vestibular apparatus, and cell bodies of the vestibulocochlear nerve.

5. Laboratory studies are an essential aid to neurological diagnosis. Such studies should be ordered *to answer specific questions* that cannot be answered by the physical and neurological examinations. In this case the initial diagnosis is infarction of the pons due to thrombosis of the penetrating arteries, but a

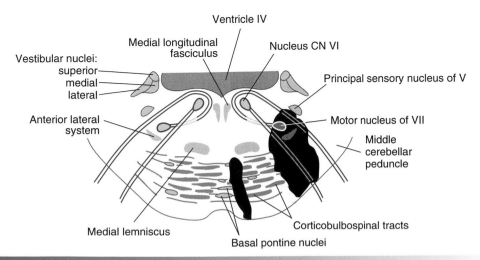

**Figure 10.33    Mr. A.M.'s lesion**

This drawing is based on inferences drawn from the neurological examination. Compare it with the lesions revealed by the MRI.

leaking aneurysm should be ruled out because treatment for thrombosis and hemorrhage are different and incompatible. The initial MRI was ordered for that purpose. It did not display any extravascular blood, an important observation that rules out intracranial hemorrhage and allows anticoagulative therapy. The MRI also revealed that in addition to these risk factors, Mr. A. M. has a tortuous basilar artery with a fusiform aneurysm. These findings constitute further risk factors for stroke, since atherosclerotic plaques and clots often form at sharp bends in arteries. Furthermore, aneurysms may leak or rupture, causing a hemorrhagic stroke (see Chapter 7). The initial MRI did not reveal a pontine infarction. Like computed tomography (CT), MRI cannot demonstrate pathological changes of stroke until about 24 hours afterward. When Mr. A. M. suddenly developed new neurological deficits (vertigo and deafness), the possibility of an intracranial hemorrhage was again presented. The second MRI was ordered to make this determination. It showed no hemorrhage. By this time, however, pathological changes could be imaged and *the second MRI confirmed the cause that had previously been deduced from the clinical evidence,* namely an infarct of the central basis of the pons in the territory of the paramedian branches of the basilar artery involving the fa-

cial motor nucleus and midline structures. The arteriogram was ordered to evaluate Mr. A. M. for surgery. Many aneurysms can be clipped, sealed, or reinforced to prevent their later enlargement or rupture. In this case the aneurysm was so large that it was deemed inoperable.

## FURTHER APPLICATIONS

Restricted lesions of the pons are not common. More commonly major branches of the basilar artery are occluded, producing large infarcts of the brainstem. For each of the arteries mentioned in the following list, sketch the expected infarct and list the sensory and motor symptoms you would expect to observe. You may want to review the brainstem circulation in Chapter 1.

**10.1.** **Posterior inferior cerebellar artery (Wallenberg's syndrome)**

**10.2.** **Anterior spinal artery at the level of the lower medulla**

**10.3.** **Vertebral circulation at the level of the lower medulla**

**10.4.** **Paramedian branches of the basilar or posterior communicating artery near the cerebral peduncle (Weber's syndrome)**

# C A S E     H I S T O R Y

## THE CASE OF THE FROZEN EYES

### HISTORY OF PRESENT ILLNESS

Mr. H. Y. is a 75-year-old white man. For the past year or two he has been having trouble with his balance. He loses his balance very easily and tumbles backward. He says that he cannot re-

cover his balance after he starts to lean backward. He senses no syncope or vertigo. He has had occasional double vision. His wife reports that his movements have generally slowed over the past 2 years. Recently he has had difficulty rising from chairs. This difficulty is apparently not due to weakness but to an inability to start the process. His speech has become soft and slurred.

## PHYSICAL EXAMINATION

Mr. H. Y. is 5 feet 10 inches tall and weighs 175 pounds. Blood pressure is 145/93; heart rate is 75. The physical examination was otherwise unremarkable.

## NEUROLOGICAL EXAMINATION

### Mental Status

Mr. H. Y. is somewhat apprehensive. He is oriented to place, time, and person. He has no memory deficits, recent or past. He could name the presidents from McKinley to the present and could recall three out of three items after 10 minutes.

### Cranial Nerves

OLFACTION: Identified methyl salicylate independently from both nostrils (see Appendix 2).

VISION: Visual fields full to confrontation (see Chapter 12).

OCULOMOTION: Mr. H. Y. could not voluntarily direct his gaze downward. He had no problem looking from side to side. When his head was rotated by an assistant, his eyes tracked in all directions (Fig. 10.34).

PUPILS: Pupils were equal in size. There was a consensual light reflex from each eye, and both eyes constricted on accommodation.

TRIGEMINAL: Sensations to pinprick and cotton were perceived from all three divisions bilaterally. Corneal reflex was present bilaterally. Jaw movements were symmetrical, and strength seemed normal.

FACIAL: Face was symmetrical upon grimace. Eyes appeared normally hydrated. Salivary production seemed normal.

AUDITION: Weber and Rinne tests were normal (see Chapter 11).

VAGOGLOSSOPHARYNGEAL: Voice was normal. Gag reflex was present bilaterally. The pharyngeal arches were high and symmetrical, and the uvula was centered.

ACCESSORY: Sternocleidomastoid and trapezius muscle strength was normal and symmetrical.

HYPOGLOSSAL: Tongue was centered on extension. There was no atrophy or any fasciculations.

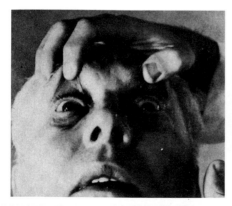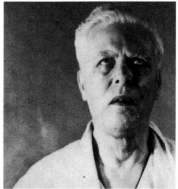

**Figure 10.34   Mr. H. Y.**

Mr. H. Y.'s eyes can gaze downward during a doll's eye maneuver (**left**) but are locked in vertical gaze when the head is stable (**right**). He cannot voluntarily direct his gaze downward. (Reprinted with permission from Rowland LP. Merritt's Textbook of Neurology. 8th ed. Philadelphia: Lea & Febiger, 1989.)

## Station and Gait

Mr. H. Y. has marked retrocollis (the neck is hyperextended, causing the head to be thrust backward). He stands on a wide base. His gait is slow and tottering. When walking he leans backward and has great difficulty correcting his balance. He falls quite frequently. During the examination he would have fallen if he had not had assistance. He has no obvious ataxia and his gait is not shuffling. He swings his arms somewhat when he walks.

## Motor Systems

STRENGTH: Strength was 5/5 at all joints in all extremities.

TONE: Muscle tone was slightly decreased in all extremities. The axial muscles were quite rigid, which accounts for the retrocollis. Examination revealed definite cogwheel rigidity in both upper extremities, greater in the left arm than in the right.

BULK: Normal for his age and symmetrical; no atrophy was noted.

ABNORMAL MOVEMENTS: Mr. H. Y. exhibits very little spontaneous movement; his face is expressionless and he seldom blinks. There were no fasciculations.

## Sensory Systems

Perception of pinprick and cotton touch were everywhere intact. Proximal and distal vibratory extinction occurred at the same time. There were no deficits in proprioception. Romberg test was negative.

## Reflexes

All MSRs were normal and symmetrical. There was no sign of Babinski from either foot.

## Coordination and Control

No abnormalities were noted.

## Parietal Functions

Mr. H. Y. had difficulty doing serial seven subtractions, but was able to spell "world" backward. There was no aphasia or any atavistic signs (see Chapter 14). OKN response demonstrated appropriate tracking and saccades in both directions.

## ANCILLARY STUDIES

MRI of the head showed atrophy of the pontine tegmentum that spared the basis of the pons. The aqueduct was enlarged. No abnormalities appeared in the cerebral cortex or the cerebellum.

## COMMENTARY

Mr. H. Y. has bradykinesia and cogwheel rigidity, is expressionless, and has a slow tottering gait. These observations all suggest parkinsonism. Several other observations, however, should alert one to the possibility that this case is a little different. First, Mr. H. Y.'s chief complaint is falling. Parkinsonism is not usually characterized by falling. Second, the patient is dystonic. His posture is affected to the point that he assumes a retrocollic position. Parkinson patients have a kyphotic (stooped forward) posture. Finally and perhaps most important, Mr. H. Y. has little voluntary control over his eyes, particularly in vertical gaze; there is definite supranuclear ophthalmoplegia.

The term supranuclear ophthalmoplegia refers to a weakness of one or more of the extrinsic eye muscles (ophthalmoplegia) that cannot be explained by involvement of the motor neurons (i.e., supranuclear). In this case, since eye movements could be proved in all directions during passive head movement (VOR), all of the nuclei of ocular motion and their nerves must be intact. Therefore, the disruption of voluntary vertical eye movement must originate in the structures that regulate the nuclei of ocular motion rather than in the nuclei themselves. Since the patient's ophthalmoplegia primarily involves downward gaze, a brainstem lesion involving the RiMLF and the pretectal nuclei should be considered; these structures are the most important in regulating vertical eye movements. These structures are not involved in parkinsonism.

In 1963 Richardson, Steel, and Olszewski described a syndrome now known as **progressive supranuclear palsy.** It is characterized by supranuclear ophthalmoplegia affecting primarily vertical gaze; dystonia of the axial muscles, especially affecting the neck and back; unsteady gait with backward falling; and diplopia. This disease is characterized by a marked degeneration of the neurons within the globus pallidus, substantia nigra, pontine tegmentum, periaqueductal gray, and neighboring pretectal nuclei. The cerebellum and the cerebral cortex are conspicuously unaffected. Mr. H. Y. displays all of the signs and symptoms of supranuclear ophthalmoplegia. The diagnosis was confirmed by the findings of tegmental and peri-aqueductal gray atrophy on MRI.

## FURTHER APPLICATIONS

10.5    Tumors of the pineal gland are asso-ciated with abnormal eye move-ments. **Consider the signs and symp-toms you would expect to see in a patient with such a tumor. How would they differ from the present case?**

10.6    **Increased intracranial pressure is a major factor with pineal tumors. What special circumstances of the pineal tumor create this problem? The symptoms associated with in-creased intracranial pressure are dis-cussed in Chapter 15.**

# C A S E     H I S T O R Y

## THE CASE OF THE EYE THAT WANTS TO STAY SHUT[12]

### HISTORY OF PRESENT ILLNESS

Mrs. P. F., a 44-year-old woman, went to the emergency department at 9:45 PM complaining of a severe headache. She described the pain as sharp and shooting into the front of her head, then aching. She also said that her left eye "wants to stay shut." She has had this pain on and off for 5 days; 4 days ago she saw her fam-ily physician, who ordered CT of the head. No abnormalities were found. She was told to take aspirin and to take it easy.

### PHYSICAL EXAMINATION

Her physical examination was unremarkable. She is 5 feet 6 inches tall and weighs 127 pounds. Her blood pressure is 131/79 with a resting heart rate of 97.

### NEUROLOGICAL EXAMINATION

#### Mental Status
She is alert and oriented to person, place, and time. She can name the presidents back to

Kennedy and can remember three out of three items after 20 minutes.

#### Cranial Nerves

OLFACTION: Identified methyl salicylate inde-pendently from both nostrils (see Appendix 2).

VISION: Visual fields were full to confrontation; no papilledema was present (see Chapter 12).

OCULOMOTION: Mrs. P. F. has weak upward and medial movements of the left eye. On forward gaze the eye is deviated slightly downward and laterally. There is mild ptosis of the left eyelid.

PUPILS: The left pupil was larger than the right (3 and 2 mm, respectively). The left eye did not demonstrate either a direct or consensual light reflex. The right pupillary responses were nor-mal. Accommodation was not tested.

TRIGEMINAL: Sensations to pinprick and cotton were perceived from all three divisions bilaterally. Corneal reflex was present bilaterally. Jaw move-ments were symmetrical and strength seemed normal.

FACIAL: Face was symmetrical upon grimace. Eyes appeared appropriately hydrated. Salivary production seemed normal.

---

[12] This case was brought to my attention by Dr. Robert King, Memorial Hospital, South Bend, IN.

AUDITION: Patient is able to hear finger rubbing in both ears (see Chapter 11).

VAGOGLOSSOPHARYNGEAL: Voice was normal. Gag reflex was present bilaterally. The pharyngeal arches were high and symmetrical, and the uvula was centered.

ACCESSORY: Sternocleidomastoid and trapezius muscle strength was 3/3 and symmetrical.

HYPOGLOSSAL: Tongue was centered on extension. There was no atrophy or any fasciculations.

### Station and Gait

Mrs. P. F. walked on a narrow base. Arm swing was present. She could walk on her heels and toes, do deep knee bends, and hop on either foot.

### Motor Systems

STRENGTH: Strength was 5/5 at all joints in all extremities.

TONE: Tone was normal.

BULK: No atrophy was noted.

ABNORMAL MOVEMENTS: No abnormal movements were noted.

### Sensory Systems

Mrs. P. F. perceived pinprick and light touch in all extremities. Extinction of vibration was equal proximally and distally. Romberg test was negative.

### Reflexes

MSRs are all normal. Toes are down going.

### Coordination and Control

Finger-to-nose and heel-to-shin movements and rapid alternating hand movements were all performed normally.

### Parietal Functions

Mrs. P. F. had no trouble with serial subtractions. There were no atavistic signs. OKN was present in both directions.

### ANCILLARY STUDIES

Mrs. P. F. was scheduled for an arteriogram the next day. It revealed a small aneurysm of the posterior communicating artery.

### SUBSEQUENT COURSE

Mrs. P. F. underwent surgery the day of the arteriogram. The aneurysm was stabilized with a clip and Mrs. P. F. recovered without incident. At a 3-month follow-up visit she was doing well.

### COMMENTARY

Mrs. P. F. had third-nerve palsy. She could not fully move her left eye upward or medially. The left pupil was larger than the right and did not react to light. A consensual light reflex was present in the right eye, proving that she was not blind in the left eye. Third nerve palsy is frequently an ominous sign. In one study of 206 cases, 25% were caused by neoplasms and 18% by aneurysms. Since the CT 4 days earlier showed no abnormalities (i.e., no neoplasm), a supraclinoid aneurysm of the carotid artery and/or the posterior communicating artery was suspected. Such vascular lesions cannot be visualized with CT.

### FURTHER APPLICATIONS

10.7  Review the course of the carotid artery. If the patient had presented with a sixth nerve palsy, where would you expect to find the aneurysm?

10.8  In this case the family physician did not pursue the patient's symptoms after the CT was found to be negative. Was this decision reasonable or an error on the part of the physician? If you believe the physician to be in error, how do you think the medical community should handle such errors? How do you think you would feel if you were that physician? Discuss these issues among your colleagues and professors.

- **Most of the cranial nerves are multimodal and are associated with more than one nucleus in the brainstem.**

  The hypoglossal (XII) and accessory (XI) nerves are exceptions to this generalization, as they are purely motor nerves with their motor neurons in correspondingly named nuclei. The hypoglossal nerve innervates the tongue; the accessory nerve innervates the trapezius and sternocleidomastoid muscles.

- **The vagus (X) and glossopharyngeal (IX) nerves can be considered together because their central connections are essentially identical; they differ primarily in their peripheral distribution.**

  The vagus and glossopharyngeal nerves have three efferent and two afferent components. The nucleus ambiguus, the largest motor nucleus, supplies the voluntary muscles of the larynx and pharynx. The dorsal motor nucleus of the vagus is the principal source of preganglionic parasympathetic fibers to the viscera (heart, lungs, and gut). The ISN supplies the preganglionic parasympathetic fibers to the otic ganglion, which supplies the parotid gland. The NST receives sensory information from the chemoreceptors and baroreceptors that detect blood oxygen tension and blood pressure. It also receives signals from the taste buds of the posterior third of the tongue. The glossopharyngeal is the principal nerve of taste. The NSTV receives pain and temperature signals from a small portion of the external auditory meatus, the oral cavity, and the posterior third of the tongue.

- **The vestibular portion of CN VIII conveys sensations of angular and linear acceleration of the head to the CNS.**

  The semicircular ducts detect angular acceleration; the maculae of the saccule and utricle detect linear acceleration. Vestibular afferent axons synapse in the vestibular nuclear complex and the cerebellum.

- **The facial nerve (VII) is a mixed nerve with both motor and sensory components.**

  The facial motor nucleus supplies the mimetic muscles of the face and the *orbicularis*

*oculi*. Motor neurons that innervate the portion of the face above the eyes are bilaterally innervated by corticobulbar axons. The motor neurons that innervate the lower portion of the face are innervated by contralateral corticobulbar fibers. The SSN supplies preganglionic parasympathetic fibers to the pterygopalatine and submandibular ganglia, which innervate the lacrimal glands and the sublingual and submandibular salivary glands, respectively. The NST receives afferent axons from the taste receptors of the anterior two-thirds of the tongue. The facial nerve also makes a minor contribution to the NSTV.

- **The trigeminal motor nucleus supplies the muscles of mastication and conveys sensations from the head.**

  The NSTV receives primarily pain and temperature signals from the face; the principal sensory nucleus receives fine tactile and proprioceptive information from the same area. The mesencephalic nucleus of V is a displaced ganglion consisting of pseudounipolar neurons of the $I_A$ trigeminal axons.

- **The oculomotor (III), trochlear (IV), and abducens (VI) are the nerves of ocular motion.**

  The abducens and trochlear nuclei supply motor axons to the lateral rectus and superior oblique muscles, respectively. The oculomotor nucleus supplies motor neurons to the remaining extraocular muscles and the levator palpebrae. Preganglionic parasympathetic axons originating in the Edinger-Westphal nucleus innervate the ciliary ganglion, which in turn innervates the constrictor muscle of the iris and the ciliary muscle of the eye. They constrict the pupil and accommodate the lens, respectively.

- **Disruptions of eye movements may manifest as paralysis of one or more of the extraocular muscles (ophthalmoplegia).**

  Muscle paralysis usually indicates nerve or nuclear damage that can be diagnosed by carefully testing the various eye muscles independently. The elevator and depressor muscles cannot be tested in forward gaze; they must be tested during slight adduction or abduction.

- **Eye movements are either tracking or saccades.**

Slow eye movements of variable velocity are achieved only when the eye is tracking an object of interest in the visual field. Saccades are fast movements of constant velocity that are used to place the image of an object of interest on the fovea. The cerebral cortex controls eye movements indirectly.

- **Nystagmus is a type of eye movement that consists of a tracking movement in one direction followed by a saccade in the opposite direction.**

Benign nystagmus may be initiated by vestibular signals (VOR) or visual signals (OKN). Spontaneous nystagmus implies damage to the labyrinth, brainstem, or cerebellum.

- **Brainstem centers independently control vertical and horizontal eye movements.**

The superior colliculus, PPRN, riMLF, and pretectal area are the major visuomotor centers in the brainstem. Lesions to the superior colliculus, riMLF, and pretectal area usually disrupt vertical eye movements; lesions to the PPRN usually affect horizontal eye movements.

- **Ophthalmoplegia may be nuclear, internuclear, or supranuclear.**

These clinical distinctions are based on involvement of the nuclei of ocular motion, the MLF or brainstem motor centers, or the cerebral cortex and corticomesencephalic pathways, respectively.

- **Pupillary constriction and lens accommodation are mediated by the pretectal nuclei and the Edinger-Westphal nucleus.**

The light and accommodation reflexes are bilateral because the fibers from the pretectal area cross the midline in the posterior commissure to synapse in the Edinger-Westphal nuclei. Light shown in the eye produces a direct light reflex in the same eye and a consensual light reflex in the contralateral eye. Bilateral accommodation and pupillary constriction normally occur during convergence.

## SUGGESTED READINGS

Friedmann I, Ballantyne J. Ultrastructural Atlas of the Inner Ear. London: Butterworth, 1984.

Lavin PJM, Weissman B. Neuro-ophthalmology. In: Bradley WG, Daroff RB, Fenichel GM, Marsden CD, eds. Neurology in Clinical Practice, vol 1. 2nd ed. Boston: Butterworth-Heinemann, 1996.

Wilson-Pauwels L, Akesson E, Steward P. Cranial Nerves: Anatomy and Clinical Comments. Toronto: BC Decker, 1988.

# The Auditory System

The hearing apparatus is a complex transducer that converts acoustic signals into coded action potentials suitable for analysis by the nervous system. By convention, the auditory system is divided into four areas: the **external ear, middle ear, inner ear,** and **central auditory pathways**. Each part plays a specific role in the transduction, neural coding, or analysis of acoustic information. This chapter describes the anatomy of the hearing apparatus, sound and sound measuring conventions, and the physiology of the transduction process. Finally, hearing impairment is discussed.

## ANATOMY OF THE HEARING APPARATUS

### The External Ear

The external ear consists of the pinna [L. *pinna,* wing] and the **external auditory meatus** [L. *meatus,* passage]. The pinna collects and funnels sound into the meatus. In some animals, such as the bat, the pinna is quite elaborate, and the animal can direct the external opening toward particular sounds. Orienting the pinna helps localize the origin of the sound. The external auditory meatus is a small tube leading from the opening within the pinna through the temporal bone (see Fig. 10.6). It is bounded internally by the **tympanic membrane**, which is protected by the deep recess of the meatus. The external auditory meatus is a warm, moist environment that is conducive to bacterial growth. **External ear infections** are common but easily treated. If such an infection remains untreated, however, bacteria can penetrate the tympanic membrane and infect the middle ear, a serious complication. Middle ear infections, as well as a number of other conditions, are discussed in more detail later in the chapter.

### The Middle Ear

The middle ear is a cavity within the temporal bone. The major chamber, the tympanic cavity, is connected with air spaces in the mastoid bone (collectively called the antrum) by a small opening, the aditus (see Fig. 10.6). The tympanic cavity is bounded on its lateral side by the tympanic membrane, which separates the middle ear from the external auditory meatus. On the medial side there are two openings into the inner ear from the middle ear, the **oval** and **round windows**. The **auditory tube** (Eustachian tube) extends from the tympanic cavity into the posterior recess of the pharynx.

Three small bones, the **ossicles**, connect the tympanic membrane with the oval window. The **malleus** [L. *malleus,* hammer] is attached to the tympanic membrane. The footplate of the **stapes** [NL. *stapes,* stirrup] is inserted into the oval window. The **incus** [L. *incus,* anvil] joins the malleus to the stapes. The three bones are articulated by tiny synovial joints. The footplate of the stapes fills the oval window and is held in place by ligaments. Two striated muscles, the stapedius and tensor tympani, are attached to the stapes and malleus, respectively.

Vibrations of the tympanic membrane are faithfully registered as vibrations of the footplate of the stapes. Therefore, anything that interferes with ossicular motion impairs hearing. For example, serous secretions from the lining of the tympanic cavity, pus from middle ear infection, or sclerosis of the ossicular joints (**otosclerosis**) all cause hearing impairment by restricting ossicular motion.

The auditory tube is a passageway through which the air pressure in the middle ear is equalized with the external environment. This equalization ensures that changes in air pressure between the middle ear and the environment do not become great enough to deform or rupture the tympanic membrane. Normally the auditory tube is closed. It opens easily, however, with movements of the pharynx, which explains why yawning is helpful to airplane passengers during periods of rapid change in cabin air pressure. If the mucous membranes of the pharynx are irritated and swollen, it may be difficult or impossible to open the auditory tube, allowing a considerable pressure difference to develop across the tympanic membrane, a painful phenomenon well known to skin divers and air travelers.

**Middle ear infections** are common, since infectious agents can easily gain entry via the auditory tube. Once an infection is established, the auditory tube becomes inflamed and closes. Continuing bacterial growth produces a large volume of pus that cannot escape the middle ear. If the infection remains untreated, the pressure increases. This not only causes great pain but may also rupture the tympanic membrane. Subsequent to infection, granulation tissue may envelope the ossicles, limiting their movement and impairing hearing. Occasionally infectious agents gain entry to the inner ear through the round or oval window. Inner ear infections can cause permanent ipsilateral hearing loss ranging from mild to profound. Finally, because of their direct connection with the tympanic cavity, the mastoid air spaces may become a repository for bacteria, resulting in chronic reinfection of the middle ear. In such cases the tegmentum tympani, the thin bone that separates the mastoid air spaces from the cranium, can eventually erode, exposing the cranium to infection that may result in bacterial meningitis. Fortunately, contemporary antibiotic treatment of middle ear infections has nearly eliminated these disastrous sequelae.

## The Inner Ear

The inner ear is the auditory portion of the membranous labyrinth (see Fig. 10.6). The inner ear consists of the cochlea [L. *coclea*, snail], a spiral structure that is entirely enclosed by the petrous portion of the temporal bone (Fig. 11.1). The cochlea is formed from three tubes, or scalae [L. *scalae*, staircase, ladder], that wind together in a circular pattern around a central core, the **modiolus** [L., the hub of a wheel]. The **scala vestibuli** begins as an opening leading from the vestibule, a large perilymphatic space (see Chapter 10) that contains the saccule. In humans, the scala vestibuli winds 2.75 turns from the **base** to the **apex** of the cochlea. At the apex it communicates with the **scala tympani** through a small hole, the helicotrema [G. *helix*, spiral, and *trema*, hole]. The scala tympani spirals from the apex to the base of the cochlea, where it dead-ends at the membrane covering the round window. The scala tympani and scala vestibuli are filled with perilymph and are continuous with the perilymphatic space of the vestibular apparatus (see Chapter 10). Between them lies the **scala media**, an endolymphatic compartment that communicates with endolymphatic space of the vestibular apparatus through the **ductus reuniens** [L. *re*, again, and *unire*, to unite].

### SCALA MEDIA

In cross-section the scala media is a triangular structure bounded at its base by the **basilar membrane** (Fig. 11.2). Superior to the basilar membrane **Reissner's membrane** separates the scala media from the scala vestibuli. The lateral wall consists of the **stria vascularis** [L. *stria*, channel, furrow]. Lying on the basilar membrane is a complex structure, the **organ of Corti**, which consists of hair cells and various types of supporting cells. In humans the hair cells are arranged in three to five rows of **outer hair cells** (OHC) and one row of **inner hair cells** (IHC). Two rows of pillar cells form the tunnel of Corti, which separates the IHC from

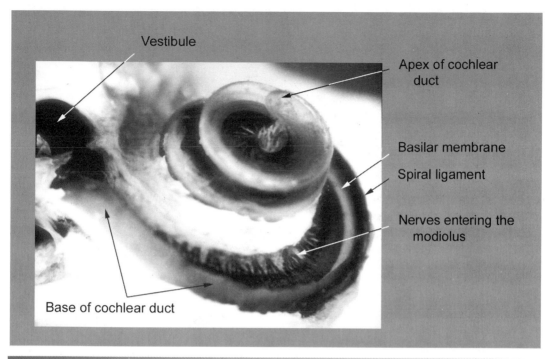

**Figure 11.1    The dissected human cochlea**

The cochlear duct free of surrounding bone. (Reprinted from Johnsson L-G, Hawkins JE Jr. A direct approach to cochlear anatomy and pathology in man. Arch Otolaryngol 1967;85:599–613.)

the OHC rows. Between the IHCs and the modiolus is a recess, the inner sulcus. The **tectorial membrane** [L. *tectorium,* overlying surface (plaster, stucco), fr. *tego,* pp. *tectus,* cover] extends from the upper lip of the inner sulcus and covers the surface of the organ of Corti. The hairs of the OHC are firmly anchored into the gelatinous material of the tectorial membrane. The hairs of the IHC are not firmly attached to it but just brush its inner surface.

COCHLEAR HAIR CELLS

Each human organ of Corti contains about 3,500 IHCs and 12,000 OHCs. Cochlear hair cells are similar to type II vestibular hair cells (see Chapter 10) but have a few key differences. Most notably, cochlear hair cells do not have a kinocilium; they retain only the basal body. Also, the stereocilia of cochlear hair cells are considerably shorter than their vestibular counterparts. Like vestibular hair cells, cochlear hair cells are polarized so that deflection of the stereocilia toward the basal body depo-

larizes the hair cell membrane. All of the hair cells are oriented in the same direction, so that movement of the hairs toward the stria vascularis is excitatory (Fig. 11.3).

THE STRIA VASCULARIS

The stria vascularis lines the lateral wall of the scala media from Reissner's membrane to the spiral prominence (Fig. 11.2). This highly vascularized, slightly pigmented epithelial tissue is composed of three layers: (*a*) a marginal layer in contact with the endolymph, derived from ectoderm; (*b*) an intermediate layer derived from the neural crest and consisting of melanocytes; and (*c*) a basal layer derived from mesenchyme. The principal function of the stria vascularis is to maintain the potassium concentration of the endolymph. As previously discussed, endolymph is rich in potassium ions (about 160 mM) with a low sodium ion concentration (less than 1 mM) (see Chapter 10). The Nernst potential for potassium (calculated from the endolymph with re-

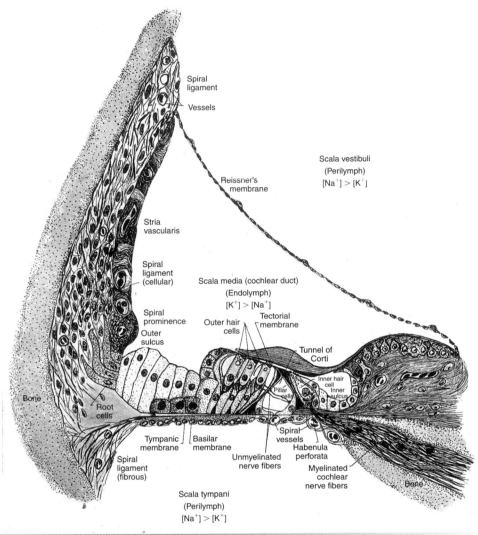

**Figure 11.2  Cross-section of the scala media**

(Reprinted with permission from Brobeck J, ed. Best & Taylor's Physiological Basis of Medical Practice. 9th ed. Baltimore: Williams & Wilkins, 1973.)

spect to the plasma) is about $+80$ mV.[1] An electrical voltage that corresponds closely with this calculated figure, the **endolymphatic potential**, can be measured between the cochlear endolymph and the plasma. The endolymphatic potential is generated by the stria vascularis. It plays an essential role in hair cell transduction (see page 406).

The neural crest origin of the intermediate layer of the stria vascularis appears to have some practical significance, as demonstrated by the consequences of the melanocytes of this layer failing to migrate into the stria vascularis. The stria vascularis fails to complete development during embryogenesis and soon degenerates; consequently, neither en-

---

[1] This figure varies between 50 and 85 mV, depending on the ionic concentration used in the calculation. These figures vary somewhat between species and among the measurements of various research groups.

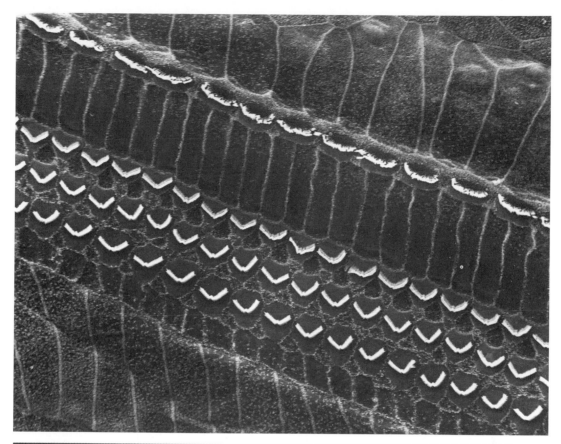

**Figure 11.3   The surface of the reticular lamina of the organ of Corti**

The tectorial membrane has been removed in this scanning electron micrograph. **Top**. The hairs protruding from the inner hair cells (*IHC*). **Bottom**. Three rows of outer hair cells (*OHC*). Between the IHCs and OHCs are the caps of pillar cells that form the tunnel of Corti. (Courtesy of Dr. C. G. Wright, University of Texas, Dallas.)

dolymph nor the endolymphatic potential is produced. For reasons that are not fully understood, the hair cells cannot survive in the absence of endolymph. The absence of hair cells, of course, produces congenital hearing loss in the affected ear.

Atrophy of the stria vascularis is frequently associated with other disorders of aberrant melanocyte migration. For example, Dalmatian dogs, whose unique spotted coat is due to melanocyte migration, frequently have severe hearing loss in one or both ears. Histological examination of the cochleas of these dogs shows that they lack a functional stria vascularis in the affected ear. Melanocyte migration disorders also affect humans. People with **heterochromic irides** (eyes of different colors) or

a white forelock are, like Dalmatian dogs, at risk for developing a severe hearing loss early in childhood, a condition known as **Waardenburg's syndrome** (incidence 2/100,000) (Fig. 11.4). Hearing loss also frequently occurs in association with other pigmentation disorders, such as **retinitis pigmentosa**, an inherited disease resulting in retinal degeneration; **hyperpigmentation**, or leopard spot syndrome; **vitiligo** [L. *vitium,* blemish, vice], or white patches on the skin due to lack of pigment; and **piebaldness** (patchy loss of pigmentation in the scalp and hair).

### Cochlear Innervation

Like the vestibular division, the auditory division of the eighth cranial nerve has both afferent and efferent components. There are two morphologically different afferent neurons, type I and type II. The cell bodies of both types of afferent neurons are in the modiolus of the cochlea. The efferent somas are in the superior olivary complex.

## AFFERENT NEURONS

There are about 30,000 afferent auditory neurons in the human; about 95% are type I. The type I neurons are true bipolar cells with a central and a peripheral axon. Both axons are myelinated over most of their length, as is the

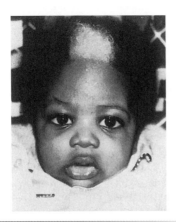

cell body. The distal axon leaves the modiolus and enters the scala media through small perforations, the habenula perforata [L. *habenula*, small strip of skin, dim. of *habena*, rein, strap, thong, strip of skin; *perforare*, pp. *perforata*, pierce] in the temporal bone, (Fig. 11.5). From the temporal bone they proceed directly to the IHCs. Each type I afferent fiber synapses with one IHC without dividing. There are more type I axons than IHCs; each IHC receives approximately 10 afferent synapses. The afferent synapses on the IHCs are clustered at the base of the cell. The afferent neurotransmitter from the IHC to the afferent axon is glutamate, which acts through an AMPA (α-amino-3 hydroxy-5-methyl-4 isoxazole propionic acid) receptor (see Chapter 3).

The type II afferent neurons are unmyelinated, and their cell bodies reside in the modiolus. These neurons are pseudomonopolar. Their single distal axon accompanies type I axons into the scala media through the habenula perforata. Once in the scala media, type II axons cross the tunnel of Corti to innervate only the OHCs. After crossing the tunnel, the type II axons divide, each axon sending collateral branches to innervate approximately 10 OHCs (Fig. 11.5). Each OHC receives afferent synapses from about four type II axons. The afferent transmitter of the OHC is unknown. Type II neurons have a central axon that terminates in the cochlear nuclei. The function of type II neurons is unknown.

## EFFERENT NEURONS

The efferent innervation of the cochlea originates in the superior olivary complex and arises from about 1500 neurons. The OHCs

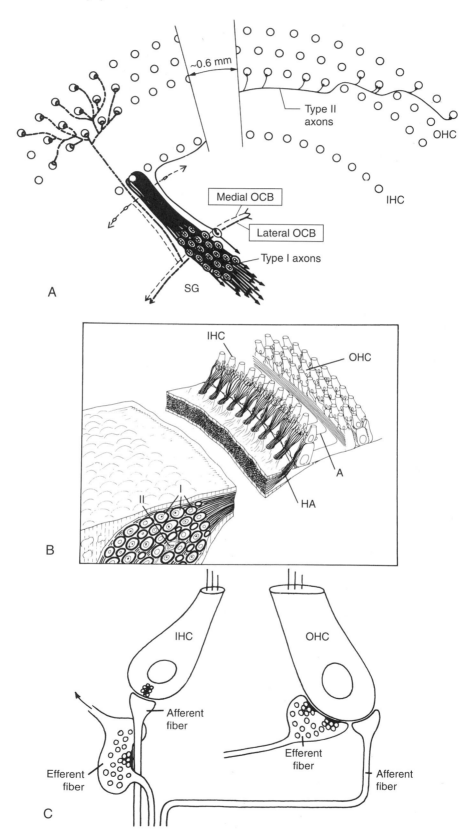

receive axosomatic synapses from efferent fibers, the majority of which originate in the contralateral superior olive. These synapses are large and highly vesiculated, and they secrete acetylcholine (ACh). The ACh receptor in the OHC is an unusual variant of the nicotinic receptor family (the 9 subunit). It has both fast (<100 msec) and slow (>20 sec) responses. In contrast, the IHCs do not receive efferent synapses. The type I primary afferent axons, however, do receive axoaxonic contacts from efferent fibers just before the efferent fibers synapse with the IHCs (Fig. 11.5C).

## THE NATURE OF SOUND

The auditory system is a highly specialized transducer that converts mechanical into electrical energy in three steps. First, the middle ear acts as a *pressure-to-displacement* transducer that converts sound into a mechanical disturbance of the basilar membrane. Second, the cochlea performs a *mechanical frequency analysis* of the signal so that different hair cells will be maximally stimulated by different frequencies. Finally, the hair cells convert basilar membrane *displacement into action potentials*. To understand these processes, we must first briefly examine the nature of sound and the conventions used to describe its physical characteristics.

### Sound Pressure Waves

Sound is the perception of pressure waves produced by mechanical disturbance in a conductive medium, which may be a gas, liquid, or solid. The energy source acts on the medium by exerting a force that compresses some of the molecules in the medium. When the force is removed, the molecules in the medium recoil. If the energy source is vibrating, a succession of compressions and rarefactions occurs among the molecules of the conductive medium. The energy induced into the medium by the vibrating energy source is propagated as a series of compression and rarefaction wave fronts. Furthermore, the compressed molecules act as an energy source to compress adjacent molecules

within the medium. In this way the wave of compression expands from the source like ripples spreading across a pond.

The *physical properties* of sound are characterized by **intensity** and **frequency. Loudness** is a psychophysical measurement of the *perception* of intensity that does not correlate well with intensity itself. Sound intensity is proportional to the velocity and the amplitude with which the stimulus compresses the transmission medium, parameters that determine the amount of energy (power) that is transferred to the medium. *The intensity of sound (i.e., its power) is measured in watts.* The frequency of sound refers to the number of compression and rarefaction events per second. The unit of frequency, measured in cycles per second, is the **hertz** (Hz).

### Intensity

It is inconvenient to express sound intensity in watts, partly because power levels of ordinary sound are very small (femtowatts per square centimeter) and partly because the range of human sound perception spans 12 orders of magnitude. Therefore, a logarithmic notation is employed. The bell (B) is a unit of measure used to express the log 10 of a ratio. For sound,

$$I_{dB} = \log \frac{P}{P_0} \qquad (11.1)$$

where IB is the sound intensity expressed in bells, P is the measured power in watts of the sound source, and $P_0$ is the power in watts of an arbitrary reference standard. The bell, however, is an inconveniently large unit, so the decibel (dB) is used instead as:

$$I_{dB} = 10 \log \frac{P}{P_0} \qquad (11.2)$$

For practical purposes it is more convenient to measure sound in terms of **pressure** rather than power. The same relative scale can be used with the substitution of a pressure reference for the power reference. However, sound intensity is still *expressed as a power* ratio despite the fact that it is *measured as pressure*. This substitution is relatively easy to do, since power (P) is proportional to the square of the pressure (p):

$$P = k \, p^2 \quad (11.3)$$

and k is a proportionality constant. Hence:

$$I_{dB} = 10 \log \frac{P}{P_0} = 10 \log \frac{p^2}{p_0^2} \quad (11.4)$$

and

$$I_{db} = 20 \log \frac{P}{P_0} \quad (11.5)$$

Table 11.1 shows some of these relations.

Since *the decibel is a relative unit of measure,* it is necessary to state explicitly the reference when expressing sound intensity. In acoustics, by agreement, the reference is 20 μPa, and sound pressures referred to this standard are noted as **sound pressure level** (SPL).[2] This reference is used because it approximates the threshold of human hearing at its most sensitive frequency (discussed later in the chapter). Note that a change of 20 dB is two orders of magnitude in power but only one order of magnitude in sound pressure.

### Table 11.1 Relations Among Decibels, Power, Power Ratios, and Pressure Ratios

| dB | Power (Wcm²) | P/P₀ | p/p₀ |
|---|---|---|---|
| 140 | $10^{-2}$ | $10^{14}$ | $10^{7}$ |
| 120 | $10^{-4}$ | $10^{12}$ | $10^{6}$ |
| 100 | $10^{-6}$ | $10^{10}$ | $10^{5}$ |
| 80 | $10^{-8}$ | $10^{8}$ | $10^{4}$ |
| 60 | $10^{-10}$ | $10^{6}$ | $10^{3}$ |
| 40 | $10^{-12}$ | $10^{4}$ | $10^{2}$ |
| 20 | $10^{-14}$ | $10^{2}$ | $10^{1}$ |
| 0[a] | $10^{-16}$ | 1 | 1 |

[a] Reference. A 10-fold increase in the pressure ratio is registered as +20 dB because sound **intensity** is expressed as **power** and power is proportional to the square of pressure. The range of sound intensity represented here approximates the range of human hearing intensity perception, although sounds at the highest levels indicated here cause damage to the cochlea.
dB, decibels; P/P, power ratio; p/p, pressure ratio.

---

## Frequency

The pressure and rarefaction waves of an acoustic signal repeat in time. The number of variations of the pattern per unit of time is perceived as **pitch** and described as the frequency measured in hertz. If the oscillation pattern is perfectly regular over time, it can be accurately described by the sine wave function (Fig. 11.6). An acoustic signal that corresponds to a perfect sine wave is perceived as a pure single tone. Pure tones are hardly ever produced by natural phenomena, so most of the sounds we hear are complex. *Arbitrarily complex sounds can be synthesized from a combination of pure tones.* The inverse is also true: a complex waveform can be decomposed into a series of pure tone components. Mathematically, the process of decomposing a complex waveform into its fundamental pure tones is called Fourier analysis, named after the French mathematician who developed the method.

The sensitivity of the hearing apparatus to sounds of different frequencies varies among animal species. *A human with perfect hearing can hear sounds ranging from about 20 Hz to about 20 kHz.* This range is fairly typical for terrestrial mammals, although cats and dogs can hear sounds up to about 50 kHz. A few animal species can hear very high frequencies, although at the expense of a reduced range at the lower end of the spectrum (Table 11.2).

## Dynamics

A third parameter of sound analysis is not a physical measurement such as intensity and frequency, but for human hearing (and probably all animals), it is critical for sound perception. Natural sounds do not instantaneously start and stop, nor do they maintain the same spectral (frequency) components and amplitude throughout their duration. The timing, intensity, and spectral variation of animal vocalizations is called the **envelope** of the sound stimulus. Anyone who is familiar with bird calls, for example, knows that the dynamic variations of the sound envelope are essential to overall perception and discrimination of the

---

[2] 20 μPa = 0.0002 dynes/cm². This is equivalent to $10^{-16}$ W/cm².

## Summation of Sin Waves

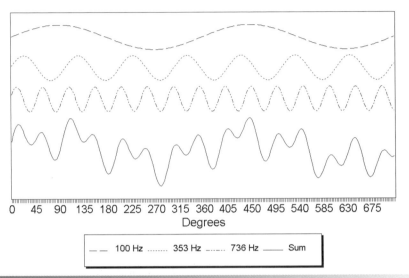

Degrees

|  | 100 Hz | ........ 353 Hz | ---- 736 Hz | —— Sum |

### Figure 11.6    Composition of complex sounds

Arbitrarily complex wave forms can be formed by the simple combination of pure sine waves of various frequencies. Conversely, Fourier analysis can be used to extract the pure sine wave components from an arbitrarily complex wave form. The top three traces are pure sine waves of the frequencies indicated in the figure. The sum of these three frequencies is shown in the bottom trace.

### Table 11.2    Range of Hearing for Selected Animals

| Species | Low (Hz) | High (KHz) |
|---|---|---|
| Human | 20 | 20 |
| Chimpanzee | 100 | 20 |
| Rhesus monkey | 75 | 25 |
| Cat | 30 | 50 |
| Dog | 50 | 46 |
| Chinchilla | 75 | 20 |
| Rat | 1000 | 60 |
| Mouse | 1000 | 100 |
| Guinea pig | 150 | 50 |
| Rabbit | 300 | 45 |
| Bat | 3000 | 120 |
| Dolphin | 1000 | 130 |
| Sparrow | 250 | 12 |
| Goldfish | 100 | 2 |

Data from Fay, R. Hearing in Vertebrates: A Psychophysics Databook. Winnetka, IL: Hill-Fay Associates, 1988.

sound. Bats spend most of their time in darkness and are nearly totally dependent on echolocation to find their way through space. The complexity of the envelope of their calls is critical to these animals' ability to identify objects as they fly (Fig. 11.7).

## SOUND TRANSDUCTION

The inner ear is derived from the lateral line of fishes (see Chapter 10) and is therefore sensitive to displacement waves in a fluid that bend the stereocilia of hair cells. Sound, however, is a pressure wave incapable of directly bending cilia. Therefore, the first step in sound transduction is the conversion of a pressure wave into a displacement wave. This step takes place in the middle ear.

### The Middle Ear

The inner ear is a fluid-filled cavity quite unlike the gaseous environment that conveys

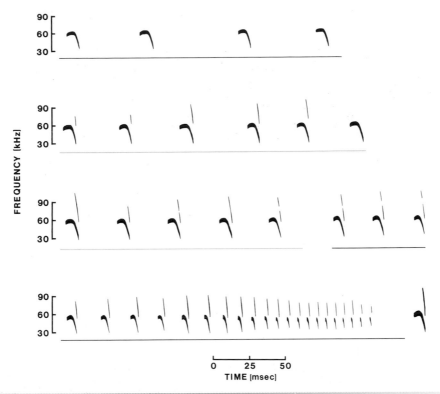

### Figure 11.7    Envelope of bat calls during hunting

Vocalizations are complex auditory signals that cannot be described simply in terms of spectral and intensity components. The timing and amplitude of the various frequency components (the envelope) are critical to its overall perception. These sound spectrographs represent vocalizations in three dimensions: frequency versus time, with intensity crudely shown by the blackness of the trace. This figure shows a continuous series of vocalizations produced by a fish-catching echolocating bat during prey detection and capture. During the search phase (*pink line*) the vocalization is a short chirp. Once the prey has been detected, the character of the chirp changes; a sharp high-frequency terminal component is added (*gray line*). During the attack phase the vocalization continuously changes as the bat makes its final attack on the prey (*black line*). (Reprinted with permission from Wenstrup J, Suthers R. Echolocation of moving targets by the fish-catching bat, *Noctilio leporiuus*. J Comp Physiol A 1984;155:75–89.)

sound to us. The interface between a gas and a liquid prevents the transfer of acoustic energy from one environment to the other because liquids are nearly incompressible. Therefore, a sound pressure wave in air is simply reflected off the surface of a liquid. Divers are quite aware of this phenomenon, for they can clearly hear sounds that are initiated within the water, such as the noise of an approaching propeller, but they are unable to hear the shouts of shipmates calling to them from the safety of the boat. The airborne sound simply bounces off water, transferring only about 2% of its energy to the water in the process.

The middle ear is a transducer that efficiently transfers airborne acoustic energy to the liquid environment of the inner ear. To understand how this transfer works, consider a balloon you have filled with air while living in Denver, the mile-high city. Since this is a thought experiment, we can consider this a perfect balloon, one that is simply a container and does not exert any forces on the gas inside it. In this situation the pressures inside and outside the balloon are equal. The skin of the balloon acts only to separate the inside and outside environments. If you take the balloon to sea level, its diameter decreases because the higher atmospheric pressure at sea level compresses the gas inside the balloon. The size of the balloon reflects the amount of compression. If you take the balloon to the top of Mount Evans, a peak in Colorado nearly 3 miles high, it expands. In other words, changing the pressure outside the balloon causes a physical displacement of its wall. The magnitude of the displacement is proportional to the magnitude of the pressure change.

The middle ear acts much like this balloon. Although most of its walls are rigid bone, the tympanic membrane and oval windows are not. Changes in pressure outside the middle ear are reflected by displacement of the tympanic membrane, just as pressure changes were reflected in displacement of the walls of our perfect balloon. In other words, *a change in pressure is transformed by the middle ear into a displacement of the tympanic membrane.*

Tympanic membrane displacements are transferred to the oval window by the action of the **ossicles**. The efficiency of the transfer is affected by two parameters, the lever action of the ossicles and the size ratio of the tympanic membrane to the footplate of the stapes. The ossicles act as a lever with a mechanical advantage that magnifies the movement of the footplate of the stapes. Although the increase in movement is small—about 1.3 times the movement of the arm of the malleus—it is nevertheless useful. The ratio of tympanic membrane area to footplate area is about 17. Combined, these factors increase the pressure exerted on the footplate of the stapes by about 22 times over the force exerted on the tympanic membrane. Even so, the transfer of energy from air to the inner ear is not 100% efficient. When all factors are taken into account, approximately 67% of the acoustic energy falling on the tympanic membrane is transferred to the inner ear. However, this amount is a great improvement over the 2% transfer that would occur in the absence of the middle ear.

## The Middle Ear Muscles

The two muscles of the middle ear, the **tensor tympani** and the **stapedius**, contract in response to loud sounds and to many non-acoustic stimuli such as swallowing, closing the eyes, adjusting the pinna, and preparing for vocalization. Contraction of the middle ear muscles decreases sound transmission through the middle ear by about 10 dB, a modest effect. Most of the attenuation is caused by the action of the stapedius muscle; the tensor tympani makes almost no contribution to sound attenuation.

The latency of the acoustic reflex contraction of the muscles varies between 150 msec and 250 msec, depending on the intensity of the stimulus. Because of this long latency period, the acoustic reflex contraction of the stapedius cannot protect the inner ear from damage caused by sudden loud noises, a claim that is often made. Nor can contraction of these muscles offer much protective benefit during prolonged loud sounds, since the attenuation factor is only about 10 dB.

## Cochlear Mechanics

The scala tympani and the scala vestibuli are a pair of tubes that communicate through the helicotrema. Lying between them is the scala media. All three tubes are normally coiled around each other like a snail shell, hence the term cochlea. To visualize how the cochlear system works, it is useful to imagine this structure uncoiled, with the scala media reduced to a thin membrane, the basilar membrane, separating the other two scalae (Fig. 11.8A).

In this uncoiled view, imagine the stapes vibrating in the oval window. As the footplate of the stapes moves into the scala vestibuli, the perilymph is displaced toward the helicotrema because the liquid perilymph is nearly incompressible. The pressure exerted on it must be relieved, in this case by an outward deformation of the round window. If the basilar membrane were a rigid structure, the perilymph displacement would have to pass the entire length of the scala vestibuli and return through the scala tympani to reach the round window. But the basilar membrane is flexible. Therefore, the displacement of the perilymph caused by inward movement of the stapes produces a deformation of the basilar membrane toward the scala tympani. In effect, the entire length of the cochlea is short-circuited, and

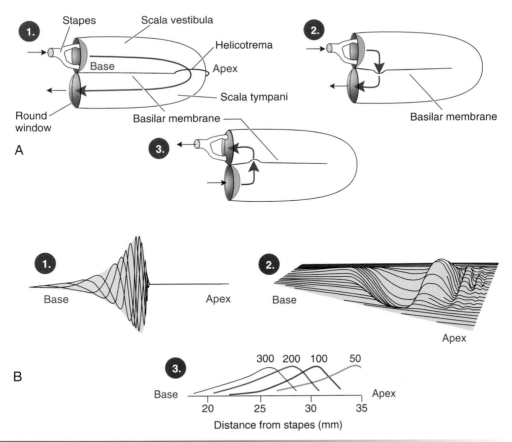

### Figure 11.8    Cochlear mechanics

**A.** The cochlea, a set of coiled tubes that can be represented by a single tube folded back on itself. The scala media is depicted as a simple boundary. *1.* If the basilar membrane were rigid, pressure caused by inward displacement of the stapes would be transferred along the entire length of the cochlea and relieved by outward displacement of the round window membrane. *2.* The basilar membrane is not rigid. Inward displacement of the stapes exerts a downward force on the basilar membrane that deforms it, transferring the pressure directly to the scala tympani and the round window membrane. In effect this pressure transfer short-circuits the system. Most pressure changes within the cochlea are limited to the basal turn. *3.* This diagram represents the reciprocal motion of the basilar membrane during outward displacement of the stapes. **B.** Displacement of the basilar membrane to a continuous pure tone stimulus. *1.* Each line indicates the membrane position at periods of one-third the stimulus period. The amplitude is greatly exaggerated with respect to natural movements of the basilar membrane. *2.* The basilar membrane position is shown at one instant during continuous pure-tone stimulation. As in **B1,** the amplitude of displacement is greatly exaggerated. *3.* The envelope of basilar membrane displacement is depicted for stimuli of various continuous pure-tone frequencies. The peak of membrane displacement varies with stimulus frequency.

the basilar membrane is deformed in the process. When the stapes moves outward, the entire process is reversed.

Once the basilar membrane has been displaced at its base, the deformation moves toward the apex of the cochlea as a **traveling wave** (Fig. 11.8*B*). As the wave moves, its ve-locity slows, causing the wave's amplitude to increase toward the apex, where it reaches a maximum, and then rapidly decreases. The location of the peak of the wave depends on the frequency of the stimulus: low frequencies peak near the apex of the cochlea; and high frequencies peak near the base.

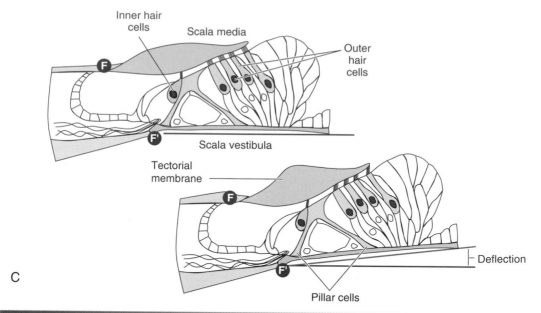

C.

**Figure 11.8    Cochlear mechanics—*continued***

**C.** Shearing of the hairs on the hair cells during displacement of the basilar membrane and tectorial membrane. Each structure flexes at a different hinge point (F and F'), a physical arrangement that creates a differential linear displacement between the base of the tectorial membrane and the reticular lamina of the organ of Corti. The hairs of the outer hair cells register this displacement because one end of the hair shaft is attached to the tectorial membrane and the other is embedded in the cuticular plate of the hair cell. The stereocilia of the inner hair cells are not embedded in the tectorial membrane but apparently brush across its undersurface during movement. (Adapted from von Békésy G. Wave motion in the cochlea. In: Wever EG, ed. Experiments in Hearing. New York: McGraw-Hill, 1960.)

The traveling wave displaces not only the basilar membrane but also the tectorial membrane. The differential movement of these two structures creates shear across the stereocilia, bending them (Fig. 11.8C). This bending of the stereocilia is the essential mechanical event that initiates hair cell depolarization.

**Cochlear Hair Cell Transduction**

The ionic mechanisms of hair cell transduction differ considerably from those of ordinary neurons. As we have noted, the stereocilia are bathed in endolymph, an environment rich in potassium ions; the hair cell body is surrounded by perilymph, a sodium ion–rich fluid. Assuming that the ionic concentration within the stereocilia is the same as in the soma, the Nernst potential for potassium ions from the endolymph to the intracellular space is about 21.8 mV. Thus, if the cilia contain potassium-selective ionophores, a strong inward gradient for potassium ions' entry into the hair cell (IHC $V_m = -40$ mV; OHC $V_m = -70$ mV) is created from the scala media through the stereocilia. The following hypothesis of IHC excitation, which is based on these considerations, generally applies to both vestibular and auditory inner hair cells (Fig. 11.9).

The stereocilia, tubelike evaginations of the cell membrane, are filled with extensively cross-linked actin, which stiffens them. They bend only at the base where they insert into the cuticular plate. The stereocilia are connected to each other by fine filaments that attach from the tip of a shorter stereocilia to the side of the adjacent, longer stereocilium. Because of these interconnections the group of stereocilia move as a unit. Furthermore, there are mechanically gated ion channels at the tips of the stereocilia, at the point of insertion of

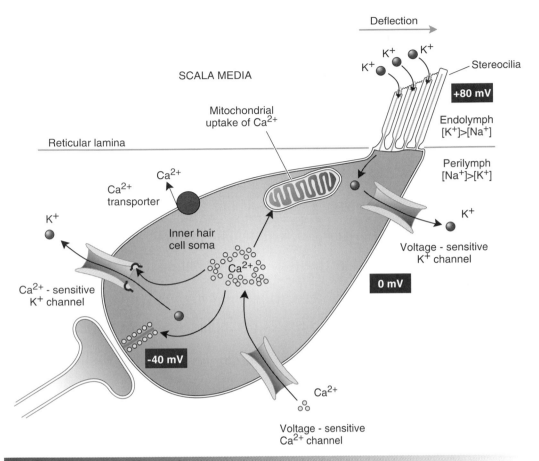

## Figure 11.9 Hair cell transduction

The various electrochemical events that are important for hair cell transduction. Bending the stereocilia opens mechanically coupled potassium channels at their tips. This initiates an *inward* flux of potassium ions because of the steep concentration gradient between the endolymph and the intracellular environment of the hair cell (endolymphatic potential about +80 mV; IHC membrane potential about −40 mV). The increasing concentration of intracellular potassium depolarizes the cell, opening voltage-sensitive calcium and potassium gates. The opening of these gates allows calcium to enter, further depolarizing the hair cell and facilitating the fusion of vesicles at the presynaptic membrane, which liberates neurotransmitter. The increase in the intracellular concentration of free calcium ions also triggers calcium-sensitive potassium gates in the soma. When they open, the electrochemical gradient between the hair cell and the perilymph allows potassium ions to leave the hair cell. The exit of potassium ions from the hair cell restores its resting polarization.

the interconnecting filament. Displacement of the stereocilia bundle toward the taller stereocilium stretches the interconnecting filament. Tension is placed on the mechanically gated ion channel, opening it. This channel is selective to potassium ions, which enter the tips of the stereocilia because of the steep electrical gradient between the endolymph and the IHC cytoplasm (about 120 mV). This *inward* potassium current depolarizes the IHC.

The depolarization of the IHC opens voltage-sensitive calcium gates in the *soma*. The rapid entry of calcium ions ($VCa^{++} \simeq +275$ mV between perilymph and the cell cytoplasm) further depolarizes the cell, and more important, increases the intracellular concentration of free calcium ions. This entry of calcium ions triggers two events. First, it opens calcium-dependent potassium gates in the *soma*, which allows potassium ions to leave the cell soma, repolarizing it. The repolarization of the cell closes the calcium gates. Second, the transient increase in the intracellular calcium concentration initiates the binding of glutamate-containing vesicles to the presynaptic membrane, prompting the release of the glutamate onto the AMPA receptors of the afferent neurons.

Stimulation of the OHC follows a similar course. Shearing of the stereocilia opens mechanically coupled ion gates in the tips of the stereocilia. The resulting inward potassium ion current depolarizes the OHC, which opens voltage-sensitive calcium ions gates in the soma, resulting in an outward potassium ion current that repolarizes the cell. Depolarization of the OHC probably does not result in the release of neurotransmitter (the afferent synapse may be nonfunctional) but rather *shortens the OHC itself.* Hyperpolarization, in contrast, lengthens the OHC. Total length changes are about 3 to 5% of the total length of the OHC.

This change in OHC length occurs cycle by cycle during an acoustic stimulus in response to the receptor potential (hyperpolarization to hypopolarization caused by the potassium ion currents) generated by the OHC itself. The cyclic change in OHC length is called the AC motor.[3] AC motor activity of the OHCs magnifies the amplitude of the traveling wave at the point of maximal deflection, resulting in much sharper frequency tuning than occurs in the absence of AC motor activity in the OHCs.

In addition to changing its shape cycle by cycle, the OHC integrates the receptor potential (which alternates in response to the stimulus) into a steady DC signal that produces a long-lasting change in OHC length called the DC motor.[4] Its effect is to change the relation between the tectorial membrane and the IHCs. Recall that the stereocilia of the OHCs are firmly embedded in the tectorial membrane; those of the IHCs are not. The tectorial membrane probably never touches the stereocilia of the IHC; rather, the sloshing of the endolymph back and forth between the tectorial mem-

brane and the reticular lamina deflects them. By lengthening or shortening, the OHCs can change the space between the tectorial membrane and the IHCs, altering the hydrodynamic forces acting on the IHC stereocilia.

The nature of the OHC motor mechanism is also unknown. It is unlike any motor mechanism previously described. It is not dependent on adenosine triphosphate (ATP) or calcium ions; it appears to derive its energy only from the endolymphatic potential. The active molecules that drive the mechanism are thought to reside in a unique subsurface structure, the **parietal lamella,** that lines the plasma membrane of OHCs. The inner leaflet of the plasma membrane contains many pits to which short pillars are attached. The pillars in turn are attached to a series of helical fibers that are probably composed of actin. These actin fibers are cross-linked by spectrin molecules, and the whole assembly lies on the first of a series of subsurface cisternae. One or more of these molecules is probably voltage sensitive, causing the helical structure to twist on itself during voltage changes. This twisting action would squeeze the cell, reducing its diameter and extending its length, much as squeezing a balloon in the fist makes it longer.

The OHCs are richly innervated by efferent fibers. Activation of these fibers produces an inhibition of auditory nerve responses. Exactly how this mechanism works is not known.

## Neural Coding

Auditory information must be encoded into action potentials in a manner that preserves the envelope, frequency, and intensity of the stimulus. This encoding can be done in a number of ways. First, intensity can be conveniently coded as a function of impulse frequency. Second, intensity can be encoded by the number of axons carrying the signal. Third, frequency can be coded by selectively exciting different axons so that each represents different frequencies. This strategy seems to be

---

[3] AC ordinarily means alternating current in electrical circuits. Its use here is slightly out of context, but it implies the same thing: a signal that alternates rapidly with time.

[4] DC ordinarily means direct current in electrical circuits. Its use here implies a steady signal that changes only very slowly with time.

an obvious outcome of the mechanical frequency tuning of the cochlea. And fourth, frequency can be coded by the synchronous firing of auditory neurons with each cycle of the stimulus. To varying degrees, all four strategies are used by the nervous system to represent auditory information.

## CHARACTERISTIC FREQUENCY

The most common way to describe the firing characteristics of auditory neurons is to determine the threshold intensity of stimuli for various frequencies and then plot the frequency versus threshold intensity (Fig. 11.10A). Such a graph illustrates two important characteris-

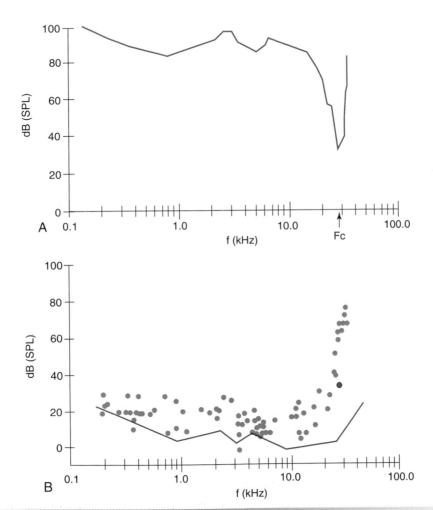

**Figure 11.10   Threshold patterns of primary auditory afferent neurons**

**A.** Tuning curve from a primary afferent neuron of the cat. *Red line,* the threshold of a single axon to auditory stimuli of various frequencies. Although it is excited by a wide range of frequencies (100 Hz to 35 kHz), it is most sensitive only to the fc, 28 kHz. Most auditory neurons have similar response curves. (Adapted from Kiang N. Stimulus coding in the auditory nerve and cochlear nucleus. Acta Otolaryngol 1965;59:186–200.) **B.** The threshold intensity at the characteristic frequency of a large number of neurons in the cat, plotted as dots. *Red dot,* the neuron in **A.** *Red line,* the hearing threshold curve for the cat as determined by behavioral responses. The hearing threshold closely follows the sensitivity of the most sensitive neurons at their characteristic frequency. (Threshold data adapted from Neff W, Hind J. Auditory thresholds of the cat. Journal of the Acoustic Society of America (JASA) 1955;27:480–483. Characteristic frequency data adapted from Busser P, Imbert M. Audition. Cambridge: MIT Press, 1992.)

tics of primary auditory nerve excitation. First, if the stimulus is intense enough, *any given axon can respond to a wide range of frequencies. Second, each axon is most sensitive to only one frequency,* its **characteristic frequency** (fc).

Plotting only the threshold of numerous primary afferent axons at their critical frequencies reveals the distribution of the spectral sensitivity of an animal's hearing (Fig. 11.10B). The hearing threshold curve revealed by these charts correlates well with the animal's behaviorally determined auditory threshold. Such charts demonstrate that individual axons code for a given frequency at their lowest threshold. This frequency coding is usually called **place coding** because the frequency sensitivity of the primary afferent auditory axons

corresponds with its origin along the basilar membrane of the cochlea.

## PHASE LOCKING

Another way of visualizing axonal responses is to display the number of action potentials versus time during the presentation of a pure tone stimulus. Superimposition of the responses to a large number of stimuli produces a pattern called a histogram (Fig. 11.11A). Histograms produced by a single auditory axon stimulated at constant intensity at various frequencies show that the action potentials occur in groups. The timing between the groups is determined by the frequency of the stimulus, a phenomenon called **phase locking**. An individual axon, however, does not

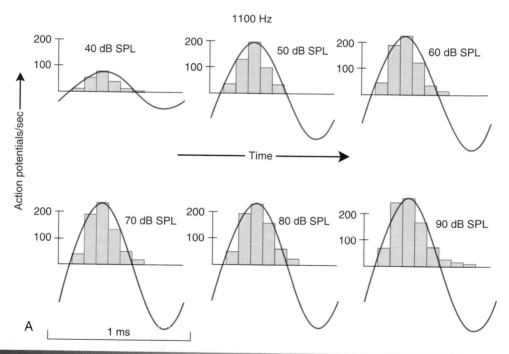

**Figure 11.11   Response characteristics of primary auditory afferent neurons**

**A.** Histograms showing a single primary afferent axon driven at different intensities at its characteristic frequency. The stimulus is superimposed on the histogram. Each bar in each histogram represents the number of spikes collected during a time interval represented by the width of the bar. Spikes occur only during one phase of the sinusoid, even when driven at very high intensities. The excitatory phase corresponds to an outward movement of the stapes and bending of the stereocilia toward the stria vascularis. Also, the total number of spikes collected is roughly proportional to intensity. (Adapted from data in Rose JE, Hind JE, Anderson DJ, et al. Some effects of stimulus intensity on the response of auditory nerve fibers in the squirrel monkey. J Neurophysiol 1971;34:685–699.)

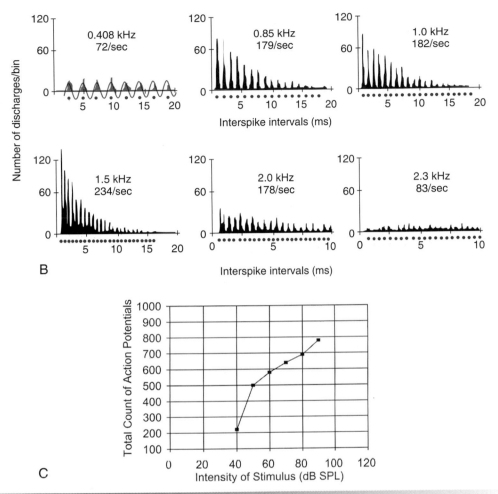

B. Histograms from a single primary auditory afferent axon driven at the same intensity (80 dB SPL) at different frequencies. The characteristic frequency of this axon is 1.6 kHz. As in **A,** the amplitude represents the number of spikes recorded at the time represented by the width of the bar. For each frequency the axon fires at an interval that is very close to the reciprocal of the stimulus frequency, that is, the period of the stimulus (marked by the *dots* below the abscissae). Although the axon phase-locks to the stimulus frequency, the rate of firing is greatest at the characteristic frequency. Axons such as these show characteristics of both volley and place coding. (Data from Rose J, et al. Patterns of activity in single auditory fibers of the squirrel monkey. In: de Reuck A, Knight J, eds. Hearing Mechanisms in Vertebrates. London: Churchill Livingstone, 1968.) **C.** Relation between the intensity of the stimulus and the number of action potentials produced by a single primary auditory afferent fiber. Data from **A.**

respond equally well to all frequencies. The axon produces the highest number of action potentials at its $f_c$ and considerably fewer action potentials at other frequencies. The action potentials produced at other frequencies are still phase-locked with the stimulus (Fig. 11.11*B*).

A careful examination of the histograms reveals that volley coding breaks down at frequencies above 2 kHz. At higher frequencies place coding predominates over volley coding, whereas at lower frequencies, volley coding dominates. This dual coding correlates well with the mechanical selectivity of the cochlea.

Low frequencies produce a traveling wave that peaks close to the apex of the cochlea, disturbing nearly the entire basilar membrane and firing almost all of the hair cells simultaneously. Place coding is therefore ineffective. Higher-frequency stimuli cause the traveling wave to peak closer to the base, stimulating fewer hair cells in the process, making place coding more selective.

Another way of looking at phase locking is to sum the number of action potentials for each cycle of the pure tone stimulus. Such interspike histograms reveal quite clearly that the axon responds only during the half of the stimulus that corresponds to the rarefaction phase of the acoustic stimulus. This phenomenon is a direct consequence of the fact that the hair cells are depolarized only when the hairs are deflected toward the basal body; hence the primary afferent axon is excited during only one phase of the stimulus.

When stimulated at the $f_c$, the intensity of the stimulus is encoded approximately by the number of action potentials produced; the greater the stimulus, the greater the probability that the axons will respond on a given cycle of the stimulus (Fig. 11.11C). These data make it apparent that the coding of the stimulus frequency and intensity is a complicated process. Individual axons simultaneously carry both frequency and intensity information. How this information is separated by the central nervous system (CNS) and appropriately interpreted is unknown.

## NEURAL PATHWAYS

The central connections of the auditory system are among the most complex in any sensory system. The ascending pathways are organized as two principal systems, the core and belt pathways. The **core pathways** are carefully organized and mapped (line labeled) according to the characteristic frequency of the neurons, creating **tonotopic maps**. Tonotopic maps are maintained at all levels, and these core pathways are the fastest and most direct in the auditory system. Surrounding the core pathways are the **belt pathways**, which are less carefully organized along tonotopic lines.

Neurons in this system are not only frequency selective but also sensitive to the timing and intensity patterns in the envelope of the signal. Some parts of the belt pathways appear to be organized to preserve binaural interactions; other areas have cells that respond only to signals with complex envelopes.

*Thus the three critical parameters of auditory signal processing—frequency, intensity, and envelope—appear to have and maintain separate information channels at all levels of the auditory system.* The following description of the central auditory pathways is greatly simplified to emphasize the core pathways within the various nuclei of the auditory system (Fig. 11.12).

As discussed earlier, physiological studies have shown that each primary afferent auditory axon responds to a wide range of auditory frequencies but has the lowest threshold for one specific frequency. Neurons in all of the auditory nuclei of the brainstem and cerebral cortex also have similar tuning curves: each responds to a wide range of frequencies but has a single characteristic frequency. In general but with many exceptions, the tuning curves of these neurons progressively narrow as they ascend the auditory system. Thus neurons at each successive level are more frequency selective than those of the previous level.

### Primary Afferent Neurons

The central axon of the afferent neurons terminates in the cochlear nuclear complex. This complex consists of three principal nuclei, the **dorsal cochlear nucleus (DCN)**, the **anterior ventral cochlear nucleus (AVCN)**, and the **posterior ventral cochlear nucleus (PVCN)**. After entering the brainstem, the primary afferent axon bifurcates. The anterior branch terminates in the AVCN; the posterior branch enters the PVCN. Before terminating, the posterior branch divides, sending one collateral to synapse in the PVCN and the other to the DCN, where it terminates (Fig. 11.12).

### Brainstem Connections

Each of the cochlear nuclei gives rise to a separate ascending pathway in the medulla, con-

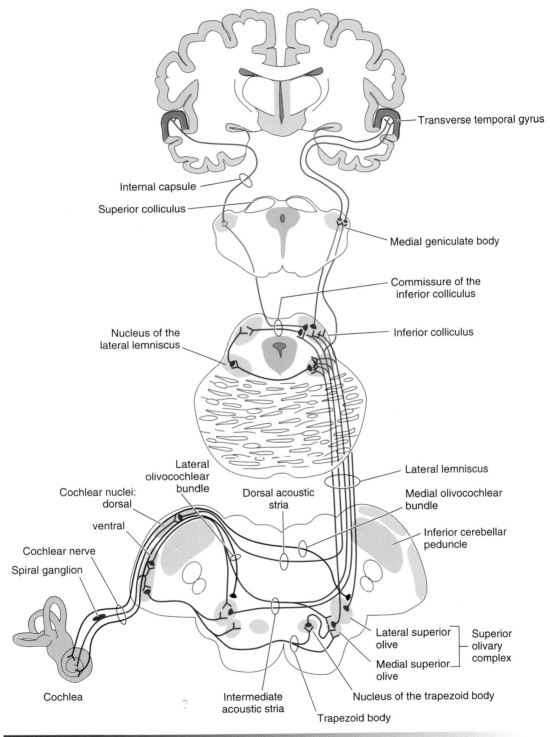

Transverse temporal gyrus

Internal capsule

Superior colliculus

Medial geniculate body

Commissure of the inferior colliculus

Nucleus of the lateral lemniscus

Inferior colliculus

Lateral olivocochlear bundle

Lateral lemniscus

Cochlear nuclei: dorsal

Dorsal acoustic stria

Medial olivocochlear bundle

ventral

Inferior cerebellar peduncle

Cochlear nerve

Spiral ganglion

Lateral superior olive

Superior olivary complex

Medial superior olive

Cochlea

Intermediate acoustic stria

Nucleus of the trapezoid body

Trapezoid body

**Figure 11.12    The principal ascending auditory pathways**

verting the single information channel of the primary afferent fibers into a multichannel system. Each channel is probably specialized to convey specific attributes of the auditory signal, and it is tempting to assume that each channel conveys one of the primary signal parameters. This correlation has been demonstrated to some degree, but our knowledge of these attributes is too incomplete to confirm this conclusion.

Axons from the DCN take the most direct route to higher auditory centers, crossing the midline as the **dorsal acoustic stria** without synapsing (Fig. 11.12). The ascending portion of these axons forms the **lateral lemniscus,** the principal ascending auditory tract of the brainstem. Fibers in the lateral lemniscus ascend to the **inferior colliculus,** where they terminate in an organized tonotopic pattern.

Axons originating primarily in the PVCN form the **intermediate acoustic stria.** Collaterals from these axons synapse in the ipsilateral and contralateral **superior olivary complex;** the main branch joins the lateral lemniscus to ascend and terminate in the inferior colliculus.

Axons originating primarily in the AVCN form the most ventral of the acoustic striae, the **trapezoid body.** This tract, which is immediately dorsal to the basis of the pons, passes through the medial lemniscus. The axons of this tract give off several collateral branches that synapse bilaterally in the superior olivary complex and the contralateral **nucleus of the trapezoid body** (NTB). Third-order fibers originating in the superior olive ascend in the lateral lemniscus to terminate in the inferior colliculus. Axons leaving the trapezoid body do not join the lateral lemniscus.

## The Superior Olivary Complex

The superior olivary complex is a collection of nuclei in the pons at the level of the facial nucleus (Fig. 11.12). The largest structures in the complex are the **lateral superior olive** (LSO) and the **medial superior olive** (MSO). Surrounding this complex are a number of small nuclei, the **periolivary nuclei.**[5] Medial to the superior olive is the nucleus of the trapezoid body. The superior olivary complex and trapezoid nuclear complex are prominent in carnivores, especially the cat, but the superior olivary complex is much smaller in the human.

The cells in the LSO and MSO have two large dendrites that extend from opposite sides of the soma. One dendrite receives projections from the contralateral cochlear nuclei, the other from the ipsilateral cochlear nuclei. This arrangement allows the olivary neurons to compare auditory information from the two ears. This system is used to determine the **spatial localization** of sound based on the interaural differences in sound intensity (LSO) and time differences (MSO) between the two ears.[6] The MSO neurons are exquisitely sensitives. These neurons can detect differences in intraaural arrival times of as little as 400 μsec, which represents a difference in path length between the two ears of approximately 5 inches. The barn owl can locate and capture foraging mice in total darkness, using the rustling sound the mouse makes as its only sensory clue.

The superior olivary complex is also the origin of the efferent axons of the auditory nerve (Fig. 11.12). This tract, the **olivocochlear bundle** (OCB), contains two classes of efferent axons: those that terminate as large vesiculated boutons on the OHCs, the **medial efferent system,** and those that make axoaxonic synaptic contact with the type I afferent axons, the **lateral efferent system** (Fig. 11.5).

Most of the 800 axons of the medial efferent system arise from the periolivary nuclei contralateral to the cochlea that they innervate. These axons branch extensively in the cochlea and ultimately innervate the entire population of about 12,000 OHCs. In contrast to the medial efferent system, most of the neurons of the lateral efferent system originate in the periolivary nuclei ipsilateral to the innervated cochlea. They also branch extensively

---

[5] They all have names, but it is not necessary for the nonspecialist to learn them.

[6] The sound from a source that is not equidistant from the two ears does not stimulate the ears equally. The ear closer to the source receives a more intensive sound stimulus with a shorter latency than the opposite ear. The brain uses both of these clues, intensity and intra-aural time difference, to determine the origin of the sound. Many animals have a mobile pinna that can be oriented toward the source, maximizing the intensity differences and therefore increasing the precision of localization.

and form synapses on most of the approximately 3,500 afferent axons; they do not terminate on any of the hair cells.

The physiological role of the efferent system in hearing is not known. It was originally hypothesized that the cochlear efferent axons sharpened the tuning curves of the primary afferent fibers, making them more frequency selective. This hypothesis does not appear to be true, as frequency sharpening seems to be an intrinsic function of the OHCs themselves (see page 408). Any neural feedback would be too slow to be effective. Experiments with trained monkeys have revealed that the efferent system may enable us to make auditory discriminations in the presence of noise, as this ability decreases after the medial OCB is lesioned. Extracting an interesting signal from environmental noise—exemplified by our ability to listen to a single person in a room full of talking people; the "cocktail party effect"—is an important attribute of our auditory system. In noisy environments humans with certain types of hearing losses have difficulty discriminating speech. Some evidence suggests that this deficit is related to loss of cochlear efferent axons. Exactly how this deficit occurs is not known.

### The Lateral Lemniscus

The lateral lemniscus is the principal fiber tract entering the inferior colliculus (Fig. 11.12). It carries fibers from the dorsal and intermediate acoustic striae and from the superior olivary complex. Many of these fibers send collaterals into the small **nucleus of the lateral lemniscus**. The commissure of the lateral lemniscus carries fibers from one nucleus to its contralateral partner. Other projections are to the inferior colliculus. Very little information is known about the function of the lateral lemniscus.

### The Inferior Colliculus

The **inferior colliculus** (IC) is a major auditory center (Fig. 11.12). Afferent fibers enter the IC from three principal areas: (*a*) the lateral lemniscus, (*b*) the contralateral inferior colliculus, and (*c*) descending connections from the ipsi-

lateral auditory areas of the cerebral cortex. Efferent axons leave the IC to innervate the ipsilateral medial geniculate nucleus, the contralateral inferior colliculus, the deep layers of the superior colliculus (SC), the pretectal area, and the mesencephalic reticular formation.

The functions of the IC remain obscure. Portions of it associated with the belt pathways are not rigorously organized tonotopically, and the underlying organizational plan is not apparent. Many cells in these regions respond to complex auditory signals. Unfortunately, the wide variety of response patterns so far precludes any generalizations.

The tonotopic organization that is characteristic of the core auditory system occurs in part of the IC. Despite this well-organized tonotopic arrangement, it would be a mistake to consider frequency analysis the principal function of the IC. Although most cells in the IC respond to binaural clues, the binaurally driven cells do not appear to be arranged so as to map the three-dimensional acoustic space. That function appears to reside in the SC, which contains cells driven by both visual and auditory stimuli (see Chapter 10). These cells are arranged so that maps of the acoustic and visual spaces are congruent. As noted in Chapter 10, the SC and its efferent projections are important in initiating movements to orient the head (and pinna if it is mobile) toward important stimuli in the visual and auditory space.

### Medial Geniculate Nucleus

The thalamic nucleus of the auditory system is the **medial geniculate nucleus** (MGN) (Fig. 11.12). The MGN is divided into four subnuclei, which receive mostly ipsilateral projections from the IC. The largest subnucleus, the lateral nucleus of the medial geniculate, is tonotopically organized. It projects to the ipsilateral primary auditory cortex (Brodmann areas 41 and 42) and constitutes the core pathway. The other subnuclei receive belt projections from the IC and project to all auditory areas of the cerebral cortex.

The MGN also receives a particularly prominent descending collection of axons that arises from the auditory cortex. The ascending axons from the IC and the descending axons from the auditory cortex converge on the dendrites of geniculate neurons, where they form complex synaptic structures called "synaptic nests." This reciprocal anatomical arrangement allows close regulation of MGN activity by the cerebral cortex.

## Auditory Cortex

In humans, most of the primary auditory cortex lies on the surface of the temporal lobe (Brodmann areas 41 and 42) buried within the lateral fissure (Fig. 11.13). This location corresponds to the **transverse temporal gyri (Heschl's gyri)**. In most persons the left transverse temporal gyri are considerably larger than the right, an asymmetry that can be seen on magnetic resonance images (MRI). The auditory cortex receives ascending afferent axons from the MGN. The auditory areas of the two hemispheres are interconnected by commissural fibers.

The core area of the auditory cortex (usually designated A-I) has prominent tonotopic organization.[7] Reflecting the pattern seen in other sensory and motor areas of the cortex, A-I is organized into vertical columns in which the cells in all of the cortical layers of a particular patch respond to the same characteristic frequency. Running perpendicular to rows of isofrequency columns are rows of columns that present binaural information. One set of columns responds if the stimulus is bilateral; another set responds to monaural stimuli. Some evidence suggests that a third level of cortical organization maps the three-dimensional auditory space.

The belt area of the auditory cortex, which surrounds A-I, has been subdivided into several areas. Although they have not been identified in humans, some anatomical equivalent probably exists. The specific functions of the belt areas remains obscure.

Studies of the cat show that *the cerebral cortex is not necessary for frequency discrimination,* which remains unimpaired after bilateral cortical ablation. However, *discrimination that is based on the timing and pattern of auditory events is severely impaired* after bilateral cortical ablation. For example, in one classic experiment, cats were trained to recognize a Morse code pattern of low-high-low pitch tone pips as signaling the safe condition. When the pattern changed to high-low-high pips, the cat had only a few seconds to move before being shocked. Normal intact cats had no difficulty learning this task. However, after cortical ablation, the cats were unable to recognize the difference in the tone patterns to avoid the shocks. Remarkably, if any auditory cortex escaped the experimenter's knife, timing and pattern discriminations remained intact. In humans, speech perception is critically dependent on timing and pattern discriminations. Speech perception is quite refractory to cortical lesions unless the infarct is very large.

One particularly useful case directly addresses this question. The patient had an infarct of the left auditory cortex and consequently some transient difficulty with speech discrimination, but he recovered fully. About 16 months later he had another infarct, this time of the right auditory cortex. This lesion left him unable to comprehend speech. His hearing threshold, as measured by pure tones, was nearly normal. He was also able to localize sounds in space. The patient's own description of his situation: "I can hear you talking, but I can't translate it."

## CLINICAL EVALUATION OF HEARING DISORDERS

The many types of hearing tests range from the simple to the specialized. Simple tests are appropriate for the routine neurological examination. Specialized examinations, which require specialized equipment and training, are useful for quantifying hearing disorders and are necessary for the fitting of hearing aids. Not appropriate for an ordinary office examination, they require the services of an audiologist. While there are numerous tests of the auditory system, only examinations most

---

[7] This discussion is based primarily on studies of the cat and monkey. Anatomical data on the human auditory cortex are sparse. In the absence of better data, conclusions based on animal studies must be extrapolated to humans.

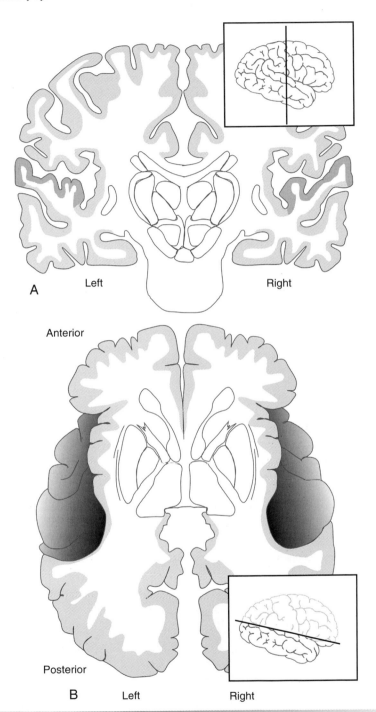

**A.** Frontal section through the cerebral cortex showing the primary auditory cortex (*gray*) on the surface of the temporal lobe. **B.** Surface of the temporal lobe with the remainder of the cerebral cortex removed. The two auditory areas are usually asymmetrical, as shown here, with the left somewhat more prominent than the right.

## Figure 11.13   The auditory cortex

relevant to primary care medicine are discussed here.

## Simple Hearing Tests

Two simple hearing tests are an essential part of the neurological examination. Both depend on the differences between **air conduction** and **bone conduction** of sound. Air conduction is the normal presentation of sound by air pressure waves impinging on the tympanic membrane. Sounds presented in this way depend critically on the transducing function of the middle ear. Bone conduction presents stimuli as oscillations in the temporal bone. Such vibrations can set the basilar membrane into motion directly, bypassing the middle ear. Bone conduction of sound is less efficient than air conduction; thresholds are about 35 dB below those of air conduction thresholds.

### RINNE'S TEST

To perform **Rinne's test**, a tuning fork (typically 512 Hz, corresponding to middle C on the piano) is set into vibration. Its stem is placed on the mastoid process to stimulate the cochlea by bone conduction (Fig. 11.14). *If the patient can hear the stimulus by bone conduction, the cochlea and central pathways are grossly functional.* The intensity of the stimulus decreases gradually as the tuning fork's vibrations diminish. The patient is asked to sig-

nal when the tone can no longer be heard. At the patient's signal the tines are placed lateral to the tragus to stimulate the ear by air conduction. *The patient with normal hearing can hear the tone for an additional 15 seconds,* since air conduction is 35 dB more sensitive than bone conduction. If the patient cannot hear by air conduction for the full 15 seconds, the middle ear is dysfunctional. Rinne's test determines only the relative sensitivity of the ear to air and bone conduction. It cannot determine the relative sensitivity of the two ears, nor can it determine a partial sensorineural hearing loss (see page 424).

### WEBER'S TEST

**Weber's test** provides a necessary adjunct to Rinne's test. In Weber's test the base of the vibrating tuning fork (512 Hz) is placed on the nasal bone[8] (Fig. 11.15). The patient is asked to localize the sound. There are two possible responses. If hearing is equal from both ears, the sound seems to come from inside the head. Otherwise, the sound is heard better from one ear. In that case the sound is louder in the more sensitive ear if the cochlea or auditory nerve is defective. Paradoxically, the sound is louder in the less sensitive ear if the middle ear is defective. This counterintuitive result is due to the fact that vibrations reach the cochlea by both air and bone conduction. These vibrations are slightly out of phase and therefore in-

---

[8] Actually, any placement on a midline structure of the skull is acceptable, but the nasal bone gives the most sensitive result.

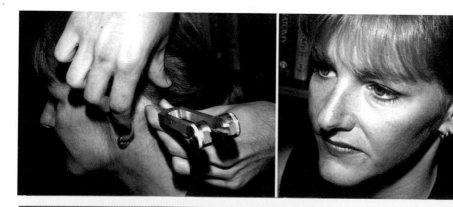

**Figure 11.14   Rinne's test**

**Left,** testing bone conduction. **Right,** testing air conduction.

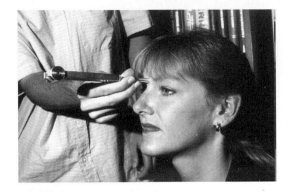

**Figure 11.15    Weber's test**

terfere with each other in the more sensitive ear. Since only bone conduction is available in the less sensitive ear, this interference does not occur. Therefore, the cochlea in the less sensitive ear receives greater stimulation. An abnormal Weber's test cannot be interpreted in isolation, as it can detect only relative differences in hearing loss between the two ears. It must be augmented by Rinne's test to determine whether or not middle ear malfunction is contributing to the hearing loss.

### Specialized Hearing Tests

#### AUDIOMETRY

Simple office hearing tests with tuning forks, while useful, cannot accurately evaluate hearing disorders. Sophisticated auditory examinations are required for accurate evaluation. Describing all of the methods of testing hearing is beyond the scope of this text; however, the primary care physician frequently must interpret the results of common hearing tests, so a few comments are appropriate. The most common hearing test is **pure tone audiometry**, which simply measures hearing thresholds at specific frequencies. In this test the patient is fitted with calibrated earphones. Pure tones are presented at various intensities and frequencies; the patient simply indicates whether or not the tone is heard. Each ear is tested separately.

Since individual hearing thresholds vary, data from thousands of young subjects with normal hearing have been averaged to provide an international standard for the hearing threshold curve (Fig. 11.16A). Several features of the normal hearing threshold curve are apparent. First, the threshold is not identical for all frequencies. Second, human hearing is most sensitive between about 500 Hz and 5 kHz. Third, although it is common to state that the normal frequency range of human hearing is 20 Hz to 20 kHz, few persons hear well below 50 Hz or above 16 kHz.

The **hearing loss curve** is a convenient method of charting a patient's hearing sensitivity. These charts, known as **audiograms**, show the *difference between the standard hearing threshold curve and the patient's threshold hearing curve.* The data are presented as hearing loss in decibels versus frequency (Fig. 11.16, *B–E*). These charts are easy to read and interpret because normal hearing is represented between 0 and −20 dB for all frequencies. However, the hearing loss curve is a threshold measured against a relative standard. Hence the absolute intensity of the 0 dB reference in the hearing loss diagram varies with frequency according to the standard threshold curve.

Other audiometric tests measure the ability to understand speech in the presence of noise and recruitment (see page 423). The **speech reception threshold** (SRT) test determines the lowest intensity at which a person can understand speech. A series of two-syllable words that have been intensity calibrated are presented to the patient through earphones. Threshold is determined when the patient can understand half of the words. The average pure tone threshold should be within 7 dB of the SRT. The **speech discrimination test** consists of presenting the patient with a series of 50 monosyllabic words that are phonetically balanced. The score is reported as the percent of words correctly understood.

#### TYMPANOMETRY

The compliance (flexibility) of the tympanic membrane can be affected by any process that restricts or enhances its movement. Two such processes are common: the accumulation of fluid in the middle ear and pathological

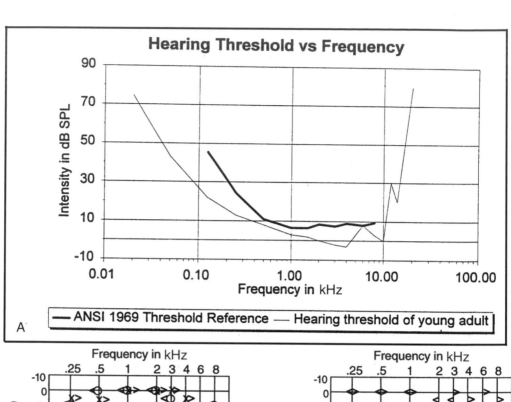

**Hearing Threshold vs Frequency**

Intensity in dB SPL

Frequency in kHz

— ANSI 1969 Threshold Reference — Hearing threshold of young adult

A

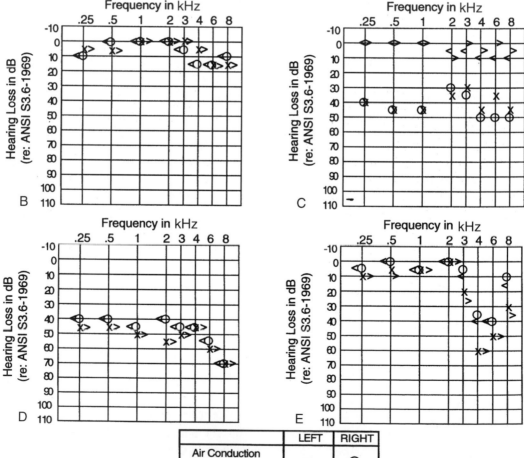

Frequency in kHz

.25 .5 1 2 3 4 6 8

Hearing Loss in dB (re: ANSI S3.6-1969)

B

Frequency in kHz

.25 .5 1 2 3 4 6 8

Hearing Loss in dB (re: ANSI S3.6-1969)

C

Frequency in kHz

.25 .5 1 2 3 4 6 8

Hearing Loss in dB (re: ANSI S3.6-1969)

D

Frequency in kHz

.25 .5 1 2 3 4 6 8

Hearing Loss in dB (re: ANSI S3.6-1969)

E

| | LEFT | RIGHT |
|---|---|---|
| Air Conduction unmasked | X | O |
| Bone Conduction unmasked | > | < |

changes in the ossicles. Middle ear compliance, often called impedance, is measured by bouncing sound waves off the tympanic membrane and analyzing the echo. If the middle ear is filled with fluid, the tympanic membrane is very stiff and its compliance reduced. Tympanometry has practical importance in diagnosing serous otitis media (see page 423) and is now routinely employed in examining children. Tympanometry is also useful in diagnosing otosclerosis and disarticulation of the ossicles.

## BRAINSTEM AUDITORY EVOKED POTENTIALS

In certain circumstances the electrical events evoked in the brainstem by auditory stimuli can be recorded from surface electrodes. To be measurable from remote sites, these signals must contain the nearly simultaneous action of a large number of closely spaced neurons. Even so, at the surface of the body these signals are so small that they usually cannot be extracted from the background noise. With special stimuli, neural signals can be extracted from background noise by computer averaging techniques.[9] Signal averaging is based on the principle that noise is random. Random noise, averaged over time, produces a signal of zero amplitude. If a *synchronized repetitive signal* is superimposed on the noise, the signal does not average to zero. Therefore, a neural signal that is smaller in amplitude than the noise itself can be extracted by the averaging process provided the timing of the signal is known.

This averaging technique has become clinically practical with the development of small, high-speed computers. These systems can digitize and average multiple recordings in real time, extracting the neural signal in the process. This method can be applied whenever a repetitive, stereotyped neural response can be elicited thousands of times. It has been applied to the auditory system: calibrated clicks (square wave auditory signals) are presented to one ear and electrical events are recorded from an electrode on the scalp. Typically some 1000 to 2000 responses are averaged, resulting in a recording of a complex waveform (Fig. 11.17) known as a **brainstem auditory evoked response** (BAER).[10]

The BAER is a powerful test because it does not require the cooperation of the patient. For example, threshold audiograms can be recorded from infants who cannot cooperate but for whom early diagnosis of hearing impairment is essential. Within the first 10 msec of the presentation of the click, five negative peaks can be identified in the BAER recording. The electrical events that contribute to these peaks originate in the brainstem auditory structures. By noting the delay or absence of the peaks, one can accurately locate brainstem lesions.

---

[9] There are two exceptions to this generality: the EEG (electroencephalogram) and the ECG (electrocardiogram). Both can be recorded without averaging because the signals are unusually large.

[10] Also known as a brainstem auditory evoked potential (BAEP) or auditory brainstem response (ABR).

---

### Figure 11.16   Pure tone audiometry

**A.** ANSI 1969 standard curve used as an approximation of the normal sensitivity of human hearing (*heavy line*). Audiogram from a young adult with normal hearing superimposed on it (*thin line*). **B.** Hearing loss diagram from a person with normal hearing. A chart such as this represents the hearing threshold at various frequencies subtracted from the ANSI 1969 standard curve at the same frequency. The difference is represented as hearing loss in decibels. Persons with normal hearing have less than 20 dB of loss at all frequencies; 35 dB is added to the bone conduction thresholds to make them congruent with the air conduction thresholds on the chart. **C.** Hearing loss curve showing conductive hearing loss from a child with serous otitis media in both ears. The loss is about the same for all frequencies for air conduction, but bone conduction is within normal limits. **D.** Hearing loss curve showing presbyacusis. In addition to the expected high-frequency hearing loss, this patient demonstrates a sensorineural hearing loss of about 40 dB. Bone and air conduction are equally affected. **E.** Hearing loss curve showing noise-induced hearing loss characterized by a sharp loss at 4 kHz with some recovery noted at 8 kHz. (Audiograms courtesy of Mary Donigan.)

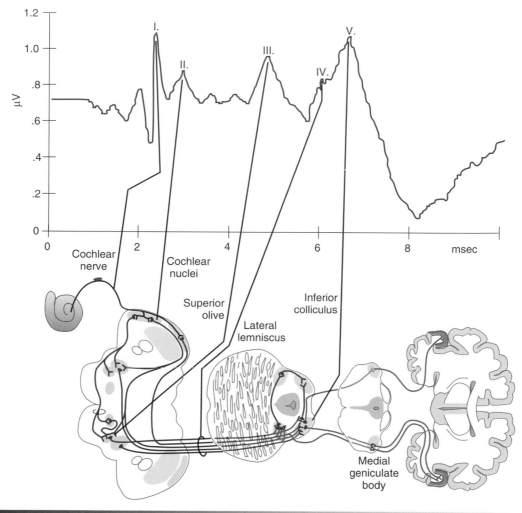

**Figure 11.17**    **Brainstem auditory evoked response**

The BAER illustrates only the first 10 msec, which corresponds to the responses obtained from the brainstem nuclei. Peaks I through V are indicated. Below the BAER the presumed origin of the various peaks is indicated. By convention, negativity is directed upward on extracellular recordings.

## COMMON HEARING DISORDERS

Hearing impairment is common. Approximately 22 million Americans have **hearing loss**, the most common form of hearing disorder. Of these, about 6 million are affected severely enough to hinder communication. Among school-aged children approximately 5% have hearing loss, and about 10% of affected children (0.57% of school-aged children) require some form of special education because of it. The United States Office of Edu-

cation estimates that only about 18% of children with hearing loss receive appropriate support.

Frequently associated with hearing loss is **tinnitus** [L. *tinnio*, ring, jingle], the objective perception of sounds that originate in the ear. Tinnitus is frequently reported as a ringing sound, but it may be a whistling, pure high-pitched tone, buzzing, roaring, or chirping. In fact, almost every type of noise has been reported. Tinnitus is very common, affecting about 37 million Americans. Its cause is unknown and there is no effective treatment. For most people it is a tolerable nuisance.

More serious than moderate hearing loss and tinnitus is **recruitment.** Normally the perception of loudness increases with intensity of sound. In certain types of hearing disorders, the perception of loudness rises faster than the actual increase in intensity. In effect the dynamic range of hearing, normally about 120 dB, is reduced to as little as 60 to 80 dB. Louder sounds, particularly speech, collapse into a cacophony of garbled noise. Thought to be caused by a loss of cochlear efferent fibers, recruitment seriously affects communication. It is treated by hearing aids with nonlinear amplifying characteristics. They amplify low-intensity but not high-intensity sounds. Some hearing aids deamplify high-intensity sound in an effort to collapse the dynamic range of the natural acoustic stimuli to fit the patient's narrow dynamic range of auditory perception.

The location of lesions affecting auditory perceptions has a significant effect on treatment; therefore, hearing disorders are frequently categorized according to the site of the lesion. The following is a brief discussion of the three principal classes of hearing impairment: **conductive, sensorineural,** and **central.**

## Conductive Hearing Loss

If the ossicles become restricted or disarticulated, acoustic energy is less efficiently passed through the middle ear. Consequently, any lesion of the middle ear produces a conductive hearing loss. Typically, all frequencies are affected, producing a relatively flat hearing loss curve at reduced sensitivity (Fig. 11.16C). Determining the presence of a conductive hearing loss is especially important, because most causes are treatable.

### MIDDLE EAR INFECTION

Middle ear infections are common in children. As the middle ear cavity fills with mucus and pus, the normal movements of the middle ear structures are impaired, resulting in a conduc-

tive hearing loss. These infections invariably cause significant pain that promptly brings the patient to medical attention. With modern antibiotic therapy, these infections are effectively treated and, as discussed on page 394, do not have the long-range implications on hearing that they once did.

### SEROUS OTITIS MEDIA

Children are also subject to **serous otitis media,** or fluid accumulation in the middle ear. This condition is *noninfectious and not painful.* Consequently, these children frequently escape medical attention. The accumulation of fluid, however, does cause hearing impairment with long-range consequences.

The cause of serous otitis media is not known. Most authorities believe that the drainage of the middle ear in children is less efficient than in the adult because the auditory tube is narrower and more horizontal than in the adult. Therefore, normal middle ear secretions may not properly drain. They become concentrated and mucoid, restricting ossicular movement and impairing hearing. Because the condition develops slowly, the loss of hearing is insidious and is rarely detected by the parents.[11] Since there is no inflammation or swelling, the condition is not painful and goes undetected by routine otological examinations. Asking parents about hearing loss may elicit a revealing comment such as, "She likes to have the TV really loud." The alert physician may detect delayed or impaired language acquisition, symptoms that suggest hearing difficulties. More frequently there are no clues. *The best routine examination is tympanometry, which immediately reveals the condition.*

Treatment is straightforward. After the middle ear is evacuated, silicone rubber tubes are placed through the tympanic membrane, a procedure that provides the middle ear with an alternative drainage path. The tubes are left in place for several years, until the head has grown sufficiently to allow proper drainage of the middle ear cavity through the auditory tube. Following middle ear evacuation, res-

---

[11] Young children do not complain of hearing loss because they are too young to appreciate normal hearing; their experience is normal to them. In addition, many children with hearing problems have yet to acquire spoken language.

toration of hearing is immediate and dramatic; children frequently awake from the anesthesia complaining of how loudly everyone is talking.

About 5% of school-aged children have impaired hearing. Such children may have retarded speech development, delayed acquisition of language, and impaired social development and academic achievement. Most do not receive any particular assistance in overcoming these difficulties, since only about 10% of them have hearing difficulties that are severe enough to qualify for special education. It seems probable that most of the less severely hearing-impaired children may have treatable disorders, such as serous otitis media. They can and should be relieved of their hearing loss by timely (preschool) diagnosis and treatment. Only the physician is in a position to provide this service.

## OTOSCLEROSIS

The most common cause of adult-onset hearing loss is **otosclerosis**. This disease is characterized by pathological growth of bone at the margin of the oval window. Initially the growth impedes only the movement of the stapes, but eventually it becomes fixed in place. Otosclerosis is an autosomal dominant genetic disorder with the defective gene on chromosome 15q and a penetrance of 25% to 40%. Surgical removal of the stapes followed by its replacement with a prosthesis restores hearing in most patients.

## Sensorineural Hearing Loss

Hearing loss associated with disease in the cochlea or the auditory nerve is **sensorineural hearing loss**. People with this type of hearing loss often benefit from the use of hearing aids.

## PRESBYACUSIS

The most common form of sensorineural hearing loss is **presbyacusis** (also spelled presbycusis) [G. *presby*, old, and *akouo*, hear], which simply means the loss of hearing with advancing age. The hearing loss primarily affects the high frequencies and correlates with loss of

hair cells in the first turn of the cochlea (Fig. 11.16D). The process is progressive and apparently begins early in life, for few persons over about age 20 have undiminished high-frequency hearing.

## OTOTOXICITY

**Aminoglycosides** are a class of antibiotic drugs that are well-known **ototoxic** agents. Aminoglycoside antibiotics are concentrated in the endolymph by the action of the stria vascularis. Therefore, over a long period (days), extremely high concentrations of the antibiotic build up in the endolymph. These high concentrations are toxic to all hair cells, both cochlear and vestibular, although some drugs affect one type of hair cell more than the other. The drugs also interfere with ATP production in the mitochondria (Fig. 11.18).

Like most antibiotics, aminoglycosides are cleared from the blood through the kidney. Therefore, any disease process that reduces renal clearance potentiates the ototoxic effect of these drugs. Some persons are genetically hypersensitive to the aminoglycosides. Ototoxic antibiotics can be used with relative safety if they are delivered as a bolus or by rapid infusion at high concentrations at long intervals (6 hours or more). Long-term infusion of these drugs at low concentrations can lead to high accumulations in the endolymph with subsequent hearing loss.

While the aminoglycoside antibiotics are among the most potent ototoxic agents, the physician must also be alert to *other iatrogenic causes of hearing impairment*. High on the list are diuretics. Quinine is moderately ototoxic. Its use as an illegal and fairly ineffective abortifacient was often the cause of "congenital" hearing loss. Aspirin is a very mild ototoxic agent. The elderly who use large quantities of aspirin to reduce the pain of arthritis may inadvertently take toxic doses.

## NOISE EXPOSURE

Intense sound kills hair cells. The more intense the sound and the longer the exposure, the greater the damage. Noise-induced cochlear damage is usually revealed by a character-

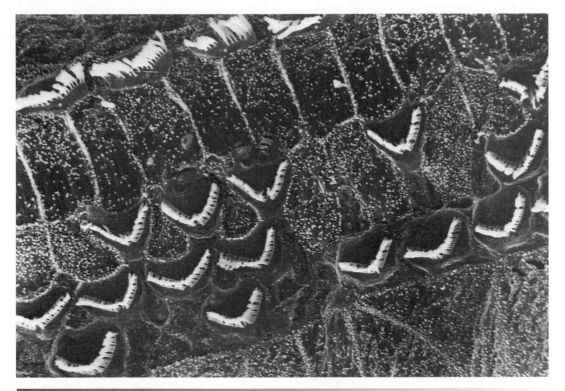

**Figure 11.18    Ototoxicity**

Ototoxic drugs kill hair cells, as in this example taken from a chinchilla treated with polymyxin. This scanning electron micrograph is taken from above the organ of Corti, looking down on the reticular lamina after the tectorial membrane is removed. The regular pattern of outer hair cells (Fig. 11.3) is clearly disrupted here. The reticular lamina remains intact, as the absent hair cells are replaced by phalangeal cells. (Reprinted with permission from Meyerhoff W, ed. Diagnosis and Management of Hearing Loss. Philadelphia: Saunders, 1984.)

istic 4-kHz notch in the pure tone audiogram (Fig. 11.16*E*) At the same time, the cochlea is remarkably resistant to damage by intense sound. Members of rock bands usually require several years of exposure during performances before they suffer the otological consequence of their art. Members of rock concert audiences usually return home with a feeling of fullness in their ears and a decrease in overall sensitivity. This phenomenon, the temporary threshold shift, resolves in about 24 hours. Enthusiastic concert goers who like to stand close to the loudspeakers usually develop a noise-induced hearing loss after only a few years. Occupational noise exposure is a well-recognized risk that can be eliminated by wearing ear protection devices (protection used by most rock stars today).

## ACOUSTIC NEUROMA

Schwannomas of the eighth nerve occur at the rate of about 1/100,000. They are called **acoustic neuromas** because their most common presenting symptom is unilateral hearing loss, although research has shown that the tumors almost always arise from the vestibular branch of the nerve. As the tumor grows, it envelops and presses on the contents of the internal auditory meatus. If left untreated, it expands into the posterior fossa and eventually involves the trigeminal nerve. In addition to unilateral hearing loss, patients frequently have vertigo, unsteady gait, facial pain, facial weakness, and tinnitus. Gadolinium-enhanced MRI can almost always confirm this diagnosis. Surgical removal is quite successful if the diagnosis is timely. Although hearing can seldom be preserved on the affected side, the facial nerve can be saved in most cases.

## Central Hearing Loss

Lesions to the auditory structures of the CNS, frequently called **retrocochlear lesions,** produce subtle hearing impairments. The subtlety is due to the number of midline crossings in the ascending auditory pathways. All auditory nuclei above the cochlear nuclei have prominent binaural representation. The clinical significance of this binaural representation is that the CNS portion of the auditory system is fairly resistant to injury. In particular, unilateral cortical lesions have very little effect on auditory thresholds; sound localization, pitch perception, and, as illustrated by the case described earlier in this chapter, even speech perception. Sophisticated audiometry may tease out the exact nature of a central auditory deficit, but such lesions usually resist treatment.

# C A S E     H I S T O R Y

## THE CASE OF THE ENTHUSIASTIC HUNTER

### HISTORY OF PRESENT ILLNESS

Mr. R. W. is a 45-year-old white man who went to see his family physician, Dr. J. P., for a life insurance examination. He had no specific complaints and said he felt in excellent health. During the course of the examination, Mr. R. W., who is an enthusiastic bird hunter, spoke of how good the hunting had been this season. He is planning a trip to Texas next year to hunt wild turkeys.

### PHYSICAL EXAMINATION

The physical examination produced unremarkable findings for a man of his age.

### NEUROLOGICAL EXAMINATION

#### Mental Status
Normal

#### Cranial Nerves

OLFACTORY: Patient identified methyl salicylate from both nostrils.

OPTIC: Visual fields full to confrontation. Fundi were normal.

NUCLEI OF OCULOMOTION: Eye movements were unrestricted in all directions. There was no nystagmus.

PUPILS: Pupils were equal and reactive to light, both direct and consensual.

TRIGEMINAL: Sensation was intact to cotton from all three divisions. Blink reflex was present bilaterally. Masseter strength was normal and symmetrical.

FACIAL: Grimace was symmetrical.

AUDITION: Rinne's test was normal for both ears, but Mr. R. W. lateralized Weber's test to the right ear. He had trouble hearing light finger rubbing with the left ear, but not with the right. Examination of the external auditory meatus revealed it to be clean and free of obstructions. The appearance of the tympanic membrane was normal.

VAGOGLOSSOPHARYNGEAL: Voice was normal. The gag reflex was present bilaterally and the pharyngeal arches were fully elevated and symmetrical.

ACCESSORY: The drape of the shoulders was symmetrical. Strength of shoulder shrug was 5/5 and symmetrical, as was head turning against resistance.

HYPOGLOSSAL: Tongue extended in the midline and was grossly normal in appearance.

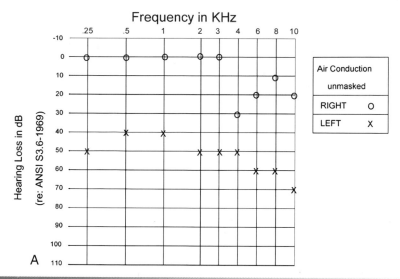

**Figure 11.19    Hearing loss data and BAER for Mr. R. W.**

**A.** Both ears demonstrate presbyacusis. There is also a 4-kHz notch in the right ear response and broadband loss in the left ear.

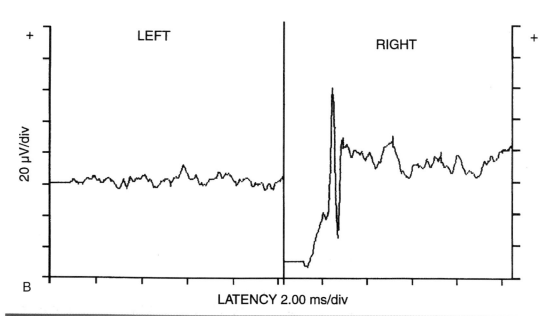

**Figure 11.19    Hearing loss data and BAER for Mr. R. W.—*continued***

**B.** This BAER was taken from a different person who has profound hearing loss in the left ear. It was elicited by a series of 1024 95-dB clicks presented to each ear separately. The right BAER is not normal, either (Fig. 11.17); peaks IV and V cannot be identified. This pattern is consistent with cochlear, auditory nerve, or auditory nuclear disease on the left and disruption of the ascending auditory pathways on the left side of the brainstem. (Courtesy of St. Joseph's Medical Center, South Bend, IN.)

## Station and Gait

Patient walked with erect posture, narrow base, and free arm swings.

## Motor Systems

STRENGTH: 5/5 and symmetrical from all extremities.

BULK: Normal and symmetrical.

TONE: Normal, with no spasticity or rigidity.

ABNORMAL MOVEMENTS: None noted.

## Sensory Systems

Sensorium was present from all extremities to cotton touch and pinprick. There was no Romberg sign.

## Reflexes

MSRs were normal. Toes were down going.

## Coordination and Control

Finger-to-nose, heel-to-shin, rapid alternating hand slapping, and thumb-to-finger tests were all performed normally.

## Parietal Functions

OKN test was present in both directions. No aphasia noted. Memory recall was intact for three items. Serial seven subtraction performed normally.

## ANCILLARY STUDIES

Mr. R. W. was referred to an ear, nose, and throat specialist, who ordered a pure-tone audiogram and speech discrimination tests (Fig. 11.19A). When these proved to be abnormal, a BAER was ordered (Fig. 11.19B). When the BAER proved to be abnormal, an MRI of the head was ordered (Fig. 11.20).

## SUBSEQUENT COURSE

MRI revealed a tumor in the posterior fossa. The tumor was removed, sparing the facial nerve, but hearing was lost on the left. Mr. R. W. continues to hunt birds but now wears a protective device in his right ear to avoid further noise-induced trauma.

## COMMENTARY

Mr. R. W. had no specific complaints about hearing difficulties. Nevertheless, Dr. J. P. was concerned that Mr. R. W. lateralized Weber's test to the right ear and that he had difficulty hearing very soft sounds from the left ear. There was no sign of external ear obstruction or damage to the tympanic membrane to explain these findings. Unexplained unilateral hearing loss in an adult suggests an acoustic neuroma, a treatable condition for which early diagnosis is essential. Therefore, Dr. J. P. referred her patient to an ear, nose, and throat specialist for a complete hearing evaluation. Since the audiogram revealed a marked hearing loss on the left and poor speech discrimination, a BAER was ordered.

The 4-kHz notch seen in the hearing loss curve from the right ear is characteristic of noise-induced hearing loss. In this case, Mr. R. W., an enthusiastic hunter, evidently hunted without hearing protection. Since he is left handed, his right ear is exposed to the report of the gun. The left ear is partially protected by the acoustic shadow provided by the head and so shows no 4-kHz notch. The left audiogram does show, however, a broadband decrease in auditory threshold both for bone and air conduction. The MRI revealed the suspected tumor, which was removed without incident.

## FURTHER APPLICATIONS

Dr. J. P. is a thorough and astute physician. This case emphasizes the need to perform a complete examination of the nervous system. It is tempting, during a routine insurance examination, to be perfunctory and to take shortcuts. Had the Rinne and Weber tests not been performed, it is quite likely that the tumor would not have been discovered until it produced symptoms associated with other cranial nerves.

11.1. What symptoms accompany well-developed acoustic neuromas?

11.2. Which cranial nerves are likely to become involved, and in what order?

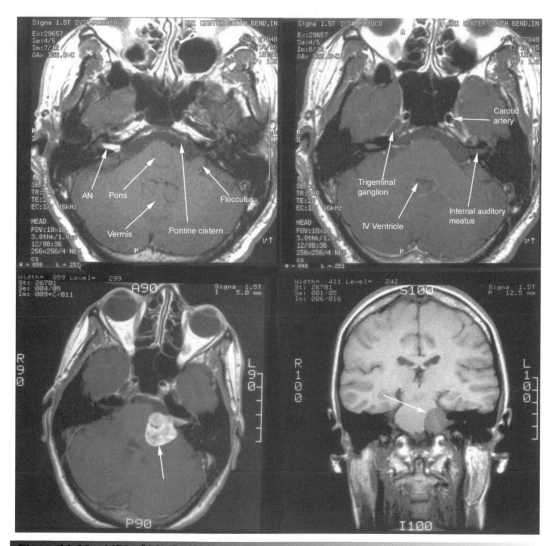

**Figure 11.20 MRI of Mr. R. W.**

**Upper left.** MRI of enhanced signal emanating from the right vestibuloacoustic nerve (*AN*), which is characteristic of an acoustic neuroma. **Upper right.** A normal external auditory meatus filled with CSF in a slightly different plane. If left untreated, acoustic neuromas (*arrows*) can grow to considerable size, as seen in the lower two MRIs from a different patient. Note the extreme compression of the pons. (Courtesy of the Magnetic Resonance Imaging Center, South Bend, IN.)

11.3. Had Mr. R. W. been right-handed, would you be justified in ordering an MRI after the hearing tests? (Assume that there was no evidence of noise-induced hearing loss in the right ear.) Defend your answer.

11.4. Look up the causes of unilateral hearing loss in a textbook of neurol-ogy. Are any of these differential diagnoses relevant in this case? If so, which?

11.5. Was Dr. J. P. justified in pursuing a tumor so quickly, or should she have performed other tests to rule out other possible causes? Defend your answer.

# S U M M A R Y

- **The auditory system consists of the external, middle, and inner ear as well as the central auditory pathways.**

The external ear consists of the pinna and the external auditory meatus. It is separated from the middle ear by the tympanic membrane. The middle ear consists of two major spaces, the tympanic cavity and the antrum, which are connected by the aditus. Three ossicles within the middle ear conduct sound from the tympanic membrane to the inner ear at the oval window. The middle ear is drained by the auditory tube.

- **The cochlea is divided into three compartments: the scala tympani, the scala media, and the scala vestibuli.**

The scala tympani and scala vestibuli, which communicate with the vestibule, are filled with perilymph. The scala media communicates with the saccule through the ductus reuniens and is filled with endolymph. Within the cochlea, Reissner's membrane separates the scala media from the scala vestibuli; the basilar membrane separates it from the scala tympani. The stria vascularis forms the lateral wall of the scala media.

- **Hair cells within the scala media are the principal transducers of the auditory system.**

The IHCs are innervated by approximately 10 type I afferent neurons that do not branch. The OHCs are innervated by approximately four type II afferent neurons that branch and innervate approximately 10 OHCs each. Efferent axons originating in the contralateral superior olivary complex form axoaxonic synapses on type I afferent axons near the base of the IHCs. They also make axosomatic synapses on the OHCs.

- **The central auditory pathways are more complex than the other sensory systems and involve multiple crossings of the midline.**

The central axons of the type I afferent neurons branch and synapse in the ipsilateral cochlear nuclear complex. From this complex three secondary pathways arise and cross the midline. Axons of the dorsal acoustic stria form the lateral lemniscus and ascend in the brainstem to synapse primarily in the inferior colliculus. Axons of the intermediate acoustic stria send collaterals to synapse in the ipsilateral superior olivary complex before joining the lateral lemniscus. Axons of the ventral acoustic stria, also known as the trapezoid body, synapse bilaterally in the superior olivary complex. From there tertiary axons join the lateral lemniscus to ascend to the IC. Neurons in the IC transmit auditory information to the MGN, from which information is transmitted to the primary auditory cortex (areas 41 and 42).

- **Sound is a pressure wave conducted in air that must be converted to a displacement wave.**

Sound pressure waves are transformed into displacements of fluid within the inner ear by the action of the middle ear. Within the inner ear, the translocation of fluids causes a displacement of the basilar membrane, which is expressed as a traveling wave. The traveling wave produces a maximal displacement of the basilar membrane at different locations depending on the frequency of the stimulus. The amplitude of the maximal displacement is amplified by the AC motor function of the IHCs.

- **Hair cells are stimulated by bending of the stereocilia.**

The differential movement between the basilar and tectorial membranes results in a shearing of the stereocilia at the apex of the cochlear hair cells. Shearing the hairs opens mechanically coupled ion gates at the tips of the stereocilia and allows potassium ions to enter the cell, depolarizing it. This depolarization opens voltage-sensitive calcium ionophores in the hair cell soma, allowing calcium ions to enter the cell. The entry of calcium ions initiates the release of a neurotransmitter at the IHC–afferent axon synapse and opens calcium-dependent potassium ionophores in the hair cell soma. The opening of these potassium ionophores repolarizes the hair cell. Depolarization causes the IHC to contract; hyperpolarization causes it to lengthen.

- **Sound is separately coded into frequency, intensity, and timing elements by the action of the cochlea.**

  Place coding is determined primarily by the cochlea, which performs a mechanical Fourier analysis that distributes acoustic information to different hair cells along the basilar membrane based on frequency. As a result of place coding, auditory neurons have a characteristic frequency at threshold. Volley coding is another method of frequency coding that is most effective for the lower frequencies. Envelope coding is apparently a function of the CNS.

- **Hearing disorders are usually classified as one of three types: conductive, sensorineural, and central.**

  Conductive hearing losses can usually be differentiated from sensorineural losses by simple tests such as Rinne's and Weber's tests. Conductive and sensorineural hearing losses can be quantified by pure-tone audiometry, speech discrimination tests, and BAER. Central hearing loss may be difficult to detect and quantify. Conductive hearing losses are due to mechanical disruption of middle ear function. Sensorineural hearing losses are caused by the loss of hair cells in the cochlea or primary afferent acoustic neurons. Central hearing losses involve the CNS auditory structures. Tinnitus and recruitment are hearing disorders of undetermined etiology. Recruitment can seriously disrupt communication and may be related to the loss of efferent innervation to the cochlea.

- **The primary care physician must be able to diagnose several common hearing disorders.**

  The most important causes of conductive hearing loss are serous otitis media, middle ear infections, and otosclerosis. The most common sensorineural disorders are presbyacusis, ototoxicity, acoustic neuromas, and noise exposure.

## SUGGESTED READINGS

Buser P, Imbert M. Audition. Cambridge: MIT, 1992.

Corey DP, Roper SD, eds. Sensory Transduction. New York: Rockefeller University, 1992.

Dallos P, Popper AN, Fay RR, eds. The Cochlea. New York: Springer Verlag, 1996.

Dallos P. The active cochlea. J Neurosci 1992; 12:4575–4585.

Edelman GM, Gall EW, Cowan WM, eds. Functions of the Auditory System. New York: Wiley, 1988.

Friedmann I, Ballantyne J. Ultrastructural Atlas of the Inner Ear. London: Butterworth, 1984.

Hallahan D, Kauffman J. Exceptional Children: Introduction to Special Education. 6th ed. Boston: Allyn & Bacon, 1994.

Hayes D, Northern JL. Infants and hearing. San Diego: Singular Pub. Group 1996. In: Northern JL, ed. Hearing Disorders, 3rd ed. Boston: Allyn and Bacon, 1996.

Northern JL, Downs MP. Hearing in Children. 4th ed. Baltimore: Williams & Wilkins, 1991.

Online Mendelian Inheritance in Man (OMIM). Baltimore: Johns Hopkins University. MIM 166800. Otosclerosis.

Online Mendelian Inheritance in Man (OMIM). Baltimore: Johns Hopkins University. MIM 124900. Sensorineural deafness.

Online Mendelian Inheritance in Man (OMIM). Baltimore: Johns Hopkins University. MIM 580000. Streptomycin ototoxicity.

Online Mendelian Inheritance in Man (OMIM). Baltimore: Johns Hopkins University. MIM 193500. Waardenburg syndrome.

*OMIM can be reached at http://www3.ncbi.nlm.nih.gov/omim/

Picton TW. Auditory evoked potentials. In: Daly DD, Pedley TA, eds. Current Practice of Clinical Electroencephalography. 2nd ed. New York: Raven, 1990.

Wilson JP, Kemp DT, eds. Mechanics of Hearing. New York: Plenum Press, 1989.

---

*Online Mendelian Inheritance in Man (OMIM). Baltimore: Johns Hopkins University. MIM 166800. Otosclerosis.

# The Visual System

The visual system consists of the eye and the central nervous system (CNS) structures associated with visual imaging. The eye is a complex sensory organ that forms an optical image on an array of sensors. The sensors transduce electromagnetic energy in the form of photons into neural signals. CNS structures interpret these signals to create our visual perceptions. The visual system has great neurological significance not only because vision plays such an important role in human behavior but also because disturbances in vision provide clues to many neurological disorders. Experimental investigations of the visual system have also provided fundamental insights into the nature of cortical information processing.

## ANATOMY OF THE EYE

The eye is a sphere approximately 24 mm in diameter. Its outer shell consists of three layers: the **corneoscleral layer**, the **uvea**, and the **retina**. Within the shell two interior spaces are separated by the **lens** [L. *lentil, bean*] (Fig. 12.1).

### The Uvea

The middle, or uveal, layer of the eye lies between the outer corneoscleral and the inner retinal layers.[1] The uvea is highly vascular and pigmented. It has three divisions: the most posterior is the **choroid** [G. *chorion,* membrane, and *oid,* like], followed by the **ciliary body** [L. *cilium,* eyelid] and finally, most anterior, the **iris** [G. *iris,* rainbow].

### THE CHOROID

The choroid lies between the sclera and the retina. It consists of a dense network of capillaries and veins derived from the ophthalmic artery. They nourish only the outermost portion of the retina.

### THE CILIARY BODY

The ciliary body (Fig. 12.2) lies near the junction of the cornea and the sclera on the inner surface of the eye. It is composed of two layers: the outer layer is an extension of the uvea, and the inner layer is an extension of the retina. The inner retinal layer is a bilaminar continuation of the embryonic optic cup (discussed later in the chapter).

In the adult the outer layer consists of connective tissue and the **ciliary muscle**. A series of 60 to 80 folds, the **ciliary process**, project into the eye from the ciliary body. The **suspensory ligaments** of the lens attach to the ciliary process and hold the lens in place under radial tension, which flattens the lens. Constriction of the ciliary muscles draws the ciliary process toward the corneoscleral junction, relieving tension on the lens. Because the lens is normally elastic, the release of radial tension allows the lens to thicken, increasing its refractive power (see Chapter 10).

### THE IRIS

The iris, like the ciliary body, is composed of two layers. The inner layer is a thin bilaminar terminal extension of the retina (discussed later in the chapter); the outer layer is

---

[1] In reference to the structures of the eye, the term *inner* refers to structures close to the center of the globe; *outer* refers to those close to the sclera.

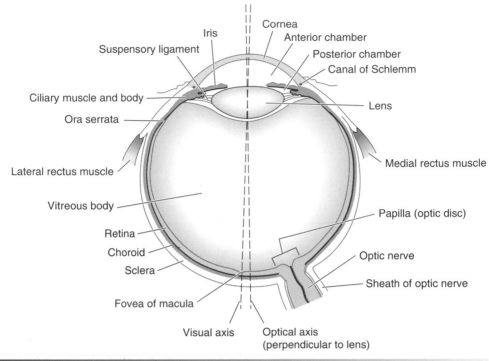

**Figure 12.1    Cross-section of the mammalian eye**

This cross-section of the human eye illustrates the major anatomical features.

the terminal extension of the uvea. The inner retinal layer is pigmented, which gives the iris a characteristic blue color. In many persons the outer layer is also pigmented, which darkens the iris, making it hazel, brown or black, depending on the amount of pigment. The pigments make the iris opaque to light.

The iris divides the space between the lens and the cornea into the **anterior chamber** and the **posterior chamber** (Figs. 12.1 and 12.2). The unattached medial edge outlines a hole, the **pupil** [l. *pupilla*, dim. of *pupa*, doll, from the doll-like image reflected from the dark, mirrorlike image of the eye]. Two muscles in the iris, the **pupillary constrictor** and the **dilator**, adjust the size of the pupil.[2] They shrink and enlarge the pupil, respectively (see Chapter 10).

The anterior and posterior chambers are filled with a clear fluid, the **aqueous humor** [L. *humor* or *umor*, moisture, a bodily fluid, fr. *umeo*,

to be moist or wet], which nourishes the avascular lens and helps hydrate both the lens and the cornea (Fig. 12.2). The aqueous humor is secreted from the ciliary process into the posterior chamber and then passes into the anterior chamber through the pupil. From there it enters a trabecular meshwork at the lateral margin of the anterior chamber, where the collagen fibers of the cornea and sclera separate. It collects in a particularly large cavity of this meshwork, the **canal of Schlemm**, before entering the venous drainage of the sclera. The aqueous humor is replaced approximately every 2 to 3 hours. Regulation of the production and reabsorption of aqueous humor determines the **intraocular pressure**, normally between 15 and 20 mmHg. This pressure maintains the shape and turgor of the eye. If the regulation becomes unbalanced and production exceeds reabsorption, intraocular pressure increases. If untreated, in-

---

[2] These smooth muscles actually migrate from the outer pigmented retinal layer and are not, as one would expect, derived from mesenchyme.

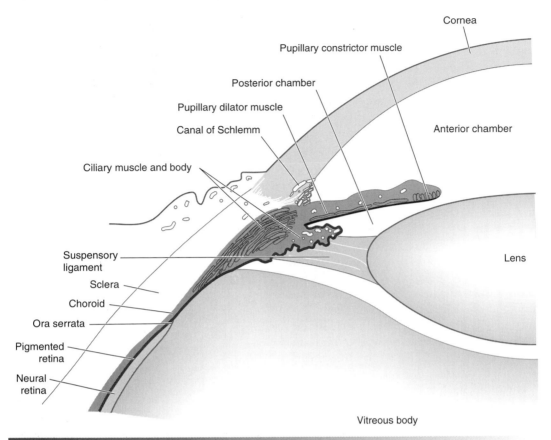

Cornea

Pupillary constrictor muscle

Posterior chamber

Pupillary dilator muscle

Canal of Schlemm

Anterior chamber

Ciliary muscle and body

Suspensory ligament

Sclera

Choroid

Ora serrata

Pigmented retina

Neural retina

Lens

Vitreous body

**Figure 12.2   The circulation of aqueous humor**

The aqueous humor is secreted continuously into the posterior chamber from the ciliary body and flows through the pupil into the anterior chamber. It is returned to the vascular space through the canal of Schlemm, which lies in the anterior chamber at the junction of the cornea and the sclera, adjacent to the ciliary muscle.

creased intraocular pressure can cause blindness by restricting blood flow to the retina, a condition known as **glaucoma** [G. *glaukos,* bluish-green].

## The Corneosclera

The corneoscleral outer layer of the eye, which consists mostly of collagen fibers, is derived from mesenchyme. The anterior sixth of the surface is the transparent, avascular cornea [L. *orneus,* horny]. The cornea consists of three layers: an outer epithelial layer, an inner endothelial layer, and a middle stroma composed almost exclusively of collagen.

The corneal endothelium is a highly active tissue that maintains a constant hydration of the corneal collagen by regulating the flow of

water into and out of the cornea. The transparency of the cornea depends on its state of hydration. Disease processes that affect the endothelium cloud the cornea. The epithelial layer of the cornea seals its anterior surface against water loss to the atmosphere.

The eye develops as an outgrowth from the prosencephalon. As it evaginates from the CNS, it carries the meninges with it. In the adult eye the meninges become the sclera [G. *skleros,* hard] and the choroid, which covers the posterior five-sixths of the eye. Therefore, the sclera of the adult eye is continuous with the dura mater and the choroid is continuous with the pia-arachnoid. Because of this continuity, the dura and pia-arachnoid form a sheath that surrounds the optic nerve and carries the subarachnoid space directly to the papilla at the posterior surface of the eye. The papilla is the internal termination of the optic nerve where it penetrates the sclera. Therefore, changes in intracranial pressure are transmitted to this weak point in the structure of the eye. Changes in intracranial pressure cause characteristic changes in the appearance of the papilla that can be seen on ophthalmoscopic examination (see page 444).

## The Retinal Layer

The innermost layer of the trilaminar shell of the eye is the **retina**. The retina is divided, anterior to posterior, into three regions. The most posterior region is the retina proper, which contains the photoreceptor cells. Anterior to it the retina loses the receptor cells and forms the inner layer of the ciliary body. The junction where the retina proper meets the ciliary retina is the **ora serrata**. The third and most anterior region of the retina forms the inner layer of the iris.

The retina itself is composed of two layers. This lamination is best understood by recalling that the retina develops from the embryonic optic vesicle. During development the outer wall of the vesicle invaginates to form a two-layered cup that protrudes from the prosencephalon. As the eye develops further, the optic cup becomes more hollow and the space that separates the two layers of the developing retina gradually disappears. However, the two retinal layers are maintained in adult life.

The outer layer of all three divisions of the retina is pigmented. That is particularly important because in the retina proper, nutrients from the vascular choroid must pass through it to reach the inner retinal layer. The pigmented layer also plays an important role in the recycling of the membrane of the outer segment of the sensory cells (see Cells of the Retina, later in the chapter).

The neural elements of the retina (photoreceptors and intrinsic neurons) develop only in the inner layer of the retina proper. However, the retinal layer continues anteriorly, without neural elements, into the ciliary and iridial parts.

Although the pigmented layer of the retina adheres firmly to the choroid, the two retinal layers are only loosely attached to each other and may separate in adult life, either spontaneously or as a result of blows to the eye. **Retinal detachment**, as it is known, causes blindness in the detached areas because the photosensitive cells degenerate when deprived of nourishment from the choroid.

## The Lens

The lens lies between the cornea and the retina (Fig. 12.1 and 12.2). Behind the lens is the **vitreous cavity** [L. *vitreus,* glassy], which is filled with a clear gelatinous material, the **vitreous body** and a serous **vitreous humor**. Like the cornea, the lens is transparent and composed of collagen fibers. Its transparency depends on its state of hydration. An opaque or partially opaque lens is said to have a **cataract**. Cataracts can be caused by prenatal rubella infection, metabolic disorders, trauma, or radiation. Most cataracts, however, develop as a natural consequence of aging. Good vision can usually be restored by surgically removing the cataract and replacing the lens with a plastic prosthesis.

## OPTICS OF THE EYE

The eye is an optical instrument. Light entering the eye through the cornea is focused by several refractive structures to form an inverted image on the surface of the retina (Fig. 12.3). The most important of these refractive surfaces is the cornea, which contributes about 42 of the 60 diopters of total refraction of the human eye.[3] The lens is also an important refractive element, providing about 18 diopters of refraction in the relaxed eye. The lens is held in place in the posterior chamber by the vitreous body that fills the main (posterior) cavity of the eye and radially by **zonal fibers** that attach it to the ciliary body. The lens is elastic, and its refraction can be in-

---

[3] The unit of refractory power is the diopter, the reciprocal of the focal length of the lens measured in meters.

creased about 12 diopters through the action of the ciliary muscles. The thickening of the lens is called **accomodation** because the eye is accommodating for near vision. The elasticity of the lens decreases with age, beginning slowly in childhood and progressing rapidly after about age 45, a condition known as **presbyopia** [G. *presbys,* old, and *ops,* eye]. By age 60 virtually no lens accommodation remains (Fig. 12.4).

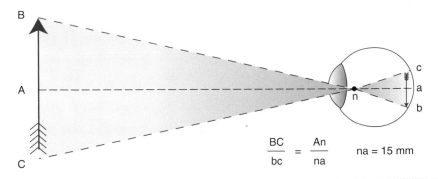

$$\frac{BC}{bc} = \frac{An}{na} \qquad na = 15 \text{ mm}$$

#### Figure 12.3  The eye as an optical instrument

There are four refractive surfaces in the eye: the two surfaces each of the cornea and the lens. This complex system can be simplified to the equivalent single-lens system, the idealized eye. A ray diagram for such an idealized eye is shown here to demonstrate the inversion and reduction of the image on the retina. The nodal point, *n*, represents the effective focal point of all refractive elements combined. The retinal image size can be computed by solving the formula shown.

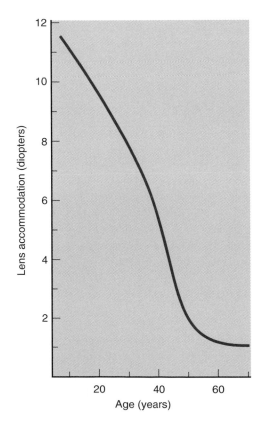

#### Figure 12.4  Presbyopia

Presbyopia, the loss of lens elasticity with age, occurs throughout life. The rate of change increases sharply at about age 40. By about age 60, the lens is essentially inelastic. The loss of elasticity is reflected in the amount of diopter change the lens can accommodate.

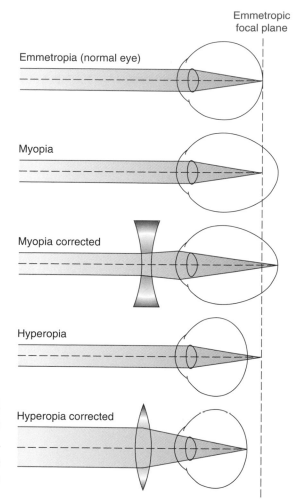

Emmetropic
focal plane

Emmetropia (normal eye)

Myopia

Myopia corrected

Hyperopia

Hyperopia corrected

**Figure 12.5   Correction of visual imper-
fections**

How abnormalities in the shape of the eye affect vision and how simple lenses, placed in front of the
cornea, bring the image to focus at the retina in the
myopic and hyperopic eye.

The normal eye is a sphere (Fig. 12.5). The term **emmetropia** [G. *emmetros,* according to measure] describes a normal, spherical eye in which distant objects are brought to focus on the retina when the ciliary muscles are relaxed. If the eyeball is elongated, the focal plane falls in front of the retina. As a result, the eye can focus only on objects close to it. This condition, **myopia** [G. *myo,* half-close] (near-sightedness), is caused by the nonuniform growth of the eye, and it usually becomes noticeable at puberty. **Hyperopia** [G. *hyper,* over, beyond] is the opposite condition (far-sightedness). The image falls behind the retina because the eyeball is flattened. Both conditions are easily corrected with appropriate lenses.

The transparent spherical cornea acts as a lens and is the most refractive element of the eye. Defects in its structure, especially its outer surface, impair visual acuity. If the curvature of the cornea is not perfect, aberrations [L. *ab,* away, and *errare,* to wander] are produced in the image. **Spherical aberrations** are produced when the surface is not perfectly spherical. In such cases light passing through different parts of the cornea is brought to focus at various distances. In the normal eye spherical aberrations of the cornea are not significant. However, in the condition known as **keratoconus** [G. *keras,* horn, and *konos,* cone] the cornea gradually thins at the center and protrudes. The spherical cornea eventually becomes cone-shaped, creating spherical aberrations that seriously impair vision. Keratoconus is probably caused by an autosomal dominant gene with variable penetrance. Although the condition is progressive, it can be treated successfully with corneal transplants.

Another aberration caused by corneal imperfections is **astigmatism** [G. *a-*, negating prefix, and *stigma*, point, mark, spot]. An astigmatic cornea has different radii of curvature at various meridians around its circumference (Fig. 12.6). As a result of this defect, a point is brought into focus over a distance between two different planes rather than on a single plane. Astigmatism can be demonstrated by viewing a Lancaster-Regan chart, which is a series of radial lines (Fig. 12.7). If the curvature of the cornea is uniform, all lines are in focus. If it is astigmatic, one line is darkest and in sharpest focus; the line perpendicular to it is lighter and out of focus.

## CELLS OF THE RETINA

Histologists identify 10 layers in the retina according to the distribution of cells and their processes (Fig. 12.8). In addition to supporting cells, there are five types of neurons: receptor, bipolar, ganglion, horizontal, and

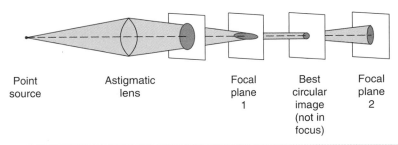

Point source · Astigmatic lens · Focal plane 1 · Best circular image (not in focus) · Focal plane 2

### Figure 12.6 Astigmatism

An astigmatic lens brings a point of light to focus not on a plane, but over a distance between two planes. At either of the two planes a distant point is focused as an ellipse. The ellipses at the two planes are perpendicular to each other. Between the planes, the distant point is focused as a large circle. Good focus cannot be achieved at any distance from the lens. The cornea is the most refractive element in the eye, and imperfections in its sphericity are the main source of astigmatism in the eye.

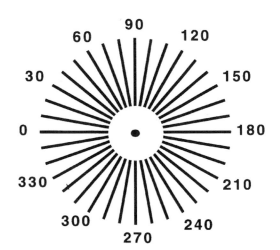

### Figure 12.7 The Lancaster-Regan chart

The set of radiating lines in this Lancaster-Regan chart appear to be evenly dense to an observer with normal vision. If astigmatism is present, some of the lines appear darker and focused; those perpendicular to them appear lighter and out of focus.

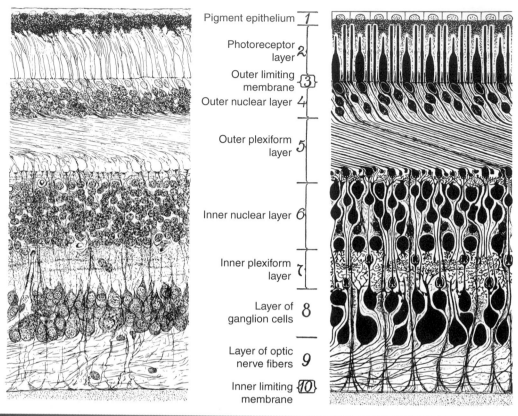

Pigment epithelium 1
Photoreceptor layer 2
Outer limiting membrane 3
Outer nuclear layer 4
Outer plexiform layer 5
Inner nuclear layer 6
Inner plexiform layer 7
Layer of ganglion cells 8
Layer of optic nerve fibers 9
Inner limiting membrane 10

**Figure 12.8    Histology of the retina**

*Left,* the 10 layers of the retina as defined by histology as they appear in routinely stained preparations. **Right.** A schematic representation of the cellular elements produced at the same magnification as the section on the **left.** In the outer plexiform layer the base of the receptor cells is greatly extended. The synapses between the bipolar cells and the receptor cells occur at the junction of the outer plexiform layer and the inner nuclear layer. The synapses between the bipolar cells and the ganglion cells occur in the inner plexiform layer. Here light reaches the retina from the bottom of the figure and must pass through 9 of the 10 layers to reach the outer segments of the receptor cells before it can be detected. (Reprinted with permission from Fawcett D, Raviola EA. A Textbook of Histology. 12th ed. New York: Chapman & Hall, 1994.)

amacrine cells (Fig. 12.9). The outermost layer of the retina, the pigment epithelium, is derived from the outer layer of the embryonic optic cup. The remaining 9 layers of the retina are derived from the inner layer of the embryonic cup. The light-sensitive **receptor cells** are closest to the pigment epithelium. All of the other neurons and the inner vascular layer lie juxtaposed between the light entering the eye and the receptor cells. This counterintuitive structure results from the development of the neural elements from the inner layer of the embryonic optic cup.

There are two types of receptors, **rods** and **cones,** named for the general shape of their outer segments (Fig. 12.9). The **outer segment** consists of a series of folded membranes. In rods these membranous folds separate to form independent disks; each disk is a closed, membrane-bound sack. In cones the membrane folding of the outer segment is considerably smaller than that of rods, and the elaborate assembly of independent disks is missing (Fig. 12.10). The photopigments necessary for phototransduction are on the interior surface of the outer segment membrane. The **inner**

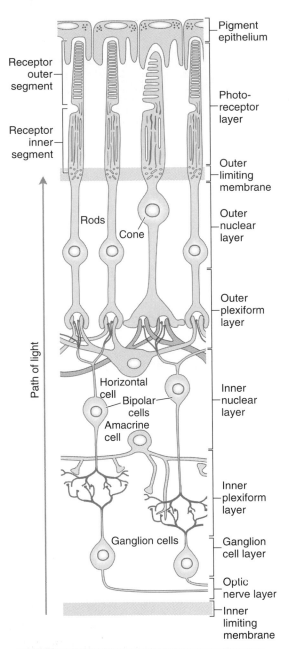

Receptor outer segment

Receptor inner segment

Path of light

Rods

Cone

Horizontal cell

Bipolar cells

Amacrine cell

Ganglion cells

Pigment epithelium

Photo-receptor layer

Outer limiting membrane

Outer nuclear layer

Outer plexiform layer

Inner nuclear layer

Inner plexiform layer

Ganglion cell layer

Optic nerve layer

Inner limiting membrane

**Figure 12.9   Synaptic connections in the retina**

The connections among the neural elements of the retina. The receptor cells synapse with bipolar and horizontal cells with chemical synapses. Some rods and cones form electrical synapses with each other.

segment of the receptors is separated from the outer segment by a narrow stalk that contains a short cilium. The outer segment membranes are continuously produced at the junction of the inner and outer segments. Membranes are sloughed from the apex of the outer segment (Fig. 12.10). Although rich in mitochondria, the inner segment does not contain the nucleus. That organelle resides in a separate bulbous segment.

The mammalian retina contains approximately $6 \times 10^6$ cones, which are concentrated in the **fovea** [L. *fovea*, pit] (Fig. 12.1). The fovea is a depression in the retina no more than 700 $\mu$m in diameter that occupies approximately the central 2° of the retina.[4] It lies at the center of the visual field on the **visual axis**, an imaginary line running from the center of the cornea to the center of the fovea. The visual axis is congruent with the straight-ahead line of sight. The fovea contains only cones, the smallest in diameter of those in the retina and the most densely packed. Cellular elements of the retina are also minimized at the fovea, which brings the cones closer to the inner retinal surface, where they can be more directly affected by light. These structural modifications greatly enhance visual acuity from the fovea. (Fig. 12.11).

Rods greatly outnumber cones; there are approximately $100 \times 10^6$ in each human eye. They are found in all parts of the retina except for the fovea and are most numerous about 3 mm from its edge, about 10 to 20° peripheral to the visual axis (Fig. 12.12).

As their name implies, **bipolar cells** have two processes. The outer process makes synaptic contact with numerous receptor cells in the outer plexiform layer. The inner process synapses with **ganglion cells** in the inner plexiform layer. The ganglion cells number about $10^6$ and are the cells of origin for all of the axons that leave the retina as the **optic nerve**.[5] There are two types of interneurons in the retina. **Horizontal cells** synapse with receptor and bipolar cells in the outer

---

[4] The retina is commonly mapped in polar coordinates with the visual axis of the eye as the center of the graph.

[5] The optic nerve is a CNS tract by virtue of its developmental history and because its axons are myelinated by oligodendrocytes. However, by convention the prechiasmatic portion of the tract is called the optic nerve and the postchiasmatic part, the optic tract.

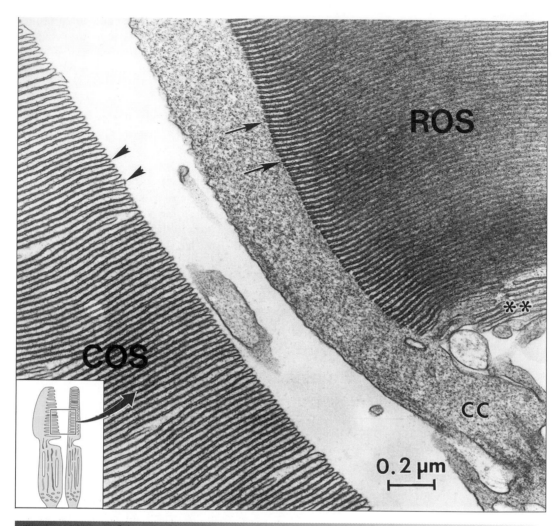

**Figure 12.10    Ultrastructure of rods and cones**

This transmission electron micrograph of a rod outer segment (*ROS*) and a cone outer segment (*COS*) from an amphibian retina shows the continuous lamellar organization and patency of the COS disk membranes (*arrowheads*) compared with the individual closely spaced membranes of the ROS (*arrows*). *Asterisks,* nascent disc membranes at the base of the ROS emanating from the connecting cilium (*cc*). Scale bar, 0.2 μm. (Courtesy of S. Fliesler, Dept. of Oph454thalmology, St. Louis University, St. Louis, MO., and J. Dant, Dept. of Molecular Microbiology, Washington University School of Medicine, St. Louis, MO.)

plexiform layer; **amacrine cells** [G. *a-; markos,* large, long; and *ismos,* fiber] synapse with the ganglion cells and the bipolar cells in the inner plexiform layer. Both types of interneurons distribute visual information laterally across the retinal surface.

The axons of ganglion cells traverse the inner surface of the retina and collect at one point, the **papilla** [L., *papilla,* nipple], or optic disk, where they penetrate the sclera to form the optic nerve. Because the papilla contains no receptor cells, no vision is possible from that portion of the visual field, the **blind spot.** Despite this name, blindness is not actually perceived because the blinded area is ignored by higher CNS structures and never brought

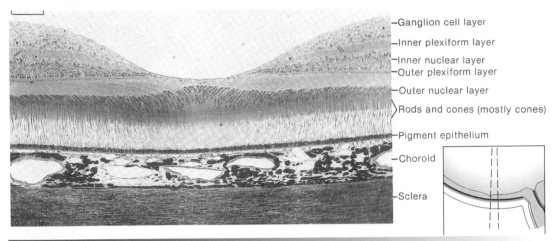

-Ganglion cell layer

-Inner plexiform layer

-Inner nuclear layer
-Outer plexiform layer

-Outer nuclear layer

Rods and cones (mostly cones)

-Pigment epithelium

-Choroid

-Sclera

### Figure 12.11   Histology of the fovea

The fovea is an area of the retina specialized for high-resolution vision. It contains only small-diameter cones. The inner layers of the retina are displaced laterally, as seen in this histological section of a monkey retina, so that light is presented to the outer segment of the receptors with as little obstruction as possible. (Reprinted with permission from Fine BS, Yanoff M. Ocular Histology. 2nd ed. New York: Harper and Row, 1979.)

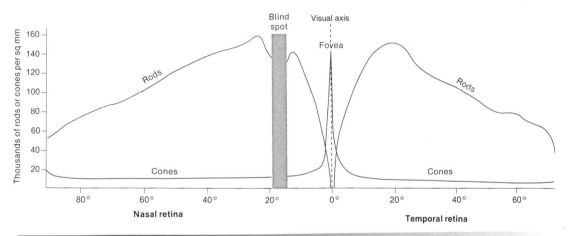

### Figure 12.12   Distribution of rods and cones in the retina

Rods and cones are not uniformly distributed across the retina. Only cones are found in the fovea. The area beyond about 10° from the visual axis contains almost no cones. The density of receptors declines rapidly beyond about 20°. (Modified from data in Østerberg GA. Acta Ophthalmol 1935; suppl 6.)

to perception. The blind spot can be demonstrated by observing an appropriately designed test figure with one eye (Fig. 12.13). Blind areas of the visual fields, known as **scotomas** [G. *skotos,* darkness], may be natural, such as the blind spot, or caused by disease. The ability of the brain to ignore and perceptually fill in blind areas in the peripheral retina is truly remarkable. Persons with very large scotomas may be totally unaware of their peripheral blindness until it is discovered during an examination of the visual fields. Scotomas in the

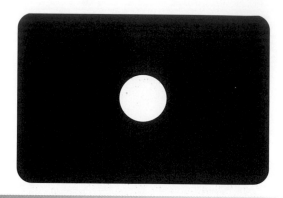

## Figure 12.13 Blind spot chart

To demonstrate the presence of the blind spot, hold this figure at arm's length and close your right eye. Focus on the white circle and slowly bring the page toward you. The crossed circle on the left disappears at about 10 inches. To find out how the brain fills in scotomas, making them imperceptible, repeat the experiment, but this time close your left eye and focus on the crossed circle. At about 10 inches the white hole in the figure will disappear.

foveal area cannot be ignored and severely interfere with vision.

The papilla is the terminus of the subarachnoid space that surrounds the optic nerve and can therefore be affected by increased intracranial pressure (see page 435). The change in the appearance of the papilla when intracranial pressure is increased is called **papilledema**. When intracranial pressure is moderately elevated, the pressure constricts the axons of the optic nerve axons like a tourniquet, restricting axoplasmic flow from the ganglion cells in the retina. A swelling is produced at the point of constriction, blurring the margin of the papilla. The increased intracranial pressure also constricts the retinal veins, producing papillary venous congestion. As the intracranial pressure increases further, the papillary congestion is exacerbated and the papilla starts to protrude

into the eye. Papilledema can be observed during examination of the eye with an ophthalmoscope (see photographs in the frontispiece). It is the most important sign of increased intracranial pressure that can be seen during a routine neurological examination.

## CENTRAL VISUAL PATHWAYS

Axons leaving the *temporal half* of the retina traverse the optic nerve to the **optic chiasm** [G. *chiasmos,* two crossed lines, fr. the letter χ(chi)], where they join the **optic tract** and project to ipsilateral structures. Axons leaving the *nasal half* of the retina cross the midline at the chiasm and terminate in contralateral structures (Fig. 12.14). This arrangement means that all the axons in one optic tract carry information about the contralateral visual field, a pattern of

## Figure 12.14 Central visual pathways

The axons of the neurons that constitute the visual pathways remain highly organized throughout their course. The projected image on the retina of the visual field is reversed by the action of the lens: the left visual fields from the eyes are both transmitted to the right LGN and visual cortex and vice versa. Also, the foveal projections are expanded in the LGN and cerebral cortex out of proportion to the amount of visual field they represent but in proportion to the number of receptor cells there. *Pink,* left visual fields; *gray,* right visual fields; the superior quadrants (*S*) are shown in lighter colors, the inferior (*I*), in darker colors. The foveal fields are shown in the darkest colors. The extreme lateral portion of temporal fields for which there is no binocular representation are shown with *stripes* or *dots.*

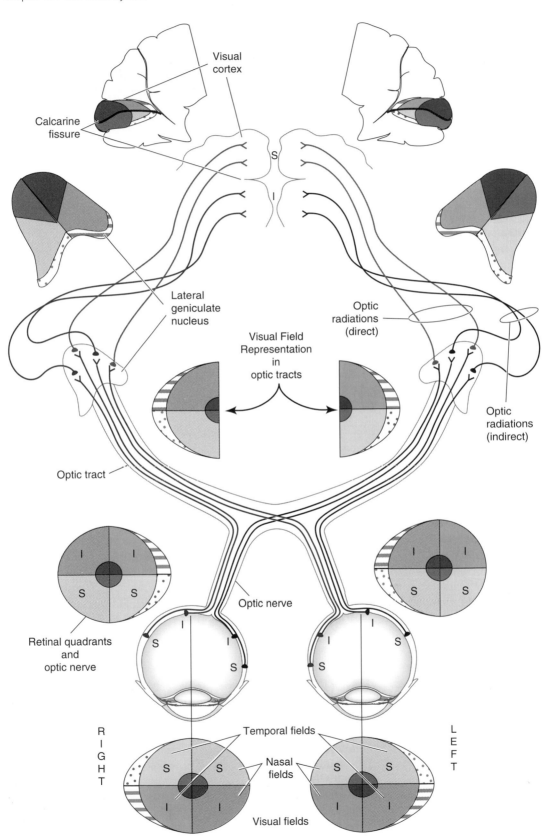

Visual cortex

Calcarine fissure

Lateral geniculate nucleus

Optic radiations (direct)

Visual Field Representation in optic tracts

Optic radiations (indirect)

Optic tract

S

I

Optic nerve

Retinal quadrants and optic nerve

S

S

I

I

R I G H T

L E F T

Temporal fields

Nasal fields

Visual fields

hemispheric reversal with respect to the external world that is consistent with the motor and somatosensory systems. Axons of the optic tract terminate in three areas of the CNS, the **lateral geniculate nucleus** (LGN), the **superior colliculus**, and the **pretectal area** (Fig. 12.15). The route through the lateral geniculate is the largest, most direct, and clinically most important pathway by which visual information reaches the cerebral cortex. A second pathway passes through the superior colliculus and the pulvinar before reaching the

cortex. The third pathway from the retina does not reach the cerebral cortex. It terminates in the brainstem pretectal nuclei that regulate eye movements, lens accommodation, and pupillary size (see Chapter 10).

About 80% of the optic tract axons synapse in the LGN (Fig. 12.16), which has six layers. The ipsilateral fibers of the optic nerve terminate in laminae 2, 3, and 5; the contralateral fibers terminate in 1, 4, and, 6. The ventral medial laminae (1 and 2) contain large cells and are therefore called the **magnocellular** [L.

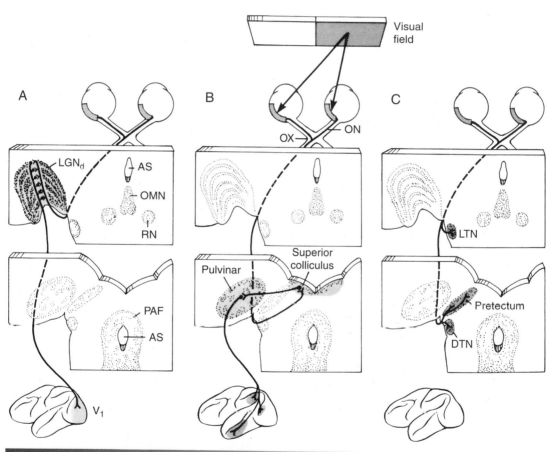

**Figure 12.15  Comparison of the three major central visual pathways**

**A.** The principal pathway, constituting approximately 80% of the optic tract axons, terminates in the LGN. LGN axons project to the primary visual cortex,V₁. **B.** Most of the remaining axons of the optic tract terminate in the superior colliculus. One efferent path from the superior colliculus projects to the pulvinar. Pulvinar efferents terminate in visual centers of the cerebral cortex other than V₁. **C.** A few optic tract axons terminate directly in brainstem nuclei, primarily in the pretectal area. *AS,* sylvian aqueduct; *DTN,* dorsal terminal nucleus; *LGN,* lateral geniculate nucleus; *LTN,* lateral terminal nucleus; *OMN* oculomotor nuclei; *ON,* optic nerve; *OT,* optic tract; *OX,* optic chiasm; *PAG,* periaqueductal gray; *RN,* red nucleus. (Reprinted with permission from Patton HD, Fuchs AF, Hille B, et al. Textbook of Physiology, 21st ed. Philadelphia: Saunders, 1989.)

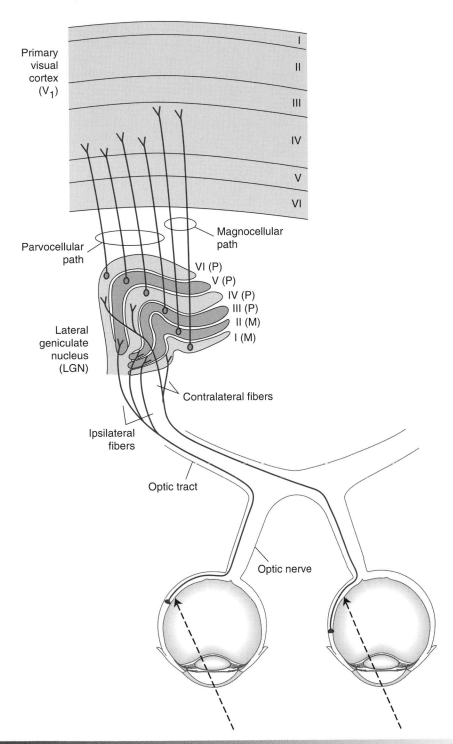

## Figure 12.16  Connections of the lateral geniculate nucleus

Ganglion cell axons from each hemiretina project to different layers of the LGN. Layers I and II of the LGN receive magnocellular retinal projections; the remaining layers receive parvocellular connections. Axons leaving the LGN remain segregated according to their magnocellular and parvocellular origins and synapse in different layers of the cortex. The left and right projections are also segregated into ocular dominance columns.

*magnus,* large] division; layers 3 to 6 are known as the **parvocellular** [L. *parvus,* small] region. Ganglion cell axons are distributed in the LGN according to their origin in the retina and in proportion to the receptor density, establishing a retinotopic organization in this structure. Because the receptors are not equally distributed within the retina, the retinotopic map on the LGN does not correlate directly with the visual space. For example, the central 20° of the visual space is optically projected to the central 20° of the retina. Although corresponding to about 10% of the total retinal area, this region contains about half of the total number of photoreceptors. The ganglion cells that receive receptor input from the central 20° of the retina send axons that synapse in about 65% of the LGN (Fig. 12.14).

Each LGN contains about 1 million neurons, all of which project to the ipsilateral occipital cortex (area 17) as the **optic radiations**. These axons fan out as they leave the LGN (Fig. 12.14). Some axons take a direct route to the occipital pole before reaching the **calcarine sulcus** and terminating in the superior gyri. Others take an indirect route through the temporal lobe, terminating in the inferior gyri. The portion of the cerebral cortex that receives LGN axons is the **striate cortex** (Brodmann area 17) or $V_1$, to designate it as the primary visual cortical area. The expanded neural representation of the fovea found in the retina and LGN is maintained in the visual cortex (Fig. 12.14). In the cerebral cortex the macula is represented at the most posterior portion of $V_1$; superior visual hemifield is projected to the inferior lip of the calcarine gyrus and the inferior visual hemifield, to the superior lip. This has some significance, since the macular area is perfused separately from the remainder of $V_1$ and is often spared by strokes that involve $V_1$.

Most of the remaining axons of the optic tract terminate in the superior colliculus. The organization of the superior colliculus is discussed in Chapter 10. To reiterate, the superficial layers of the superior colliculus receive both retinal and cortical visual information, the latter descending primarily from $V_1$. Neurons in the superficial superior colliculus project to both the pretectal area and the **pulvinar** [L. *pulvinus,* cushion], a large nucleus of the thalamus. Neurons in the pulvinar project back to the cerebral cortex. Unlike those from the LGN, thalamocortical connections from the pulvinar do not synapse in $V_1$.[6] Instead, the pulvinar innervates a number of extrastriate cortical areas, including areas 18 and 19 and the temporal lobe, particularly the superior temporal gyrus. These regions are important for processing highly abstracted visual perceptions (discussed later in the chapter).

## PHOTOTRANSDUCTION

The conversion of photon signals into neural signals, called phototransduction, takes place in the receptor cells. Phototransduction is a three-stage process. First, a pigment absorbs a photon and is isomerized; second, the isomerization triggers a biochemical cascade; and finally, sodium ionophores are altered, modulating ionic current within the receptor. As in other neurons, alteration in ion current flow leads to neurotransmitter release and information transfer to other neurons.

### Stage 1: Photochemical Events

The stacked disks in the outer segment of rods contain a membrane protein, **rhodopsin** [G. *rhodon,* rose, rose-colored, and *opsis,* vision]. Rhodopsin is composed of two subunits. The larger subunit (384 amino acid residues) is a membrane-spanning protein, **opsin** (Fig. 12.17A). Attached to residue 296 is a smaller molecule, **retinal**, a 6-carbon ring with a side chain (Fig. 12.17B). In the absence of light the side chain is bent at the $11^{th}$ carbon atom. In this form it is called **11-*cis* retinal**. When retinal absorbs a photon, it undergoes photoisomerization, forming the straight chain version called **all-*trans* retinal**.

This subtle alteration in the retinal fragment triggers a cycle of changes in the opsin fragment that ultimately recreates the unactivated rhodopsin (Fig. 12.18). The initial iso-

---

[6] Area 17 ($V_1$) is innervated by the pulvinar in the cat and probably other carnivora. Most authorities do not report connections from the pulvinar to $V_1$ in primates.

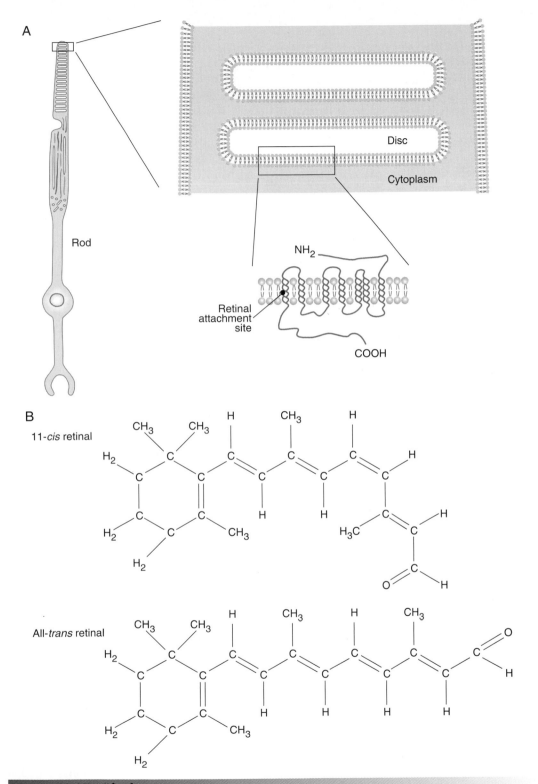

## Figure 12.17  Rhodopsin

**A.** Rhodopsin is a protein in the membrane of the rod outer segment disks. **B.** Retinal consists of a six-member ring with a nine-carbon side chain. In the dark the side chain is bent (11-*cis* retinal). After absorbing a photon, 11-*cis* retinal undergoes isomerization that straightens the side chain, forming all-*trans* retinal.

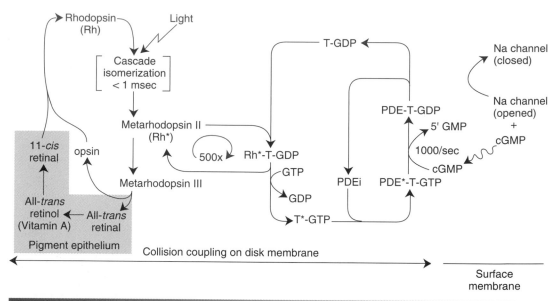

## Figure 12.18   The photochemical cascade

The biochemical events in the membranes of the outer segment of the photoreceptors. The absorption of a photon activates rhodopsin, allowing it to couple with the G-protein transducin (*T*). Transducin is activated by the replacement of GDP with GTP, allowing its α-subunit (*T\*-GTP*) to activate a phosphodiesterase. The activated phosphodiesterase (*PDE\*-T-GTP*) catalyzes the conversion of cGMP to 5' GMP. The loss of cGMP from the sodium ionophore closes it, reducing the inward flux of sodium. PDEi, inactive phosphodiesterase.

merization steps occur in less than a millisecond and produce metarhodopsin II, the activated form of rhodopsin. The half-life of metarhodopsin II is several minutes, allowing it to interact repeatedly with a G-protein, transducin. The next stage in the cycle is the transformation of metarhodopsin II into metarhodopsin III, which rapidly dissociates into opsin and all-*trans* retinal.

All-*trans* retinal diffuses out of the outer segment of the receptor into the pigmented layer of the retina, where it is reduced to all-*trans* retinol, or **vitamin A**. Finally, all-*trans* retinol is synthesized into 11-*cis* retinal, which reassociates with opsin in the outer segment, completing the cycle. The metabolic substrate for this cycle, vitamin A, cannot be synthesized by humans; it must be supplied in the diet. Consequently, dietary vitamin A deficiency causes visual impairment because the rhodopsin cycle cannot be completed. Chronic retinol deficiency leads to degeneration of the receptor outer segments and permanent blindness.

### Stage 2: Biochemical Cascade

Metarhodopsin II, the active form of rhodopsin, initiates an elaborate biochemical cascade, the second stage of the phototransduction process (Fig. 12.18). The activated rhodopsin (metarhodopsin II) collides with and activates the G-protein **transducin**, inducing the exchange of guanosine diphosphate (GDP) for guanosine triphosphate (GTP) within the transducin α-subunit. The α-subunit is immediately transferred to a **phosphodiesterase**, which hydrolyzes cytoplasmic cyclic guanosine monophosphate (cGMP) to 5′-GMP. The decrease in the concentration of cytoplasmic cGMP in the rod's outer segment releases bound cGMP from cGMP-gated sodium ion channels in the outer segment membranes. Dissociation of cGMP from the channels prompts the final stage in the phototransduction process, the closing of the sodium ion channel in the outer segment.

This complex, multistage process seems cumbersome. How much simpler it would be if the photon directly affected the sodium channel. The principal advantage of this indirect photochemical process is the degree of amplification it affords. One molecule of rhodopsin can absorb only a single photon. However, activated rhodopsin activates approximately 500 transducin molecules before it is inactivated. Each resulting phosphodiesterase-transducin-GDP molecule produces approximately 1000 cGMP molecules every second. Therefore, *a single photon can hydrolyze some 500,000 cGMP molecules per second* (Fig. 12.18). This biochemical amplification is directly responsible for the remarkable sensitivity of the retina to

light. Research has shown that humans can consciously detect the absorption of a single photon of light by a rod.

### Stage 3: Ionic Currents

In the dark, receptor cells have a resting potential of about −40 mV. This relatively small potential is due to a steady current flow through the cell, the **dark current**, that is carried by sodium and potassium ions (Fig. 12.19). First, sodium ions enter the outer segment through **cGMP-gated ionophores** that remain open as long as they bind cGMP. In the dark the continuous inward flow of sodium partially depolar-

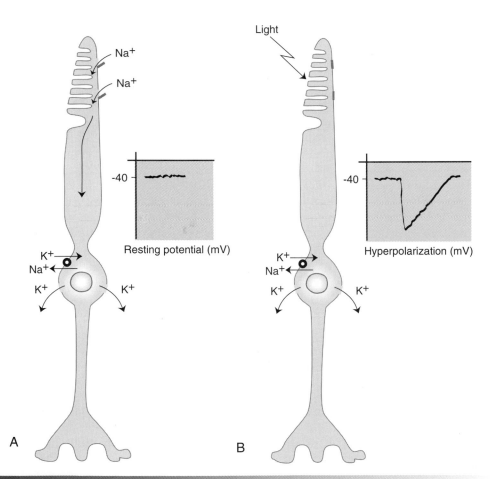

**Figure 12.19   Ionic currents in photoreceptors**

**A.** In the dark, ionic currents continuously flow through the receptors. Sodium ions enter the outer segment through cGMP-gated ionophores. The current leaves the body of the cell as a potassium ion current. A sodium ion–potassium ion exchange pump maintains the ionic balance within the cell. **B.** Light striking the receptor closes the cGMP-gated sodium ionophore, reducing the sodium current. Because of the equilibrium potential, potassium ions continue to leave the cell, hyperpolarizing it.

izes the receptor cell, producing the resting potential of about −40 mV. This steady depolarization continuously drives potassium ions out of the cell at the inner segment. To maintain homeostasis between sodium and potassium ions, an adenosine triphosphate (ATP) dependent exchange pump restores the ionic milieu.

As we have seen, when light strikes the receptor cell, the cytoplasmic concentration of cGMP is decreased in the outer segment of the receptor. The decrease in cytoplasmic cGMP concentration favors the diffusion of cGMP from the sodium ion channel into the cytoplasm. Without the bound cGMP, the sodium channel closes, reducing the inward flow of sodium ions.

Thus, when light strikes the receptor, the sodium gates in the outer segment close, reducing the dark current and allowing the cell to become hyperpolarized by the unopposed potassium efflux. Therefore, the dark current is modulated in proportion to the number of photons, hence the intensity of light, absorbed by the outer segment. The ionic current flowing through the receptor is an analogue of the photic signal. *The modulated dark current is the receptor potential in the photoreceptor cells.* As we have seen in other neurons, the flow of current through the cell affects the membrane potential, which in turn determines the degree of binding of vesicles at the presynaptic membrane (see Chapter 3). In photoreceptors modulation of the dark current regulates the release of neurotransmitter (probably glutamate) at the base of the rods and cones.

Because the dark current flows continuously in rods and cones, these cells remain in a continuous state of partial depolarization. In contrast to "ordinary" neurons, in which a neurotransmitter is released from the bouton as a discrete event in response to an action potential, *in photoreceptor cells neurotransmitter is continuously released from the synapses,* even in the dark. Therefore, modulation of the dark current *modulates the release of neurotransmitter* from the receptor cells. The modulation of neurotransmitter release would offer no benefit if the bipolar cells responded to the neurotransmitter with action potentials. All of the subtle changes in neurotransmitter concentra-

tion above and below threshold would be lost in the all-or-nothing response. Therefore, except for the ganglion cell, none of the retinal cells display action potentials. Instead, *all of the signaling within the retina is performed by graded potentials.* Visual information is converted to a digital form (action potentials) only when the information must be conveyed a considerable distance from the retina.

## Differences Between Rods and Cones

The photochemical and biochemical events in rods and cones are believed to be essentially the same. Nevertheless, there are important physiological differences between the two receptors. Perhaps the most conspicuous difference is that rods are about 30 times as sensitive to light as cones. At low ambient light levels the cones are too insensitive to be stimulated and vision is entirely dependent on the rods. Vision mediated by rods in low light is called **scotopic vision.** At high levels of ambient light the rhodopsin in the rods is completely converted to the all-*trans* state. Therefore, the rods cannot contribute to visual perception and vision depends entirely on the cones. Vision mediated by cones under high ambient levels of light is called **photopic vision.** Together, rods and cones can detect light over approximately five orders of magnitude of light intensity. The iris can affect the light intensity falling on the retina by approximately one order of magnitude. Combined, the rods, cones, and iris provide for a total range of sensitivity of approximately six orders of magnitude.

As discussed earlier, acute vision is possible only if the image falls on the fovea. Because the fovea contains only cones, high-resolution imaging can take place only in photopic conditions. In contrast, highly sensitive vision can occur only in the extrafoveal retina. Lateral to the fovea the density of cones diminishes rapidly until at the periphery of the retina, only rods are found. Rods are not only more sensitive to light than cones; they are larger and less densely packed. Consequently, rod-mediated vision, although highly sensitive, has poor resolution. The sensitivity of rod vision can be demonstrated on a dark night by viewing the Pleiades, a cluster of stars in the northern winter sky. It is difficult to see all of the "seven sisters" within the cluster when looking directly at it because the fovea has no rods and the cones are not sensitive enough to detect the light from dim stars. Looking a few degrees away directs starlight onto the rod-rich perifoveal retina, and all seven daughters of Atlas come into view.

Rods and cones also differ from each other in their spectral sensitivity. The differences arise from the incorporation of different opsin proteins with 11-*cis*-retinal, which alters the absorption characteristics of the molecule. In humans there are four types of opsin molecules. One type is found only in rods, and the other three are found only in cones. The cone opsins have absorption characteristics that respond maximally to the wavelengths that are perceived as blue, green, and red light. Each cone produces only one type of opsin, so the signals transmitted to higher centers by the cones carry spectral as well as intensity and spatial information (Fig. 12.20). Although there is considerable overlap in their spectral sensitivity, particularly between the green and red cones, the combination of signals from these three types of cones is sufficient to account for our perception of colors.

## NEURAL CODING IN THE RETINA

One way to conceptualize visual information is as a collection of points or pixels of light, each pixel derived from an individual receptor cell. In this scheme each pixel contains spatial, spectral, and luminance information about one spot of the visual image. Attractive as this

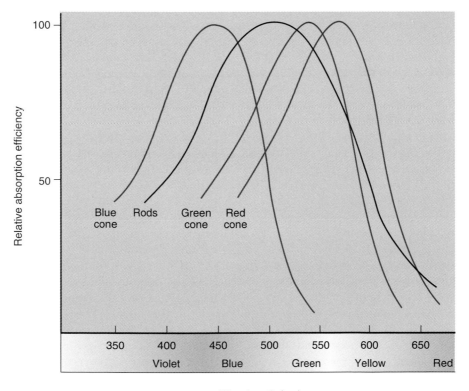

### Figure 12.20 Spectra of photopigments

The spectral absorption curves of the four photopigments. The ordinate is a normalized relative scale; the four pigments do not all have the same absorption efficiency.

model is, it is too simple. The retina transforms the 100 million or so pixels of light into about 1 million packets that convey more than spatial, spectral, and luminance data. The following paragraphs briefly discuss some aspects of retinal function.

Information from receptors is transferred both across (radial pathway) and through (transretinal pathway) the retina (Fig. 12.9). The transretinal pathway passes from the receptors through the bipolar cells to the ganglion cells. Because the retina contains well over 100 million receptor cells but only about 1 million ganglion cells, considerable convergence takes place along the transretinal pathway. For example, in the cat fovea, approximately 200 receptor cells affect a single ganglion cell. In addition to convergence along the transretinal pathway, horizontal and amacrine cells provide the mechanism for radial spread of information across the retina. The radial pathway ensures that a single receptor cell can affect several adjacent ganglion cells.

Action potentials can be recorded from a single ganglion cell in response to light stimuli applied to the retina. Ganglion cells respond to light that strikes a restricted locus in the retina, the **receptive field** of the ganglion cell. One type of ganglion cell responds by increasing its firing rate when a small spot of light shines on the retina within its receptive field. If the spot enlarges, the ganglion cell's response also increases (Fig. 12.21). If the size of the illuminated spot enlarges beyond a certain point, the ganglion cell's response decreases. Past a certain size further increases in the size of the spot have no more effect on ganglion cell output. These observations lead to the conclusion that the ganglion cell's responses reflect the influence of a large number of adjacent receptors. Receptors in the center of the illuminated field converge on and excite the single ganglion cell. Receptors outside this central core of synergistic receptors (the surround) inhibit the ganglion cell. Another type of ganglion cell has inverse receptive properties; the center must be dark and the surround, illuminated.

Thus the *pattern* of illumination that maximally excites this ganglion cell looks like a doughnut. The doughnut hole is the center; the doughnut itself is the surround. This **center-surround receptive field**, or **anulus**, is typical of almost all of the ganglion cells in the retina. The two types, on-center and off-center ganglion cells, are represented in almost equal numbers in the mammalian retina. The most effective size of the center varies with its location on the retina. In the cat fovea the center is about 30+ of a degree; at the periphery it may be as large as 8°. By comparison, the size of an individual cone in the fovea is about 4+ of a degree.

What are the advantages of representing an image as a field of anuli as opposed to a field of simple pixels? Chapter 4 discusses the principle of **lateral inhibition** as a computational mechanism to enhance the detection of boundary conditions (see Fig. 4.12). The center-surround response characteristics of retinal ganglion cells are simply the visual manifestation of that same principle. The lateral inhibition of retinal center-surround receptive fields enhances the boundary between the light and dark areas of the image; these areas are emphasized in the neural signaling of the ganglion cells. Therefore, *receptive field representation of an image carries information to central visual structures not inherent in a simple pixel representation of an image.*

Although virtually all ganglion cells respond to the center-surround pattern, they can be subdivided into three classes based on their temporal responses to stimuli. Classified in this way, they are named **X**, **Y**, and **W** cells. In the most general terms X cells synapse on the parvocellular cells in the LGN. They have small receptive fields (about 1°) and for the most part carry information from the central area of the retina. They respond to light roughly in proportion to its intensity. Y cells synapse in the magnocellular laminae of the LGN. They have larger receptive fields (about 3°), and most originate in the peripheral portions of the retina. Y cells generally respond at the onset and termination of the stimulus and prefer stimuli moving quickly across the visual field. W cells are not as well characterized as X

A

Light stimulus

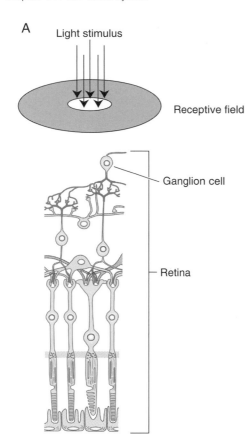

Receptive field

Ganglion cell

Retina

### Figure 12.21    Response properties of ganglion cells

**A.** Light is presented to the retina in the form of an anulus with a bright center and a dark surround. This pattern stimulates numerous rods and cones in the retina (*below*). **B.** As the radius of the light spot increases (light color in the *left column*, top to bottom), the firing rate of a typical on-centered retinal ganglion cell increases (*next column to the right*) up to a certain spot size. Further increases in spot size reduce the firing rate of the ganglion cell to a point beyond which ganglion cell responses do not change. Off-center ganglion cells (*next column*) have the opposite response when presented with a dark-centered anulus. Y-type cells (*far right column*) signal the temporal boundaries of the stimulus presentation.

## Ganglion cell responses

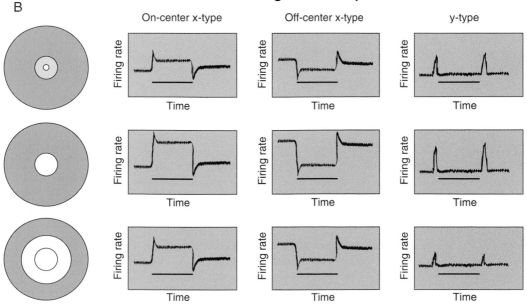

B

On-center x-type

Off-center x-type

y-type

and Y cells because they have unusual response requirements that do not correspond to the center-surround receptive fields of the X and Y cells. Their conduction velocities are slow. Many respond to general levels of illumination and are apparently important in regulating the iris. The most numerous central connections of W cells are with the superior colliculus and the pretectal area.

## CENTRAL PROCESSING OF VISUAL INFORMATION

The visual system has been studied extensively for several decades. Although relatively little is known about transformation of information in the LGN, certain features of information processing in the visual cortex shed light on neocortical function in general. Therefore, central visual processing can serve as a framework for studying cortical function.

### Serial Processing in the Visual Cortex

Properties of cortical cells in the visual system can be studied as retinal ganglion cells are studied: visual stimuli are presented to the retina, and the activity of the cortical cells is recorded. Just as with ganglion cells, it is possible to determine the most effective stimulus shape for the cortical cells and map their receptive fields. From these experiments it has been found that the most effective stimulus shape for individual neurons in the primary visual cortex, $V_1$, is different from the center-surround that is so effective in driving ganglion cells in the retina and LGN. In the visual cortex neurons respond best to rectangles. Neurons in $V_1$ are divided into two broad classes, simple cells and complex cells.

**Simple cells** in $V_1$ respond best to a moving bar of light oriented to a particular angle in the visual field. The bar must be presented within a receptive field that is also rectangular. Stimuli that have excitatory centers and inhibitory surrounds or vice versa (Fig. 12.22) elicit the most responses from simple cells. The effective stimuli and receptive fields for simple cortical cells are analogous to the anulus fields of the ganglion cells except for their shapes and preference for moving stimuli. One attractive explanation for the bar-shaped receptive fields of simple cells suggests that the output of several geniculate neurons with "typical" anular receptive fields that overlap in the shape of a bar converges on a single cortical cell. The simultaneous activity of all of these converging geniculate cells would be required to cause the cortical cell to fire.[7]

**Complex cells** have response properties similar to those of simple cells, but their response fields are much larger, approaching, in some cases, the entire visual space. The preferred stimulus for a complex cell is a properly oriented moving bar of light, but the bar may appear anywhere in the large receptive field of the cell (Fig. 12.23). In other words, *complex cells respond to an abstracted version of the stimulus that excites simple cells.* The quality that is abstracted, or generalized, is the angle of the bar within the visual space. The behavior of complex cells can be explained by assuming that all simple cells with the same orientation but with receptive fields in different parts of the visual space synapse with a single complex cell. Each simple cell can fire the complex cell.

### Columnar Organization of the Visual Cortex

Like the other cortical regions discussed, the visual cortex is organized into functional columns (see Chapter 5). Like the columns in other parts of the cerebral cortex, the different columns are activated by various types of stimuli. For example, the cells in one cortical column respond to stimuli of a particular orientation that is presented to the ipsilateral eye. The cells in an adjacent column respond to a stimulus rotated about 10° from its neighbor. The cells in the next adjacent column are activated by a stimulus rotated about 20° from the first (i.e., 10° from its immediate neighbor), and so forth across the cortex. This pattern repeats until all orientations, encompassing 360°, are represented by separate cortical **orientation columns.**

[7] This is the neural equivalent of a Boolean logical AND function.

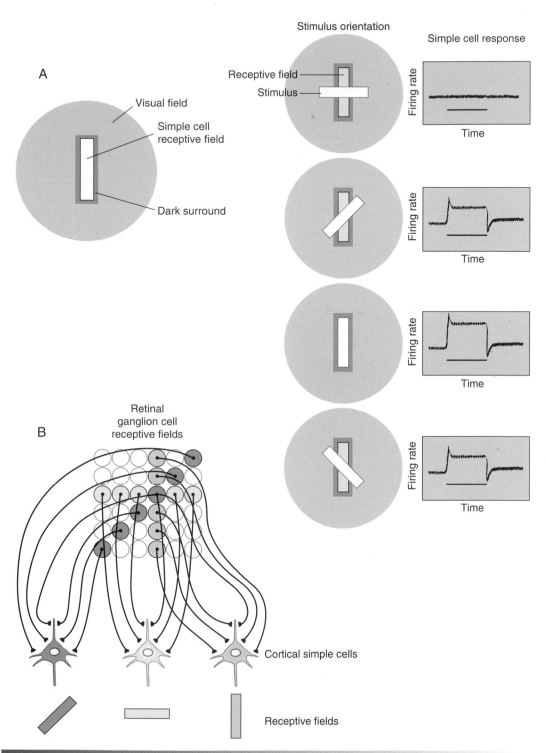

**Figure 12.22 Simple cells**

**A.** Simple cells have rectangular receptive fields. *Right,* the firing rate of a simple cell in response to differing stimuli. **B.** The receptive fields of LGN cells (*circles*) with connections going to simple cortical cells. A single LGN cell can contribute to more than one cortical cell. The response of the simple cells is in proportion to the number of active LGN cells that synapse with the cortical cell. *Shading,* the contribution of the LGN cells to three simple cortical cells.

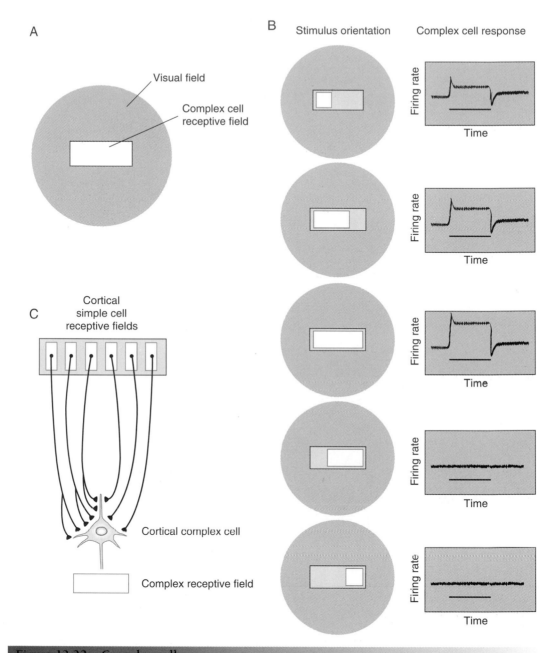

## Figure 12.23   Complex cells

**A.** Complex cells have large receptive fields. **B.** Complex cortical cells have multiple stimulus requirements, some of which are generalizations of simple cell response requirements. A properly oriented edge facilitates the cell no matter where in the response field it is, as long as the illumination is greater on the left than on the right. Otherwise the cell is inhibited. *White area,* stimulus within the receptive field (*large gray box*). **C.** The synaptic drive for complex cells is thought to be derived from the output of many simple cells. Extra synapses are shown from the left simple cells to account for the asymmetry of the complex cell's response. *White boxes,* simple cell receptive fields within the complex cell's receptive field (*large gray box*).

Columns can also be defined on the basis of which eye excites their cells. These **ocular dominance** columns exhibit a regular pattern of excitation that alternates from left eye to right eye to left eye, and so on. Each ocular dominance column contains all of the orientation columns associated with one eye (Fig. 12.24). Ocular dominance is based on the projection of the LGN on the cortex. One dominance column receives input from LGN laminae 2, 3, and 5 (ipsilateral eye); its neighbor receives afferents from LGN laminae 1, 4, and 6 (contralateral eye).

A pair of ocular dominance columns and all of the associated orientation columns within them are collectively called a **hypercolumn.**

Hypercolumns are organized across $V_1$ in a retinotopic pattern that maps the visual field onto the visual cortex. Dispersed among the ocular dominance columns are **blobs**, cylindrical areas within an ocular dominance column that receive parvocellular LGN afferents. Blobs appear to be exclusively devoted to processing color information and do not have orientation requirements (Fig. 12.24).

The cerebral cortex also has a horizontal structure. Pyramidal cells within cortical layers 3 and 5 send axons horizontally across the cortex for several millimeters. These axons extend vertical arborizations at intervals that correspond to the width of a hypercolumn. Physiology studies have shown that color

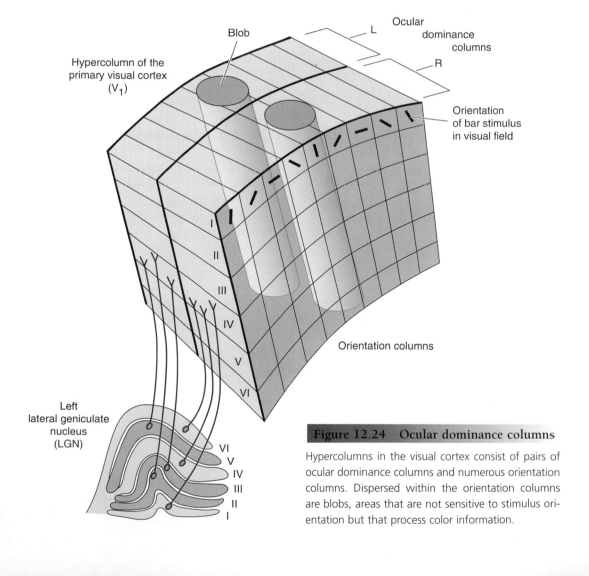

**Figure 12.24  Ocular dominance columns**

Hypercolumns in the visual cortex consist of pairs of ocular dominance columns and numerous orientation columns. Dispersed within the orientation columns are blobs, areas that are not sensitive to stimulus orientation but that process color information.

blobs and orientation columns of the same angle are interconnected across hypercolumns. This horizontal structure provides an anatomical basis to account for observed interactions between the left and right ocular dominance columns (discussed later in the chapter).

## Parallel Processing in the Visual System

The visual system also processes information along separate parallel pathways. Four parallel channels of information—one scotopic (monochromatic) for the rods and three photopic (red, green, and blue) for the cones— are extracted from the visual signal by the receptors. The parvocellular (X cell) and magnocellular (Y cell) pathways divide the visual space into two paths. X is a high-acuity path with static properties; Y is a low-acuity path that is very sensitive to movement. This visual information is segregated according to position within the visual field. All of these channels are segregated at the level of the retina.

Further divisions occur at the level of the thalamus. Visual information passing through the LGN is directed to $V_1$ of the cortex. A separate parallel path through the pulvinar innervates all other visual areas in the cortex *except* $V_1$. Within the LGN and cerebral cortex, the parvocellular and magnocellular channels remain segregated. The parvocellular path synapses in the deepest part of layer 4; the magnocellular path synapses more superficially in layer 4. The parallel distribution of information is further elaborated by the output pattern from the cortical columns. The upper layers (3 and 2) of the cortex project to other cortical areas through intracortical association fibers. The deeper layers project to the superior colliculus, pulvinar (from layer 5), and LGN (from layer 6).

## Poststriate Processing

Feature abstraction continues beyond $V_1$ in the extrastriate visual areas. As many as 20 retinotopically mapped areas have been discovered. In broad terms the anatomical organization of these areas appears to extend the serial and parallel organizational schemes just described. At least two parallel information channels leave $V_1$ (Fig. 12.25). The magnocellular Y pathway appears to extract information about motion, interocular disparity (necessary for depth perception), and spatial relations. This path proceeds serially through several individually mapped regions into the posterior parietal cortex. The parvocellular X pathway analyzes form, color, and interocular disparity. It projects in serial stepwise fashion to the temporal lobe. The *blob system,* a subset of the parvocellular system, seems to be exclusively associated with color analysis and may be yet a third parallel path. These parallel pathways are not strictly separated; they interact at several levels.

Because the various extrastriate visual areas apparently individually abstract certain global attributes from the visual image, it seems reasonable to hypothesize that *abstractions of the visual scene are analyzed and individually brought to conscious perception by anatomically separate parts of the cerebral cortex.* This hypothesis predicts that appropriately placed lesions produce perceptual losses of specific attributes while preserving other attributes. This hypothesis is supported by some clinical data.

Lesions that produce a defect in recognition or meaning without losses in objective sensations are termed **agnosias** [G. *a-* and *gnosis,* knowledge]. Agnosia is not a sensory loss in the same way that blindness and lack of vibratory sensations are sensory losses. Agnosia is the *inability to recognize or attach meaning to perceived stimuli.*

Several visual agnosias have been correlated with specific cortical lesions. For example, **object agnosia** is the inability to recognize familiar objects by visual means alone. Patients can readily recognize objects by tactile manipulation, auditory cues, sometimes even odor. Visual recognition is not possible because visual sensations, although consciously perceived, hold no meaning for the patient. Object agnosia can be quite specific. For instance, one form of object agnosia, called **prosopagnosia** [G. *prosopone,* face], is the inability to recognize faces. Such patients cannot recognize people from their faces but have no difficulty recognizing them by body movement or the

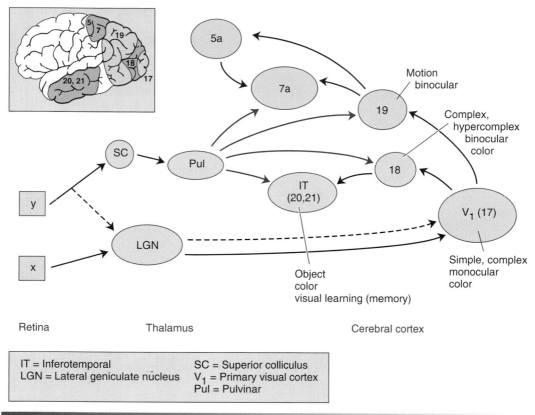

**Figure 12.25    Poststriate visual processing**

A few of the interconnections between some of the visual areas of the cerebral cortex suggesting some discrete functions served by each area. *Broken lines,* magnocellular paths; *numbers,* Brodmann areas.

sound of their voice. Object agnosias are associated with bilateral lesions to the ventral medial portion of the occipitotemporal cortex (Brodmann's areas 20 and 21).

One possible physiological explanation for such bizarre syndromes as prosopagnosia is found in the monkey, whose inferotemporal cortex is remarkable for its collection of neurons that respond only to the most esoteric of stimuli. Within it are single cells that respond only to visual stimuli in the shape of a simian hand (the subject was a monkey) or the outline of a simian face. These rare cells have been dubbed "grandmother cells," a term used apocryphally to suggest that certain cells may be so specific that they respond only to one's grandmother. Discovery of these cells has provided a possible physiological explanation for such bizarre syndromes as prosopagnosia.

**Achromatopsia** [G. *a-* and *chroman,* color] is the inability to make color hue discriminations. People with this condition report that everything looks gray. Not to be confused with color blindness, which is a retinal defect due the absence of one or more sets of color-sensitive cones, achromatopsia is a type of agnosia. Color information is sent to the brain, but it holds no meaning for the patient. Without meaning, discriminations cannot be made. Achromatopsia is associated with bilateral lesions to area 37 (and perhaps also to area 18), a transition zone between the occipital and temporal lobes.

Motion plays a critical role in visual perception. For example, many subprimates have considerable difficulty attaching meaning to nonmoving objects. A dog has difficulty seeing a rabbit that remains motionless, but once the rabbit starts to run, the dog is in hot pursuit. Primates are less dependent on movement for visual perception. Nevertheless, a separate specialized region of the cerebral cortex is necessary to perceive motion. Recent experiments on monkeys show that artificially stimulating a small number of cells in the movement perception area of the cortex can alter the monkey's *perception* of the direction of a moving target. The monkey makes errors while reaching for moving targets during stimulation that he does not otherwise make, even though motor areas of the brain are not stimulated. In humans, a bilateral lesion of the posterior part of the middle temporal gyrus and the adjacent lateral occipital gyrus results in the inability to perceive motion. Visual perception is otherwise normal. A description of this phenomenon, as documented by the experience of one patient, follows:

> The visual disorder complained of by the patient was a loss of movement vision in all three dimensions. She had difficulty, for example, in pouring tea or coffee into a cup because the fluid appeared to be frozen, like a glacier. In addition, she could not stop pouring at the right time since she was unable to perceive the movement in the cup (or a pot) when the fluid rose. Furthermore the patient complained of difficulties in following a dialogue because she could not see the movements of the face and, especially, the mouth of the speaker. In a room where more than two other people were walking she felt very insecure and unwell, and usually left the room immediately, because "people were suddenly here or there but I have not seen them moving." The patient experienced the same problem but at an even more marked extent in crowded streets or places, which she therefore avoided as much as possible. She could not cross the street because of her inability to judge the speed of a car, but she could identify the car itself without difficulty. "When I'm looking at the car first, it seems far away. But then, when I want to cross the road, suddenly the car is very near." She gradually learned to "estimate" the distance of moving vehicles by means of the sound becoming louder.[8]

## DEVELOPMENT OF CEREBRAL FUNCTION

How are the synaptic connections of the cerebral cortex determined? Obviously, the principal organization is determined by the genetic code. The LGN is always connected by the optic radiations to the cerebral cortex of the calcarine fissure; the visual cortex is never seen straddling the lateral fissure. The ocular dominance columns are always arranged retinotopically. But what about the synaptic connections within and among the cortical columns? Are they determined genetically, or can experience influence the nature of the final synaptic arrangement of the cerebral cortex in a way that ultimately determines function? The columnar structure of the cerebral cortex has allowed for the design of a number of important experiments that probe these questions.

Investigators have divided cells in the visual cortex into seven classes according to how strongly they are driven by either eye. Cells in category 1 are driven exclusively by the contralateral eye; those in category 7, by the ipsilateral eye. Category 4 contains cells driven about equally by both eyes. The other categories indicate intermediate levels of lateralization. The degree to which a cell is driven by both eyes is determined by the strength of the horizontal circuits that interlink the ocular dominance columns. If the horizontal connections do not develop, all of the cells in a column are driven monocularly.

If a newborn kitten is deprived of visual input to one eye by suturing the eyelids together, the effect of that monocular deprivation on cortical development can be observed because most of the cortical synapses in cats form during the second through fifth weeks of life. The pattern of ocular dominance shifts away from the unstimulated eye after only 10 days of monocular deprivation, which ultimately results in a permanent loss of vision in the unstimulated eye. The ability to shift the pattern of ocular dominance depends on the age of the kitten. By the time the animal is 4 months old, the cortical synapses are sufficiently estab-

---

[8] Quoted with permission from Zihl JD, von Cramon D, Mai N. Selective disturbance of movement vision after bilateral brain damage. Brain 1983;106:313–340.

lished that monocular deprivation barely disrupts the ocular dominance pattern. In adult cats, even 3 months of monocular deprivation does not seriously affect the binocular pattern.

The orientation columns are also affected by perinatal experience. Kittens raised in a visual environment consisting of vertical or horizontal stripes develop orientation columns in $V_1$ that correspond to the orientation of the visual stimulus. The wide range of orientation columns representing all angles that is so characteristic of the normal $V_1$ is absent. One can only speculate how this adaptive transformation of cortical function affects the actual perceptions of these animals in their visual world.

The difference in effect between depriving adult and neonatal cats suggests that there is a perinatal **critical period** during which cortical synaptic relations are indeterminate. After the critical period the synaptic structure of the cortex is sufficiently established to be permanent. *Experience is the force that ultimately determines adult cortical synaptic structure.* In cats this critical period lasts for approximately the first 100 to 120 days of life. The critical period for humans cannot be established with certainty. Some insight is provided by children with **strabismus** [G. *strabismos,* squint], a condition in which the eyes do not track together. Frequently caused by a weakness of one or more of the muscles of ocular motion, strabismus results in **diplopia**, or double vision, since the two retinal images cannot be fused by movement of the eyes. If it persists, diplopia is resolved by a neurological suppression of one of the two images. If the condition begins during infancy and persists into the fifth or sixth year, vision is permanently lost in the suppressed eye, just as with the monocularly deprived kittens. Treatment consists of surgically correcting the muscle weakness causing the strabismus. If surgery fails to correct the problem, vision in both eyes can usually be salvaged by alternately patching the eyes during the critical period. Alternate patching forces the child to use both eyes but avoids diplopia. After the child reaches age 5 or 6, the patching is discontinued. Thereafter vision in one eye is suppressed, probably by inhibition in the cerebral cortex, not by failure of synapses to develop. Later in life, if vision is lost in the good eye, as

for example through trauma, vision from the suppressed eye is often restored.

## LESIONS TO THE VISUAL PATHWAYS

Lesions to the visual pathways produce characteristic deficits in the visual fields. These deficits can be documented during the neurological examination and are extremely useful in reaching a proper diagnosis. For these reasons, the visual field losses associated with specific visual pathway lesions (Fig. 12.26) should be memorized.

Visual fields are tested at the bedside or during an office examination by a **confrontation test.** The examiner faces the patient, who covers one eye with one hand and fixes the gaze on the examiner's nose. The examiner then places objects in the visual field of the open eye. Moving targets, such as twitching fingers, should be avoided, since the patient may respond to the motion without having a good perception of the visual image. Showing one or two fingers and asking the patient to name the number of fingers showing is a better test of vision. At a minimum, the examiner should determine that vision is present in all four quadrants of each eye separately and that the visual fields extend nearly 90° from forward gaze, except where blocked by the nose. If necessary, the visual fields can be accurately mapped by a specialist using computer-assisted perimetry. It is customary to describe visual deficits in terms of the *visual fields,* not the retinal fields. The visual fields are, of course, the opposite of the retinal fields because of the inverting action of the lens.

**Monocular blindness**, or total blindness in one eye, can be caused by *total failure of the retina or loss of the entire optic nerve.* More common, however, is partial monocular blindness, in which the retina has punctate lesions that leave scotomas in the visual fields, much like the blind spot associated with the papilla. **Glaucoma** is manifested by a shrinking of the visual fields from the perimeter in a more or less symmetrical pattern. If the optic nerve is the primary site of the lesion, one eye may have acute blurring or haziness. In some cases a scotoma is present. If the optic nerve is involved near the papilla, the disk margin may

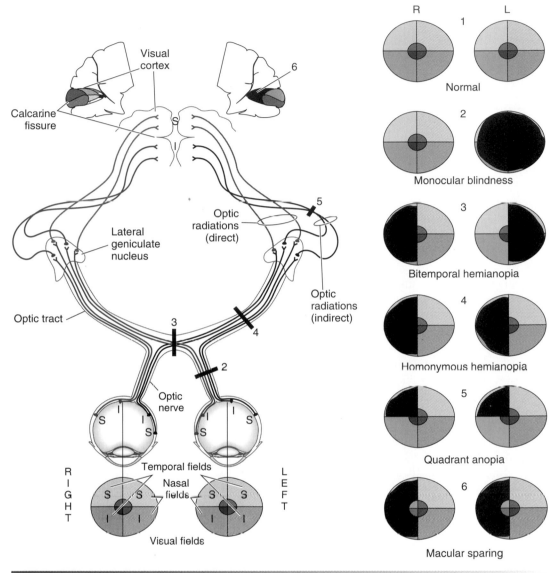

**Figure 12.26  Visual system lesions**

Lesions to the visual pathway produce various patterns of blindness (*dark areas*).

be swollen or blurred, a condition known as **papillitis.** Papillitis is differentiated from papilledema because the latter usually does not produce visual disturbances.

**Homonymous hemianopia** [G. *homos,* same; *nomos,* law; *hemi,* half; *a-,* not] is the loss of vision in half of the visual field divided by the vertical meridian. As the name implies, the same hemifield is affected in both eyes. Homonymous hemianopia may be **complete**

or **incomplete,** depending on whether the entire half of the visual field is affected. It can be produced by almost any lesion more central than the optic chiasm. This characteristic deficit is explained by the crossing pattern of the optic nerve axons at the optic chiasm. Since the axons arising from the nasal half of one retina cross the midline to join the axons arising from the temporal half of the opposite retina, all of the axons in the optic tract receive light from the same visual hemifield. Lesions producing homonymous hemianopia are contralateral to the visual field defect.

Complete homonymous hemianopia can be produced if the entire *optic tract, LGN, optic radiations, or primary visual cortex* ($V_1$) is destroyed. It is not possible, however, to differentiate which of these structures is affected from visual field data alone. It is useful to know that lesions to the optic tract and LGN are rare but infarctions of the optic radiations are relatively common. Furthermore, because the optic radiations are a large tract, most lesions involving it are partial, producing incomplete homonymous hemianopia. As discussed previously, about half of the axons in the optic radiations take an indirect course from the LGN to the calcarine fissure, passing around the lateral ventricle in the temporal lobe. Axons taking the indirect path terminate in the inferior lip of the calcarine fissure, and their loss produces **superior-quadrant homonymous hemianopia.** Loss of the axons taking the direct path causes **inferior-quadrant homonymous hemianopia.**

Occipital cortex lesions can be expected to produce complete homonymous hemianopia. As a practical matter, occlusion of the *calcarine artery,* a branch of the posterior cerebral artery, usually spares the macular portion of the visual field. This **macular sparing** is probably due to perfusion of the occipital pole by anastomotic collateral circulation, which reaches it from the terminal branches of the middle cerebral artery.

Lesions to the optic chiasm may produce almost any type of visual field disturbance, since all of the optic fibers are present in that structure. The most characteristic deficit is **bitemporal hemianopia,** which is caused by severing only the crossing fibers, sparing the uncrossed fibers. Such visual field deficits are fairly common. They may be caused by a pituitary tumor, aneurysm in the circle of Willis, or neoplasm at the base of the third ventricle. Division of all of the axons at the optic chiasm, as may occur with bullet wounds following unsuccessful suicide attempts, results in **total blindness.**

C A S E     H I S T O R Y

## THE CASE OF THE MALIGNANT MERRY-GO-ROUND[9]

### HISTORY OF PRESENT ILLNESS

Ms. C. F. is a 41-year-old woman who had intermittent vertigo during the past summer. She would have overwhelming sensations of the room spinning as if she were on a merry-go-round. There were no precipitating factors, such as changes in head position, or any association with viral infections or other illnesses. The inter-

mittent vertigo continued for several months. Her primary care physician ordered an ENG (electronystagmogram),[10] which indicated a CNS lesion. The symptoms gradually abated.

In the autumn she began to have episodes of poor coordination of the right hand. She had trouble with fine motor control, which manifested in poor handwriting. She also had dysarthria and difficulty with her balance, which gave her a tendency to stumble. She fell to the ground twice. She had no loss of vision, diplopia, dysphagia, lateralized weakness, numbness, or bowel or bladder symptoms.

---

[9] This case was given to me by Paula Toth-Russell, South Bend Neurology, South Bend, IN.
[10] A recording of nystagmus induced by caloric stimuli.

## MEDICAL HISTORY

About 6 months prior to this examination, Ms. C. F. had blurred vision in her right eye that she described as "spots in front of my eye." Her vision was moderately disturbed. Worried, she saw an optometrist, who told her that it was papillitis and would probably clear up in a few weeks; it did. She has had no other serious illnesses. Her mother has had a stroke, but otherwise there is no family history of neurological disease.

## PHYSICAL EXAMINATION

Unremarkable.

## NEUROLOGICAL EXAMINATION

### Mental Status
She is awake, alert, and oriented to person, place, and time.

### Cranial Nerves

OLFACTION: She correctly identified methyl salicylate from each nostril.

VISION: Visual fields were full to confrontation. Disks were flat bilaterally.

OCULOMOTION: Extraocular movements were full. A left lateral nystagmus was noted on left lateral gaze.

PUPILS: Pupils contracted briskly from 4 mm to 2 mm to direct and consensual light reflex.

TRIGEMINAL: Perception to light cotton touch was symmetrical and equal over all three divisions. Masseter and temporalis bulk and strength were within normal limits.

FACIAL: Face was symmetrical; grimace was full and symmetrical. Frontalis muscles contracted symmetrically.

AUDITION: Finger rubbing was perceived in both ears. Air conduction was more sensitive than bone conduction for 12 seconds. The Weber test was perceived midline.

VAGOGLOSSOPHARYNGEAL: The palate elevated symmetrically; gag reflex was present bilaterally.

ACCESSORY: Sternocleidomastoid and trapezius bulk and strength were within normal limits.

HYPOGLOSSAL: The tongue extended in the midline. No atrophy or fasciculations were noted.

### Station and Gait
She walks on a narrow base with normal arm swings. She had difficulty with tandem gait but is able to heel-and-toe walk without assistance.

### Motor Systems

STRENGTH: Muscle strength (5/5) and bulk were within normal limits throughout.

TONE: Tone was normal everywhere except in the right arm, where some spasticity was noted in the brachioradialis.

BULK: Muscle bulk was symmetrical. No atrophy was observed.

ABNORMAL MOVEMENTS: No abnormal movements were observed.

### Sensory Systems
Sensorium was intact to light touch, pinprick, vibration, and proprioception throughout. The Romberg sign was absent.

### Reflexes
MSRs were brisk (+) at the right biceps, triceps, and brachioradialis; normal at the left biceps, triceps, and brachioradialis; and normal bilaterally at the patella and ankle. Toes were down going to plantar stimulation bilaterally.

### Coordination and Control
Slight ataxia was noted on finger-to-nose testing in the right arm; the left was normal. Rapid alternating movements were normal. No rebound was noted.

### Parietal Functions
There was no aphasia, agnosia, or disorientation as to left and right. Optokinetic reflex was present in both directions. There were no atavistic signs.

## ANCILLARY STUDIES

An evoked potential study (somatosensory evoked potential [SER]), brainstem auditory evoked response (BAER), and visual evoked response (VER) were ordered. Results of all three were within normal limits. Examination of the cerebrospinal fluid (CSF) obtained by spinal tap revealed 9 oligoclonal bands (0 to 1 normal) by isoelectric focusing. Magnetic resonance imaging (MRI) (Fig. 12.27) of the head revealed 10 periventricular areas of signal enhancement.

## SUBSEQUENT COURSE

Ms. C. F. was counseled extensively with her husband about her papillitis and her treatment options.

## COMMENTARY

The initial episode of papillitis is a significant finding in this case. Papillitis is a swelling and blurring of the papilla caused by an inflammation of the optic nerve close to its insertion into the eyeball. Papillitis produces disturbed vision and is frequently associated with scotomas. The eyeball may also be tender to touch and painful during normal eye movements. Usually no cause is determined, and two-thirds of patients have restoration of normal vision within a few weeks. The remainder are left with some permanent visual disturbance ranging from very slight to total blindness. Although at the time of examination no cause for the papillitis can usually be determined, approximately 75% of these patients develop **multiple sclerosis** (MS) within 15 years.

Following the episode of papillitis, Ms. C. F. had two other symptoms that can be explained by CNS lesions. The first was intermittent vertigo, which was followed a few months later by poor coordination and dysarthria. The two episodes appear to affect different parts of the CNS, and she had a nearly complete recovery between each episode. None of her symptoms can be ascribed to lesions in the peripheral nervous system. *The pattern of recurring multifocal CNS lesions with intervening recovery is the hallmark of MS.*

MS is a *demyelinating disease of the CNS.* In MS, demyelination is the principal pathological event; almost all neurological diseases ultimately cause secondary demyelination. Although there is no accepted etiology of MS, accumulating evidence suggests that it is caused by an infectious

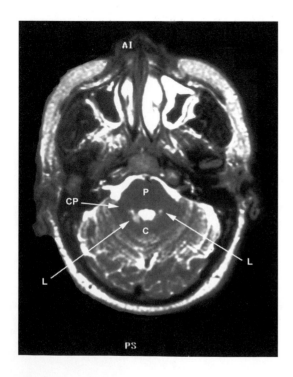

**Figure 12.27  MRI of Ms. C. F.**

(Courtesy of the Magnetic Resonance Imaging Center, South Bend, IN.)

agent. Susceptibility to this agent seems to occur between ages 11 and 45 years; 6 to 12 years after the initial infection, the presumed infectious agent provokes an autoimmune response directed against *CNS myelin. Peripheral myelin is spared.*

During the immunological attack, inflammation, edema, and demyelination interfere with axonal function, producing *symptoms restricted to the CNS.* The attack is aggravated by nitric oxide, which is produced by cytokine-induced immune cells. The released nitric oxide can form complexes with certain amino acids and make them immunogenic, exacerbating the acute illness. Antibodies to the nitric oxide–amino acid complexes are found in patients with MS. Eventually the inflammation and edema subside, but the demyelination remains.[11] Although acute symptoms decrease, a residual deficit usually remains.

For reasons that are not understood, after an indeterminate period the patient may undergo repeated autoimmune attacks followed by remissions. Each exacerbation leaves the patient more compromised. Each immunological attack strikes the CNS randomly, resulting in multifocal lesions. Therefore, MS is characterized by *periods of exacerbation and remission, with symptoms disseminated in space and time and following a relentlessly progressive course.* The progression of MS is highly variable. Some people have one or two exacerbations followed by a life-long remission. In others the disease follows a malignant course, causing death within a few months with no remissions.

No specific laboratory studies can unequivocally diagnose MS; the diagnosis ultimately rests on the long-term picture of exacerbations, remissions, multifocal CNS lesions, and the exclusion of other possible diagnoses. The most useful procedures are the immunoglobulin-$\gamma$ (IgG) index, demonstration of oligoclonal IgG bands

on CSF electrophoresis, and MRI. The IgG index compares the ratios of IgG and albumin in the CSF and serum.[12] A ratio greater than 1.7 in conjunction with the demonstration of oligoclonal bands is found in about 90% of patients with clinically diagnosed MS. MRI can usually demonstrate multifocal white-matter lesions.

There is no specific treatment for MS. Anti-inflammatory therapy with adrenocorticotropic hormone (ACTH) or methylprednisolone can sometimes hasten recovery from acute episodes, but there is no evidence that it alters the course of the disease or lessens the number or severity of subsequent relapses. Immunosuppressive therapy has not been proved to be beneficial at this time.

Recently introduced drugs have been effective in well-controlled blinded clinical trials. Two of these drugs are different forms of recombinant interferon-$\beta_1$. Both appear to decrease the rate of exacerbations and the progression of disability. Their mode of action in MS is uncertain, but $\beta$-interferon is known to inhibit the production of $\gamma$-interferon by T-helper cells and delayed-type hypersensitivity (DTH) effector cells. Decreasing the availability of $\gamma$-interferon attenuates both the immunological response to antigens and the effector mechanisms recruited to attack the antigen.[13] Interferon's effects can all be explained by suppression of the immunological attack. There is no evidence of a cure, since exacerbations continue to occur, albeit more slowly, and the disease continues to progress.

## FURTHER APPLICATIONS

**12.1.    A neurological diagnosis seeks to account for all of the patient's signs and symptoms with as simple an explanation as possible. If a patient's situation can be explained by two widely separated lesions or a single**

---

[11] Recall the structure of the oligodendrocyte and its inability to regenerate lost processes (see Chapter 3).

[12] $IgG\ index = \dfrac{CSF\ IgG/serum\ IgG}{CSF\ albumen/serum\ albumen}$

[13] $\beta$-Interferon also has antiviral properties, but no virus has been causally associated with MS. If the causative agent is a virus, the virus does not appear to still be present by the time the immunological attack commences. Therefore, the beneficial effects of $\beta$-interferon therapy are probably not due to the antiviral properties.

lesion, the single lesion is most likely the correct diagnosis. MS challenges this approach, at least in the long run. However, most exacerbations of MS are explained by a single lesion. Identify the location of the lesion in the present case following each attack. Can all attacks be explained by the same lesion? Make a drawing of the appropriate areas to illustrate your hypotheses.

12.2.	Explain how papillitis can be a sign of MS, since MS signs must be referable to the CNS.

12.3.	Explain why MRI is successful in demonstrating CNS demyelination

but computed tomography almost always fails to image white matter plaques caused by MS.

12.4.	In this case, after the diagnosis of papillitis, the ophthalmologist suspected that Ms. C. F. had MS. He did not reveal his suspicions to her at that time. She learned of her diagnosis only after the neurological consultation ordered by her primary care physician. With a friend or in a small group, debate the pros and cons of telling Ms C. F. after the first examination that she probably had MS. Ask physicians you know what they do in this situation.

## S U M M A R Y

• **Light is transformed into coded electrical signals by the eye.**

The optical elements of the eye, the cornea and lens, focus images on the transducer cells of the retina, the rods and cones. Photons are absorbed by the visual pigments in the receptors and induce a series of G-protein-mediated biochemical reactions that affect the availability of cGMP to the sodium ion channels in the receptors. The availability of cGMP modulates the sodium current, which in turn modulates the release of neurotransmitter (probably glutamate) from the receptor's synapses.

• **There are five principal neuronal cells in the mammalian retina.**

Receptor cells synapse on bipolar and horizontal cells in the retina. The bipolar cells synapse on ganglion and amacrine cells. Although the synapses are chemical, only the ganglion cell supports action potentials; intraretinal signaling is accomplished by graded local potentials.

•**The retina performs the first stage of transformation of information in the visual pathways.**

Visual information transduced into electrical form by the 6 million cones and 100 million rods converges on 1 million ganglion cells. In the process the pixels of photic information detected by the receptor cells are combined into more complex center-surround patterns. Retinal processing enhances the detection of boundary conditions in the visual image.

• **Postretinal processing of visual information takes place in three noncortical areas of the CNS.**

Ganglion cell axons carry visual information from the retina to the LGN, the superior colliculus, and the pretectal area of the brainstem. The axons in the optic nerve are rearranged at the optic chiasm in such a way that the visual image from one half of the visual field is carried to contralateral central structures, regardless of the eye of origin. The visual fields are mapped onto the receiving structures in a precise retinotopic organization. The optic radiations in the occipital lobe transmit visual information from the LGN to the striate cortex, $V_1$. Visual information from the superior colliculus is transmitted to the pulvinar, among other places, from which it is sent to extrastriate visual cortical areas.

- The first stages of cortical processing of visual information occur in hierarchical levels.

In $V_1$, simple cells are sensitive to bars of light oriented in a particular direction. Simple cells have relatively small receptive fields. The response of simple cells is an abstraction of the properties of many LGN cells. Complex cells are also sensitive to particularly oriented moving bars of light; however, they have large receptive fields. The response of complex cells is an abstraction of the response of many simple cells with the same orientation.

- Later stages of visual processing occur in the poststriate visual cortex and follow parallel pathways.

From the striate cortex visual information is processed by at least two parallel cortical systems, each of which is composed of several serially linked, independently mapped visual processing areas. In very broad terms, the parallel paths abstract information about movement, color, shape, and spatial relations from the visual image. Damage to these higher-order processing centers leads to specific visual agnosias that correspond to the visual quality abstracted by that center.

## SUGGESTED READINGS

Kaas JH. Theories of visual cortex organization in primates. Cereb Cortex 1997;12:91– 125.

Katz L, Callaway, E. Development of local circuits in mammalian visual cortex. Annu Rev Neurosci 1992; 15:31– 56.

Kaupp UB, Koch KW. Role of cGMP and $Ca^{2+}$ in vertebrate photoreceptor excitation and adaptation. Annu Rev Physiol 1992;54:1992.

Kurtzke JF. Epidemiologic evidence for multiple sclerosis as an infection. Clin Microbiol Rev 1993;63:82.

Legothetis NK, Sheinberg DL. Visual object recognition. Ann Rev Neurosci 1996;19:577– 621.

Merigan WH, Maunsell JHR. How parallel are the primate visual pathways? Annu Rev Neurosci 1993;16:369– 402.

Miyashita Y. Inferior temporal cortex: where visual perception meets memory. Annu Rev Neurosci 1993;16:245– 263.

Moore KL, Persaud TVN. The developing human: clinically oriented embryology. 6th ed. Philadelphia: Saunders, 1998.

Ohzawa I, DeAngelis GC, Freeman RD. The neural coding of stereoscopic depth. Neuroreport 1997;10:iii– xii.

Online Mendelian Inheritance in Man (OMIM). Baltimore: Johns Hopkins University. MIM 148300. OMIM can be reached at http://www3.ncbi.nlm.nih.gov/omim/

Sengpiel F, Blakemore C. The neural basis of suppression and amblyopia in strabismus, part 2. Eye 1996;10:250– 258.

Uhl R, Wagner R, Ryba N. Watching G-proteins at work. Trends Neurosci 1990;13.64– 70.

# 13

# The Autonomic Nervous System

By convention, the nervous system is divided into *voluntary* and *involuntary* divisions, the latter known as the **autonomic nervous system** (ANS). Although this dichotomy is too simple, the concept of an independent or autonomous portion of the nervous system is useful. The ANS regulates many physiological functions, such as the cardiovascular and digestive systems, temperature, and reproduction. Some of these functions are entirely autonomous, such as the regulation of body temperature, over which we exert no conscious control. Others are semiautonomous, having both conscious and autonomous elements. For example, we have some conscious control over sexual arousal—initiation of sexual activity and copulation, for instance—yet we cannot control some aspects of sexuality, such as orgasm. This chapter gives a brief overview of some of the clinically significant aspects of the autonomic nervous system.

## ANATOMY OF THE ANS

The ANS is composed of three sections: the **sympathetic, parasympathetic,** and **enteric** divisions. The sympathetic and parasympathetic divisions are composed of central and peripheral neurons. The central neurons are called **preganglionic** because they synapse with peripheral **postganglionic** neurons either in discrete **autonomic ganglia** or in a peripheral target organ. The preganglionic neurons of the ANS reside in brainstem and spinal cord nuclei. Their axons leave the central nervous system (CNS) in the cranial nerves or ventral roots. The postganglionic neurons synapse with the target organ (Fig. 13.1). The enteric

division resides entirely within the layers of the gut and its closely associated organs, the gallbladder and the pancreas. Because it receives both sympathetic and parasympathetic fibers, it comes under some central regulation, but it also can function autonomously.

## Parasympathetic Division

Preganglionic parasympathetic axons, which are generally long, synapse in ganglia in or near the target organ. These axons originate in brainstem nuclei (Edinger-Westphal, salivatory, dorsal motor nucleus, nucleus ambiguus) or in the sacral spinal cord (S2 to S4) (Fig. 13.2). Those originating in the brainstem travel with specific cranial nerves (CN III, VII, IX, or X); those originating in the spinal cord form the **pelvic splanchnic nerves** [G. *splancna*, internal organs, viscera] and are distributed to the pelvic structures via the inferior hypogastric plexus and the hypogastric nerve and its branches.

## Sympathetic Division

The preganglionic neurons of the sympathetic nervous system originate in the **intermediolateral nucleus** of the thoracic and lumbar spinal cord. The sympathetic preganglionic axons are generally short and myelinated, synapsing in ganglia that are close to the CNS (Fig. 13.2). The preganglionic axons leave the CNS in the ventral root but soon separate from it as the **white ramus** [L. *ramus*, branch]. Most of the axons of the white ramus enter a chain of **paravertebral ganglia** that are close to and segmentally associated with all of the thoracic and the first two or three lumbar spinal seg-

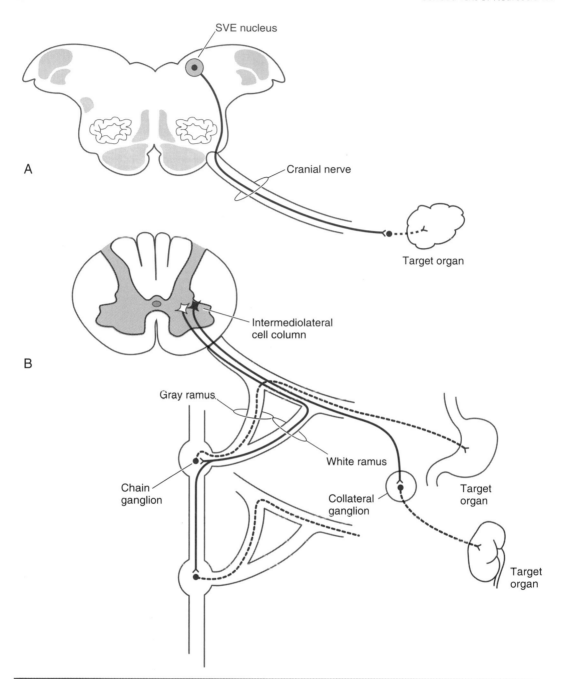

**Figure 13.1    Peripheral plan of the autonomic nervous system**

**A.** The parasympathetic nervous system has a long preganglionic axon that originates in motor neuron nuclei in the brainstem or spinal cord. The preganglionic axon synapses in a peripheral ganglion close to or within the target organ. **B.** The sympathetic nervous system has a short preganglionic axon that originates in the spinal cord. The axon synapses in a peripheral ganglion remote from the target organ.

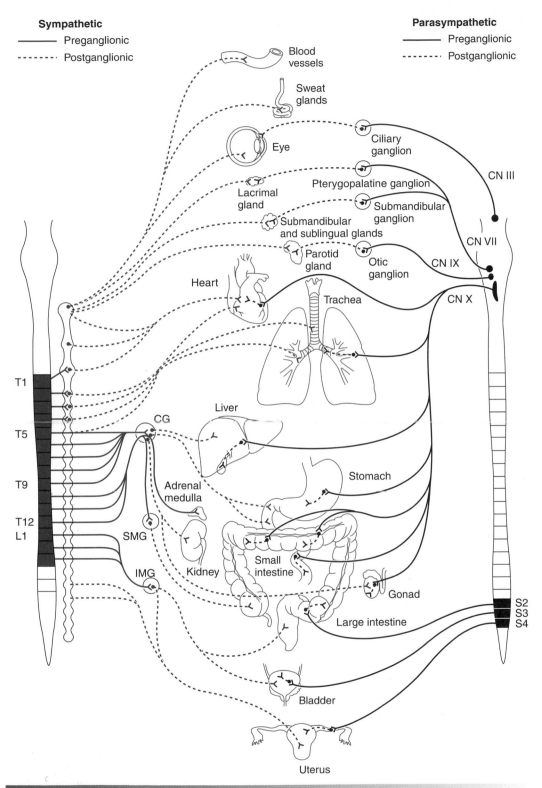

**Figure 13.2    The peripheral components of the autonomic nervous system**

**Left**. Sympathetic components. **Right**. Parasympathetic components. *CG*, celiac ganglion; *SMG*, superior mesenteric ganglion; *IMG*, inferior mesenteric ganglion.

ments. Three ganglia in the cervical region, the **inferior**,[1] **middle**, and **superior cervical ganglia**, are connected to this chain but have no direct segmental connections with the spinal cord. The chained paravertebral ganglia are interconnected, and preganglionic axons may synapse, via collateral fibers, in more than one ganglion.

Postganglionic sympathetic axons are unmyelinated. They leave the chain ganglia as the **gray ramus** to rejoin the spinal nerves. Axons from the gray ramus typically innervate the body wall and blood vessels. Structures in the face are innervated by axons that arise from cell bodies in the inferior and superior cervical ganglia. They follow the carotid and vertebral arteries to their targets. The eyes and glands of the head and the large internal organs, including the heart and lungs, are innervated by axons arising from neurons in the chain ganglia.

In addition to the paravertebral chain ganglia, there are several **collateral sympathetic ganglia**; the **celiac**, the **superior mesenteric**, and the **inferior mesenteric** are the most prominent. These collateral ganglia are independent of the paravertebral chain. The preganglionic axons destined to synapse in the collateral ganglia arise from neurons in the spinal cord and pass through the paravertebral ganglia without synapsing. Postganglionic axons leaving the collateral ganglia form the splanchnic nerves that innervate the viscera. An exception to the usual pattern of preganglionic and postganglionic innervation of visceral organs is found in the innervation of the adrenal medulla, which receives preganglionic axons directly from the spinal cord without an intervening ganglionic synapse.

### The Enteric Division

The enteric division of the ANS lies entirely outside of the CNS. It is composed of two nets of interconnected neurons, the **myenteric plexus** [G. *mys*, muscle, and *enteron*, small intestine; L. *plexus*, pl. plexus, braid] and the **submucosal plexus** (Fig. 13.3). Together they con-

tain as many as $10^8$ neurons. The myenteric plexus lies between the longitudinal and circular muscle layers of the gut; the submucosal plexus lies between the circular muscle layer and the mucosa. Each layer contains a multitude of ganglia. The ganglia of the two plexus are interconnected by axons that form an intricate network. Some of the neurons are sensory, registering distention of the gut and the chemical environment of the mucosa. Other neurons affect the smooth muscle walls, the tone of the vasculature, and the secretory activity of the glands. The enteric system maintains the rhythmic and coordinated contractions of the intestinal tract. Although it can function independently of the CNS, it is normally regulated by both sympathetic and parasympathetic innervation.

## SUPRASPINAL REGULATION OF THE ANS

Despite its name and apparent autonomy, the ANS is closely regulated by supraspinal structures. The hypothalamus (see Chapter 14) is the principal integrating center for ANS activity. To exert this control the hypothalamus is connected with brainstem and spinal cord autonomic nuclei through three principal pathways: the **dorsal longitudinal fasciculus (DLF)**, **the mammillotegmental tract**, and the **medial forebrain bundle** (MFB) (Fig. 13.4).

The DLF is the principal tract that connects hypothalamic nuclei with the sympathetic and parasympathetic preganglionic nuclei in the brainstem and spinal cord. This tract originates in cells in the medial hypothalamus, adjacent to the third ventricle. The fibers descend into the brainstem, pass through the periaqueductal gray (PAG) and reticular formation, and terminate in the dorsal motor nucleus of the vagus, the nucleus ambiguus, the reticular formation, and probably also in the salivatory and Edinger-Westphal nuclei. From the brainstem the DLF continues into the spinal cord, where it terminates in the intermediolateral cell column and the sacral autonomic nucleus.

---

[1] The inferior cervical ganglion is usually fused with the first thoracic ganglion, forming a large, star-shaped structure, the stellate ganglion.

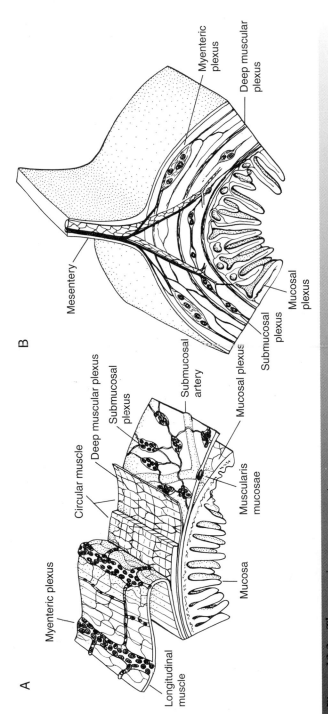

**Figure 13.3 The enteric nervous system**

**A.** The two layers of the enteric plexus along with a dissection of the layers of the gut. **B.** Cross-section of a segment of the gut showing the relation of the enteric plexus and the mesentery. (Reprinted with permission from Kandel E, Schwartz JH, Jessell TM. Principles of Neural Science. 3rd ed. New York: Appleton & Lange, 1991;767.)

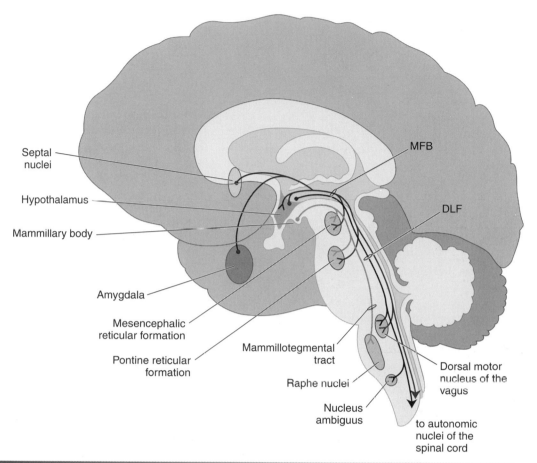

**Figure 13.4    Connections of the hypothalamus with brainstem structures**

The three principal tracts connecting the hypothalamus with the brainstem and spinal autonomic motor nuclei are the dorsal longitudinal fasciculus (*DLF*), mammillotegmental tract, and medial forebrain bundle (*MFB*).

The mammillotegmental tract originates in the mammillary body and descends into the brainstem, where it synapses in the mesencephalic and pontine reticular formation and the raphe nuclei.

The MFB is bidirectional and more diverse in its connections than the aforementioned tracts. Descending fibers originate not only in the medial hypothalamic nuclei but also in the amygdala and septal nuclei (see Chapter 14). They synapse in the dorsal nucleus of the vagus, preganglionic autonomic nuclei of the brainstem and spinal cord, locus ceruleus, and reticular formation, including the raphe nuclei. The most important ascending fibers arise from the brainstem reticular formation, especially the raphe nuclei, and terminate in the septal nuclei, hippocampus, cingulate gyrus, and prefrontal lobes.

Although it is known that sensory information reaches the hypothalamus, the pathways other than the MFB are poorly understood. Most sensory information reaching the hypothalamus seems to originate from a variety of cell types that may express catecholamines, serotonin, or acetylcholine (ACh). The information appears to arrive indirectly at the hypothalamus by way of the brainstem reticular formation.

## INNERVATION OF SPECIFIC ORGANS

ANS dysfunction is a common sign in neurological diseases. Knowing the specific autonomic innervation of the major organs is therefore helpful in understanding certain disease processes and reaching appropriate diagnostic conclusions. Many of the following descriptions depend on a thorough grasp of the autonomic components of the cranial nerves, which are presented in Chapter 10.

## Peripheral Blood Vessels and Skin

The skin and peripheral vasculature receive only postganglionic sympathetic innervation. The sympathetic axons arise from the chain ganglia and accompany the peripheral somatic nerves that are distributed to the *sweat glands, pilomotor muscles,* and the *smooth muscles of the arterioles* in skin and deep muscles. Stimulation of the sympathetic fibers *increases sweat production and causes cutaneous vasoconstriction and vasodilation of the deep muscle vasculature.*

## Structures of the Face and Orbit

The parasympathetic innervation of the muscles in the iris[2] originates in the **Edinger-Westphal nucleus.** The preganglionic axons leave the brainstem in the oculomotor nerve (CN III) and terminate in the **ciliary ganglion.** Postganglionic fibers synapse on the circular muscles of the iris. Contraction of the circular muscle *constricts the pupil.* Other axons synapse on the ciliary muscle. Stimulation of the ciliary muscle allows the lens to thicken, *accommodating the eye to near vision* (see Chapter 12).

The sympathetic preganglionic innervation of the eye and face arises in the spinal cord (T1 to T3) and reaches the **superior cervical ganglion** without synapsing. Postganglionic fibers originating in the ganglion ascend into the cranium as the internal carotid nerve by following the internal carotid artery (Fig. 13.5). The internal carotid nerve has two branches. The lateral branch forms the internal carotid plexus; the medial branch continues to follow the carotid artery into the cavernous sinus, where it forms the cavernous plexus. A large branch leaves the cavernous plexus to course briefly with the abducens nerve before joining

the ophthalmic branch of the trigeminal nerve. The remainder of the cavernous plexus joins the ophthalmic artery into the orbit as the ophthalmic plexus.

The upper face and orbit are innervated by three sympathetic nerves. Sympathetic fibers make their way from the ophthalmic nerve to the nasociliary nerve and finally reach the eye via the long ciliary nerves. These fibers synapse on the radial muscle of the iris.[3] Contraction of this muscle *dilates the pupil.* A second set of sympathetic fibers leaves the ophthalmic nerve to join the frontal and finally the supraorbital nerve to innervate the sweat glands of the supraorbital area. A third group of sympathetic fibers arises from the cavernous plexus and joins the oculomotor nerve to innervate the smooth muscles of the levator palpebrae muscle.

The sympathetic innervation of the lower face also arises from the superior cervical ganglion but takes a different course from the fibers that innervate the supraorbital region. Sympathetic fibers destined for the lower face follow the distribution of the external carotid artery. These axons innervate the sweat glands, vasculature, and pili erector muscles of the lower face.

Loss of sympathetic innervation to the eye by destruction of either the preganglionic or postganglionic axons produces **Horner's syndrome,** a characteristic triad of signs including **miosis** [G. *meion,* less], **ptosis** [G., falling, dropping, collapse], and **anhidrosis** [G. *an,* without; *hidros,* sweat; and -osis, abnormal condition]. *Pupillary constriction (miosis) is caused by the* unopposed action of the parasympathetic fibers on the circular muscle of the iris. *Drooping of the eyelid (ptosis) is caused by loss of the* sympathetic innervation to the levator palpebrae muscle. *Lack of sweating on the affected half of the face (anhidrosis) is caused by the* loss of sympathetic innervation to the sweat glands of half of the face. Without sympathetic innervation the sweat glands fail to function.

Horner's syndrome may be caused by interruption of the DLF, the principal brainstem

---

[2] The innervation of the choroid is derived from the superior salivatory nucleus via the pterygopalatine ganglion.

[3] Authorities differ on the path the sympathetic fibers take to the iris. For a thorough review of the subject, see Watson and Vijayin, Suggested Readings list.

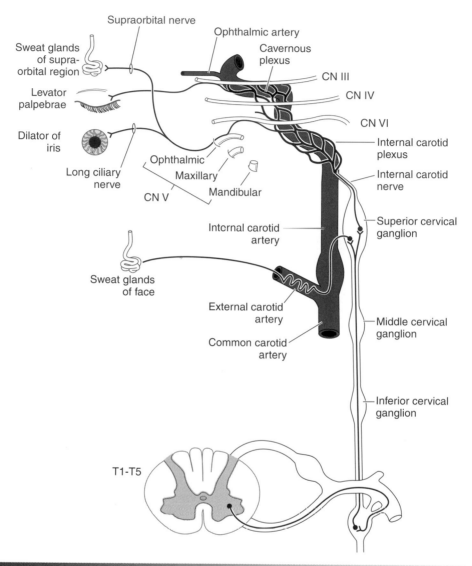

**Figure 13.5   Sympathetic innervation of the head**

The sympathetic innervation of the head follows the vasculature into the cranium and then various cranial nerves to the peripheral targets. The sympathetic nerves to the iris and sweat glands of the forehead follow the abducens and then the ophthalmic nerves, and the sympathetic innervation of the levator palpebrae follows the oculomotor nerve. The sweat glands of the lower face are innervated by sympathetic fibers that follow the external carotid artery.

tract that connects the hypothalamus to the spinal cord. It can also be caused by interruption of any part of the extensive peripheral path of the sympathetic nerves supplying the head. Horner's syndrome is an important neurological sign, and its cause must be identified. In this regard, the somewhat complicated distribution of sympathetic fibers to the face is

clinically significant. For example, dissecting aneurysms below the bifurcation of the carotid artery often produce a complete Horner's syndrome (ipsilateral miosis, ptosis, and anhidrosis) *over the entire half of the face.* A similar aneurysm central to the carotid bifurcation produces ipsilateral miosis and ptosis but *anhidrosis only of the supraorbital region.* Common causes of Horner's syndrome that may elude casual observation are mediastinal tumors, apical lung tumors, aneurysms of the aorta and carotid arteries, and abscesses in the neck.

The **lacrimal gland** [L. *lacrima,* tear] receives both sympathetic and parasympathetic innervation. The **superior salivatory nucleus** provides the parasympathetic preganglionic innervation. Parasympathetic preganglionic axons from this nucleus follow the facial nerve (CN VII) to innervate the **pterygopalatine ganglion.** The sympathetic innervation is similar to that of the orbital structures. Sympathetic fibers probably innervate only the blood vessels of the gland, since sympathectomy does not appear to interfere with lacrimation. In contrast, loss of the parasympathetic fibers can inhibit tearing to the point that the integrity of the cornea may be compromised (see Bell's palsy in Chapter 10).

## The Heart

The preganglionic parasympathetic innervation of the *heart* arises from the **nucleus ambiguus** [L. *ambiguus,* obscure, doubtful, disputed]. The axons follow the vagus nerve (CN X) into the thoracic cavity and then separate from it as the **cardiac nerve** before innervating the heart. Within the heart these axons synapse on scattered postganglionic neurons at the base of the atria. The postganglionic axons synapse in the **sinoatrial** [L. *sinus,* bay, hollow, and *atrium,* entranceway] (SA) and **atrioventricular nodes.** The *activity of the postganglionic axons slows the heart rate.*

The preganglionic sympathetic neurons affecting the heart reside at approximately T1 to T5 in the spinal cord. The preganglionic axons synapse in the corresponding thoracic ganglia and all of the cervical ganglia. Postganglionic axons from the cervical ganglia travel to the heart in the superior, middle, and inferior cardiac nerves; the thoracic cardiac nerve carries the axons from the thoracic ganglia. The postganglionic fibers synapse on the SA node, myocardium, and coronary vessels. Activation of the sympathetic system *increases the heart rate and strength of contraction and dilates the coronary arterioles* of the heart muscles.

## The Respiratory System

The *nasal mucosa* receives its preganglionic sympathetic innervation via the superior cervical ganglion with axons that follow the vascular supply into the mucosa. The parasympathetic supply arrives via the facial nerve and the pterygopalatine ganglion (see lacrimation in the section Structures of the Face and Orbit). The *larynx* receives its parasympathetic innervation via the laryngeal nerve, a branch of the vagus nerve. Autonomic fibers of the laryngeal nerve synapse on scattered postganglionic cells in the walls of the larynx. The sympathetic innervation arrives via the middle cervical ganglion. The autonomic innervation of the nasal mucosa and the larynx is believed to be primarily vasomotor: the *sympathetic innervation produces vasoconstriction; the parasympathetic innervation causes vasodilation.*

The *trachea, bronchi,* and *lungs* receive parasympathetic innervation from the vagus nerve. These axons synapse on postganglionic neurons in the trachea and bronchi that supply the glands and smooth muscles of the bronchial tree. The sympathetic innervation is supplied by the inferior cervical ganglion and the first four thoracic ganglia. Postganglionic fibers are distributed to the smooth muscles and glands of the bronchi. *Parasympathetic stimulation produces bronchial constriction and increases secretion from the glands; sympathetic stimulation produces bronchial dilation and decreases secretion.* The autonomic effect on pulmonary vessels apparently is slight.

## The Digestive System

The *submandibular* and *sublingual glands* receive their preganglionic parasympathetic supply from the facial nerve (CN VII); the *parotid gland* is supplied by the glossopharyngeal nerve (CN IX). The postganglionic fibers arise from the **submandibular** and **otic ganglia,** respectively. The sympathetic innervation of these glands originates in the superior cervical ganglion and reaches the glands by following the vasculature. The *parasympathetic stimulation dilates the blood vessels in the glands and increases the production of serous saliva. Sympathetic stimulation constricts the blood ves-*

*sels of the glands and increases the production of mucous saliva.*

The vagus nerve, which provides the parasympathetic preganglionic innervation to the *gut,* extends from the lower, smooth-muscle portion of the esophagus to the junction between the transverse and descending colon. The remainder of the colon, the rectum, and the internal anal sphincter receive preganglionic innervation from neurons located in the sacral spinal cord (S2 to S4). The preganglionic parasympathetic fibers synapse on neurons in the myenteric plexus and submucosal plexus of the enteric nervous system. These plexus act as the postganglionic neurons for the gut. Neurons in the myenteric plexus innervate the smooth muscle of the gut; those in the submucosal plexus innervate the secretory glands.

The preganglionic sympathetic innervation of the gut arises from the thoracic and lumbar spinal cord (T5 to L2). These axons do not synapse in the chain ganglia but innervate collateral ganglia (celiac, superior, and inferior mesenteric), from which the postganglionic axons are distributed to the gut via the splanchnic nerves. *Digestion is aided by parasympathetic activity, which increases motility and secretions and dilates the vasculature of the gut; sympathetic activity reduces motility, secretions, and blood flow.*

The extrinsic organs of digestion, the *liver* and *pancreas,* are innervated in a manner similar to that of the gut. The only difference is that scattered postganglionic parasympathetic neurons substitute for the enteric plexus. As in the gut, *parasympathetic activity generally aids digestion by increasing pancreatic secretion (acinar and islets cells) and inducing glycogenesis in the liver. Sympathetic activity decreases pancreatic islet secretion and induces glycogenolysis and gluconeogenesis in the liver.*

## The Urogenital System

The splanchnic nerve supplies the kidneys with sympathetic innervation; the kidneys appear to lack parasympathetic innervation. Autonomic regulation of the kidney and urine production is minimal. The preganglionic sympathetic innervation to the urogenital or-

gans arises from neurons in T10 to L2 of the spinal cord. After forming the **lumbar splanchnic nerve**, they synapse in the **inferior mesenteric ganglion**. The postganglionic fibers from this ganglion are distributed to the organs through the hypogastric nerves and plexus.

The preganglionic parasympathetic neurons are in the ventral horn of the sacral spinal cord (S2 to BS4) in the intermediolateral cell column. The parasympathetic efferent axons leave the spinal cord in the ventral roots and immediately separate as **pelvic splanchnic nerves**, which join the inferior hypogastric plexus. Small twigs of nerves leave this plexus and are distributed to the pelvic viscera and urogenital organs via the pelvic and pudendal nerves, where they synapse on neurons in the walls of these target organs.

## MICTURITION

**Micturition** [L. *micturire,* to urinate], the controlled elimination of urine, is a complex and well-organized function. Micturition can be divided into two phases. During the **filling phase**, the **detrusor muscle** [L. *de,* down, and *trudo,* thrust, force, compel to go] in the wall of the urinary bladder is relaxed and the urinary sphincter muscle is contracted. During the **emptying phase**, the reverse occurs: the detrusor actively contracts while the sphincter relaxes. The emptying phase can be controlled by voluntary action.

### The Micturition Reflex

Reflex micturition, the storage and release of urine without conscious control, normally occurs only in infants. During the filling phase, sympathetic activity actively inhibits the detrusor muscle of the bladder. This inhibition keeps the detrusor in a nearly flaccid state, which allows the bladder to increase in size without a concurrent increase in bladder wall tension. With the detrusor muscle in this relaxed state, the base of the bladder is flattened. As a result, the urethra is pulled upward, which constricts its orifice and impedes the flow of urine. Urine flow is further restricted by the urethral sphincter muscle, which contracts under a steady background stimulation by sympathetic fibers during the filling phase. Thus, sympathetic activity has two effects: relaxation of the detrusor muscle and contraction of the urethral sphincter.

The switch from the filling to the emptying phase is triggered by tension in the bladder wall. As the bladder reaches capacity, it can no longer passively expand. Tension in the wall rapidly increases, which stimulates stretch receptors (slowly adapting mechanoreceptors) within the bladder wall. Signals originating in the stretch receptors are carried by Aδ afferent fibers from the bladder to the sacral spinal cord via the pelvic nerves. The axons of these afferent fibers are distributed over several segments (approximately L4 to S4) in the dorsolateral fasciculus (Lissauer's tract) before synapsing in laminae I, V, VII, and X. From the spinal cord signals conveying bladder tension ascend to the brainstem, where they synapse in the PAG. Signals descending from the PAG synapse in a small nucleus in the pons, the **pontine micturition center** (PMC). Finally, axons originating in the PMC descend to the lumbosacral spinal cord, where they synapse on the preganglionic sympathetic and parasympathetic neurons. Therefore, the reflex loop moves from the spinal cord to the pons and back to the spinal cord (Fig. 13.6).

The descending activity from the PMC inhibits the preganglionic sympathetic neurons. This inhibition releases the active contraction of the urethral sphincter and removes the inhibition from the detrusor muscle, preparing the system for emptying. A few seconds after the sympathetic activity is inhibited by the PMC, an increase in parasympathetic activity actively contracts the detrusor muscle. Contraction of the detrusor not only squeezes the body of the bladder but also extends its base, giving it a funnel shape. This change in shape enlarges the urethral orifice, facilitating the flow of urine.

## Supraspinal Control of Micturition

The smooth coordination that characterizes the switch between the filling and emptying phases of micturition is brought about by the PMC and PAG (Fig. 13.6). The PAG, which receives information from the spinal cord that signals bladder fullness, also receives descending information from the preoptic area of the hypothalamus. Although the nature of the hypothalamic signal is unknown, the supraoptic-PAG connection probably represents the final common descending pathway for a number of factors that modify the fundamental micturition reflex. One of these factors is, of course, voluntary control. In humans, voluntary control is a necessary social function. Other animals control micturition to mark areas of their territory with urine. Another factor that affects the control of micturition is the emotional state of the animal. For example, micturition is strongly suppressed during sexual arousal and copulation but may occur involuntarily during moments of extreme fright. Also, some animals, such as the dog, micturate as a sign of submission. Therefore, the PAG appears to be an important area in the brainstem where the descending signals controlling micturition are integrated with the ascending sensory signals.

Voluntary micturition is also regulated through a small pontine nucleus lateral to the PMC. Simply called the **L region**, this nucleus sends axons to the sacral spinal cord. Here they synapse in the **nucleus of Onuf**, the motor nucleus in lamina IX that controls the voluntary striated muscles of the urethral sphincter. A number of cortical areas have been implicated in the control of micturition and presumably the innervation of the L region, but the relevant pathways have yet to be discovered.

## Disruption of Micturition

Four distinct alterations in micturition can be caused by lesions to the nervous system. First, lesions to the lumbosacral spinal cord that destroy the preganglionic sympathetic and parasympathetic neurons or their axons abolish the micturition reflex. Furthermore, loss of sympathetic efferent fibers greatly diminishes sphincter tone, producing incontinence. Finally, since the pons can no longer communicate with the spinal cord, the patient has no voluntary control over micturition. This areflexia is temporary, however, because denervation of the peripheral autonomic ganglia stimulates reorganization of the peripheral

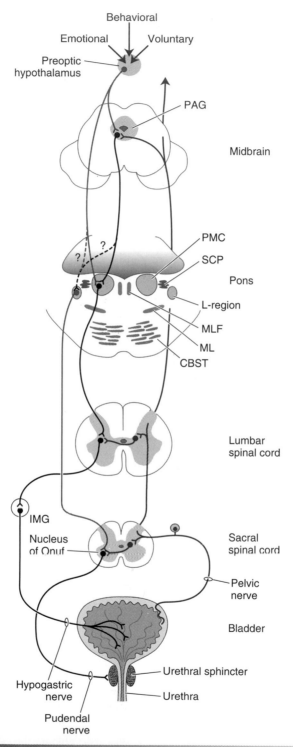

## Figure 13.6  Pathways that control micturition

The principal reflex pathway is indicated with *heavy lines;* sensory pathways are shown in *pink,* motor in *black.*
*PAG,* periaqueductal gray; *PMC,* pontine micturition center; *MLF,* medial longitudinal fasciculus; *ML,* medial
lemniscus; *CBST,* corticobulbospinal tract; *SCP,* superior cerebellar peduncle; *IMG,* inferior mesenteric ganglion.

innervation of the bladder and sphincter. Denervation of the parasympathetic postganglionic neurons that reside in the bladder stimulates the up-regulation of α-receptors in the detrusor smooth muscle. Denervation also prompts axons of sympathetic postganglionic neurons to sprout new collateral fibers that are attracted to the new α-receptors in the muscle and that fill the synaptic voids on the postganglionic parasympathetic neurons created by denervation. Thus the bladder and sphincter become overdriven by sympathetic fibers, which increases tension in the detrusor muscle and the sphincter simultaneously. Voiding becomes difficult or impossible; frequent catheterization is required. Internal bladder pressure can also increase, leading to increased pressure throughout the entire urinary tract that can result in serious kidney damage.

Second, lesions between the lumbar spinal cord and the pons produce an areflexic bladder and a permanent loss of voluntary control of micturition. The areflexia is temporary, however. Synapses reorganize, shifting the balance between local, spinal, and pontine control. Eventually reflex micturition emerges, but it is poorly regulated because of the lack of signals from the PMC and L region. However, the greatest difficulty that stems from this type of lesion is caused by the loss of supraspinal control of the urethral sphincter muscle, which remains contracted when the detrusor muscle contracts. This sustained urethral contraction results in incomplete bladder emptying. Not only does the sphincter not fully relax during voiding, but it frequently relaxes and contracts rhythmically and involuntarily, producing an interrupted stream. Since bladder emptying is incomplete, cystitis and urinary tract infections are common.

Third, lesions between the hypothalamus and the pons make voluntary delays of micturition difficult or impossible. The micturition reflex itself and the desire to regulate its timing remain intact. However, loss of forebrain control severs the link between desire and accomplishment. Patients feel an extreme urgency to urinate that they often cannot delay.

Fourth, lesions to the prefrontal lobes often result in incontinence. Again, the micturition reflex is intact. However, the *desire* to control micturition seems to be absent with the loss of the prefrontal lobes.

## SEXUAL RESPONSE

The physical responses to sexual arousal require both sympathetic and parasympathetic innervation. In general, parasympathetic activity increases the secretions from the glands associated with the genital tract and promotes the engorgement of erectile tissue with blood. Sympathetic activity stimulates smooth muscle contraction.

Men require penile erection for copulation, and failure to achieve erection is a common and disturbing medical condition. Erection is due to increased blood flow into the corpus cavernosum, which causes it to swell and become rigid. Stimulation of the genitalia or erotic stimuli descending to the spinal cord from supraspinal levels increase the parasympathetic activity in the pudendal nerves that supply the penis. The parasympathetic activity causes the release of nitric oxide in the region of the precapillary sphincter muscles of the afferent arterioles in the penis. Nitric oxide is a potent vasodilator because it causes smooth muscle relaxation. Blood flow to the erectile tissue increases, producing erection.

Continued tactile and erotic stimuli also increase sympathetic activity, which contracts the smooth muscles of the vas deferens and seminal vesicles. This contraction brings **seminal fluid** into the posterior urethra, a process known as **emission**. At the same time, parasympathetic activity causes the prostate and bulbourethral glands to produce secretions that mix with the seminal fluid in the urethra to form **semen** [L. *semen,* seed]. Sympathetic activity facilitated by the continued tactile stimulation of the penile shaft and glans penis, together with continued supraspinal erotic stimuli, culminates in abrupt, spasmatic contractions of the periurethral, bulbocavernosus, and ischiocavernosus muscles and perineal musculature, causing **ejaculation** [L. *ejacto,* shoot out] of semen from the penis. These muscles are thought to be under both sympathetic and parasympathetic control. Parasympathetic activity subsides after ejaculation. The production of nitric oxide ceases, allowing the precapillary sphincter muscles in the penis to contract in response to noradrenaline (NA) released by the still-active sympathetic fibers that also supply the penis. Detumescence follows rapidly as blood drains from the corpus cavernosum.

Like micturition, the coordination of the various stages of the male sexual response requires careful coordination between the parasympathetic and sympathetic autonomic systems. The CNS structures responsible for this coordination are not well understood. Much of the coordination is assumed to occur in the lumbar and sacral spinal cord. But higher centers must also be involved, since erotic stimuli play such an important role in the sexual response. The location of these centers and the pathways by which they are interconnected remain to be elucidated.

Female sexual responses are very similar to those in the male. Although the neurophysiological basis for the female sexual response is presumed to be similar to that of the male, it is far less well studied.

### The Adrenal Medulla

The autonomic innervation of the adrenal medulla deserves special consideration because the **chromaffin cells** of the adrenal medulla are derived from the neuroectoderm of the neural crest. Chromaffin cells are highly modified neurons that secrete catecholamines directly into the bloodstream. The adrenal medulla is innervated by preganglionic sympathetic fibers that originate in the intermediolateral cell column at T8 to T11 and synapse directly on the chromaffin cells. Since the chromaffin cells of the adrenal medulla develop from the neural crest and migrate into the periphery, as do the cells that become the postganglionic neurons of the chain ganglia and collateral ganglia, *chromaffin cells are homologous to the neurons in the chain and collateral ganglia.* As such, these secretory cells of the adrenal medulla mark an interface between the nervous system and the vasculature whereby the nervous system can secrete its neurotransmitters directly into the bloodstream. The neurotransmitters epinephrine and norepinephrine thus act both as hormones and as neurotransmitters.

## AUTONOMIC AFFERENTS

The ANS also contains sensory axons. Some of these axons are nociceptors that are responsible for pain referred from the viscera (see Chapter 5). Another form of visceral pain that is often overlooked is pain derived from nociceptors in blood vessels, especially the arteries. Vascular nociceptors respond to ischemia (for example, ligation of an artery or an arterial thrombosis is painful) and to the injection of certain irritating substances. **Raynaud's syndrome** is characterized by a reflex vasoconstriction that results in severe ischemic pain in the affected extremities, usually the hands. The reflex vasoconstriction may be triggered by exposure to cold or emotional stress, or it may be caused by systemic disease that affects the peripheral nerves.

## PHYSIOLOGY OF THE ANS

The discussion of the autonomic innervation of the various organs reveals that sympathetic and parasympathetic activity usually produce antagonistic physiological effects. For example, sympathetic activity increases the heart rate and strength of contraction; parasympathetic activity decreases both.

Autonomic effects on target organs are not always consistent from one tissue to another. For example, sympathetic activity reduces blood flow to the gut and skin but increases blood flow to the deep muscles. Both parasympathetic and sympathetic activity increase salivation. Although it is tempting to generalize about autonomic activity, most such statements have significant exceptions. Despite these exceptions, it is fairly safe to say that the parasympathetic and sympathetic systems have contradictory actions, and thus *the net physiological effect of autonomic activity rests on the balance of activity between the two systems.*

As previous chapters show, the nervous system functions primarily through the essential competition between excitation and inhibition. In the voluntary nervous system this competition occurs at the synaptic interfaces between neurons. The ebb and flow of postsynaptic currents reflects the inhibitory-excitatory competition. In the ANS competitive interaction takes place at the effector organ, where the struggle is resolved not through postsynaptic potentials but in the final physiological effect on the organ itself.

The dichotomy of autonomic function is reflected in the types of neurotransmitters used by the sympathetic and parasympathetic systems. Although the preganglionic axons of each system use ACh and the postganglionic parasympathetic axons also liberate ACh, the postganglionic fibers of the sympathetic system secrete catecholamines. In addition to these classic neurotransmitters, preganglionic fibers corelease a number of neuroactive peptides that modulate the postganglionic cell's response to ACh. To complicate matters fur-

ther, there are a number of receptors for ACh and norepinephrine, each producing quite different physiological effects. The two major classes of cholinergic receptors, **nicotinic** and **muscarinic** [L. *musca,* key], are so named because they were originally differentiated by their ability to bind these chemicals. Today subcategories of each of these receptors are now recognized. The two main classes of norepinephrine receptors, **α-receptors** and **β-receptors**, also contain subcategories.

In autonomic ganglia, nicotinic cholinergic receptors are found on all of the postganglionic neurons. By opening sodium ion channels, ACh binding to these receptors produces in the postsynaptic cell a fast (about 20 msec) excitatory postsynaptic potential (EPSP) that usually results in an action potential (Fig. 13.7). If this receptor is blocked with a competitive antagonist, transmission through the ganglion ceases.

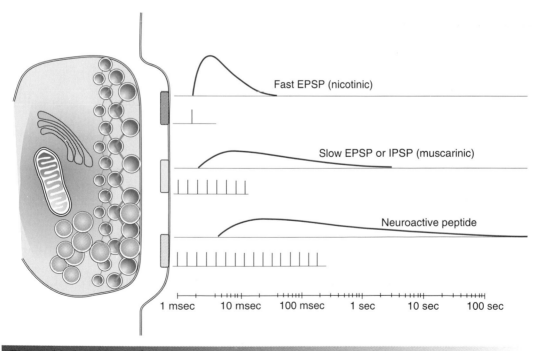

**Figure 13.7 PSPs in the autonomic nervous system**

The PSPs evoked in a postganglionic cell vary greatly according to the available neurotransmitter and receptor. Acting through nicotinic receptors, ACh develops fast, short-acting EPSPs in response to a single afferent action potential. Acting through muscarinic receptors, ACh develops a longer lasting EPSP but requires a train of action potentials to activate the synapse. Neuroactive peptides develop very long-lasting PSPs and usually require long trains of stimuli to activate. The time course of the PSPs vary over approximately five orders of magnitude.

In contrast to the fast nicotinic ACh receptor, muscarinic ACh receptors produce slow (about 2 seconds) postsynaptic potentials (PSPs). Since muscarinic receptors function through second-messenger systems (see Chapter 3), their effects are usually slower to develop and longer lasting than those produced by nicotinic receptors. The PSPs produced by muscarinic receptors may be excitatory or inhibitory, depending on the type of receptor expressed on the postsynaptic cell. In either case the PSPs are produced only in response to trains of incoming action potentials; isolated action potentials have little effect on the muscarinic receptors.

High-frequency trains of action potentials are also required to promote the release of neuroactive peptides, which produce very slow (about 4 minutes) EPSPs in the postsynaptic neuron. Peptides used as neurotransmitters are not inactivated immediately after their release; they diffuse within the interstitial space and affect other postsynaptic neurons as paracrines. This paracrine effect (see Chapter 3) is a common feature of neuropeptide signaling in autonomic ganglia. Finally, within the autonomic ganglia, chromaffin cells act as dopamine-releasing interneurons.

These cells, which are activated by incoming preganglionic axons, inhibit the postganglionic neurons.

The target organs contain a variety of receptors, most commonly among the adrenergic receptors. Some of the diverse effects of sympathetic activation can be explained by the type of receptors expressed. For example, sympathetic neurons, by releasing norepinephrine, cause vasoconstriction in the visceral organs and the skin because the smooth muscle of the arterioles express α-receptors. The blood vessels in the deep muscles, however, express β-receptors, and sympathetic activity dilates them. Heart muscle also expresses β-receptors. The effects of sympathetic stimulation on heart rate and contractility can be selectively inhibited by so-called β-blockers, pharmacological antagonists that specifically bind to the β-receptors. Finally, any tissue that expresses adrenergic receptors can respond to circulating catecholamines. Through its ability to control secretions from the adrenal medulla, the ANS can function as an endocrine organ. The adrenal medulla in turn can rapidly and globally reinforce the neuronal sympathetic effect by enhancing its secretion of NA.

## SUMMARY

- There are three divisions of the ANS: sympathetic, parasympathetic, and enteric.

The peripheral components of the parasympathetic system are composed of a long efferent preganglionic axon that originates in certain cranial nerve nuclei or in the intermediolateral cell column in the sacral spinal cord.

- The preganglionic axon synapses in or near the target organ, from which a short postganglionic axon innervates the target tissue.

The peripheral components of the sympathetic system are composed of a short efferent preganglionic axon that originates in the intermediolateral cell column in the sacral spinal cord.

- The preganglionic axon synapses either in the spinal chain ganglia or a collateral ganglion from which a long postganglionic axon emerges to innervate the target tissue.

Preganglionic neurons secrete ACh; postganglionic parasympathetic neurons secrete ACh, but postganglionic sympathetic neurons secrete NA. There are several different receptors for each transmitter.

- The ANS is closely regulated by CNS structures.

The hypothalamus is the principal CNS division that regulates autonomic function. Three tracts carry information from the hypothalamus to the brainstem and spinal ANS motor neurons pools: the DLF, mammillotegmental tract, and MFB.

- All of the organ systems of the body receive both sympathetic and parasympathetic innervation.

ANS lesions often produce specific dysfunctions and syndromes. Among the most important are pupillary dysfunction, cardiac dysrhythmias, gastric motility dysfunction, dysfunction of micturition, dysfunction of sexual performance, and Horner's and Raynaud's syndromes.

- ANS functions are based on the balance of antagonistic functions between the sympathetic and parasympathetic divisions.

In ANS, the balance between excitation and inhibition occurs at the organ level in contrast to the CNS, where it occurs at the cellular level.

## SUGGESTED READINGS

Burnett AL. Nitric oxide control of lower genitourinary tract functions: a review. Urology 1995; 45:1071–1083.

Blok BFM, Holstege G. The neuronal control of micturition and its relation to the emotional motor system. Prog Brain Res 1996;107:113–126.

deGroat WC, Kruse MNC, Vizzard MA, et al. Modification of urinary bladder function after spinal cord injury. Adv Neurol 1997;72:347–364.

Watson C, Vijayan N. The synaptic innervation of the eyes and face: a clinicoanatomic review. Clin Anat 1995;8:262–272.

# The Hypothalamus
# and Associated Systems

The **hypothalamus** [G. *hypo-*, under, and *thalamos*, bedchamber] is a small division of the diencephalon. It has connections with many parts of the central nervous system (CNS), including the pituitary gland, hippocampus, amygdaloid nuclei, thalamus, brainstem, spinal cord, and the frontal lobes of the cerebral cortex, to name just the most important areas. Although the diverse structures with which the hypothalamus makes connections have equally diverse functions, they share one feature: all play important roles in maintaining a stable internal environment, or homeostasis. The hypothalamus coordinates the homeostatic activity of these diverse structures.

The constancy of the internal milieu is maintained by *local, nervous, hormonal,* and *behavioral* mechanisms. The interplay of these four mechanisms is essential to the long-range survival of the organism. The regulation of blood flow provides an excellent example of this interplay. Blood flow in capillary beds is regulated by precapillary sphincters. These muscles are influenced by a number of *local*, or **paracrine**, factors, including local pH and oxygen, carbon dioxide, and nitric oxide tension. Blood flow may be shunted from one large capillary bed to another by the action of the *nervous system*, as for example when blood flow to the digestive organs is reduced in favor of the deep muscles and vice versa. Circulating *hormones*, such as angiotensin II, influence blood pressure in the organism by causing massive peripheral vasoconstriction. Finally, *behavioral*

*responses*, such as lying down on feeling faint, help to restore blood flow to the brain.

The hypothalamus organizes whole-body homeostasis by means of three of the four mechanisms. First, through its descending connections with the brainstem and spinal cord, the hypothalamus *controls and regulates the autonomic nervous system* (ANS). Second, the hypothalamus itself *is an endocrine organ*. Substances released from hypothalamic neurons into the bloodstream control and regulate a number of physiological and endocrine functions. Finally, through its connections with forebrain structures, the hypothalamus *plays an important although poorly understood role in regulating the behavior of the organism*. This chapter considers each of these three functions, the associated anatomy of the hypothalamus, and its connections with other regions of the nervous system.

## GROSS ANATOMY OF THE HYPOTHALAMUS

The hypothalamus, a subdivision of the diencephalon, lies on either side of the most ventral reaches of the third ventricle. It is separated from the thalamus by the **hypothalamic sulcus** (Fig. 14.1). At its rostral pole the hypothalamus is bounded by the **lamina terminalis** [L. *lamina*, a plate, leaf, layer, and *terminalis*, marking a boundary], a thin sheet of nervous tissue that constitutes the remains of the anterior pole of the neural tube and in the adult, separates the

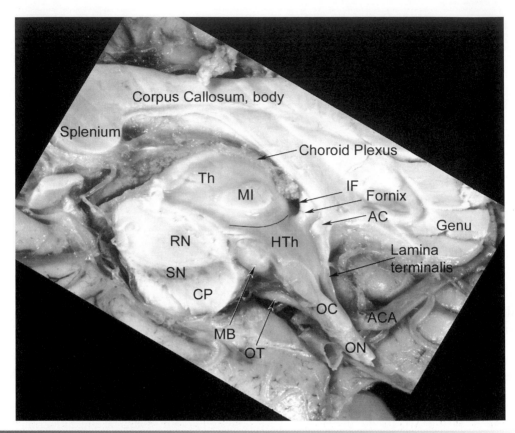

**Figure 14.1    The hypothalamus**

The midline structures of the brain are viewed in this midsagittal section through the third ventricle. *AC*, anterior commissure; *ACA*, anterior cerebral artery; *CP*, cerebral peduncle; *HTh*, hypothalamus; *IF*, intraventricular foramen (leading into the lateral ventricle); *MI*, massa intermedia; *MB*, mammillary body; *OC*, optic chiasm; *ON*, optic nerve; *OT*, optic tract; *RN*, red nucleus; *SN*, substantia nigra; *Th*, thalamus.

diencephalon from the telencephalon. The optic chiasm and optic tracts cradle the anterior portion of the hypothalamus and serve as important landmarks by which many hypothalamic structures are identified. The **mammillary bodies** [L. *mammila,* breast, nipple] mark the most posterior extent of the hypothalamus. Internally, the hypothalamus is bounded to the posterior by the subthalamus.

The inferior portion of the hypothalamus narrows to a small neck, the **tuber cinereum** [L. *tuber,* protuberance, swelling, and *cinereum,* ash-colored ointment]. The most inferior portion of the tuber cinereum, the **median eminence** [L. *emineo,* stick up, stand out, project, protrude], which is slightly swollen, underlies the third ventricle. The median eminence blends into the **infundibular stalk** [L. *in-*

*fundibulum,* funnel], which is continuous with the posterior lobe of the **hypophysis** [G. *hypo-,* under, and *phyein,* grow], or **pituitary gland** [L. *pituita,* phlegm or mucus].

The hypophysis is composed of an anterior and a posterior division. The median eminence, infundibulum, and posterior division of the pituitary gland are known as the **neurohypophysis.** The neurohypophysis is not composed of glandular tissue but is actually an extension of the CNS (see Appendix 1). The anterior portion of the pituitary gland is called the **adenohypophysis** [G. *adenos,* gland]. It is composed of two major divisions, the **pars tuberalis,** which has no endocrinological function, and the **pars distalis,** the secretory portion of the gland. Between these two divisions of the hypophysis lies the **pars intermedia,** a portion of the gland that is poorly developed in humans (see Appendix 1).

The hypothalamus can be divided into a number of regions. Imaginary frontal planes divide the hypothalamus into three regions (Fig. 14.2) The most rostral is the **anterior region**. It is composed of the area of the hypothalamus immediately superior to the optic tracts and chiasm. The **tuberal region** lies over the tuber cinereum; the **posterior region** includes the mammillary bodies and the part of the hypothalamus immediately superior to them. The hypothalamus can also be divided into a **medial** and **lateral** part by an imaginary sagittal plane passing through the **fornix** [L. *fornix,* arch] (Fig. 14.3). Consequently, each

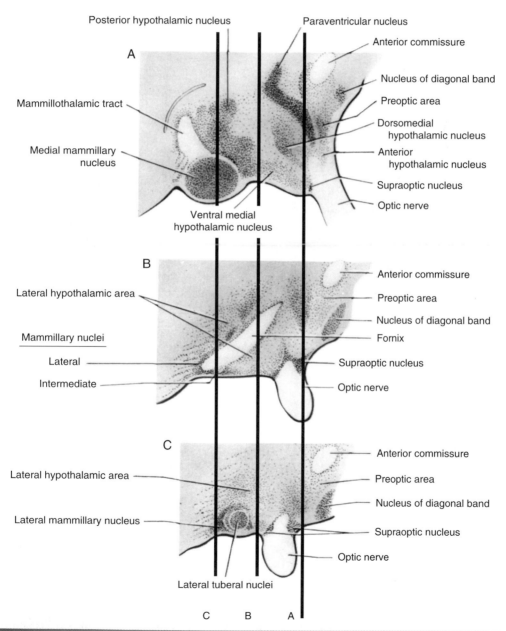

**Figure 14.2   Sagittal view of the nuclei of the hypothalamus**

Lines *A, B,* and *C* correspond to the planes shown in Figure 14.3. (Reprinted with permission from Carpenter MB, Sutin J. Human Neuroanatomy. Baltimore: Williams & Wilkins, 1983.)

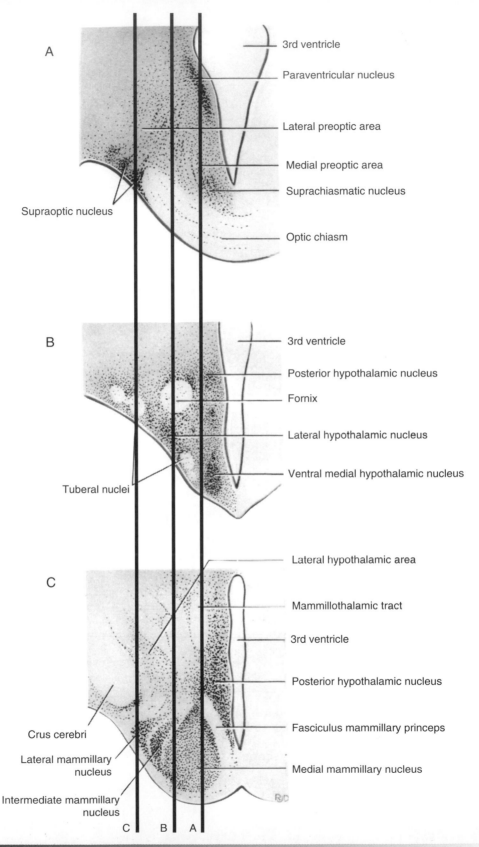

A

3rd ventricle
Paraventricular nucleus
Lateral preoptic area
Medial preoptic area
Suprachiasmatic nucleus
Supraoptic nucleus
Optic chiasm

B

3rd ventricle
Posterior hypothalamic nucleus
Fornix
Lateral hypothalamic nucleus
Ventral medial hypothalamic nucleus
Tuberal nuclei

C

Lateral hypothalamic area
Mammillothalamic tract
3rd ventricle
Posterior hypothalamic nucleus
Crus cerebri
Fasciculus mammillary princeps
Lateral mammillary nucleus
Medial mammillary nucleus
Intermediate mammillary nucleus

C   B   A

**Figure 14.3   Frontal view of the nuclei of the hypothalamus**

Lines *A, B,* and *C* correspond to the planes shown in Figure 14.2. (Reprinted with permission from Carpenter MB, Sutin J. Human neuroanatomy. Baltimore: Williams & Wilkins, 1983.)

**Table 14.1  Principal Nuclei of the Hypothalamus**

| Region of the Hypothalamus | Nuclei |
| --- | --- |
| Anterior | Preoptic |
| | Suprachiasmatic |
| | Supraoptic |
| | Anterior |
| | Paraventricular |
| Tuberal | Dorsomedial |
| | Ventral medial |
| | Arcuate |
| Posterior | Posterior |
| | Mammillary |

half of the hypothalamus can be divided into six compartments. Most of the named nuclei of the hypothalamus lie in the medial compartments. The principal named nuclei in each region are listed in Table 14.1.

## HYPOTHALAMIC CONNECTIONS WITH THE ENDOCRINE SYSTEM

The distinctions traditionally drawn between the endocrine and nervous systems have become increasingly blurred as our understanding of their physiological roles broadened. Both systems are regulatory. The endocrine system generally regulates the internal milieu by means of blood-borne chemical signals that modify metabolism, reproductive states, digestion, and electrolyte balance. These hormonal signals reach every cell in the body; the specificity of their action depends on the receptors expressed by the target cells. The nervous system regulates these same physiological systems by means of electrical signals that reach their targets by nerve axons. Although widely distributed, individual neurons do not reach every cell in the body. Nervous system specificity relies on the anatomical relations between neurons and target cells. Both endocrine and nervous systems depend on delicately balanced negative feedback mechanisms to achieve their regulatory goals.

The primary criterion for distinguishing between the two systems, electrical versus chemical signaling, breaks down when it is realized that neurons are essentially secretory cells. All neurons secrete neurotransmitters as a means of signaling other neurons and regulating secretory glands. Most neurons secrete neurotransmitters that affect only the cell on which they are released, although some neurotransmitters diffuse beyond the synaptic cleft and affect nearby neurons, as in the autonomic ganglia (see Chapter 13). A few neurons secrete neurotransmitters directly into the bloodstream, in which case the neurotransmitter can exert its influence in the manner of a hormone. Chapter 13 discusses one example, the secretion of norepinephrine from the chromaffin cells of the adrenal medulla. Other examples are discussed later in this chapter.

It is often assumed that the CNS is beyond the reach of the endocrine system because of the blood-brain barrier, which isolates the CNS from certain blood-borne substances. Recent evidence, however, refutes this assumption. The circumventricular organs (CVOs) (see Chapter 1) are specific areas in the brain where the blood-brain barrier is greatly modified or simply does not exist. Cells in these organs are endowed with special receptive properties that enable them to serve as hormonal-neuronal transducers. Furthermore, secretion directly into the cerebrospinal fluid (CSF) provides yet another means by which the brain can be affected by circulating chemical signals. The brain's ability to secrete regulatory chemicals into the bloodstream and CSF and its ability to respond to chemical signals in the blood and CSF clearly qualifies the brain, at least in part, as an endocrine organ.

It is convenient to define a **hormone** [G. *hormon*, urging one, fr. *hormao*, urge, stir up, excite] as a chemical signal that is conveyed to its target by the bloodstream or the CSF; a **neurotransmitter** is a chemical signal that is restricted in its extracellular distribution to the synaptic cleft or interstitial fluid space. According to these definitions, certain secretory products, such as norepinephrine and enkephalin, can be both a hormone and a neurotransmitter, depending on their mode of release.

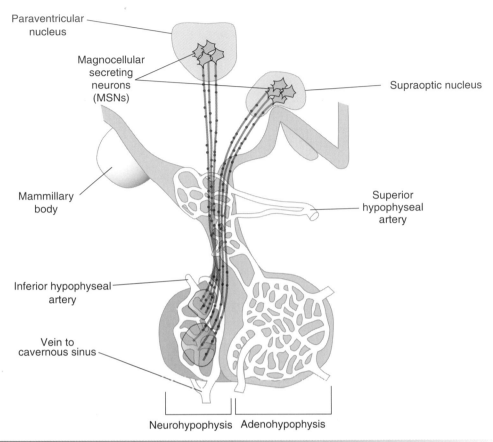

Paraventricular nucleus

Magnocellular secreting neurons (MSNs)

Supraoptic nucleus

Mammillary body

Superior hypophyseal artery

Inferior hypophyseal artery

Vein to cavernous sinus

Neurohypophysis    Adenohypophysis

**Figure 14.4    The neurohypophysis**

Location of MSNs in the hypothalamus and their association with the posterior hypophysis. The posterior hypophysis is not an endocrine gland; it is simply a specialized capillary bed that receives the hormones delivered to it from the hypothalamus to be released into the general circulation.

The endocrinological role of the brain is an enormous topic that can be presented here only in abbreviated form. A more extensive discussion of this subject can be found in the suggested readings. By means of introduction, the endocrine role of the brain is most clearly demonstrated in the relation between the hypothalamus and the hypophysis. A brief discussion of this topic follows.

**The Neurohypophysis**

Two nuclei in the hypothalamus, the **supraoptic** and **paraventricular nuclei**, contain large cells that send axons into the neurohypophysis (Fig. 14.4). These cells, known as **magnocellular-secreting neurons** (MSNs), produce **antidiuretic hormone** (ADH) and **oxytocin** [G. *oxys*,

sharp, keen, and *tokos*, birth, and -*in*, a suffix denoting an activator] from precursor peptides. Synthesized as a prohormone that is packaged in large 1200- to 2000-Å diameter vesicles, the precursor peptide is cleaved into the active hormone and a related peptide, **neurophysin**, within the vesicle as it is transported along the axon. Some of the MSNs produce oxytocin and its companion peptide neurophysin I. Others produce ADH and neurophysin II. None of the MSNs produce both sets of hormones simultaneously. The hormone-containing vesicles are transported along the magnocellular axons to the neurohypophysis. In response to electrical activity, the axons release the hormones into the perivascular space of the neurohypophysis. From there the hormones diffuse into the bloodstream by passing through fenestrated capillaries.

## OXYTOCIN

The circulating hormone oxytocin has two principal physiological effects: it initiates milk letdown from the mammary glands and causes contraction of the uterine muscles during parturition. Oxytocin effects the release of milk by inducing the contraction of the myoepithelial cells of the mammary glands. Suck-

ling by the infant produces tactile stimuli that reach the hypothalamus by neuronal pathways that have not been clearly delineated (Fig. 14.5). The suckling stimuli produce bursts of electrical activity in MSNs that cause the release of oxytocin into the neurohypophysis, where it enters the bloodstream. Approximately 13 seconds after oxytocin is released into the neurohypophysis, intramammary pressure increases as milk enters the ducts of the gland.

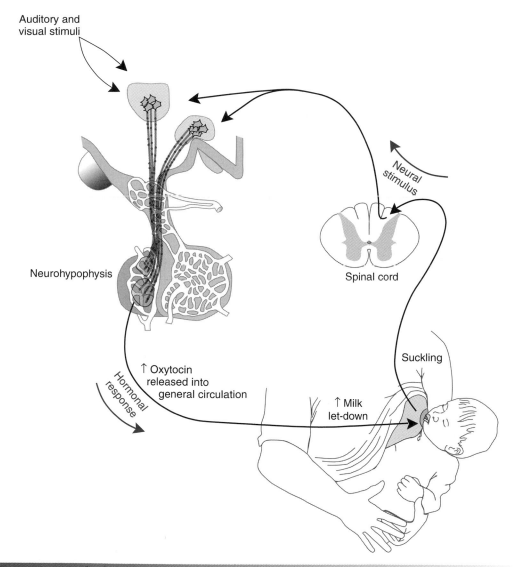

Auditory and visual stimuli

Neural stimulus

Neurohypophysis

Spinal cord

Suckling

↑ Oxytocin released into general circulation

Hormonal response

↑ Milk let-down

**Figure 14.5   The lactation reflex**

The lactation reflex is a mixed neuronal and endocrinological reflex. The afferent side of the reflex loop is neural; the efferent side is endocrinological.

The afferent path of the milk letdown reflex is neural, which makes it possible for other neural signals to interact in the hypothalamus and modify the reflex. For example, the reflex is facilitated by specific auditory and visual cues. Every lactating mother has experienced milk ejection in response to the cry of her hungry child. The reflex can also be inhibited by anxiety, a fact that sometimes interferes with initiation and full development of lactation.

Oxytocin also stimulates powerful contractions of the myometrium. Evidence suggests that the initiation and progression of labor are closely related to biochemical events associated with the fetus, placenta, and chorionic membranes. Oxytocin itself does not initiate labor, but its release during parturition enhances the strength and frequency of uterine contractions. This release is controlled by a positive feedback loop. Pressure on the cervix is transmitted by neurons to the hypothalamus. This signal prompts the secretion of oxytocin, which is carried to the uterus by the bloodstream. Oxytocin increases the strength of uterine contractions, which in turn increases the pressure on the cervix.

## ANTIDIURETIC HORMONE

ADH is a circulating hormone that increases the permeability of the collecting duct cell membranes in the kidney. This increased permeability allows water and electrolytes to be reabsorbed into the circulation. Without ADH the kidney produces copious amounts of a very dilute urine, a condition known as **diabetes insipidus** [G. *diabetes,* passing through, and L. *insipiens,* unsavory, lacking flavor or zest]. ADH is only one of many factors that are important in the closely intertwined mechanisms of blood volume regulation, electrolyte balance, and blood pressure regulation. The MSNs neurons that release ADH into the bloodstream are influenced by several feedback systems that control the firing rate of these neurons and consequently the release of ADH. Three of these systems are described next (Fig. 14.6).

First, although the MSNs in the hypothalamus appear to be directly sensitive to plasma osmolarity, they also receive afferent connec-tions from the **organum vasculosum** (OV) [G. *organon,* instrument, organ of the body, and L. *vasculum,* small vessel]. This CVO is exquisitely sensitive to plasma osmolarity because of its unusually permeable capillaries. Axons leaving the OV stimulate the secretion of ADH from MSNs. Increased plasma osmolarity also causes the sensation of thirst and induces drinking behavior. Experimental destruction of the OV in rats decreases their ADH secretion and renders them **adipic** [G. *a,* negative prefix, and *dipsa,* thirst]. The diabetes insipidus causes them to excrete a very dilute urine. Without compensatory drinking, the animals become chronically hypernatremic [G. *hyper-,* above, and L. *natrium,* sodium].

Second, another CVO, the **subfornical organ** (SFO), is sensitive to circulating levels of the hormone **angiotensin II**, which causes an increase in the secretion of ADH by acting through connections between the SFO and the MSNs of the supraoptic and paraventricular nuclei. Angiotensin II plays a key role in blood pressure regulation, electrolyte balance, and maintenance of blood volume. It is the product of a chemical cascade that is initiated by the release of the hormone renin from the kidney in response to a decrease in perfusion pressure of the glomerulus, decreased sodium at the macula densa, or a decrease in extracellular fluid volume. Angiotensin II causes peripheral vasoconstriction, which dramatically increases blood pressure; it is the most potent pressor hormone. It also causes the release of aldosterone, the mineralocorticoid that facilitates sodium ion absorption by amiloride-sensitive sodium channels. In the hypothalamus angiotensin II facilitates the release of ADH. Together, all of these mechanisms constitute an appropriate response to the decrease in blood pressure and blood volume that results from hemorrhage.

Third, blood pressure and oxygen tension affect the release of ADH. Signals from the carotid bodies and aortic arch reach the hypothalamus from the nucleus of the solitary tract (see Chapter 10). These peripheral cardiovascular signals reach the MSNs of the hypothalamus, where the information they convey is integrated with the other relevant signals just discussed.

## The Adenohypophysis

Unlike the neurohypophysis, the adenohypophysis is a true endocrine gland. Cells within the gland secrete a variety of hormones directly into the bloodstream. The release of these hypophyseal hormones is regulated by hormones that are secreted by **parvocellular-secreting neurons (PSNs)** of the hypothalamus. Hence the adenohypophysis not only se-

cretes hormones but also is under direct hormonal control.

The adenohypophysis receives the hypothalamic hormones that regulate it via a specialized vascular system called the **hypophysioportal** [L. *porta,* gate, opening; concerning the portal system of the pituitary gland] **system** (Fig. 14.7). Arterial branches from the internal carotid arteries and from the circle of Willis

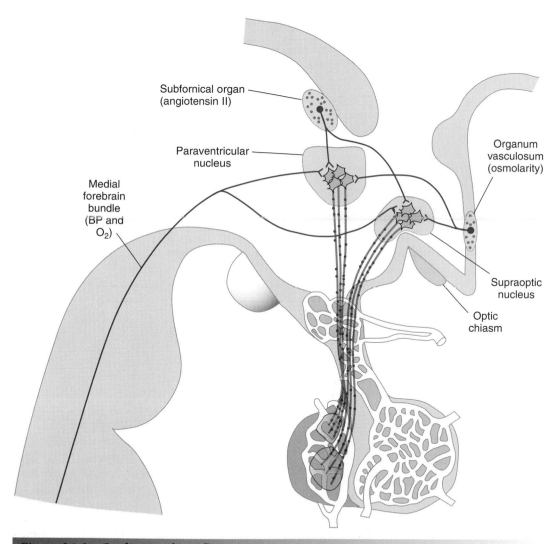

**Figure 14.6   Cardiovascular reflexes**

The release of ADH is regulated by at least three mechanisms. The subfornical organ is sensitive to plasma osmolality; the organum vasculosum detects circulating levels of angiotensin II. Both CVOs facilitate the release of ADH from the supraoptic and paraventricular nuclei. These nuclei are further regulated by ascending signals from the carotid bodies and aortic arch receptors. Therefore, ADH is under neural, endocrino*logical,* and osmolar regulation.

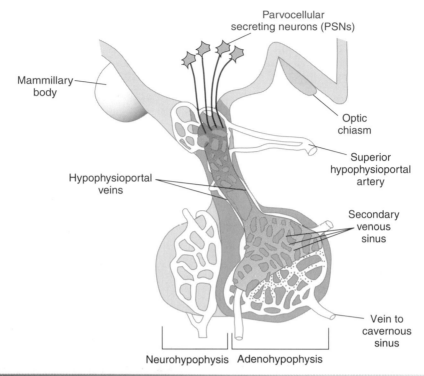

Parvocellular
secreting neurons (PSNs)

Mammillary
body

Optic
chiasm

Hypophysioportal
veins

Superior
hypophysioportal
artery

Secondary
venous
sinus

Vein to
cavernous
sinus

Neurohypophysis   Adenohypophysis

### Figure 14.7   The adenohypophysis

The adenohypophysis, a true endocrine gland, contains secretory cells regulated by hormones secreted into the blood by PSNs in the hypothalamus; these hormones are delivered to the anterior hypophysis by this restricted circulatory portal pathway.

### Table 14.2   Source of Hypothalamic-Releasing Hormones

| Nucleus | Releasing Hormones |
|---|---|
| Supraoptic | Oxytocin, ADH |
| Paraventricular | Oxytocin, ADH, CRH |
| Preoptic | GnRH |
| Septal | GnRH |
| Arcuate | GnRH, GHRH, PRIH |
| Periventricular | TRH, GHIH |

form a *primary capillary network* in the median eminence of the hypothalamus. Hypophyseal portal veins from this capillary network traverse the surface of the pars tuberalis to reach the pars distalis, where they form a *secondary venous sinus* within the gland. Emis-

sary veins from this secondary sinus drain into the cavernous sinus. PSNs of the hypothalamus send axons into the median eminence, where they *terminate on the primary capillaries of the hypophysioportal system.* Secretions from the hypothalamic neurons are carried by the bloodstream from the median eminence into the pars distalis, where these **hypothalamic-releasing hormones** diffuse from the secondary sinus bed to reach the secretory cells of the adenohypophysis (Table 14.2). The hormones of hypothalamic origin may inhibit or facilitate the release of hormones from the adenohypophyseal cells. Hormones secreted by the hypophyseal cells enter the emissary venous sinus of the gland and are carried into the general circulation.

Adenohypophyseal hormones are grouped into three classes based on their chemical structure: the **glycoprotein** hormones, the mammosomatotropic [G. *mamma*, breast; *soma*, body; and *trope*, turning] hormones and the **opiomelanocortin** [G. *opion*, opium; *melanos*, black, dark colored; and L. *cortex*, bark, covering] hormones. These hormones and their various releasing and inhibiting hormones are briefly considered next.

## THE GLYCOPROTEIN HORMONES

The **glycoprotein hormones**—thyroid-stimulating hormone (TSH), luteinizing hormone (LH), and follicle-stimulating hormone (FSH) consist of two protein subunits, each about 100 amino acids long. One subunit, the α-chain, is essentially identical in all three hormones. The β-chain is variable and accounts for the physiological specificity of the three hormones. Glycoprotein hormones also contain carbohydrate segments that not only are variable between hormones but can vary within the same hormone. For example, there are at least eight FSH molecules that differ only in their carbohydrate moieties. The significance of this variability is not known.

### Gonadotrophins: Luteinizing Hormone and Follicle-Stimulating Hormone

Although the names of the two gonadotrophins reflect their actions in the female, these hormones affect the reproductive organs in both males and females. **Follicle-stimulating hormone** (FSH) promotes the growth of follicles in the ovary. After the follicle matures, a surge of FSH secretion accompanied by an even greater surge of **luteinizing hormone** (LH) [L. *luteus*, yellow] secretion induces ovulation. Following ovulation, FSH and LH secretion return to baseline levels. In addition to promoting the development of the follicle and causing ovulation, FSH and LH induce the corpus luteum to produce steroid hormones, particularly **progesterone** and **estrogen** [G. *oistros*, mad desire, and *gennan*, to produce]. In the male, LH stimulates the interstitial (Leydig) cells[1] of the testes to produce testosterone, which is necessary for spermatogenesis and other male reproductive functions.

The secretion of LH and FSH is stimulated by **gonadotropin-releasing hormone** (GnRH) [G. *gone*, seed ], a small, 10-amino-acid protein produced in scattered parvocellular neurons of the **preoptic** and **septal** regions and in the **arcuate nucleus** [L. *arcuatus*, bowed, arc shaped] of the hypothalamus (Fig. 14.8). Axons from these areas descend into the median eminence, where they liberate GnRH into the capillary bed of the hypophysioportal system.

### Thyroid-Stimulating Hormone

**Thyroid-stimulating hormone** (TSH) acts on the follicular cells of the thyroid gland. Its secretion from the pituitary gland is stimulated by **thyrotropin-releasing hormone** (TRH). TRH, only three amino acids long, is perhaps the smallest peptide hormone. It is produced in the **periventricular nucleus**.

## THE MAMMOSOMATOTROPIC HORMONES

The second class of hormones, the **mammosomatotropic hormones** (growth hormone and prolactin), consist of an α-helical chain about 200 amino acids long.

### Growth Hormone

**Growth hormone** (GH) acts throughout the body to stimulate the growth of bone and affect the metabolism of cells. Its secretion is regulated by two hypothalamic hormones. **Growth hormone–releasing hormone** (GHRH) is produced in the arcuate nucleus (Fig. 14.9) and effects the release of GH from the anterior pituitary. **Growth hormone–inhibiting hormone** (GHIH, also known as **somatostatin**) is primarily produced in the periventricular nucleus, although it is also present in the supraoptic and paraventricular nuclei. As its name implies, GHIH inhibits the release of GH.

### Prolactin

**Prolactin** promotes the development of breast tissue and prompts milk production. Unique among the anterior pituitary hormones, prolactin appears to be exclusively regulated

---

[1] LH is sometimes called *interstitial–cell–stimulating hormone* (ICSH) when referring to the male reproductive system.

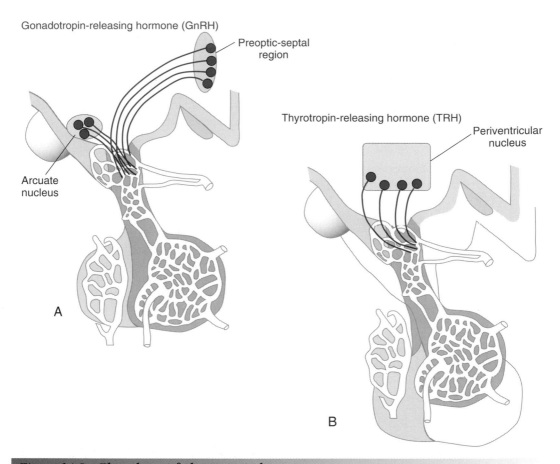

**Figure 14.8    The release of glycoprotein hormones**

Location of PSNs that synthesize GnRH (**A**) and TRH (**B**), hypothalamic hormones that regulate the secretion of the glycoprotein hormones.

by a release-inhibiting hormone, **prolactin release–inhibiting hormone** (PRIH). PRIH is not a protein; it is probably **dopamine**. It is secreted into the portal system by diffuse neurons in and near the arcuate nucleus.

## OPIOMELANOCORTIN HORMONES

The **opiomelanocortin hormones** (adrenocorticotrophic hormone [ACTH], melanocyte-stimulating hormone [MSH], β-lipotropin, and β-endorphin) are cleaved from a common prohormone, pro-opiomelanocortin. β-Endorphin is a neurotransmitter, and neurons secreting it are important in modulating the perception of pain (see Chapter 5). Only ACTH is normally secreted by the adenohypophysis. The physiological role of β-lipotropin and β-endorphin as hormones is not understood.

The adrenal cortex is an endocrine gland that produces several types of steroids, including **androgens, estrogens, progesterones**, and the major classes of **mineralocorticoids** and **glucocorticoids**. The secretion of mineralocorticoids is controlled and regulated primarily by the renin-angiotensin system. The secretion of glucocorticoids falls under the regulation and control of the adenohypophysis. ACTH is the pituitary hormone that affects the adrenal cortex by stimulating steroid synthesis. The release of ACTH is controlled by **corticotropin-releasing hormone** (CRH), a hormone produced in parvocellular neurons of the **paraventricular nucleus** and released in the capillary bed of the median eminence (Fig. 14.10). This nucleus also contains magnocellular neurons that secrete oxytocin and

ADH. Interestingly, the ability of CRH to effect the release of ACTH is potentiated by ADH, and the correlates of these hormones from the parvocellular neurons has been reported.

## Regulation of Hormone Secretion

Like the nervous system, the endocrine system is carefully regulated by negative feedback mechanisms that limit the effects of its actions within a very narrow range. Four types of negative feedback signals regulate the release of hormones from the adenohypophysis (Fig. 14.11). They are designated according to the nature of the feedback loop as long loop, short loop, or ultrashort loop. The long-loop systems are either direct or indirect.

### LONG-LOOP FEEDBACK

With the exception of prolactin, adenohypophyseal hormones all stimulate the release of circulating hormones or metabolic products that can affect the hypothalamus. For example, estrogen inhibits the release of GnRH by acting on the hypothalamus. Somatomedins, which are secreted by the liver in response to GH, facilitate the release of GHIH, which inhibits the further release of GH. This indirect signaling system (*hypothalamic releasing hormone→ hypophyseal hormone→circulating hormone→ hypothalamic releasing hormone*) is **indirect long-loop feedback**. This indirect signaling system is the principal means by which the adenohypophyseal hormones are regulated.

The secretion of hypophyseal hormones can also be regulated by the circulating hormone

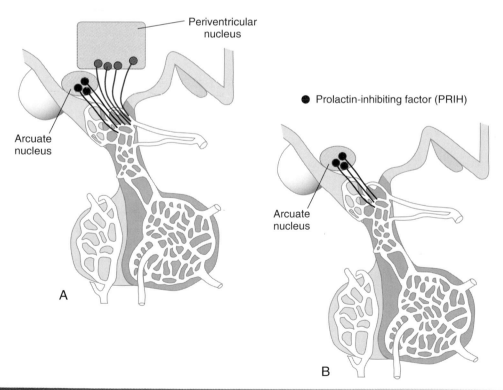

● Growth hormone-inhibiting hormone (GHIH)
● Growth hormone-releasing hormone (GHRH)

● Prolactin-inhibiting factor (PRIH)

Periventricular nucleus

Arcuate nucleus

A

Arcuate nucleus

B

**Figure 14.9   The release of mammosomatotropic hormones**

Location of PSNs that synthesize GHRH, GHIH (somatostatin) (**A**), and PRIH (probably dopamine) (**B**), hypothalamic hormones that regulate the secretion of the mammosomatotropic hormones.

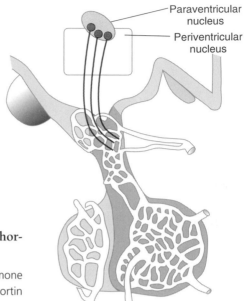

● Corticotropin-releasing hormone (CRH)

Paraventricular
nucleus

Periventricular
nucleus

**Figure 14.10   The release of opiomelanocortin hormones**

Location of PSNs that synthesize CRH, the hypothalamic hormone that regulates the secretion of ACTH, the only opiomelanocortin hormone secreted by the anterior hypophysis.

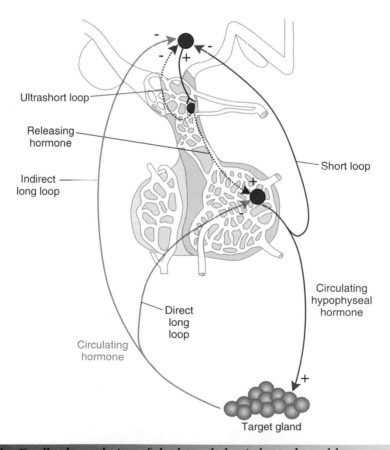

Ultrashort loop

Releasing hormone

Indirect long loop

Short loop

Circulating hypophyseal hormone

Direct long loop

Circulating hormone

Target gland

**Figure 14.11   Feedback regulation of the hypothalamic-hypophyseal hormone systems**

directly (*hypothalamic releasing hormone→ hypophyseal hormone→circulating hormone→ hypophyseal hormone*) by **direct long-loop feedback** to the adenohypophysis. For example, estrogen acts not only at the hypothalamus but also at the hypophysis to inhibit the release of LH and FSH. Direct feedback mechanisms appear to work by reducing the responsiveness of adenohypophyseal cells to releasing hormones rather than by limiting their intrinsic secretory capabilities. In effect, the circulating hormones "blind" the secretory cell to the releasing–hormone signal provided by the hypothalamus.

## SHORT-LOOP FEEDBACK

Under certain hydrodynamic circumstances, blood flow in the hypophysioportal system can reverse. When this occurs, hypophyseal hormones are carried back to the hypothalamus, where they can inhibit the secretion of releasing hormones. Therefore, hypophyseal hormones themselves are feedback signals that can affect the hypothalamus (*hypothalamic releasing hormone→hypophyseal hormone→ hypothalamic releasing hormone*). Such signaling is termed **short-loop feedback** because *it does not involve the general circulation*. Part of the regulation of gonadotrophins involves this short-loop inhibition of hypothalamic neurons. In another form of regulation, **ultra-short-loop feedback**, the presence of releasing hormones in the median eminence provides negative feedback paracrine regulation by inhibiting their own release from the hypothalamic neuron bouton.

## CONNECTIONS WITH FOREBRAIN STRUCTURES

The hypothalamus lies at a crucial place in the neuraxis. Descending influences from cortical areas converge at the hypothalamus to affect the most primitive survival functions of the organism, such as cardiovascular and temperature regulation, respiration, defense mechanisms, digestion, and reproduction. The hypothalamus also serves as a relay point from which ascending information relating to these survival functions can be distributed appropriately throughout the nervous system to be integrated with descending commands. These connections therefore incorporate behavioral mechanisms into the physiological homeostatic mechanisms of survival. For example, feeding behavior is an essential component of digestion. Seeking shade or digging a hole to uncover cooler earth, accompanied by panting, is an essential facet of temperature regulation. Foreplay (courtship) is essential to reproduction in many animals.

The role of the hypothalamus in the interplay between sensory experience and behavior is not understood, although much detail is known about its anatomy and physiology. Some of the more interesting experiments performed in this century have demonstrated how lesions to or stimulation of hypothalamic structures can trigger survival behavior. Results of these experiments should not be interpreted to mean that the hypothalamus is the "center" for behavioral motivation in the brain but rather that hypothalamic structures are intimately associated with other neural structures that can act together to release stereotypical behaviors. The hypothalamus probably affects behavior through reciprocal connections with cortical structures. Research has focused on the relations among the hypothalamus and the associated archicortex, paleocortex, and neocortex. The most important of these telencephalic structures are the amygdala, the hippocampal formation, the septal nuclei, and the cingulate and prefrontal cortices (see Figs. 1.9 and 1.12).

The following paragraphs describe the principal connections of the hypothalamus with these important telencephalic areas. A brief discussion of some of the more important behaviors associated with these structures follows.

### The Amygdala

The **amygdala** [G. *amygdale*, almond] lies within the temporal lobe, deep to the uncus [L. *onkos*, hook], a swelling on its medial aspect (see Fig. 1.12). The amygdala is a heterogeneous region of the brain. It consists of three

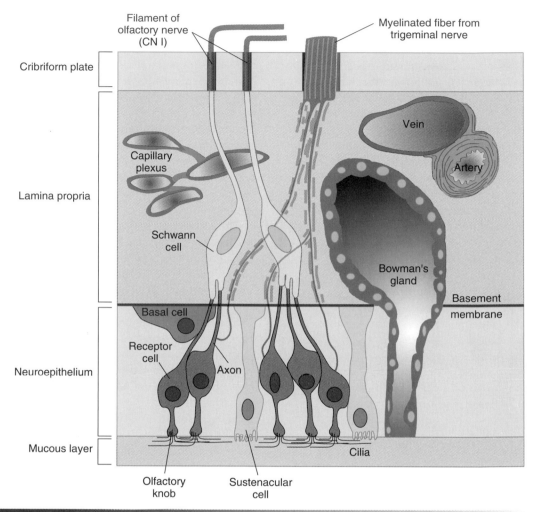

Filament of olfactory nerve (CN I)

Myelinated fiber from trigeminal nerve

Cribriform plate

Lamina propria

Vein

Capillary plexus

Artery

Schwann cell

Bowman's gland

Basement membrane

Basal cell

Receptor cell

Axon

Neuroepithelium

Mucous layer

Cilia

Olfactory knob

Sustenacular cell

**Figure 14.12    The olfactory epithelium**

principal divisions: **olfactory, autonomic**, and **cortical**. The connections between these divisions and the CNS are not well defined, so their functions also remain poorly defined. Since the largest portion of the amygdala and its overlying cerebral cortex constitute the principal cortical target for the central olfactory projections, the essential features of the olfactory system are presented here.

## OLFACTORY SYSTEM

The sense of smell is fundamentally important to many animals. Without it their food-gathering and reproductive capacities would be severely limited. For example, many species se-

crete specific odors that trigger reproductive behavior in other members of the species. The ability to detect these molecules, known as **pheromones**, is remarkable. In many animal species, olfactory competence is essential for food gathering. Although not trivial, the role of olfaction is much smaller in human behavior. Reflecting their diminution of importance, the olfactory structures in humans are relatively modest.

The human **olfactory epithelium** lies in the olfactory cleft within the roof of the nasal cavity. It has a surface area of approximately 10 cm². The olfactory epithelium contains **sustentacular, basal**, and **bipolar receptor cells** (Fig.

14.12). The surface of the epithelium is coated with thick mucus secreted by the secretory epithelium that lines the entire nasal cavity and by the specialized sustentacular cells and **Bowman's glands** in the olfactory epithelium. The mucus is secreted continuously and flows over the olfactory epithelial surface, cleansing the receptors of odoriferous molecules about every 10 minutes. The olfactory epithelium rests on a basement membrane that separates the superficial neuroepithelium from the deep lamina propria. The distal pole of the bipolar receptor cell terminates as a knob from which a variable number of cilia extend onto the surface of the olfactory epithelium. Fully differentiated receptor cells exist for only about 30 to 60 days before they die and are sloughed from the epithelium. They are continuously replaced by differentiating basal cells.

Like those found in vestibular and cochlear hair cells, the cilia of the olfactory receptor cell are arranged in the typical 9 + 2 configuration of microtubules. Receptor sites, probably composed of membrane proteins, are located on the cilia. The binding of a single appropriate molecule to one receptor site in the receptor cell causes depolarization sufficient to generate an action potential. It is hypothesized that different receptor sites on the cilia bind different classes of molecules, and that each class has certain steric and/or charge characteristics that distinguish one class from another. The perception of different odors may be explained on the basis of different receptor cells expressing different receptor molecules. The combination of different receptor cells activated by specific odoriferous molecules creates a pattern of excitation that can encode the full spectrum of perceived odors. This process is similar to our perception of color hue from only three types of photoreceptors in the retina.

Unmyelinated axons emerge from the proximal pole of each receptor cell. The axons penetrate the basement membrane of the olfactory epithelium, where they become myelinated by Schwann cells in the laminae propriae. Bundles of axons pass through the **cribriform plate** [L. *cribrum,* sieve, and *forma,* form] of the **ethmoid bone** [G. *ethmos,* sieve, and *eidos,* form] as the **olfactory nerve** (CN I). Somatosensory information is carried by branches of the anterior ethmoidal nerve, which also passes through the cribriform plate before joining the trigeminal nerve. The trigeminal sensory fibers provide nociceptive sensitivity to the olfactory epithelium.[2] The cribriform fenestrations in the ethmoid bone, which are necessary for the passage of axons, also provide a potential pathway by which infectious agents may gain entry into the cranium. Once inside, they can form abscesses in the frontal lobes.

After entering the cranium, the olfactory nerve axons immediately penetrate the **olfactory bulb,** within which they synapse with **mitral cells** [L. cap, miter] and **tufted cells** in a complex structure, the **olfactory glomerulus** (Fig. 14.13*A*). The olfactory bulb contains several types of interneurons that provide for a rich lateral interaction between the primary neurons of the olfactory nerve and secondary mitral and tufted neurons. Axons from mitral and tufted neurons form the olfactory tract, which lies in the **olfactory sulcus** of the overlying frontal cortex. On reaching the **anterior perforated substance,** the olfactory tract divides into the **lateral** and **medial olfactory striae.** The medial olfactory stria contains mostly axons from the **anterior olfactory nucleus,** a collection of cells in the olfactory tract that receive mitral and tufted cell axon collaterals. The medial stria joins the anterior commissure to cross the midline. On the contralateral side the axons enter the olfactory tract and terminate in both the anterior olfactory nucleus and olfactory bulb. Containing primarily axons from the olfactory bulb, the lateral olfactory stria passes lateral to the anterior perforated substance before entering the **piriform cortex** [L. *pyrum,* pear]. There the axons collateralize extensively, forming branches that terminate in the piriform cortex, the **entorhinal cortex** [G. *entos,* within, and Gr. *rhis,* nose], and the olfactory division of the amygdala. The piriform cortex lies immediately over the amygdala and extends medially from the **rhinal sulcus** to the medial extent of the temporal lobe.

---

[2] The remainder of the nasal cavity is supplied by branches of the anterior ethmoidal nerve that enter the nasal cavity through the ethmoidal fissure after crossing the cranial surface of the cribriform plate.

Caudal to the piriform cortex, lying between the **collateral sulcus** and the **hippocampal sulcus**, is the entorhinal cortex (Fig. 14.13B). It extends caudally to the **isthmus of the cingulate gyrus** [L. girdle, fr. *cingo*, surround].

## CONNECTIONS OF THE AMYGDALA

Fibers leave the amygdala by two major pathways (Fig. 14.14). The most prominent path-

way is the **stria terminalis**, a macroscopic fiber bundle that courses along the wall of the lateral ventricle. It follows the caudate nucleus to the rostral portion of the ventricle before entering the septal nuclei and the hypothalamus. Within the hypothalamus most of the axons terminate in the preoptic and ventral medial areas. A second amygdalofugal [L. *fugio*, flee; i.e., away from] pathway proceeds along

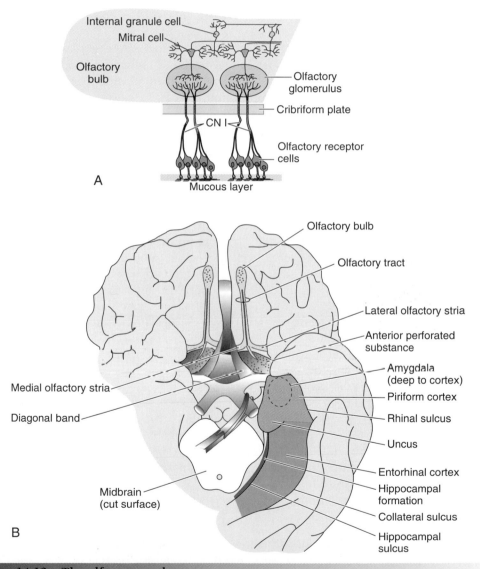

A. Principal arrangement of synapses in the olfactory bulb. **B.** Ventral view of the brain illustrating the principal olfactory areas (*pink*). The optic chiasm and nerves have been displaced to reveal the olfactory trigone and the diagonal band of Broca.

**Figure 14.13   The olfactory pathways**

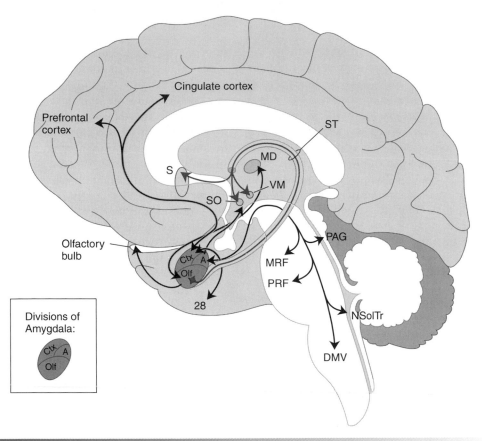

**Figure 14.14   Principal connections of the amygdala**

*MRF,* mesencephalic reticular formation; *PRF,* pontine reticular formation; *PAG,* periaqueductal gray; *DMV,* dorsal motor nucleus of the vagus; *NSolTr,* nucleus of the solitary tract; *MD,* dorsomedial nucleus; *SO,* supraoptic nucleus; *S,* septal nuclei; *VM,* ventral medial nucleus; *ST,* stria terminalis. Divisions of the amygdala: *Olf,* olfactory; *Ctx,* cortical; *A,* autonomic.

the base of the brain and spreads out to innervate the dorsomedial nucleus of the thalamus, the prefrontal and entorhinal cortex, and the brainstem.

The olfactory division of the amygdala projects through the stria terminalis to the hypothalamus and the septal nuclei. These connections strongly influence reproductive and defense behaviors. It also projects to the **dorsomedial nucleus** of the thalamus, an area thought to influence one's affect towards sensory stimuli. The dorsomedial nucleus is reciprocally connected with the frontal lobes. Finally, the olfactory division of the amygdala makes reciprocal connections with the autonomic and cortical divisions.

As might be expected, the autonomic division of the amygdala makes extensive connections with the autonomic regions of the hypothalamus. It also has direct connections with major brainstem autonomic centers, including the mesencephalic and pontine reticular formation, the periaqueductal gray (PAG), the nucleus of the solitary tract, and the dorsal motor nucleus of the vagus.

As its name implies, the cortical division makes reciprocal connections with the cerebral cortex, particularly from the frontal, temporal, and cingulate areas. It sends fibers to the autonomic area of the amygdala and to the caudate, putamen, and nucleus accumbens of the basal ganglia.

## FUNCTIONS OF THE AMYGDALA

The functions of the amygdala are related to its three divisions. Knowledge about the functions of the amygdala is based on animal experiments and human lesions. These data are subject to a variety of methodological difficulties. Nevertheless, *experimental evidence suggests that the amygdala plays an important role in determining one's affective perception of sensory stimuli,* particularly stimuli with survival value. The cortical and olfactory divisions of the amygdala send axons into the autonomic division, which directly drives both the autonomic parts of the hypothalamus and the brainstem autonomic centers. Therefore, under appropriate circumstances sensory stimuli passing through the amygdala can evoke a strong autonomic response. In addition, the amygdala makes both direct and indirect connections with the frontal and cingulate cortices through the dorsomedial nucleus of the thalamus. These cortical areas are associated with the interpretation or attachment of meaning to stimuli. Other major connections of the amygdala are made with the temporal lobe, especially with the hippocampus (discussed later in the chapter), which is very important in memory. Although the mechanism is not understood, it seems likely that amygdaloid connections with these temporal lobe structures is important in using the memory of past events to shape the interpretation of a sensory stimulus. Thus, the amygdala apparently contains the necessary neural mechanisms to provide both psychic and physiological responses to stimuli. This combination of *psychic* and *physiological* responses to a stimulus is called *emotion.*

The best-studied neurological response to emotion is *fear conditioning,* in which an innocuous conditioned stimulus, such as a flash of light or a tone, is paired with a noxious unconditioned stimulus. The unconditioned stimulus produces a natural response to a threatening condition that the conditioned stimulus alone does not produce. When pairing the conditioned and unconditioned stimuli, the conditioned stimulus alone produces the same response as the unconditioned stimulus, and the animal is said to be fear conditioned. This type of conditioning may occur after only a single pairing of the conditioned and unconditioned stimuli. Fear conditioning has been demonstrated in numerous animals, including humans.

The amygdala is required for both the acquisition of fear conditioning and the expression of the behavioral response to the conditioned stimulus. Its central role in fear conditioning is based on its anatomical position between the sensory association areas of the cerebral cortex and the deep forebrain structures that regulate autonomic (hypothalamus) and hormonal (septum and hypothalamus) responses. The amygdala also feeds back to the cerebral cortex through the basal ganglia, a pathway that may explain the psychic aspects of fear.

Abundant evidence suggests that the amygdala plays a central role in the affect of fear and fear conditioning in humans. For example, humans with a form of epilepsy (see Chapter 15) that causes abnormal discharges in the amygdala often describe a feeling of intense fear or dread just before an epileptic attack. Patients may also experience abnormal gastric sensations or olfactory hallucinations of a particularly disagreeable nature. In contrast, lesions of the anterior temporal lobe that include the amygdala[3] produce a diminished capacity for fear conditioning.

### The Hippocampal Formation

The **hippocampal formation** [G. *hippocampos,* seahorse], a complex structure that lines the medial aspect of the temporal lobe (see Fig. 1.12), extends from the amygdala to the isthmus of the cingulate gyrus. In cross-section it resembles the seahorse from which its name is derived (Fig. 14.15). The hippocampal formation consists of three divisions: the **dentate gyrus** ($CA_4$);[4] the **hippocampus proper** ($CA_1$, $CA_2$, and $CA_3$); and the **subiculum** [L. *subex,* layer]. The dentate gyrus is a bulge of cortex bounded to the inferior by the **hippocampal**

---

[3] The anterior portion of the temporal lobe is commonly amputated in patients with intractable epilepsy that originates in the temporal lobe.

[4] The designations $CA_1$ through $CA_4$ are based on histological differences that are unimportant to the physician. They are used here only for purposes of anatomical reference. *CA* is derived from *cornu ammonis,* an archaic eponym for the hippocampus.

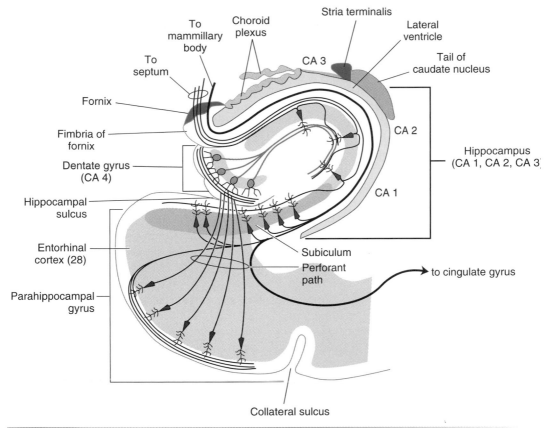

**Figure 14.15   The hippocampal formation**

sulcus and to the superior by the **fimbria** [L. *fimbria*, fringe] of the fornix. Wrapping around the concave side of the dentate gyrus is the hippocampus proper. It is bounded on its lateral surface by the lateral ventricle. The hippocampus proper curves around the inferior aspect of the dentate gyrus, gradually becoming wider as it merges with the entorhinal cortex (area 28). This transition area is the subiculum.

The dentate gyrus and hippocampus are phylogenetically the oldest portion of the cerebral cortex, generally designated **archicortex**. They are composed of only three cell layers. The subiculum, which has more recent phylogenetic origin, consists of three to five layers. The subiculum, piriform cortex, and cingulate gyrus are designated **paleocortex**. The remain-

der of the cerebral cortex, the **neocortex**, consists of six layers. These designations, based on comparative anatomical studies, concern the physician only as terms of reference.

## CONNECTIONS OF THE HIPPOCAMPAL FORMATION

Pyramidal cells in the entorhinal cortex supply most of the fibers that enter the hippocampal formation (Fig. 14.15). These axons pass through the subiculum to reach the dentate gyrus, where the majority terminate. This pathway is called the **perforant path** because of the way it penetrates the subiculum. Axons from cells of the dentate gyrus innervate the adjacent portion of the hippocampus proper $(CA_3)$.[5] Pyramidal cells leaving this area di-

---

[5] The dentate gyrus and hippocampus are subdivided into several areas labeled $CA_1$ through $CA_4$, which reflect certain histological differences.

vide; one branch enters the fornix; the other branch innervates the more distal portion of the hippocampus ($CA_1$). Pyramidal cells from $CA_1$ innervate the subiculum. Axons leaving the subiculum innervate two areas, the adjacent entorhinal cortex and, via the fornix, the mammillary body of the hypothalamus. In addition to the principal afferents from the entorhinal cortex, a small number of axons from the septum innervate the hippocampal formation. These enter via the fornix, and most are cholinergic.

The largest number of efferent connections of the hippocampal formation project from the subiculum to the adjacent entorhinal cortex (Fig. 14.15). A large number of connections are also made with the cingulate gyrus. Although massive in number, the axons that make these connections are diffuse and carry no specific name. Nevertheless, it is important to know that the *principal efferent connections of the hippocampus are with cortical structures*.

The second efferent path from the hippocampal formation is the fornix. This pathway is formed from axons of pyramidal cells of the hippocampal formation. These axons collect on the ventricular surface, forming a white structure, the **alveus** [L. *alveus,* cavity, trough]. Tiny strands of axons leave the alveus as the fimbria, traverse the third ventricle, and collect as a compact bundle on the superior wall of the ventricle as the fornix. The fornix follows the ventricle, passing out of the temporal lobe, where it joins the inferior aspect of the septum near the midline. It then proceeds anteriorly to the anterior commissure, where it divides into **precommissural** and **postcommissural** segments. Axons originating in the hippocampus proper follow the precommissural fornix and terminate in the **septal nuclei**. Axons originating in the subiculum follow the postcommissural fornix into the hypothalamus, where they terminate in the ipsilateral mammillary body.

The physio*logical* role of the hippocampal formation is much debated. Although a great deal of evidence suggests that it is essential for certain types of memory tasks, the hippocampal formation is certainly not a memory bank in the same sense that information is stored in specific locations, as in computers or libraries.

Human memory is much more complicated. An adequate discussion of neuron-based memory would fill a book (see Suggested Readings list). A brief introduction to the subject as it relates to the hippocampus is presented here, because memory disorders are an important part of neurology.

## MEMORY

When an organism modifies its behavior in response to experience, we usually consider that modification to be a learned response. It is apparent, however, that this type of learning depends on the organism being able to retain memory over a long period. Therefore, memory and learning are intimately intertwined. It is the ability of the nervous system to associate present experience with the memories of similar past experiences and to project future consequences that enables the organism to respond appropriately to a situation. The more complex the nervous system, the richer and more varied the memory associations and the more accurate the projection into the future. Therefore, the development of memory systems that enable complex learning behavior has strong survival value.

Mammals have at least three types of memory systems. The simplest system is the reflex, for example the muscle stretch reflex. While we generally do not consider reflexes a memory, they can be considered a kind of memory developed by evolution. They are *hard-wired systems that have evolved to respond to certain stereotyped experiences that require stereotyped responses.* They are skills learned by the species and incorporated into the structure of the nervous system. To invoke a computer analogy, reflexes are analogous to read-only memory (ROM).

The next level is a type usually called **procedural memory**. Procedural memory is *skills learned by the person* that are so well incorporated into the mind that the person calls on them subconsciously. Walking, riding a bicycle, and using language are examples of this type of memory. The cerebellum is the neural structure most closely associated with procedural memory. In our computer analogy, procedural memory is probably best represented by program subroutines of the operating system that are called on to perform routine tasks such as reading a sector from a disk or sending data to a printer.

Finally, there is **declarative memory**, the type that we usually mean when we say we are remembering things. In this case, declarative memory is the *conscious recall of experiences, facts, or events*. In the computer analogy the recalled events are represented by the variable data operated on by the programs and stored in random-access memory (RAM) or magnetic memory (disks). The distinctions among the three types of memory are important because each uses different neurological mechanisms and brain structures. Here we are concerned only with declarative memory.

Declarative memory mechanisms are composed of three functional elements: **acquisition, storage**, and **retrieval** (Fig. 14.16). The acquisition of sensory experiences and their internal representation as a neurological signal has been discussed in the previous chapters. We have seen how various abstractions of sensory experiences are prepared by various parts of the cerebral cortex (see Chapter 12). Highly abstracted information from all parts of the cerebral cortex converges on the temporal cortex (see Chapter 15).

Human memory is bimodal; that is, there are two types of storage mechanisms. The first phase is **recent memory** (sometimes called *short-term memory*) because events stored by this mechanism can be recalled only for a few minutes after they occur. Unless some significance is attached to the event, we soon forget it. This type of memory is equivalent to RAM

in our computer analogy, since information in RAM, although relatively persistent, is easily lost unless transferred to magnetic memory. The inability to retain in memory most occurrences of daily life is important, for without this gift of forgetting, our minds would be burdened with all the trivial happenings of a lifetime. Furthermore, selective forgetting is essential because it is doubtful that the brain has enough capacity to retain all the information we receive in our lifetimes.

The second storage phase is **long-term memory**. Events to which we attach particular importance can be remembered, essentially indefinitely. After events become incorporated into recent memory, additional neuronal processing incorporates them into long-term memory. Long-term memory is sometimes called permanent memory, but no memory is really permanent, as any student taking an examination can attest! We gradually forget, over the years, most events committed to long-term memory (Fig. 14.17). Some memories, particularly those with a strong emotional association, are permanent. To continue our computer analogy, long-term memory is analogous to hard-disk storage.

The permanence of memory depends on the context in which the events are presented. Strong emotional or humorous associations help to sear experiences into long-term memory. Furthermore, long-term memory is an ongoing, active process. Permanence largely depends on subsequent events. Frequent recollection aids retention. Also, making new as-

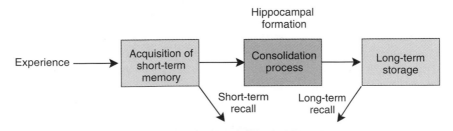

**Figure 14.16    Functional elements of declarative memory**

Black box relation between long- and short-term memory mechanisms and their readout systems. The Korsakoff amnesic state is caused by a malfunction of the process of long-term memory consolidation. Previously stored memory is available for recall. Similarly, recent events can be appreciated and remembered, but only for a limited time.

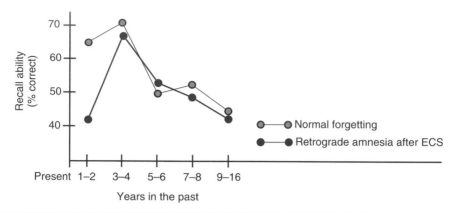

Figure 14.17   Typical rate of forgetting

The rate of forgetting in subjects who have had electroconvulsive shock compared with that of control subjects. Normally, although less is remembered from the distant past than from the recent past, distant memories are more resistant to loss in the face of functional disturbances of the brain. (Adapted from data in Marler P, Terrace HS, eds. The Biology of Learning. New York: Springer-Verlag, 1984.)

sociations with a remembered event can extend and enhance the ability to recall it.

The bimodal model of memory implies that a neurological mechanism consolidates events from short- to long-term memory. That mechanism is not understood. It is clear, however, that *the hippocampal formation is absolutely required for long-term memory consolidation.* The anterior and dorsomedial nuclei of the thalamus, septal nuclei, and nucleus accumbens have also been implicated, but their direct role in memory consolidation is less certain.

The role of the hippocampal formation in memory consolidation is illustrated by patients with bilateral lesions of the hippocampus.[6] These patients have no trouble remembering past events. They also have no trouble solving current problems or functioning in everyday life. However, they *cannot consolidate current events into a permanent memory that can be recalled later.* All of life's experiences between the time of the lesion and the present vanish.[7] Time ceases except for the immediate present and the remote past. This deficit carries no immediate emotional strain, since the problem cannot be

recognized by the patient. With time, however, patients become more baffled and confused. To their bewilderment, their environment changes instantly the moment they leave familiar surroundings ("How did these trees get so huge overnight?" "How could the Jones's house vanish overnight?"). As long as these patients can be maintained in a familiar environment, they can function nearly normally. Thrust into the present world, they become disoriented and confused. An elegant description of such a patient has been provided by Oliver Sacks (see the Suggested Readings list).

The inability to remember events that occurred prior to the onset of illness is called **retrograde amnesia**; the inability to incorporate new information into memory is known as **anterograde amnesia**. The combination of limited retrograde amnesia with anterograde amnesia in a person *who has otherwise normal cognitive abilities,* as has just been described, is called **Korsakoff's amnesic state**, after the Russian physician who first described it. This condition is much more common than one might suppose, since it is frequently *caused by thiamine (vitamin*

---

[6] Unfortunately for our understanding of memory mechanisms, these lesions invariably include the inferomedial temporal lobe and parts of the amygdala.

[7] Some retrograde amnesia also occurs; that is, some amnesia of events before the time of the lesion. The amount of time lost varies among patients.

Chapter 14 / The Hypothalamus and Associated Systems

*B1) deficiency.* It is most common in people who abuse alcohol, because their thiamine reserves can be rapidly depleted. Other neurological signs that commonly accompany this condition include ophthalmoplegia, ataxia, and occasionally atrophy of the anterior lobe of the cerebellum. These signs may appear in the absence of Korsakoff's amnesic state. If there is no cerebellar atrophy, the motor symptoms are promptly relieved, usually within hours, by the administration of thiamin, but the amnesic state persists despite treatment.

The hippocampal formation is necessary for memory consolidation. It receives information via the entorhinal cortex from all of the association areas of the neocortex—areas on which multimodal forms of sensory information converge. This information passes serially through a three-neuron feed-forward path (dentate gyrus→CA$_3$→CA$_1$→subiculum) in the hippocampal formation and then returns to these same neocortical association areas. The reinforcement of the neuronal signal by hippocampal efferents is presumed to be the process by which permanent memory traces are formed. The critical dependence of memory consolidation on the hippocampus is dramatically illustrated in a patient who developed a lesion that involved only CA$_1$ but that was sufficient to interrupt the neocortex→ hippocampus→neocortex loop. This patient exhibited all the manifestations of Korsakoff's amnesic state[8] (Fig. 14.18).

Another aspect of memory is familiarity. We all recognize places we have been before—a form of memory recollection. Associated with this recognition is a sense of comfort that accompanies knowledge of one's immediate environment. When placed in a strange environment, animals and humans explore their surroundings until a certain level of familiarity and comfort are achieved. Animal studies show that the hippocampal formation plays a role in achieving this sense of familiarity about one's surroundings. Individual hippocampal cells have been observed to fire only if the animal is in a specific place in a familiar environment. These place cells are very particular

---

[8] Many textbooks assert that the mammillary bodies are important in long-term memory consolidation. These assertions are based on the connections between the subiculum and the mammillary bodies via the fornix and the frequent association of mammillary atrophy with Korsakoff's amnesic state. However, recent animal studies clearly show that transection of the fornix does not dramatically impair memory. The role of the fornix and the mammillary bodies in memory consolidation has been greatly overstated.

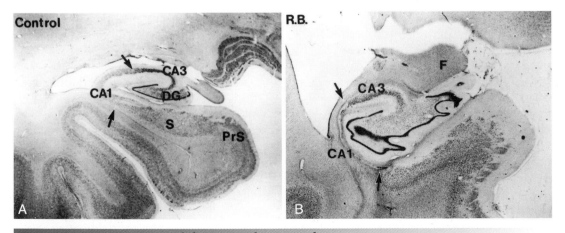

**Figure 14.18  Hippocampal damage and memory loss**

**A.** Histology of a normal hippocampal formation. The CA$_1$ region is labeled (between *arrows*). **B.** Histology of a similar view of the hippocampal formation from a patient with pronounced Korsakoff's amnesia. CA$_1$ (between *arrows*) is nearly devoid of cells. This bilateral lesion, which extended the full length of the hippocampus, was caused by an ischemic event. It was the only significant lesion observed in this patient's brain. (Reprinted with permission from Squire L. Memory and Brain. New York: Oxford University, 1987.)

about the environmental cues that cause them to fire. In this regard they are reminiscent of the face-sensitive cells discovered in the inferior temporal cortex (see Chapter 12). The importance of the place cells is suggested by the experience of humans who have epileptic seizures originating in or near the hippocampus (see Chapter 15). Just before an attack, these patients often report a sense of unfamiliarity with their surroundings, a feeling often accompanied by great fear. This sense of unfamiliarity exists even if the patient objectively understands that she knows the surroundings and that they ought to be familiar.

## The Septal Nuclei

The lateral ventricles are divided at the midline by a sheet of tissue called the **septum pellucidum** (see Chapter 1). In most mammals a few neurons occupy this sheet, but in humans it is essentially devoid of cells. A small group of cells, the **septal nuclei**, occupy the rostral portion of the septum, near the midline and anterior to the anterior commissure and fornix (Fig. 14.19). This group is usually divided into three subnuclei, the medial, lateral, and dorsal septal nuclei. Several other collections of cells are variously included in the generic structure called the septum by some authors. The most prominent of these structures are the **nucleus of the diagonal band**, the **bed nucleus of the stria terminalis**, and the **bed nucleus of the anterior commissure**. The anatomy of this region is not well understood.

The septal nuclei receive afferent connections from the hippocampus proper via the precommissural fibers of the fornix. The only other connection between the septal nuclei and the cerebral cortex is with the anterior portion of the **cingulate gyrus** (area 24). The septal nuclei also receive fibers from the amygdala via the diagonal band. The septal nuclei receive afferents from the brainstem through the **medial forebrain bundle**. The most prominent of the brainstem nuclei that send axons to the septum are the **locus ceruleus**, the **dorsal raphe**, and the PAG.

Efferents from the septal complex descend through the hypothalamus in the medial forebrain bundle and continue into the brainstem. Fibers in the medial forebrain bundle termi-

nate throughout the hypothalamus, particularly in the mammillary bodies. In the brainstem they synapse in the locus ceruleus, the dorsal raphe, and the PAG. Efferents from the septum also synapse in all parts of the hippocampal formation, entering it by way of the fornix. Similarly, septal efferents also innervate the amygdala. Septal efferents also project to area 24 of the cingulate gyrus.

The physiological significance of the septum is not clear. In some of the most intriguing experiments relating to septal function, stimulating electrodes have been placed in the septum or the medial forebrain bundle of rats. The rats can press a lever that delivers an electrical stimulus to the medial forebrain bundle. The stimulus is apparently perceived to have great significance to the rat, because it will press the lever to the exclusion of all other activity, including feeding and sex. The results are more variable in similarly equipped humans, but many have reported a feeling of profound well being. These experiments must be interpreted with caution, since stimulation of the medial forebrain bundle affects many structures, from the brainstem to the cingulate gyrus. They do nothing to elucidate septal function per se. However, the septal nuclei are strategically placed and may be an important link between the hippocampal formation, amygdala, hypothalamus, and the cerebral cortex, in particular the cingulate gyrus.

## The Cingulate Gyrus

The cingulate gyrus wraps around the external border of the corpus callosum (see Fig. 1.9). Wrapping around its genu, the cingulate gyrus becomes the **subcallosal gyrus.** At the posterior portion of the corpus callosum the isthmus of the cingulate gyrus blends into the parahippocampal gyrus. Deep to the cingulate gyrus is the **cingulum**, a large bundle of association fibers that connect the cingulate gyrus with many distant areas of the brain.

The subiculum of the hippocampal formation provides the most prominent connections with the cingulate gyrus (Fig. 14.20). Two pathways, one direct, one indirect, connect the subiculum with the cingulate gyrus. The direct path, which is reciprocal, is via the cingulum. The indirect path involves the subicular

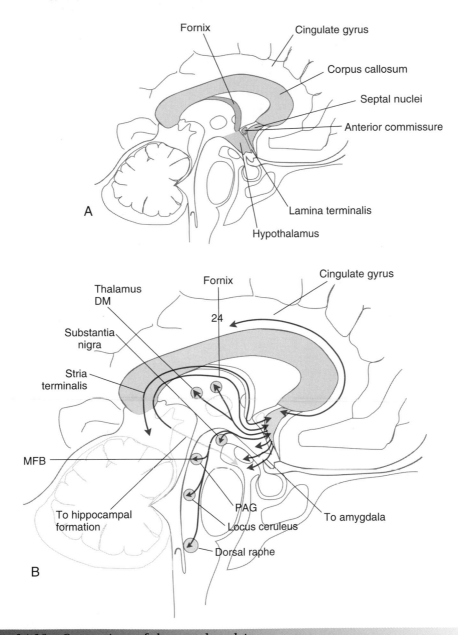

**Figure 14.19    Connections of the septal nuclei**

*DM,* dorsomedial nucleus; *MFB,* medial forebrain bundle; *PAG* periaqueductal gray; *24,* Brodmann area 24.

fibers of the fornix that innervate the mammillary bodies in the posterior hypothalamus. From there the **mammillothalamic tract** carries information to the anterior nucleus of the thalamus. The anterior thalamic nucleus in turn projects to most areas of the cingulate gyrus, with the heaviest innervation to the anterior region (area 24). A second indirect path from the hippocampal formation to the cingu-

late gyrus originates from the hippocampus proper. These axons project to the septal nucleus via the fornix. From the septum axons innervate Brodmann's area 24.

Like all parts of the cerebral cortex, the cingulate gyrus makes important connections with specific thalamic nuclei. As mentioned earlier, area 24 receives fibers from the anterior thalamic nucleus; however, cingulate in-

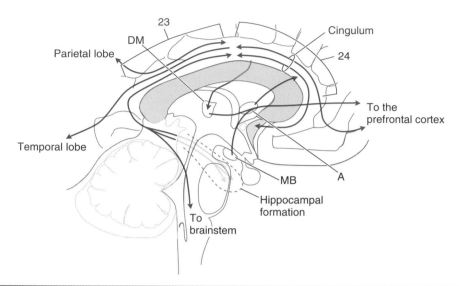

**Figure 14.20    Connections of the cingulate gyrus**

*A*, anterior nucleus; *VA*, ventral anterior nucleus; *DM*, dorsomedial nucleus; *MB*, mammillary body. Numbers indicate Brodmann areas.

formation is returned to the anterior nucleus from the posterior region (area 23). The two cingulate regions, 23 and 24, are interconnected by numerous short association fibers in the cingulum. The anterior region (area 24) also projects, apparently unidirectionally, to the dorsomedial thalamic nucleus. This link is significant because the dorsomedial nucleus projects heavily to the prefrontal lobes of the cortex and seems to be important in the affect of perception (see page 507 and Chapter 15).

In addition to the well-documented reciprocal connections of the cingulate gyrus with the subiculum, it also projects to and receives information from the **temporal, parietal,** and **prefrontal lobes** of the cerebral cortex. These connections are with regions of the cerebral cortex commonly called association areas. This term is imprecise and has various meanings to various authors. Generally, association areas of the cerebral cortex are not primarily motor or sensory. They usually receive secondary or tertiary projections from primary motor or sensory regions.

Finally, the anterior region of the cingulate gyrus projects to the amygdala. This connection provides two indirect paths by which the

cingulate gyrus can influence the prefrontal cortex. First, the amygdala projects directly to the prefrontal lobes via the uncinate fasciculus. Second, it makes reciprocal connections with the dorsomedial nucleus of the thalamus, the principal thalamic nucleus associated with the prefrontal lobes.

The function of the cingulate gyrus is not known. Stimulation in experimental animals seems to evoke the same sort of behavioral changes that occur as a result of stimulating the amygdala. Bilateral ablation of the anterior region has been claimed to decrease aggressiveness in animals, although the opposite has also been reported. Cingulotomies and ablation of portions of the cingulate cortex and cingulum have been performed in humans in an effort to modify socially unacceptable behavior associated with certain psychic disorders. This type of psychosurgery has met with varying results. Some evidence suggests that cingulotomy can relieve chronic pain in selected cases. These results have led some researchers to hypothesize that the cingulate gyrus and/or those brain structures closely connected with it are important in attaching emotional quality or meaning to sensory signals, functions that have also been ascribed to the amygdala.

## Behavioral Correlates

Knowledge of the behaviors that can be affected by lesions to the hypothalamus and closely related structures is clinically useful, so a brief synopsis is presented here.

### FEEDING BEHAVIOR

Certain hypothalamic lesions alter feeding behavior. Roughly speaking, ventral medial lesions produce **hyperphagia** [G. *phagein,* eat]; lateral lesions produce aphagia. Experiments based on hypothalamic lesions should be interpreted with caution because the hypothalamus is a small structure, and fibers of passage are freely intermingled with the cell bodies of neurons. Therefore, no lesion is limited to a single structure. Nevertheless, the clinical implications of these experiments are clear: eating disorders commonly accompany hypothalamic tumors and lesions.

### RAGE

More dramatic, perhaps, are reactions commonly called **sham rage**. Experimentally, removal of the neocortex causes an animal to display unusually violent responses to stimuli. The animal demonstrates poorly directed attack behavior against almost any stimulus. If the hypothalamus is removed, this rage reaction can no longer be provoked. In intact animals, rage can be evoked by stimulating various structures, including the septal nuclei and the anterior hypothalamus. These observations suggest that neocortical structures suppress primitive behaviors by acting through hypothalamic centers. When disconnected from neocortical elements, primitive behaviors are released or at least very poorly regulated. Humans with lesions affecting hypothalamic structures or their connections may exhibit bizarre attack behaviors and may even become physically violent (see the case of Ms. P. R.).

### SEXUAL BEHAVIOR

The behavioral manifestations of reproduction are similarly affected by the hypothalamus. Stimulation of anterior regions often produces poorly directed mounting behavior. In one classic experiment, goats would mount and attempt to copulate with the nearest object when the anterior hypothalamus was stimulated electrically by a chronically placed electrode. Slightly different stimulus parameters or electrode placement would cause the goats to begin drinking as soon as the stimulus began and to continue drinking until it ceased.

# C A S E   H I S T O R Y

## THE WOMAN WHO BIT HER DOCTOR[9]

### HISTORY OF PRESENT ILLNESS (12 NOV 1962)

Ms. P. R., a 20-year-old bookkeeper, was admitted to the hospital complaining of polydipsia, polyuria, and bitemporal headaches.

### MEDICAL HISTORY

She is taking no medications and has had no previous medical problems. There is no family history of neuromuscular disorders.

### PHYSICAL EXAMINATION

She has had no menses for the past 10 months. She is 5 feet 5 inches tall and weighs 134 pounds.

[9] This case was originally reported in Reeves AG, Plum F. Hyperphagia, rage, and dementia accompanying a ventral medial hypothalamic neoplasm. Arch Neurol 1969;20:616–624.

## NEUROLOGICAL EXAMINATION

### Mental Status

Ms. P. R. was alert and knew who she was, where she was, and why she had come to the hospital. She gave a coherent and concise history. At the end of the examination, she remembered the three items she was asked to memorize.

### Cranial Nerves

All cranial nerve functions were normal.

### Station and Gait

Her gait was balanced, smooth, and on a narrow base.

### Motor Systems

STRENGTH: Strength was 5/5 in all extremities and all joints.

TONE: There was no spasticity or rigidity.

BULK: Appropriate and symmetrical for a woman of her age.

ABNORMAL MOVEMENTS: None noted.

### Sensory Systems

She could perceive light touch to cotton and pinprick in all extremities, including the face. Proprioception was intact at the fingers and toes. Romberg test was normal.

### Reflexes

MSRs were present and normal at all extremities. Toes were down going.

### Coordination and Control

Finger-to-nose and heel-to-shin tests were accomplished without difficulty. Rapid alternating hand slapping and finger touching were easily accomplished.

### Parietal Functions

Optokinetic reflex was present in both directions. There was no aphasia or atavistic signs.

## ANCILLARY STUDIES

### Laboratory Studies

URINE PRODUCTION: After 10 hours of water deprivation, her urine specific gravity was 1.003. Urine output (volume unspecified) remained unchanged after a 45-minute infusion of 2.5%

saline; however, urine production was inhibited by injection of 0.1 units of ADH.

HORMONE ANALYSIS: Urine gonadotropins were 0 units in 24 hours.

CSF EXAMINATION: Protein content 43 mg/dL, glucose 47 mg/dL, and opening pressure 70 mm CSF.

### Imaging Studies

A pneumoencephalogram (see Appendix 4) could not outline the third ventricle.

## SUBSEQUENT COURSE

The diagnosis of diabetes insipidus was made based on the ability of ADH to inhibit urine production. The failure of the pneumoencephalogram to show the third ventricle suggested a hypothalamic tumor that subsequent craniotomy failed to confirm. She recovered from surgery uneventfully. Her diabetes insipidus was controlled with ADH and she was discharged. Her headaches persisted, however.

Ms. P. R. returned to the hospital September 8, 1964. Since the previous July her behavior had undergone a remarkable transformation. Although withdrawn most of the time, she sometimes burst out with unprovoked laughter, crying, or rage. At times she became confused and was found sleeping in the wrong bed. She occasionally conversed with imaginary people and had several times disrobed in public. Her physical examination was unremarkable except that she was overweight and her pubic hair was sparse.

A neurological examination could not be performed because of the patient's aggressive and uncooperative behavior. At times she would strike out and attempt to hit, scratch, or bite the examiner. She was frequently disoriented as to place and time. Her memory was variable; sometimes she could not remember past events and at other times her memory seemed normal. Occasionally she was pleasant and cooperative and expressed regret for her aggressive behavior. Her body temperature fluctuated, sometimes reaching 104° F. No source of infection was found. Laboratory studies at this time revealed decreased thyroid, adrenal cortical, and gonadal function in addition to the previously noted diabetes insipidus. CSF examination revealed protein content 73 mg/dL, glucose 82 mg/dL, and an opening pressure of 220 mm CSF.

A second pneumoencephalogram failed to outline the suprachiasmatic recess. Craniotomy revealed a tumor at the base of the third ventricle, but no attempt was made to remove it because of its critical location. The patient recovered from surgery without complications, but her behavioral symptoms deteriorated. To quote from the original report:

> In spite of the sedation and the correction of her metabolic and hormonal deficits, the patient continued to display frequent outbursts of directed violence, consisting of hitting, biting, scratching, and throwing objects at attendants. Although these initially appeared to be unprovoked, we subsequently noted that the withholding of food, which she consumed in quantities of 8,000 to 10,000 calories per day, invariably evoked aggressive behavior. Near the end of her hospitalization, continuous feeding was found to be the only method which succeeded in maintaining the patient in a reasonably tractable state. . . . Her hyperphagia was unabated and by the end of her second month of hospitalization she had gained 24 kg (52.8 lb).[10]

The patient died on December 23, 1964. Autopsy revealed a tumor in the ventral medial portion of the hypothalamus that spared the dorsal and lateral regions and the mammillary bodies but included the fornices and the median eminence (Fig. 14.21).

## COMMENTARY

In this case the tumor was probably initially limited to a small region in the posterior medial region of the hypothalamus. The tumor involved the arcuate nucleus and the magnocellular axons entering the neurohypophysis, the former an important source of GnRH. As the tumor expanded to involve the median eminence, almost any endocrinological dysfunction would be expected. This patient showed decreased function of several endocrine systems.

## FURTHER APPLICATIONS

14.1. Cases such as this, although rare, are instructive because they reveal the close correlation between anatomical structure and function. Identify the lesioned structures that produced the following symptoms in this case: diabetes insipidus, unstable body temperature, decreased en-

---

[10] Reprinted with permission from Reeves AG, Plum F. Hyperphagia, rage, and dementia accompanying a ventral medial hypothalamic neoplasm. Arch Neurol 1969;20:616–624.

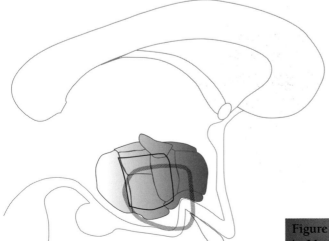

**Figure 14.21   Location of the tumor found in Ms. P. R.**

docrinological function, hyperphagia, and rage reactions.

14.2. No adequate explanation of the derangements in the patient's mental status is as yet possible. The waxing and waning of the patient's emotional state—the incontinence of emotions, disrobing in public, lapses in memory, and at the end of her illness, frank dementia—are symptoms that have not been directly associ-

ated with hypothalamic function. Speculate on the structures involved in this case that might be responsible for the observed behaviors.

14.3. At the time of this case (1962), modern imaging techniques were not available. What mode of imaging would be most appropriate in this case? Had it been available in 1962, how would it have affected the way this case was handled?

# C A S E    H I S T O R Y

## A FALL DOWN THE STAIRS

### HISTORY OF PRESENT ILLNESS

Mrs. M. O. arrived unconscious at the emergency room on 22 Oct. Her daughter said that she was visiting and apparently got out of bed in the middle of the night, became disoriented, and stepped into the stairwell, thinking that it was the bathroom.

### MEDICAL HISTORY

Mrs. M. O., an 80-year-old woman, was in good health until one evening she fell down a flight of stairs at her daughter's home, striking her head against the wall at the foot of the stairs. Before the accident Mrs. M. O. lived alone, drove her car, and led an independent life. About 15 years previously she had a transient ischemic attack. After that incident, on the advice of her physician, she gave up smoking. She has had no recurrences. She had a hysterectomy in 1945.

### PHYSICAL EXAMINATION

Her blood pressure was 154/95. Heart rate was 112. Respiration was steady at 11. Radiographs taken in the emergency department revealed no

broken bones. A limited neurological examination at that time revealed conjugate doll's-eye maneuvers, normal pupillary reflexes, normal MSRs from all test points, and flexor plantar responses. Computed tomography (CT) revealed minimal high densities in the right parietal cortical area consistent with a right parietal contusion. After about 2 hours she began to regain consciousness but was disoriented. She was hospitalized.

### NEUROLOGICAL EXAMINATION (23 OCT)

#### Mental Status

Mrs. M. O. was disoriented and confused. She communicated very little but was basically cooperative.

#### Cranial Nerves

Most of the cranial nerves could not be tested because the patient was confused and at times stuporous and could not cooperate. Tests that could be performed demonstrated normal doll's-eye responses. Pupils reacted to light from 3 mm to 2 mm, both directly and consensually. There was no ptosis or nystagmus. The face appeared symmetrical, with no obvious paresis.

#### Station and gait

Could not be tested.

## Motor Systems

STRENGTH: Could not be tested.

TONE: There was no spasticity or rigidity.

BULK: Appropriate and symmetrical for a woman of her age.

ABNORMAL MOVEMENTS: None observed.

## Sensory Systems
Could not be tested.

## Reflexes
MSRs from the left biceps, brachioradialis, and quadriceps muscles were brisker than from the right. The sign of Babinski was present on the left, absent on the right.

## Coordination and Control
Could not be tested.

## Parietal Functions
There was no apparent aphasia or atavistic signs.

## SUBSEQUENT COURSE

In the hospital, Mrs. M. O. became febrile. She was found to have pneumonia, probably caused by aspiration. The infection responded rapidly to antibiotic therapy. Although her general confusion and disorientation improved during the first few days of hospitalization, it never fully resolved. On the fourth day she became delirious and then unconscious. Plasma sodium levels were found to be 108 mEq/L and urine osmolality, 523 mosmol/kg. Her fluid intake was restricted to 500 mL/day. Over the next 24 hours her plasma sodium increased to 119 mEq/L. She regained consciousness and her confusion and disorientation gradually improved. During the next 2 weeks her plasma sodium levels fluctuated from 105 mEq/L to 129 mEq/L; her confusion and disorientation fluctuated in concert with the sodium levels. Eventually she stabilized and was discharged to a rehabilitation unit, where she remained for 4 weeks. At that time she was discharged to a nursing home, where she lived until her death from unrelated causes.

## COMMENTARY

Blood volume and osmolality are carefully regulated within narrow limits by hormonal and be-havioral mechanisms that are coordinated by the nervous system. It follows, therefore, that insult to the nervous system can disrupt this homeostatic mechanism. Closed head injury, brain surgery, meningitis, encephalitis, stroke, subarachnoid hemorrhage, and neoplasms can all interfere with hypothalamic function and lead to the **syndrome of inappropriate secretion of ADH** (SIADH). Although the causative mechanisms are unknown, SIADH is common and well recognized.

This case is typical. Following a closed head injury, ADH secretion continues inappropriately. Water loss through the kidney decreases, resulting in expansion of the blood volume and consequent dilution of the plasma sodium (**hyponatremia**) and reduction in blood osmolality. Normally, hyponatremia and decreased blood osmolality suppress drinking and ADH secretion. However, in SIADH, ADH secretion and thirst continue unabated. As plasma sodium levels fall below about 120 mEq/L, higher cortical functions become increasingly compromised. Loss of alertness, drowsiness, coma, convulsions, and eventually death can occur. Treatment of SIADH is aimed at restoring sodium levels, which is usually accomplished by restriction of water intake rather than by infusing sodium. For unknown reasons sodium infusion frequently results in central pontine myelinolysis (degeneration of myelin).

## FURTHER APPLICATIONS

14.4.  **Considering what you know about the ionic mechanisms of action potentials and synaptic transmission, speculate about the possible mechanisms involved in SIADH that can lead to cortical function compromise.**

14.5.  **What parts of the nervous system are involved in maintaining osmolality of the blood? How could the diverse set of causal factors in this case affect these structures?**

# C A S E    H I S T O R Y

## AN UNEXPECTED SHIVER

### HISTORY OF PRESENT ILLNESS

Mr. B. T., a 52-year-old man, was taken to the hospital by his family after he became delirious and confused at the family Fourth of July picnic. Although the temperature was in the 80s, Mr. B. T. felt cold and asked for a blanket. Thinking he was joking, the family ignored his request. Later they found him wrapped in a blanket, shivering and delirious. In the emergency department Mr. B. T. was no longer delirious. He was shivering violently and wrapped in the three blankets he had asked for from the nurses.

### PHYSICAL EXAMINATION

Blood pressure was 132/82, pulse was 97, and temperature was 103° F. He was not perspiring.

### NEUROLOGICAL EXAMINATION

#### Mental Status
Mr. B. T. was awake, alert, and oriented to date, time, and place. He stated that his family thought he was delirious because he had asked for a blanket. He said that he just was very cold. He was aware that it was a hot July day. He said he didn't know why he was cold. He could perform serial 7 subtractions and recall the presidents in reverse order from the present to Truman. At the end of the examination he was able to remember the three items he had been asked to memorize.

#### Cranial Nerves

OLFACTION: He could detect and correctly identify methyl silicate from both nostrils.

VISION: There was a dense bitemporal hemianopsia on confrontation testing.

OCULOMOTION: He could track the examiner's moving finger in all directions. There was no obvious weakness of any of the muscles of ocular

motion or nystagmus. Pupillary responses were present and consensual from both eyes. There was no ptosis.

TRIGEMINAL: Sensations to cotton and pinprick were present and symmetrical from all divisions. Corneal reflex was present. Masseter muscles were equal.

FACIAL: Grimace was symmetrical and full. Eyes appeared normally hydrated.

AUDITION: Hearing was grossly normal to finger rubbing.

VAGOGLOSSOPHARYNGEAL: Voice was normal. Pharyngeal arches were high and symmetrical. Uvula was midline. Gag reflex was present.

ACCESSORY: Sternocleidomastoid and trapezius muscles seemed to have normal strength and were symmetrical.

HYPOGLOSSAL: Tongue protruded in the midline. There were no fasciculations or atrophy.

#### Station and Gait
Gait was normal. Tandem walk, hopping, Romberg test, heel-to-shin and finger-to-nose were all performed without difficulty.

#### Motor Systems

STRENGTH: Strength was 5/5 in all extremities and joints. There was no drift.

TONE: There was no spasticity or rigidity.

BULK: Muscle bulk was symmetrical and appropriate.

ABNORMAL MOVEMENTS: None noted.

SENSORY SYSTEMS: Perception of pinprick and cotton were present and symmetrical in all areas. The Romberg test was normal.

#### Reflexes
All MSRs were within normal limits and symmetrical. Plantar signs were flexor.

## Coordination and Control

Finger-to-nose, heel-to-shin, rapid alternating hand slapping, and finger touching were all accomplished without difficulty.

## Parietal Functions

There was no aphasia or atavistic signs.

## COMMENTARY

Finding Mr. B. T. shivering and wrapped in three blankets on a hot July day may suggest that he is delusional or hysterical. However, a psychiatric illness is less likely in light of the bitemporal hemianopia revealed during the neurological examination and the lack of sweating despite his elevated body temperature. CT of the head revealed a large mass at the level of the optic chiasm.

## SUBSEQUENT COURSE

A craniotomy was performed and the mass successfully removed. Mr. B. T. recovered from surgery without complication. He subsequently moved from the Indianapolis area and was lost to follow-up.

### FURTHER APPLICATIONS

14.6. Explain how the major findings in this case—bitemporal hemianopia and lack of sweating—can be explained by a single-locus lesion. Where is the lesion and what structures are involved?

14.7. Explain how the patient could be shivering and wrapping himself in a blanket despite his abnormally high body temperature. What nonneurological cause for increased body temperature ought to be considered?

14.8. Compare the three cases presented in this chapter. All three patients have lesions located within a few millimeters of each other, yet their presentations are completely different. Explain the reasons for these differences in presentation.

## S U M M A R Y

- **The hypothalamus is associated with the three principal homeostatic regulatory systems through its neural connections.**

  The hypothalamus regulates the autonomic nervous system, the endocrine system, and behavioral homeostatic responses.

- **Nuclei in the hypothalamus are the main source of the descending signals that control the parasympathetic and sympathetic divisions of the ANS.**

  Signals that regulate autonomic functions descend in the dorsal longitudinal fasciculus, mammillotegmental tract, and medial forebrain bundle. The anterior region of the hypothalamus is closely associated with parasympathetic functions (slowing of the heart rate, decrease in blood pressure, peripheral vasodilation, increased gastric motility, salivation, and sweating). The posterior and lateral hypothalamic regions are associated with sympathetic functions (increased heart rate and blood pressure, peripheral vasoconstriction, decreased gastric motility, lack of salivation and cessation of sweating). Micturition is regulated through mesencephalic nuclei that project to spinal sympathetic and parasympathetic nuclei.

- **The neurohypophysis, an extension of the hypothalamus, is the interface between the nervous system and the vascular system.**

  Neurosecretory granules containing prohormones for ADH or oxytocin are produced by MSNs in the anterior hypothalamus. Axons from these neurons pass into the neurohypophysis and release the active form of these hormones into the perivascular space, from which they diffuse into the bloodstream.

- **The adenohypophysis, a true endocrine gland, is partially controlled by hormones produced in the hypothalamus.**

  These regulatory hormones are synthesized by parvocellular-secreting hypothalamic neurons, transported along axons, and released into the hypophysioportal system, which transports them to the adenohypophysis. Within the adenohypophysis they regulate the release of the circulating hormones TSH, LH, FSH, GH, prolactin, and ACTH. The release of these hormones and the hypothalamic releasing hormones is partially regulated by long-loop and short-loop negative feedback systems.

- **Endocrine signals can reach the hypothalamus by means of the circumventricular organs.**

  For example, the subfornical organ senses circulating angiotensin II; the organum vasculosum senses the circulating sodium concentration. The median eminence senses circulating hormones for the indirect, short, and ultra-short loop feedback regulation of hormone release.

- **The hypothalamus affects behavior through its connections with forebrain structures, principally the amygdala, the hippocampal formation, the septal nuclei, and the cingulate and prefrontal cortices.**

  These structures are interconnected by complex reciprocal pathways. Fibers from the amygdala enter the hypothalamus via the stria terminalis. The principal efferent connections of the hippocampal formation are with the cingulate gyrus via fibers originating from the subiculum and adjacent entorhinal cortex. Axons also leave the hippocampal formation via the fornix and synapse in the mammillary bodies (from the subiculum) and the septal nuclei (hippocampus proper). The septal nuclei send axons into the hypothalamus via the MFB. Hypothalamic connections with the cingulate gyrus are indirect, being mediated by the anterior and dorsomedial nuclei of the thalamus, the hippocampal formation, the amygdala, and the septal nuclei. These connections are important because the cingulate cortex is connected with the prefrontal, temporal, and parietal lobes of the cerebral cortex.

- **Stimulation of or lesions to various parts of the hypothalamus directly affect certain primitive behaviors.**

  Ventral medial lesions to the hypothalamus disrupt feeding to the point of hyperphagia.

Lesions to lateral areas produce the opposite effect, aphagia. Unprovoked rage-like reactions can be produced by stimulation to the septal nuclei or the anterior hypothalamus. Depending on electrode placement, anterior hypothalamic stimulation can also produce inappropriately directed sexual mounting behavior or unceasing drinking.

## SUGGESTED READINGS

Armony JL, LeDoux JE. How the brain processes emotional information. Ann N Y Acad Sci 1997; 821:259–270.

Davis M. The role of the amygdala in fear and anxiety. Annu Rev Neurosci 1992;15:353–375.

Ito M, Nishizuka Y. Brain Signal Transduction and Memory. London: Academic Press, 1989.

LeDoux JE, Muller J. Emotional memory and psychopathology. Trans Royal Soc Lond 1997;352: 1719–1726.

LeVay S. The Sexual Brain. Cambridge, MA: MIT, 1993.

Pitkänen A, Savander V, LeDoux JE. Organization of intra-amygdaloid circuitries in the rat: an emerging framework for understanding functions of the amygdala. Trends Neurosci 1997;20:517–523.

Sacks O. The lost mariner. In: Sacks O, ed. The Man Who Mistook His Wife for a Hat. New York: Harper & Row, 1987.

Simpson JB. The circumventricular organs and brain barrier systems. In: Patton HD, Fuchs AF, Hille B, et al. eds. Textbook of Physiology. Philadelphia: Saunders, 1989.

Squire LR. Memory and Brain. New York: Oxford University Press, 1987.

Squire LR, Knowlton B, Musen G. The structure and organization of memory. Annu Rev Psychol 1993;44: 453–495.

Swanson LW, Petrovich GD. What is the Amygdala? Trends Neurosci 1998;21:323–331.

Watson C, Vijayan N. The synaptic innervation of the eyes and face: a clinicoanatomic review. Clin Anat 1995;8:262–272.

Zola-Morgan S, Squire LR. Neuroanatomy of memory. Annu Rev Neurosci 1993;16:547–564.

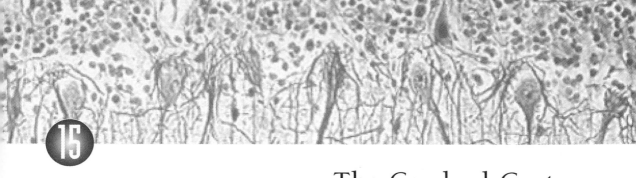

# The Cerebral Cortex

The cerebral cortex is perhaps the most enigmatic part of the mammalian nervous system. Although its essential structure is quite simple, it performs the most complex functions of any living tissue. The functional entities attributed the cerebral cortex include learning, perception, self-awareness, free will, and the most mysterious of all neuronal functions, consciousness. How these complex cortical functions are achieved is not known. The simple structure of the cortical column seems to be an essential feature that enables the cerebral cortex to perform complex transformations of information. This chapter briefly examines the electroencephalogram, altered states of consciousness, the properties of cortical columns acting in concert, and finally, some of the clinically pertinent functions associated with the cerebral cortex.

## THE ELECTROENCEPHALOGRAM

A cortical column is a self-contained information processing unit (see Chapter 5). However, columns also make connections with adjacent columns, adjacent gyri, lobes, hemispheres, and subcortical structures, such as the thalamus and brainstem. Thus columns do not function in isolation but rather as an *ensemble*. Working together, the columns have *ensemble properties* that are characteristic of the group, much as an orchestra has properties that differ from those of its individual instruments.

Although the activity of single neurons can be accurately monitored with intracellular and extracellular electrodes, there are no satisfactory methods for measuring the activity of neuron ensembles. A crude method for measuring the electrical activity of ensembles of columns is to record the electrical potentials from the cortical surface (**electrocorticogram** [ECoG]) or from the surface of the scalp (**electroencephalogram** [EEG]). The ECoG is used during surgery; the noninvasive EEG is routinely used in the clinic.

A typical EEG is recorded from 19 electrodes attached to the scalp and 1 attached to each ear (Fig. 15.1). Amplifiers detect the electrical difference between pairs of electrodes, and this potential is amplified and displayed on a polygraph (typically 16 to 20 individual channels) as a graph of voltage versus time. Because each channel of the recording indicates the electrical difference between pairs of electrodes, the activity displayed in each channel of the polygraph recording is derived from a relatively isolated portion of the cerebral cortex. Before the advent of modern imaging techniques, the EEG was the only noninvasive way of localizing brain dysfunction. It is still useful for this purpose, particularly when the underlying lesion cannot be visualized by computed tomography (CT) or magnetic resonance imaging (MRI).

Nevertheless, the EEG is not a good measure of cortical activity because it primarily reflects the activity of pyramidal cells, which are large and oriented vertically with respect to the cortical surface. When active, pyramidal cells create large electrical dipoles that are aligned perpendicular to the cortical surface. Their parallel arrangement permits these extracellular electrical fields to sum. In contrast, most cortical interneurons are small and symmetrical. Because they are symmetrical, they do not produce strong electrical dipoles. Their

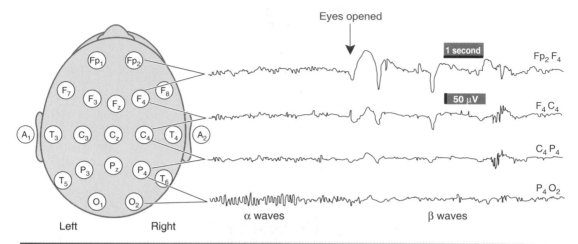

## Figure 15.1    The electroencephalogram

**Left.** Standard placement of electrodes for recording the EEG is shown with their labels. Odd-numbered electrodes are on the left; even-numbered ones, on the right. Pairs of electrodes lead to differential amplifiers that amplify the potential difference between the electrodes. Each potential difference is displayed simultaneously as a separate channel on a polygraph. **Right.** Four channels from an EEG record taken from a relaxed but awake subject with examples of α- and β-waves. Alertness, indicated by the opening of the eyes, extinguishes the α-waves.

electrical fields tend to be oriented randomly, which cancels out their electrical activity.

Another limitation of the EEG is its narrow frequency range. For a number of technical reasons the EEG is restricted to a frequency range of about 0.5 to 30 Hz. Therefore, it indicates the activity of postsynaptic potentials, not action potentials. An EEG recording is divided into four frequency bands for ease of description and analysis. These are the **β-band**, 13 to 30 Hz; **α-band**, 8 to 13 Hz; **θ-band**, 4 to 8 Hz; and **δ-band**, 0.5 to 4 Hz. An awake but quiet normal person produces α- and β-waves. Characterized by high frequency and low amplitude, β-waves are produced by multiple **asynchronous** postsynaptic potentials (PSPs). Because they are asynchronous, PSPs occur randomly over time and consequently sum to a small average amplitude (destructive interference). **Synchronization** of the PSPs magnifies the recorded amplitude of the waveform because the extracellular currents occur more or less at the same time and therefore sum constructively. Transient periods of synchronization signaled in the EEG as a series of waxing, then waning, low-frequency waves develop during periods of relaxed wakeful-

ness. The waxing and waning waves indicate a sequence of increasing, then decreasing synchrony among PSPs in pyramidal cells. Since α-waves are associated with a relaxed but awake state, sensory stimulus, such as opening the eyes or hearing a novel sound, extinguishes the α-waves and reestablishes an EEG dominated by β-waves, which are therefore associated with an alert state (Fig. 15.1).

## ALTERED STATES OF CONSCIOUSNESS

The EEG is a useful clinical and research tool. It can be used to determine the overall activity of the cerebral cortex and to some extent to localize abnormal activity to relatively small cortical areas. *The EEG is an essential ancillary method of diagnosing disorders of sleep and epilepsy and for differentiating coma from cerebral death.*

### Sleep

The human brain alternates between periods of wakefulness and periods of **sleep**. If deprived of sleep, many animals die within weeks. This observation has not been confirmed in humans,[1] but the human brain deprived of sleep does become increasingly dysfunctional. Sleep-deprived humans first become irritable and fatigued, with difficulty concentrating. Motor skills then deteriorate, and sustained thinking becomes impossible. Eventually sensory disorientation develops and the person begins to hallucinate. The need for sleep is absolute. The reasons we need sleep are unknown.

## STAGES OF SLEEP

The EEG undergoes characteristic transitions during the course of sleep (Fig. 15.2). The sleep EEG can be categorized into various stages that differ in the degree of synchrony, represented by the increasing dominance of θ- and δ-waves. As one enters sleep, the EEG becomes more and more synchronized. Moderate postsynaptic inhibition of the α-motor neurons in the brainstem and spinal cord re-

sults in skeletal muscle relaxation. The parasympathetic division of the autonomic nervous system (ANS) dominates; gastric motility increases; heart rate and blood pressure decrease; and temperature regulation becomes erratic. During the most synchronized phase of sleep the EEG suddenly assumes a highly desynchronized pattern that is indistinguishable from the EEG pattern seen in the wakeful state. During this desynchronized period of sleep there is intense postsynaptic inhibition of the α-motor neurons and presynaptic inhibition of all of the sensory systems. The person is difficult to arouse because of the massive inhibition of motor and sensory systems. In effect, the nervous system disconnects itself from the exterior world; internally generated signals dominate cortical activity. These internally generated signals are impressed on consciousness as dreaming, which

---

[1] Fatal familial insomnia is a prion disease that causes degeneration of the ventral anterior and dorsomedial nuclei of the thalamus and perhaps other CNS structures.

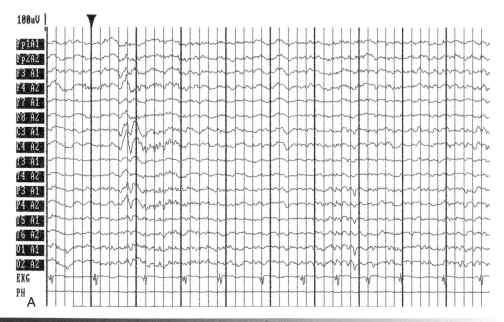

## Figure 15.2 EEG record showing the stages of sleep

Typical 16-channel records taken while the subject was in various stages of sleep. The pair of electrodes connected to the differential amplifier driving each channel is indicated in the *black box* to the left of each trace. See Figure 15.1 for identification of electrodes. Note the ECG trace at the bottom of each record. The PH trace monitors photic stimulation, not used here. **A.** Stage 1 sleep is characterized by a low-amplitude, high-frequency record. The REM stage (not shown) is indistinguishable from stage 1 except for rapid eye movements.

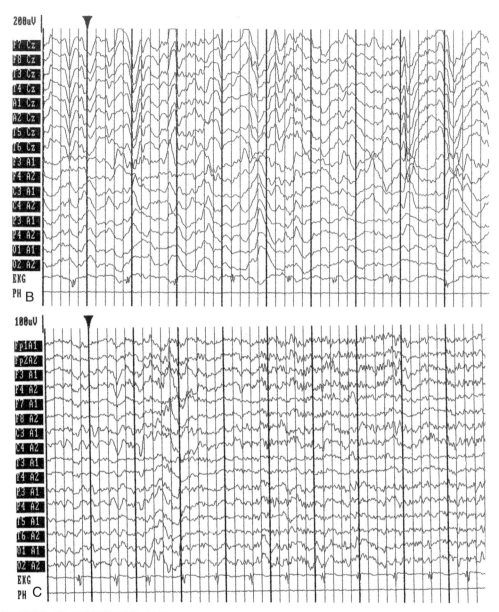

**Figure 15.2    EEG record showing the stages of sleep—*continued***

**B.** Stage 2 is signaled by the development of high-amplitude, low-frequency sleep spindles, 13- to 16-Hz waves superimposed on a β-wave background. **C.** Stage 3 is similar to stage 2 but with the addition of Δ-waves.

is signaled externally by characteristic rapid eye movements (REM) and twitching of the muscles of the face and upper extremities.

## SLEEP CYCLES

Clinicians and researchers break down sleep into five stages labeled 1 to 4 and REM. Stage

1 is "light" sleep characterized by a desynchronized EEG; stages 2, 3, and 4 are characterized by increasing synchronization of the EEG. Each successive stage is considered to be "deeper" than the previous one. The stages progress in order. Stage 1 is reached approximately 10 minutes after retiring, and it is fol-

lowed by stages 2, 3, and 4. The order reverses until stage 1 is reached and followed by REM. This completes one full **sleep cycle.**

A typical person completes three to five cycles during the night, each cycle taking approximately 90 minutes (Fig. 15.3). Early in the night sleep is dominated by slow-wave sleep (stages 2, 3, and 4). REM bouts are brief and widely spaced. By morning there is little slow-wave sleep, and REM bouts become more frequent and longer lasting. However, this description is only a generalization, as sleep patterns vary with age. Children have more synchronized sleep than the elderly, but

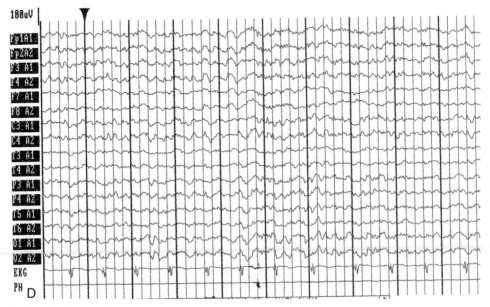

**Figure 15.2    EEG record showing the stages of sleep—*continued***

**D.** Stage 4 is dominated by Δ-waves with no spindling.

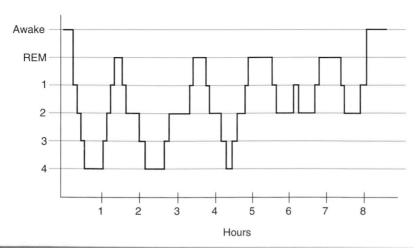

**Figure 15.3    The sleep cycle**

The amount of time an adult spends in each stage during one period of sleep. Several cycles occur during the night, and time spent in REM toward the end of the sleep period increases at the expense of time spent in stages 3 and 4.

the total amount of REM sleep each night remains fairly constant throughout life, accounting for about 20% of total sleep time.

EEG records reveal that *the brain is not quiescent during sleep*. Quite the contrary, as recorded by EEG, neuronal activity is prominent during sleep. Metabolic studies also show that brain metabolism is as high during sleep as it is during wakefulness. Sleep involves the entire brain. Much evidence supports the hypothesis that the thalamus, the principal subcortical source of cortical afferents to the brain, establishes the major states of brain activity and in turn is driven by a number of brainstem nuclei. Among these nuclei the reticular formation, raphe nuclei, periaqueductal gray (PAG), and pedunculopontine and lateral dorsal tegmental regions are particularly important in sleep.

It now seems certain that *brainstem nuclei regulate the sleep-wakefulness cycle* through their action on the thalamus. In animals, if the diencephalon and telencephalon are isolated from the brainstem, activity in the cerebral cortex becomes highly synchronized and the EEG assumes a pattern identical to that of the synchronized phase of sleep. However, the desynchronized phase of sleep and REM episodes fail to develop. The sleep cycle is broken. In humans, lesions affecting the PAG and some tumors of the diencephalon have a similar effect. Nuclei in the brainstem associated with specific neurotransmitters, most notably the locus ceruleus (norepinephrine), raphe nuclei (serotonin), and ventral tegmental area (dopamine) also project widely to parts of the cerebral cortex and may help to regulate its major activity states (wakefulness or stages of sleep). However, their exact roles remain elusive.

## DISORDERS OF SLEEP

Disturbances of sleep fall into three categories: disorders of initiating and maintaining sleep during normal sleeping periods (**insomnia**), disorders of excessive sleep during normal waking periods (**hypersomnia**), and disorders of the sleep cycle and other nonsleep dysfunctions associated with sleep (**parasomnia**). A full description of the various sleep disorders can be found in the references. Only the most prominent examples of each class are discussed here.

### Insomnia

Difficulty in initiating or maintaining sleep is very common, affecting perhaps as many as 40% of the population. However, few people seek professional help for this disorder. Most forms of insomnia are psychophysiological and transient, reflecting periods of stress or emotional disturbances.

A physiological form of insomnia is **central sleep apnea** [G. *a-*, negative prefix, and *pnoe*, breathing]. It is characterized by hypopnea due to a diminished central respiratory drive that results in diaphragmatic arrest lasting more than 10 seconds. The resulting hypoxemia and hypercapnia arouse the patient repeatedly during the night.

All forms of insomnia result in excessive sleepiness during normally wakeful periods. However, excessive sleepiness during normal waking periods can be caused by sleep disorders other than insomnia. One of the most common problems, **obstructive sleep apnea**, is caused by an excessive relaxation of the pharyngeal muscles, which results in snoring and restriction or collapse of the upper airway during sleep. That problem is most prevalent in people over the age of 40 and is 20 times as common in men as in women. It is exacerbated by obesity. The airway obstruction can continue for several minutes at a time. Although oxygen saturation may drop to as low as 50%, the person usually does not awaken. The duration of sleep stages 3 and 4 are, however, greatly diminished, causing excessive daytime somnolence. The problem can be relieved by tracheostomy; continuous positive airway pressure maintained by a nasal mask is a nonsurgical alternative that is also very effective.

### Hypersomnia

**Narcolepsy**, which is inherited as an autosomal recessive trait, affects about 4/10,000 persons. Narcolepsy is a form of hypersomnia characterized by uncontrollable napping during the day, cataplexy, hallucinations while falling asleep, and sleep paralysis. Cataplexy is a brief loss of muscle tone without loss of consciousness. It often occurs during periods of emotional excitement. Hypnagogic [G. *hypnos,* sleep, and *agogos,* leading into] hallucinations occur during the onset of sleep and may take the form of a dream. Sleep paralysis, which is profound, overtakes the narcoleptic person while she is falling asleep or awakening. The person is fully aware of the paralysis and remembers it in detail. Any sensory stimulus, such as a light touch from a bed partner, is sufficient to terminate it, or it spontaneously subsides after a few minutes. Narcolepsy is thought to be a fragment of REM sleep that inappropriately penetrates the wakeful state. People with narcolepsy fall asleep almost immediately after retiring and enter REM sleep without passing through the other stages of sleep. This rapid REM onset is considered diagnostic for narcolepsy.

Disturbances of the normal sleep-wakefulness cycle are thought to be associated with the biological clock. In humans, certain biological functions, such as body temperature, hormone secretions, and psychological performance, vary during the day. If a person is kept in isolation without external clues, these biological functions free-run on an approximately 25-hour cycle. Various triggers, especially light cycles, entrain these biological clocks to the 24-hour period of the earth's rotation. The inability to entrain these systems to the rhythm of the earth leads to sleep disturbances. For most people these disturbances are caused by sociological events such as jet travel across several time zones or work shift changes. After a day or two, one's internal biological clocks become resynchronized with the earth. Some people, however, appear to have an error in the entrainment mechanism. Their clocks free-run and are only occasionally synchronized with the earth. Their lives can be seriously disrupted, since they are also not synchronized with the daily life pulse of society.

## Parasomnia

A variety of other disturbances, the parasomnias, are associated with sleep but are not disturbances of the sleep cycle itself. For example, sleepwalking (**somnambulism**) is common in children (incidence about 15%). Sleepwalking occurs during stages 3 and 4 but not during REM, and the sleepwalker seldom recalls the event when awakened. Therefore, sleepwalking is not acting out of a dream, as commonly supposed or a manifestation of epilepsy (discussed later in the chapter). Children usually outgrow sleepwalking, and it is considered a benign condition. The onset of sleepwalking in an adult may be a sign of psychiatric disease and should be investigated.

In contrast to sleepwalking, which is almost always a childhood phenomenon, a **REM-associated sleep disorder** is almost never seen except in adults. As its name implies, this disorder occurs exclusively during REM and appears to be an acting out of threatening dreams. Sleeping persons become violent and dangerous, often injuring themselves and their bed partners. The condition responds well to anticonvulsant drugs.

### Brain Injury and Consciousness

Injury to the brain frequently causes alterations in consciousness. A strong blow to the head may jar the brain enough to cause a temporary loss of consciousness. Brain injury may be a simple **concussion** [L. *concussio,* shake violently] or if part of the brain is bruised, a **contusion** [L. *contusio,* fr. *contundre,* bruise]. The loss of consciousness following a concussion or contusion is brief and never lasts more than a few minutes. Longer-term alterations of consciousness that result from more serious brain insult include **confusion, stupor, coma,** and **cerebral death.**

### CONFUSION

Confusion, a clouding of consciousness, is the least disturbed alteration of the conscious state. In this condition a patient's thinking processes are slowed. The patient has difficulty integrating contemporary experiences into the thought processes and carrying out simple commands; he may be inattentive and disoriented to time and place. Speech may be slow, sentences incomplete, and vocabulary limited.

## STUPOR

Stupor is a disturbance of consciousness that is more profound than confusion. Stuporous patients are minimally conscious and can be brought to awareness only by strong sensory stimuli. Even then they may not be able to respond to simple commands, although they may seem conscious and aware of the examiner. They easily lapse back into stupor.

## COMA

A patient who cannot be aroused by strong sensory stimuli, such as a sternal rub,[2] is in coma [G. *komoa*, deep sleep], an unconscious state in which *the metabolic activity of the brain is reduced from normal levels.*

Coma is unlike sleep. During sleep the brain's metabolic activity is equal to or may even exceed that of the waking state; in coma it is depressed. Furthermore, some level of awareness seems to be present during sleep, since dreaming reflects at the very least a distorted form of consciousness. Consciousness is also suggested by the preservation of the sense of time during sleep. One is always aware of the passage of time, even after a period of the soundest slumber. On recovery from coma the patient has no recollection of events that occurred during the coma. This amnesia is generally complete, with no sense of time having passed, and in that regard coma is much like the anesthetic state. Finally, sensory stimuli can terminate sleep and bring one fully awake; the comatose patient cannot be aroused. Sleep is a natural facet of normal brain activity; coma is a depressed disease state.

Some alterations in brain metabolism produce **metabolic coma**. Metabolic coma can be caused by impaired production of neurotransmitters because of disturbances in protein metabolism, impaired synaptic transmission as a result of hypoxia, or even widespread but incomplete impairment of neuronal function because of exposure to toxins. Toxins may be from industrial sources (carbon monoxide poisoning), felonious intent (cyanide, arsenic), self-induced (barbiturates), or iatrogenic [G. *ia-tros*, physician, and *gennan,* produce] (prescribed drugs). A few other common causes of metabolic coma include hypoxia, hypoglycemia, disturbance in cerebral or blood pH, and electrolyte imbalances, particularly those affecting potassium and sodium. Determining the cause of coma can be a major challenge.

## CEREBRAL DEATH

Advances in medicine have improved methods of resuscitation to the point that the body may be alive and functional but the brain is not. Under such circumstances the body can remain viable as long as proper nursing care is provided. The coma, however, is irreversible. This condition has been termed cerebral death, or brain death. Whether a person in such a condition is living or dead is a legal and ethical question (discussed later in the chapter). This issue grows more pressing as the need for donor organs and issues related to allocation of medical resources becomes more acute.

### Brainstem Injury and Consciousness

Alterations in consciousness can be caused by lesions to the cerebral cortex, the thalamus, or the brainstem. Lesions to the cerebral cortex do not produce alterations of consciousness unless they are massive and usually bilateral. However, profound and irreversible coma can be produced by small, highly localized lesions to the thalamus or reticular formation, because these lesions interfere with the thalamus's ability to regulate cortical activity. Thalamic regulation can be lost if the thalamus either is damaged directly or is disconnected from the brainstem structures that regulate it.

Coma can also be caused by disruption of the connections between the brainstem and the thalamus. These connections pass through the **tentorium** [L. *tentorium*, tent], the meningeal structure that separates the superior from the inferior cranial fossa. The thalamus, basal ganglia, and cerebral cortex lie in the superior cranial fossa; the brainstem lies in the inferior cranial fossa. The tentorial notch is

---

[2] Pressing and rubbing vigorously on the sternum with a knuckle. It is very painful.

the ridge of dura that circles the brainstem approximately at the level between the mesencephalon and the diencephalon. Consisting of dura mater, the tentorium is tough and unyielding. Therefore, brain structures passing through the tentorial notch can be trapped and injured. Because of this anatomy, expanding lesions superior to the tentorium have different symptoms from those that develop inferior to it. Lesions that affect consciousness are therefore categorized as either **supratentorial** or **infratentorial** to reflect the location of the primary pathology. It is essential to differentiate supratentorial from infratentorial causes of altered consciousness. Many supratentorial causes can be successfully treated; the prognosis for infratentorial lesions is more ominous.

## SUPRATENTORIAL LESIONS

*Lesions that occupy the supratentorial space frequently affect consciousness slowly, in a stepwise fashion.* This stepwise effect on consciousness is due in part to the enclosure of the brain, cerebrospinal fluid (CSF), and blood of the cerebral circulation within a rigid structure, the skull. Expansion of one of these elements or introduction of a new element (e.g., a tumor) is borne at the expense of blood and CSF volume. For example, a slowly expanding mass (tumor or hematoma) displaces brain tissue and squeezes blood and CSF out of the cranial vault. As a result, the ventricles diminish in size and the intracranial contents shift position to make room for the mass. As the mass expands further, additional compression of the ventricles becomes impossible, and intracranial pressure increases rapidly.

When intracranial pressure exceeds diastolic blood pressure, cerebral perfusion is diminished. The first effect on consciousness is confusion. Stupor follows as the mass expands and intracranial pressure continues to increase. The pressure, transferred to the brainstem, frequently stimulates emetic centers, causing vomiting that can be dramatically violent (**projectile vomiting**). A large supratentorial mass can displace other structures, commonly the uncus and part of the hippocampus, through the tentorial notch. Uncal herniation shifts the position of the brainstem and

stretches the ipsilateral oculomotor nerve over the posterior clinoid process, creating a third-nerve palsy and loss of the light reflex from the ipsilateral eye (see Chapter 10). Pressure can also be exerted on the cerebral peduncles, which manifests as upper motor neuron signs in the extremities (Fig. 15.4).

The displacement of supratentorial structures through the tentorial notch can also constrict the posterior cerebral artery, leading to ipsilateral occipital lobe infarction and a contralateral homonymous hemianopia (see Chapter 12). Uncal herniation also restricts blood flow to the upper brainstem, causing local brainstem ischemia. The loss of perfusion renders the upper brainstem dysfunctional. Since brainstem activity drives the thalamus, coma ensues because the thalamus is deprived of the essential brainstem activation necessary for consciousness.

Further expansion of the mass may force the lower brainstem and cerebellar tonsils into the foramen magnum. This compromises the cardiovascular and respiratory centers of the medulla, which typically raises blood pressure and decreases the heart rate. **Cheyne-Stokes respiration** soon develops. This pattern of breathing is characterized by a gradual increase in depth and sometimes in rate of respirations up to a maximum, followed by a gradual decrease to the point of apnea. The duration of these cycles and the period of apnea usually increases until respiration eventually ceases. The consequent total collapse of the respiratory and cardiovascular centers brings death.

## INFRATENTORIAL LESIONS

In contrast to the slow, ominous progression of symptoms associated with supratentorial lesions, *expanding infratentorial lesions first produce dramatic symptoms associated with the cranial nerves.* Vertigo, nausea, deafness, facial paralysis, nuclear ophthalmoplegia, and projectile vomiting may be early signs, depending on the placement of the lesion. If the lesion affects the upper pons before the medullary respiratory centers, coma may develop without the preceding signs of confusion and stupor. Since the cerebral cortex is still alive, the EEG

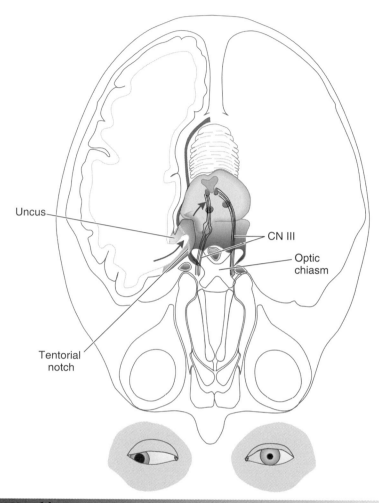

Uncus

CN III

Optic chiasm

Tentorial notch

**Figure 15.4    Uncal herniation**

An expanding supratentorial mass can herniate the uncus through the tentorial notch, displacing the upper brainstem and stretching the ipsilateral oculomotor nerve (CN III) over the posterior clinoid process. This ominous condition is signaled by confusion, stupor, or coma combined with unilateral third-nerve palsy.

of such patients is not isoelectric but displays the patterns associated with slow-wave sleep. If the lesion is reversed, recovery is possible. If the lesion remains stable, the patient may remain in the coma–sleep state indefinitely.

### Seizures

Under certain conditions the ensemble of cortical neurons fails to function in a coordinated and purposeful manner. The uncoordinated neuronal activity is described as a **seizure** [OF. *seisir,* to take possession of] when the activity is highly synchronized. Therefore, *seizures are*

*characterized by a prolonged synchronous discharge of large numbers of cortical neurons.* This neuronal state brings about disturbances of perception, inappropriate motor functions, and alterations in awareness and consciousness. **Epilepsy** [G., *epi,* on upon, and *lambenein,* overtake, seize, take by violence], an illness affecting about 1% of the U.S. population, is characterized by repeated seizures that continue intermittently throughout life unless successfully treated. Seizures are classified as **general** or **partial**, based on the area of the brain initially involved and the manner in which the seizure spreads to other areas. Partial seizures account for about two-thirds of epilepsy cases. **Febrile seizures** are a special class outside the general illness of epilepsy.

## PARTIAL SEIZURES

Seizures that are initiated in a small, local part of the brain are termed partial or focal seizures to suggest involvement of only part of the brain. The initial symptoms of a partial seizure are appropriate to the restricted location of the epileptogenic activity, known as a **focus** [L., hearth, meeting place (of light rays)]. The patient feels these symptoms as an **aura** [L., air in gentle motion, vapor, gleam]. For example, if the focus is in the somatosensory cortex (areas 3, 1, and 2), the patient experiences paresthesias in the corresponding body area. Similarly, a focus in the motor cortex (area 4) produces myoclonic twitching from the appropriate muscles. If the temporal lobe is the focus, particularly in the region of the uncus, the aura may be an unpleasant odor. Psychic auras are common manifestations of foci in the temporal lobe. For example, the patient may have feelings of great fear or dread because of the involvement of the amygdaloid nuclei (see Chapter 14). Abnormal premonition, **déjà vu** [F., *déjà vu*, already seen], or unfamiliarity, **jamais vu** [F., *jamais vu*, never seen], are common. These auras may indicate hippocampal activity. Autonomic signs, such as pupillary dilation, pallor, flushing, or palpitations, may also accompany the onset of partial seizures originating in the temporal lobe. These autonomic auras reflect the intimate connections of the temporal lobe with the hypothalamus. Partial seizures frequently progress, becoming tonic-clonic seizures after a few seconds (discussed later in the chapter).

Partial seizures can be further described as either simple or complex, depending on whether they affect general consciousness. In **simple partial seizures**, general consciousness remains unaffected. The seizure remains confined to the focus, and symptoms are limited to the aura. In **complex partial seizures**,

which constitute approximately 75% of partial seizures, consciousness is affected. Immediately after the aura the patient usually performs some type of simple automatonlike activity, such as arranging objects at hand (clothing, objects on one's desk, dishes) or walking aimlessly about the immediate environment. More rarely the patient may undress or leave the immediate environment (e.g., walk outdoors into traffic). Simple automatisms, such as lip smacking, chewing, and swallowing, are most common. After the seizure abates, the patient does not remember the automaton activity.

## GENERAL SEIZURES

In contrast to partial seizures, general seizures are thought to involve the entire brain immediately. No aura or other sign occurs to indicate that only a particular part of the brain is involved. There are two major types of general seizures, **absence seizures** and **tonic-clonic seizures.**

Absence seizures[3] are characterized by loss of awareness without loss of muscle tone. The person suddenly loses awareness for several seconds. Absence seizures occur repeatedly and may number several to several hundred a day. There are no obvious motor signs. Some persons flutter their eyelids or make minor chewing movements. Although fully aware and mentally alert immediately after the seizure, the patient has no recollection of the passage of time or of events that occurred during the seizure. Absence seizures usually begin between ages $2\frac{1}{2}$ and 20. About half have occasional tonic-clonic seizures. Only a few have other neurological problems. Absence seizures are readily diagnosed by a 3-Hz spike-wave complex recorded by EEG.

Tonic-clonic [G. *tonikos*, tense, fr. *tonos*, stretching, contraction, tension, and *klonos*, confused motion, turmoil, tumult] seizures are dramatic events.[4] The patient loses consciousness and falls. The onset of the seizure is characterized by general stiffening of the body as all

[3] These seizures used to be known as *petit mal seizures*. This term is falling into disuse because it has been applied to so many unrelated types of seizures that it has become medically meaningless.
[4] The term *grand mal* is no longer applied to tonic-clonic seizures.

muscles contract (**tonic phase**). The initiation of the seizure is frequently heralded by a vocalization as air is involuntarily expelled through the larynx. During the tonic phase, which lasts about a minute, breathing ceases and the patient may become cyanotic. Rhythmic symmetrical muscle jerking (**clonic phase**) follows the tonic phase. During this phase, which lasts for about another minute, the tongue may be lacerated, increased salivation may cause frothing at the mouth, and urinary incontinence may occur. Following the clonic phase are several minutes of postictal stupor and confusion. On full recovery the patient has no recollection of the seizure.

## FEBRILE SEIZURES

Febrile seizures occur in about 4% of children aged 6 months to 4 years. Febrile seizures, which are almost always general, are associated with a rapidly rising fever. The probability of a second attack is much greater if the first attack occurs at an early age, and the risk of recurrence drops rapidly with maturity. True febrile seizures are considered a benign event of infancy. They are not a predictor of childhood or adult epilepsy. The principal difficulty for the physician is separating febrile seizures from true epilepsy and seizures having a treatable cause. Consequently, the diagnosis of all seizures in infants must be vigorously pursued.

## CAUSES OF SEIZURES

Seizures may be initiated by a number of factors, not all of which are understood. However, all seizures seem to be related to cortical damage. Seizures may be caused by isolated events that temporarily disrupt cortical function, such as concussion, hypoglycemia, meningitis, and encephalitis. Such seizures are usually one-time occurrences that are directly related to the insult. Seizures can also be the unwelcome herald of brain tumors, brain abscesses, intracranial vascular lesions, and metabolic disease. They can be caused by taking certain drugs; withdrawal from other drugs, primarily barbiturates and alcohol; and neurotoxins, particularly carbon monoxide.

Perhaps the best-documented cause of seizures is "scarred" brain tissue. After brain injury, neurons and glia die, and they are phagocytized and replaced by proliferating astrocytes. The distal part of the axons of the damaged and dying neurons separate from the soma. These distal axons degenerate, which removes synaptic boutons from other neurons; that is, the neurons are deafferented. Undamaged axons in the vicinity sprout new processes, many of which form new synapses to replace those lost. The regrowth of new processes and the formation of new synapses may upset the balance between excitation and inhibition in the deafferented neurons. Some of these neurons become chronically depolarized, so that they spontaneously fire in the manner of a cardiac pacemaker, forming an **epileptic focus.**

By itself an epileptic focus is not a seizure, nor is it necessarily a sign of epilepsy. Many people have an identifiable focus and never have seizures. In other cases, for reasons that are not understood, the epileptic focus transiently expands, recruiting additional neurons in a wider and wider area of the cerebral cortex. If the epileptic focus is near the central sulcus, for example, the expansion of the focus can be tracked by observing the advance of rhythmic motor contractions that correspond to the somatotopic organization of the precentral gyrus. The advancing contractions, first noted by the 19th-century neurologist John Hughlings Jackson, are known today as the Jacksonian march.

Many forms of epilepsy have no identifiable focus. In many of these cases an epileptic focus probably does exist but does not register on EEG. In other cases there may be no focus, and the initiating mechanism is unknown.

## HEMISPHERIC SPECIALIZATIONS

The most obvious fact about the gross anatomy of the brain is that it is a bilaterally symmetrical paired organ. The left and right hemispheres have only minor structural differences. Among other findings, the left temporoparietal junction contains slightly more brain tissue than the right, and in some persons the surface of the left temporal lobe posterior to Heschl's gyri is somewhat larger than the right temporal lobe. These differences are so subtle that one would not expect to find major functional differences between the left and right hemispheres.

Animal studies and clinical evidence, however, suggest that there are indeed important differences between the hemispheres. For example, strokes affecting the right hemisphere produce left hemiparesis and left homonymous hemianopia but usually spare the personality, intellect, and consciousness. Strokes involving the right hemisphere do not usually affect speech, reading, or writing. In contrast, left-hemisphere strokes produce right hemiparesis and right homonymous hemianopia and can destroy the ability to use language. Large lesions to the left hemisphere can abolish a person's essence as a human being by destroying normal consciousness.

About 90% of the human population prefers to use the right hand for most delicate motor activities. The association of right-handedness and left hemispheric language function is almost universal. Only about 4% of the population have language representation in the right hemisphere. The reasons for the prevalence of language skills in the left hemisphere are not known. Many people with language skills in the right hemisphere had neonatal or perinatal brain damage to the left hemisphere. It is presumed that language development was transferred to the opposite hemisphere to compensate for the injury. However, brain injury does not explain all instances of right-hemisphere language development. For example, language representation has been found to be bilateral in bilingual interpreters (people who verbally translate language as it is being spoken), which suggests that if the linguistic pressures are great, the right hemisphere can be recruited. There are so many exceptions to these observations that generalizations are difficult to justify.

Differences between the left and right hemispheres other than language have only recently been systematically studied in the human. These studies are possible in patients whose corpora callosa were divided as a treatment for intractable epilepsy. Because these patients appear neurologically normal, it took many years to develop specific tests that elucidated the effects of hemispheric isolation. These tests take advantage of the fact that visual images can be presented to the two hemispheres independently (Fig. 15.5A). An image presented only to the right visual hemifield is perceived by the left hemisphere and accurately reported verbally. An image presented only to the left visual hemifield is perceived by the right hemisphere but cannot be accurately reported verbally; either the verbal report is a confabulation (made up without regard to facts) or the patient says that nothing was presented. The left hand, however, which is controlled by the right hemisphere, can correctly convey what was seen by pointing at a picture or picking up an appropriate object.

In addition to documenting the almost total lateralization of language in most persons, these isolated-hemisphere (split-brain) experiments have also provided insight into the lateralization of functions to the right hemisphere that could not be uncovered by other means. In general, functions relating to spatial problem solving are lateralized to the right. These problems are solved holistically, by what seems to be an intuitive approach. Examples of such problems are recognition of music and faces, three-dimensional puzzle solving, and map reading. The left hemisphere is more adept at solving problems that require a linear, stepwise, logical solution. Spoken language and mathematics are examples of such problems.

The left hemisphere also has a particular need to bring all observations into logical unity. After division of the hemispheres, the left hemisphere often invents a rationalization of the behavior of the left hand over which it has no control. One famous example occurred in an experiment in which a person with separated hemispheres was shown two pictures (Fig. 15.5B). The right hemisphere saw a house in a snowstorm; the left hemisphere saw a chicken claw. The patient was asked to select with his hands items that were logically related to the picture. The right hand picked out a chicken head; the left hand picked out a shovel. When asked why he made those particular choices, the patient replied that the chicken head obvi-

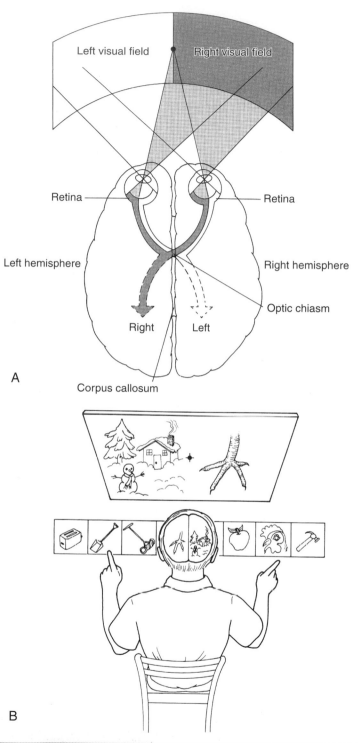

## Figure 15.5  Isolated hemisphere experiments

**A.** In persons with isolated hemispheres (split brain), the two hemispheres can be separately presented with information by taking advantage of the contralateral mapping of the visual hemifields on the primary visual cortex. The patient must gaze at the center spot and the stimulus must be brief (less than 100 msec) to ensure that the stimulus reaches only one hemisphere. **B.** Using the left and right hands independently, the subject points to a figure that correlates with what has been seen.

ously went with the claw; the shovel was needed to clean up after the chicken.

The need for communication between the hemispheres is dramatically revealed by the puzzle-solving paradigm. One patient with isolated hemispheres, when asked to use both hands to solve a three-dimensional block puzzle, demonstrated an amazing display of interhemispheric competition. The right hand (left hemisphere) grabbed all of the pieces of the puzzle and placed them at the far right end of the table. It then attempted to put the pieces together and failed. The left hand (right hemisphere) furtively grabbed two or three pieces and placed them at the extreme left side of the table, where it assembled them correctly. The left hand tried to grab another piece, but when the right hand (left hemisphere) became aware that some of the pieces were at the left side of the table, it grabbed all of the pieces and returned them to the right side, disassembling the partially completed structure in the process. The puzzle was never solved.

## DISORDERS OF THE CEREBRAL CORTEX

A wide variety of neurological disorders can be attributed to lesions in the cerebral cortex. Examples already discussed include spastic hemiparesis, hemiparesthesia, hemihypoesthesia, homonymous hemianopia, and central hearing losses. These disorders are directly related to the sensory or motor systems.

The cerebral cortex is essential for a number of important functions that are not directly related to the sensory or motor systems. Foremost among these functions is *the attachment of meaning to symbols in our minds or objects in our environment*. For example, the Platonic notion of dogness is the meaning and recognition we attach to one class of four-legged animals and to no others. An extension of this crucial function is language, because the essence of

language is the attachment of meaning to symbols. The symbols may be physical objects in our environment (the letters on the page), patterns of pressure waves in the air (sounds of spoken words), or patterns of neuronal activity that represent our thoughts.

A few of the more important nonsensorimotor disturbances of cortical function are discussed in the following paragraphs.

### Aphasia

Language is the use of complex abstract symbols to represent one's perception of the world to another. The symbols are related to each other by specific rules of *syntax* that help to organize and clarify the underlying *semantics*. Language is a function unique to the human cerebral cortex and the quintessential feature of the human mind.[5] Language is expressed outside the brain in multiple forms. In human society, one form, verbal (oral and written) language, is universal. It is commonly expressed in writing or speech but can also be expressed in other ways, such as by gestures in American Sign Language or by use in Braille, which is tactile. **Aphasia** [G. *a-; phasis*, speaking; and *-ia*, abnormal condition] is the inability to transform the internal mental representation of verbal language into its external spoken and written forms and vice versa, the inability to transform the external spoken or written forms into a meaningful internal verbal form.[6] Aphasia must be differentiated from **dysarthria** [G. *dys*, bad, difficult; *arthroun*, speak distinctly], speech loss due to a motor disorder; **dysphonia** [G. *phone*, voice], disorders of the larynx; and speech disorders secondary to **dementia** [L. *de*, down from, decrease in, and *mens*, mind] (discussed later in the chapter).

### ANATOMICAL CORRELATES OF LANGUAGE

The verbal language areas of the brain are restricted to a narrow band of tissue, the oper-

---

[5] A few chimpanzees and gorillas have been taught to sign with their hands or to use computer interfaces in an effort to determine whether they are capable of linguistic expression. The interpretation of these experiments is hotly debated. Regardless of these experiments, humans remain the only animals who have evolved as language users.

[6] The definition of aphasia includes all transformations of language, including Braille and American Sign Language. Documentation of these cases is sparse, but see the article by Bellugi et al. in the Suggested Readings list for a review of language deficits in deaf people following cortical lesions.

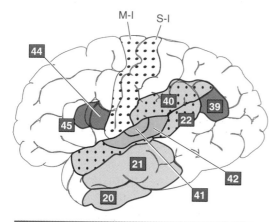

**Figure 15.6 Language areas of the left hemisphere**

Areas of the left hemisphere, identified by Brodmann number, that are associated with spoken and visual language.

culum on the lateral surface of the left hemisphere,[7] which surrounds the lateral sulcus (Fig. 15.6). The primary auditory cortex (areas 41 and 42) lies deep within the lateral fissure. Surrounding the primary auditory cortex is area 22, an auditory association area. Located in the parietal cortex, area 39 and its surrounding cortex mark the posterior boundary of the region of higher-order language. The frontoparietal operculum, which includes area 40, extends along the lateral fissure from area 39 to its anterior limit at area 44. Areas 44 and 45 mark the anterior limit of the superior opercular structures associated with higher language function. The arcuate fasciculus connects the posterior (area 39) region with the anterior (areas 44 and 45).

The language area is strategically located. The temporal operculum is connected by many association fibers to the primary auditory cortex and to the lateral temporal lobe (areas 20 and 21), a relation that is presumed to link spoken language with memory (see Chapter 14). To the posterior, area 39 is connected by association fibers to the visual association cortex, which is presumed

to link language with its visual representation in the cortex. The anterior region (areas 44 and 45) is linked by short association fibers with the motor areas of the face, tongue, and larynx. Lesions to each of these areas produces specific deficiencies in language, discussed next.

## EXPRESSIVE APHASIA

**Expressive aphasia** (formerly called Broca's aphasia) is the inability to transform one's thoughts into speech. Patients with this disorder have an essentially unimpaired mental concept of language. They can understand both spoken and written language. The frustration of understanding language but being denied linguistic expression usually causes the patients to attempt to speak. Such efforts produce only the most rudimentary forms of vocal expression. Unfortunately, the ability to write is usually impaired as well.

The nature of expressive aphasia is made apparent to the informed observer when the patient demonstrates good control over the muscles of the face and mouth. These patients can chew, swallow, and vocalize nonverbally, such as humming melodies (but not songs with the words). Depending on the size of the lesion, mild motor deficits of the right arm and face may be observed, but these deficits are not paralyzing and are not the cause of the language impairment. *Expressive aphasia is the inability to initiate vocal motor commands in response to the internal knowledge and will to do so.*

As might be expected, a wide range of disability is shown by patients with expressive aphasia. The least affected may be able to speak slowly and with difficulty. In some cases speech improves rapidly to nearly complete recovery. Most evidence suggests that in these cases only areas 44 and 45 are affected. In more serious cases the frontoparietal operculum, extending nearly the entire length of the lateral sulcus, may be affected. CT shows that the insula is rarely spared, although this finding may be incidental. Areas that are always

---

[7] As already discussed, in about 4% of the human population spoken language is lateralized to the right hemisphere. To simplify this discussion, however, spoken language is treated as if it were the exclusive province of the left hemisphere.

spared in expressive aphasia are area 39 and the inferior temporal operculum.

## RECEPTIVE APHASIA

Another language disturbance, **receptive aphasia** (formerly called Wernicke's aphasia), interferes with a person's ability to understand language. These patients have no apparent understanding of either spoken or written language and cannot extract meaning from linguistic symbols. Despite this deficiency, they verbalize effortlessly. The speech they produce is generally understandable in the sense that most of the words can be recognized. However, the vocalizations have *no syntactical or semantic meaning*. It is as if the word-generating part of the language system were connected to a random phrase generator. Since the patient cannot communicate effectively, there is no way to determine whether the internal representation of language is intact or also has been deranged. The only clue, perhaps, is that such persons seem to show no particular anxiety or distress as a result of their condition, unlike those with expressive aphasia, who display considerable frustration, distress, and anxiety.

Receptive aphasia is usually caused by a lesion of area 39. Frequently receptive aphasia is accompanied by a quadrantanopia because of the involvement of the indirect optic radiations that pass through the temporal lobe and lie deep to this area (see Chapter 12). Like expressive aphasia, many variations of receptive aphasia can be distinguished by the extent and the exact location of the lesion. Some patients can read but cannot comprehend spoken language. As with most insults to the cerebral cortex, receptive aphasia usually improves with time, although full recovery is not common.

## CORTICAL LANGUAGE PROCESSING

Observation of aphasic patients has led to certain theories about the representation of verbal language processing in the human brain. These theories recognize that *language is not a single process and that various aspects are relegated to different parts of the brain.* Auditory and visual association areas are thought to parse the sensory input into generic linguistic abstractions specific to each of these modalities. The abstractions are integrated into a universal language representation that endows the generic abstractions with meaning; this integration probably occurs in area 39. The frontoparietal operculum transforms the universal representation into generic motor commands that are specified more explicitly into vocal motor patterns by areas 44 and 45. Some evidence suggests that a similar premotor area adjacent to the hand area in the motor cortex governs writing.

The parceling of linguistic functions suggests that specific lesions should produce linguistic dissociations. For example, if only visual or auditory association areas are lost, the complementary language skill should be preserved if area 39 remains intact. Loss of the arcuate fasciculus, an association tract that connects the parietal with the frontal lobe, should leave comprehension of spoken and written language intact while disrupting the ability to speak intelligibly. Loss of only area 39 should devastate all language skills. While this scheme is oversimplified, to some degree these dissociations have been observed in patients who had infarctions restricted to these sites. The interpretation of these "accidental experiments" is open to considerable debate, since the lesion is seldom precisely defined. In addition, the few patients who have been systematically observed were not subject to controlled protocols.

## OTHER LANGUAGE REPRESENTATIONS

As we have noted, language is an abstraction and representation of the world in a symbolic form and is governed by syntactical rules designed to elucidate the underlying semantics. Symbols and syntax are not limited to the spoken and written forms that are so prominent in human society. For example, mathematics is a symbolic representation of the world with its own syntax. It is a highly developed and profoundly expressive language. Those who are skilled in its use can express and develop ideas that cannot be adequately expressed and developed with other forms of language. The language of mathematics does not, however, have a unique phonetic structure. Mathematical ideas can be verbalized only with the ordinary spoken language. Cortical lesions to the left parietal association areas, especially those close to area 39, severely disrupt mathematical functions.

Leonard Bernstein, in a particularly insightful series of lectures, proposed that music is a language in the same sense that English, German, and Chinese are languages. He argues persuasively that music has a *phonetic, syntactical,* and *semantic* structure that is analogous to that of verbal language. Music, of course, does not have the ability of verbal language to literally transcribe the external world into symbolic expression. Rather, music can powerfully express nonliteral symbolic meaning, much as poetry does. Like poetry, Bernstein argues, the power of musical expression depends on its *ambiguity,* a property that endows both poetry and music with multiple parallel meanings.

Unlike mathematics, music has independent phonology that makes possible the dissociation of musical expression from verbal expression. Most aspects of musical cortical function are associated with the right hemisphere, so lesions to the right parietotemporal lobes produce severe disruptions in the perception, appreciation, and expression of music while sparing verbal language. In contrast expressive verbal aphasia, because it is associated with left-hemisphere lesions, usually leaves musical expression relatively intact. If Bernstein's hypothesis is correct, our usual concept of language as exclusively a verbal abstraction of the world is too narrow. A more accurate concept of language would acknowledge that it is verbal, mathematical, and musical, with the right hemisphere's potential for linguistic processing having been appropriated for musical processing.

## Agnosia

To function normally, humans must be able to attach "meaning"—significance to the mind—to sensory stimuli. For humans, significance is usually brought about by relating sensory experiences to one's mental reference system. A person's reference system includes a *personal schema* of oneself, *memories* of similar experiences, *analogies* to stimuli derived from other

sensory modalities, and *expectations* derived from experience. **Agnosia** [G. *a-* and *gnosis,* perception] is the clinical term applied to disorders in which a patient is unable to attach meaning or significance to perceived sensory stimuli. *Agnosia is caused by a lesion that leaves the primary sensory pathways intact.* The sensory stimuli reach the brain and are perceived as stimuli, but they cannot be integrated into the mental system of reference.

## ASOMATOGNOSIA

Patients with parietal lesions of the nonspeaking hemisphere frequently manifest dramatic inability to attach meaning to stimuli coming from the contralateral half (usually left) of their field of perception. Despite intact vision, they may pay little or no attention to visual stimuli on the contralateral side. Neglect is usually seen as *left-sided* because the nondominant hemisphere is usually on the right; lesions to the dominant, speaking hemisphere are usually so devastating that the neglect cannot be demonstrated. The neglect disorder is known as **asomatognosia** [G. *a,* and *soma,* body]. These patients are unaware of tactile stimuli from the left side of the body. Furthermore, when asked to move the left extremity, they may move the right or not move at all. When shown their own left extremity, they may seem surprised. Asked to identify it, they may deny that it is their own arm or leg and assign its possession to the examiner or to God or simply express total bewilderment.

The inability to incorporate left-sided stimuli into the mental frame of reference also extends to self-directed activity. When asked to bisect a line, patients with right parietal lesions invariably mark the midpoint far to the right of center. If asked to draw the petals on a daisy or to number the face of a clock, they place all of the objects on the right half of the drawing (Fig. 15.7). Patients with this lesion frequently have a very difficult time dressing themselves, because they often fail to clothe the left side of their body. Women may apply lipstick only to the right side of the mouth, and men may shave only the right side of the face.

Patients with right parietal lesions have more than left-sided neglect; most cannot

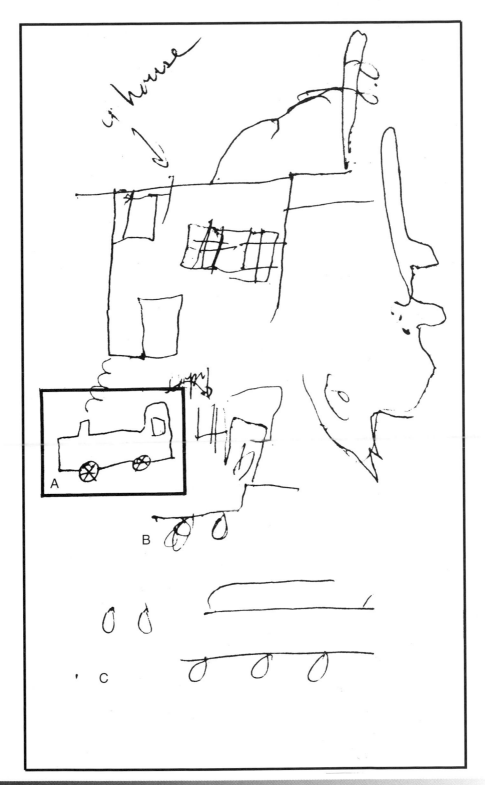

**Figure 15.7  Asomatognosia**

Patients with certain lesions to the right posterior parietal cortex are unaware of the left half of their world. When they attempt to draw figures, as in this example, they exhibit constructional apraxia. **A.** Figure drawn by the examiner. **B** and **C.** The patient's attempts to copy the figure. *Top.* Attempts by the patient to draw a house or the examiner are at the top of the figure. (Reprinted with permission from Curtis BA, Jacobson S, Marcus EM. An Introduction to the Neurosciences. Philadelphia: Saunders, 1972.)

solve spatial problems. Clothing presents particular difficulties, for these patients may be unable to figure out the orientation of a shirt and for example put their arm through the neck opening. With such a bad start, further attempts at dressing result in hopeless entanglement. They also have difficulty reading maps and relating them to the real world. They cannot follow routes and frequently get lost.

While asomatognosia is usually discussed in relation to the right (nonspeaking) hemisphere, it has also been observed to follow lesions in the parietal lobe of the left (speaking) hemisphere. Many cases of left-hemisphere asomatognosia are undoubtedly obscured by the associated aphasia, which makes effective communication with the patient impossible. When observable, however, the neglect syndrome is quite prominent when the left parietal lobe is affected.

## VISUAL AGNOSIAS

There are a number of visual agnosias, all of which are fairly rare but instructive. Two have already been discussed: **prosopagnosia** [G. *posopon,* face], the inability to recognize previously familiar faces, and visual motion agnosia (see Chapter 12). **Object agnosia** is the inability to identify familiar objects by sight even though ordinary vision is intact and there is no aphasia. The object can be immediately recognized by touch, sound, or smell, as appropriate. **Achromatopsia** [G. *a; chroma,* color; and *opsia,* sight] is visual agnosia limited to color perception. Patients cannot distinguish objects by color, although other aspects of vision are relatively normal. Achromatopsia must be differentiated from **color blindness**, an inherited disorder related to the loss of one or more of the visual pigments (see Chapter 12). The visual agnosias are more or less related to bilateral lesions of the inferior medial portion of the occipital lobe where it blends with the temporal lobe. The visual agnosias may appear independently or in combination.

The presence of visual agnosias that are independently related to different aspects of visual perception—motion, color, object recognition, and so on—implies that physically separate areas of the cerebral cortex are devoted to extracting specific information from the visual stimulus. Furthermore, information from these separate sensory processing centers must be integrated at other remote areas of the brain, usually called association cortex, before **perception** is realized. This hypothesis is difficult to verify from human lesions because few patients fulfill all the theoretical criteria for agnosia (loss of perception while all sensory, linguistic, and mental faculties are intact). The behavioral deficits of humans with various agnosias do seem to support the notion that multimodal integration is an essential component of the attachment of meaning to sensory phenomena. Animal studies also offer some validation for this idea. As discussed in Chapter 12, considerable physiological data support the hypothesis that the extraction of specific features of sensory signals is parceled to different physical regions of the cerebral cortex. However, animal studies cannot elucidate the nature of perception.

## Disorders in Personality and Motivation

In 1848, Phineas P. Gage, a shrewd, patient, and energetic railroad foreman, was tamping dynamite into a drill hole in rock. The dynamite exploded, driving the tamping rod through his left orbit. The rod, 3.5 feet long and 1.25 inches in diameter, emerged from the superior surface of his skull anterior to the coronal suture near the midline, destroying most of the frontal lobes in the process. J. M. Harlow, a physician, treated Gage, daily cleansing the wound by scraping away pustulant and necrotic brain tissue until the defect closed and healed. Harlow followed this patient for a number of years and published his findings in 1868. The most remarkable feature of the Gage case other than his initial recovery[8] was that he had few obvious neurolog-

---

[8] Such a recovery is not unprecedented. An elderly retired physician told me that soon after he left medical school, he was called to a farm where there had been a terrible accident. A 2-year-old child had been kicked in the head by a horse. Upon arriving at the scene, the physician observed that the right hemisphere had been almost entirely removed by the horse's hoof. The wound had clotted but was contaminated with straw, dirt, and manure. He advised the family to prepare for the child's imminent death, but much to his surprise, the boy survived, grew to manhood, graduated from college, and led a full and productive life.

ical deficits. However, in addition to the relatively minor motor and sensory deficits, Mr. Gage did suffer a marked change in personality. To quote from Harlow:

> Previous to his injury . . . he possessed a well-balanced mind, and was looked upon by those who knew him as a shrewd, smart business man, very energetic and persistent in executing all his plans of operation. [After his recovery] the equilibrium . . . between his intellectual faculties and animal propensities seems to have been destroyed. He is fitful, irreverent, indulging at times in the grossest profanity (which was not previously his custom), manifesting but little deference for his fellows, impatient of restraint or advice when it conflicts with his desires, at times pertinaciously obstinate yet capricious and vacillating, devising many plans of future operation, which are no sooner arranged than they are abandoned in turn for others appearing more feasible. A child in his intellectual capacity and manifestations, he has the animal passions of a strong man. . . . In this regard his mind was radically changed, so decidedly that his friends and acquaintances said he was "no longer Gage". (Harlow, 1868)

Gage lived for many years but never recovered his original personal qualities. The changes observed by Harlow have now become recognized as **prefrontal lobe syndrome**, which results from lesions to the portion of the frontal lobes anterior to the premotor area (anterior to area 6). The most important features of the syndrome are (*a*) personality changes, (*b*) deficits in strategic planning, (*c*) perseveration, (*d*) release of "primitive" reflexes, and (*e*) **abulia**.

Personality changes accompany the apathetic state. Patients with prefrontal lobe lesions frequently exhibit lack of compassion and sensitivity to social conditions. They are usually uninhibited and may make inappropriate jokes or comments that are hurtful to others. They seem to have no concept of social restraint.

Persons with lesions to the prefrontal lobes also exhibit certain mental deficiencies that are usually thought to be associated with strategic thinking and planning. They may not be able to solve problems that require planning. This deficiency is not a memory defect, because they can describe the problem. They cannot apply that knowledge or abstract the problem in ways that suggest options for a solution.

Another characteristic feature of frontal lobe lesions is perseveration, the constant repetition of an action in response to a situation. Perseveration may manifest in a number of ways. When asked to name objects, for example, a patient may correctly identify a pen that is presented for identification. The patient identifies the next object, a set of keys, as a pen; likewise a handkerchief. In other words, once the idea of "pen" has been established, the patient gets stuck on it and cannot free the thought processes so as to entertain a new idea. In a different, more subtle context, the patient may devise a correct solution to a problem, but if the problem is changed to require a new solution, the patient doggedly sticks to the original strategy despite its ineffectiveness.

Abulia [G. *a,* and *boule,* will] refers to a general slowing of the intellectual faculties. The patient is apathetic, speech is slow, and spontaneous participation in social intercourse is decreased almost to the point of nonparticipation. The profoundly apathetic patient may lie motionless and mute for weeks, despite intact sensory modalities and the ability to speak and move. This condition is sometimes called akinetic mutism.

A more objective sign of prefrontal lobe lesions is the emergence of "primitive" infantile reflexes that are suppressed with development. A good example is the suckling reflex evoked by touching the cheek. The head turns reflexively to the side of the stimulus and the mouth attempts to find and suckle the nipple. Scratching the palmar surface of the hand evokes a reflex closure of the fingers, allowing the infant to grasp whatever touches the hand. Normally suppressed in the adult, these reflexes are released with loss of prefrontal lobe function. The elicitation of primitive reflexes is an important part of the examination, as it may provide the only objective evidence of frontal lobe involvement.

## Dementia

Dementia is a general term that describes the global loss of higher cortical functions, especially memory, personality, and language. Dementia can be caused by any process that interferes with cortical function, including disease, hydrocephalus, toxins, and multiple cerebral infarcts. The most common cause of dementia is **Alzheimer's disease**, a degenerative disorder that constitutes about half of diagnosed dementias. Dementia secondary to vascular disease accounts for another 25% of presentations.

Alzheimer's disease causes a loss of neurons in the telencephalon, particularly the large pyramidal cells of the cerebral cortex. The remaining neurons contain less RNA and are smaller than normal. The loss of neurons is accompanied by proliferation of astrocytes and thinning of the outer cortex that widens the gyri, a marker that can be visualized with CT or MRI. **Senile** or **neuritic plaques** are found scattered throughout the cortical gray matter at autopsy. These plaques contain an **amyloid protein** [G. *amylon,* starch, and *eidos,* like] and fragments of degenerated dendrites, terminals, and lysosomes. **Neurofibrillary bodies** composed of twisted pairs of tubules are found within many neurons. The loss of neurons and the number of plaques and neurofibrillary bodies correlate quite closely with the degree of dementia. Although these pathological changes occur throughout the cerebral cortex, the temporal, frontal, and parietal lobes are usually the most severely affected. The most severely damaged parts of the brain are $CA_1$ of the hippocampus and the subiculum. It is presumed that loss of these areas causes the distinctive memory deficits associated with Alzheimer's disease.

Alzheimer's disease usually begins after the sixth decade of life but can occur sooner. Its frequency increases with age (Fig. 15.8). The incidence of onset for ages 30 to 59 is 0.02%. It rises about 10-fold to 0.3% between ages 60 and 69. Another 10-fold increase occurs during ages 70 to 79, when the rate is 3.2%. The 80- to 89-year-old population runs a risk of 10.8%. Alzheimer's is partly hereditary; an autosomal dominant gene on chromosome 21 has been associated with it. The expression of the gene, however, is not determined by hereditary influences alone. Although first-degree descendants of a person with Alzheimer's disease have a risk about 4 to 5 times that of unrelated persons, only about half of identical twin children of an affected person develop the disease. The related risk factors are not known. Nearly all persons with Down's syndrome (trisomy 21) develop amyloid plaques and neurofibrillary bodies after age 40.

The clinical picture of Alzheimer's disease is relentlessly progressing dementia with rela-

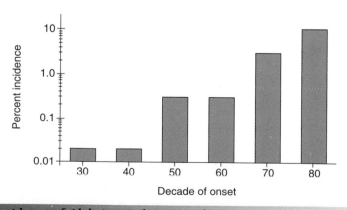

**Figure 15.8   Incidence of Alzheimer's disease with age**

tive sparing of other neural functions until the later stages of the disease. For example, motor skills remain relatively intact. The muscle stretch reflexes remain normal, and the plantar signs are flexor. The most characteristic symptoms are loss of memory, loss of spatial orientation, and personality changes.

Memory deficits are frequently the first symptoms to appear. Initially, the deficit manifests as simple forgetfulness, the inability to recall a name or think of a word. Later, Alzheimer's patients have difficulty incorporating the present into long-term memory, a situation that is similar to Korsakoff's amnesic state (see Chapter 14). Patients also begin to have speech difficulties, particularly aspects that require memory. For example, because they have difficulty finding the right word, patients with Alzheimer's disease have halting speech interspersed with pauses. Eventually the patient falls mute. As the cerebral cortex continues to deteriorate, the effects on the language areas become more profound. Language comprehension also becomes defective, affecting not only verbal comprehension but reading and writing.

When the loss of neurons involves the parietal lobes, particularly on the right side, the patient becomes increasingly disoriented (see discussion of agnosia earlier in the chapter). They get lost easily and cannot follow even a simple map. They have trouble dressing because they cannot correlate the spatial arrangement of the clothing with their bodies. They may display any of the agnosias associated with parietal lobe injury. Involvement of the frontal lobes can produce personality changes associated with prefrontal lobe syndrome (discussed earlier in the chapter). In the later stages of the disease, primitive reflexes appear and are followed by bowel and bladder incontinence. The incontinence appears to be more related to apathy than to lack of motor control.

New drugs appear to slow the progression of the disease in some cases, but the process itself remains refractory to medical intervention. It is important, however, to diagnose Alzheimer's disease accurately to differentiate it from treatable causes of dementia. The most common non-Alzheimer's dementias are secondary to depression, normopressure hydrocephalus, operable intracranial masses, nutritional deficiencies, endocrinological disorders that affect general metabolism, and drug intoxication.

## ETHICAL ISSUES OF DEATH

Mrs. C. B., a 25-year-old woman, entered the hospital for a routine prenatal ultrasound examination. Unfortunately, the examination revealed an anencephalic fetus. Mrs. C. B. and her husband were counseled and advised of their options, which included carrying the infant to term (with a 65% probability of stillbirth) or termination of the pregnancy. The parents' religious beliefs precluded abortion. After considerable deliberation, they asked that if born alive, the baby could be declared brain dead at birth so that the organs could be donated for transplant. The health care providers could not grant the parent's request because anencephalic babies are born with a functional brainstem and do not meet the legal requirements of brain death. The parents petitioned the courts and were denied their request. The baby was carried to term and was born alive, but by the time she died of natural causes, her internal organs had deteriorated to the point that organ donation was no longer possible.

One of the unintended consequences of modern medical advances has been to blur the line between life and death. Before the second half of the 20th century, death was marked by the rapid and nearly simultaneous collapse of all organ systems. Now, with medical intervention, organ systems do not necessarily cease to function simultaneously. The need for a formal definition of death compatible with a partly functioning body gave rise to the concept of brain death in the 1960s. The *1980 Uniform Determination of Death Act* and the *1981 Report of the President's Commission* have set a legal and practical foundation for establishing death in the United States. Unfortunately, much debate still surrounds both documents, and there is little agreement among physicians, philosophers, and the legal profession about the presuppositions those authors brought to the discussion or with the conclusions they drew.

The legal questions related to determining death are not settled. Criteria for determining death vary from nation to nation, and within the United States they vary from state to state. Hospitals set their own standards for determining death in accordance with the ethical and legal environment in which they operate. Therefore, it is not possible in these few pages to describe a protocol for establishing death. In general no single criterion can be used to determine death. For example, electrocerebral silence as determined by EEG is one criterion. It is an imperfect tool, however, since drug-induced reversible metabolic coma can produce electrocerebral silence. To provide a reasonable assurance of death, most protocols require some evidence of *brainstem death* as well as *cerebral death*. The former is often determined by documenting sustained apnea or by the demonstration of an isoelectric BAER (see Chapter 11).

What exactly constitutes brain death? The general notion is that someone without a functioning brain is dead even if other bodily functions are present. The original, practical approach to brain death was that loss of brain function served as a reliable *predictor* of collapse of all other organ system functions. Collapse was certain if the brainstem ceased to function, since respiration depends on brainstem integrity. A more recent approach to brain death rests on the presumption that human life may be divided into cognitive (human consciousness and cognition) and biological (all other organic functions, such as digestion and respiration) forms. Assuming that this division is valid, the loss of cognitive capability signals the loss of human capacity and therefore *the extinction of the person as a human being*. Since consciousness and cognition appear to reside exclusively in the cerebral cortex, the loss of cortical function alone would be sufficient to signal the end of human capacity even if the brainstem remained viable.

The anencephalic infant brings these issues into sharp focus. These babies have no cerebral cortex but do have a functioning brainstem. They clearly have biological life. They respond to touch, sound, and light. Many of them have eye movements and even follow an object with their eyes. All of these responses can be associated with brainstem function alone, and as long as any part of the brainstem is functional, they cannot be declared brain dead in most countries. The ethical debate centers on how much cognitive capability they have. Those who define death in cognitive terms argue that anencephalic infants cannot have human cognitive capacity. Without cognitive potential they do not and can never exist as a human being. They are therefore brain dead. Consequently, supporters of the cognitive definition of brain death argue that the laws are not consistent with our understanding of brain function. Others argue that since the neurological capacity of an anencephalic infant is comparable with that of intact normal infants for at least the first 2 months of life, they should be accorded the same rights and protections that are afforded normal infants. They argue that the laws should remain conservative, notwithstanding the need for organ donors and other practical considerations.

The ambiguity of death is forcing society to reexamine its beliefs about the essence of humanity. What really separates humans from other life forms? Is it our consciousness? If so, what defines and differentiates human consciousness from animal awareness? Is human consciousness a unique consequence of human brain function? Without consciousness, have we lost our human qualities? Can we be alive as *human* beings if we have no conscious awareness? Of course, none of these questions can be answered definitively. Knowledge of the structure and function of the brain does have a bearing on how we think about these questions. Struggling with these questions is necessary if one is to find a morally acceptable as well as practical way of facing the problems that the ambiguity of death has thrust upon modern society and the medical practitioner.

# C A S E   H I S T O R Y

## THE VENGEFUL TREE[9]

### HISTORY OF PRESENT ILLNESS

Mr. G. P., a 36-year-old landscaper, was seen in the emergency department because a large tree branch fell on his head as he was cutting down the tree with a chain saw. The branch pushed his chest onto the handle of the chain saw, and the blade of the saw got stuck in the ground. He complained of chest and back pain and headache. The 8-cm laceration on his occipital scalp was repaired. A cervical spine radiograph and neurological examination produced normal findings. He was discharged.

Then, 48 hours later, Mr. G. P. took approximately 12 200-mg ibuprofen tablets over a brief period because of worsening interscapular pain. About 4 hours later, 52 hours after the initial injury, he complained of sudden worsening of the back pain, which radiated to the anterior chest and shoulders. He fell to the floor unable to move his legs and complained of numbness in his legs. He was able to move his arms and his left toes. As he was brought to the emergency department by ambulance, he lost all motor activity of his lower extremities and noted tingling of his arms. Over 2 hours in the emergency department and radiology suite he developed weakness of hand grip.

### PHYSICAL EXAMINATION

Blood pressure 160/95; respirations 12 and labored.

### NEUROLOGICAL EXAMINATION

#### Mental Status
Mr. G. P. is awake, alert, and oriented to person, time, and place.

#### Cranial Nerves
No abnormalities in cranial nerve function were observed.

#### Station and Gait
Not tested.

#### Motor Systems

STRENGTH: Strength was 0/5 in all muscle groups in both lower extremities; strength of hand grip and wrist flexors, 4/5.

TONE: Muscle tone was flaccid in both lower extremities. The upper extremity tone was normal.

BULK: Muscle bulk was normal for a laboring man of his age. There was no atrophy.

ABNORMAL MOVEMENTS: None were observed.

#### Sensory Systems
There is a complete sensory loss to pinprick and light cotton touch from the C7-T1 level down.

#### Reflexes
MSRs from the brachioradialis, biceps, and triceps are normal bilaterally. The gastrocnemius and quadriceps MSRs are absent bilaterally. There is no response to plantar stimulation. Cremasteric and abdominal reflexes are absent bilaterally. There is paradoxical abdominal motion with breathing. There is no rectal tone and the anal wink reflex[10] is absent.

#### Coordination and Control
Not tested.

#### Parietal Functions
Not tested.

#### ANCILLARY STUDIES

Both radiography and CT of the thoracic spine produced normal findings. CT of the cervical spine suggested an epidural hematoma at C6 to

---

[9] This case was provided to me by Mark Walsh, St. Joseph Medical Center, South Bend, IN.
[10] Scratching the skin adjacent to the anus elicits a reflex contraction of the anal sphincter.

C7. A myelogram revealed a long circumferential epidural hematoma extending from C2 to T3 with a nearly complete block at C6 to C7 (Fig. 15.9).

## SUBSEQUENT COURSE

The patient was immediately taken to surgery, where a laminectomy from C3 to T3 was performed to relieve the pressure on the spinal cord and evacuate the hematoma. In the recovery room Mr. G. P. noted normal movement of his arms and fingers. Over the next 2 weeks he regained complete recovery of his motor and sensory functions in the reverse order of the ascending paralysis.

## COMMENTARY

In Mr. G. P.'s case the extreme and rapid flexion of the spine over the handle of the impaled chain saw probably stretched the spinal cord over the anterior bodies of the vertebrae, contusing the venous plexus from approximately C6 to C7 and causing some relatively minor bleeding. The large quantities of ibuprofen the patient took caused platelet dysfunction, which resulted in significant bleeding from the already compromised venous plexus. The resultant bleeding caused strangulation of the spinal cord. The sudden weakness of the lower extremities followed by the gradual onset of partial motor and sensory loss of the upper extremities dramatically demonstrates the sequential compression of the corticospinal tract fibers: those that extend to the lumbar cord are superficial to those serving the thoracic region; the fibers that terminate in the cervical spinal cord lie deepest in the tract (see Chapter 7). Therefore, slow strangulation of the spinal cord produces *ascending paralysis*. Despite its classification as an UMN lesion, the acute presentation is flaccid paralysis due to spinal shock. After the pressure on the spinal cord was relieved, the return of motor function

mirrored the pattern of motor losses, with function returning first to the deepest corticospinal fibers serving the upper extremities and then to the more superficial fibers serving the chest, abdomen, and lower extremities. The excellent recovery obtained in this case is attributed to the prompt diagnosis and rapid decompression. Prolonged compression of the spinal cord normally results in permanent paralysis.

## FURTHER APPLICATIONS

**15.1.** This patient's initial injury was head trauma, yet he had a spinal hemorrhage. What key observations should direct your attention to spinal trauma rather than cerebral trauma?

**15.2.** If Mr. G. P. had an intracranial bleed, how would you differentiate between an epidural and a subarachnoid intracranial hematoma? Is this distinction important? Would bleeding from the external auditory meatus be significant in making this distinction? Explain.

**15.3.** Describe the pattern of paralysis that you would expect if the bleed were intracranial. How does this pattern differ from Mr. G. P.'s?

**15.4.** What pattern of sensory losses, if any, would you expect to observe if the lesion were intracranial? How does this pattern differ from that of the present case?

**15.5.** If the lesion were intracranial, would you expect cranial nerve involvement? If so, which nerve or nerves? What would you see? Explain. What were the cranial nerve findings in this case?

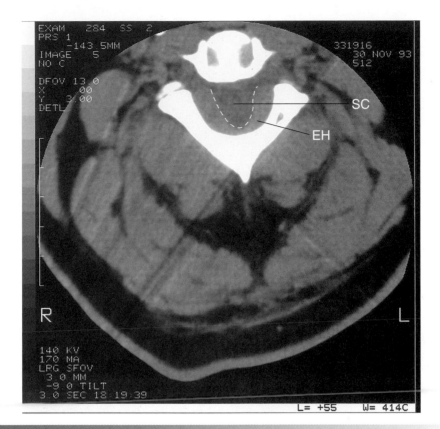

**Figure 15.9   Spinal CT from Mr. G. P.**

The *broken lines* outline the spinal cord (*SC*), which is surrounded by an epidural hematoma (*EH*). The spinal cord is somewhat misshapen by compression. The dense white areas are the vertebrae.

# C A S E   H I S T O R Y

## THE SLEEPY MAN WITH BUGGY EYES[11]

### HISTORY OF PRESENT ILLNESS

Mr. C. V. was a 70-year-old Baptist minister. His wife took him to the emergency department with the complaint, "My husband's eyes be buggy and he be sleepy." The patient was in good health until an hour prior to admission, when he suddenly began to have a waxing and waning level of consciousness associated with widening of the palpebral fissures and extension of the neck when attempting to look at objects.

---

[11] This case was given to me by Mark Walsh and Janet Peterson, St. Joseph Medical Center, South Bend, IN.

## MEDICAL HISTORY

Mr. C. V. has a history of hypertension, congestive heart failure, and insulin-dependent diabetes mellitus.

## PHYSICAL EXAMINATION

Temperature, 97° F; heart rate 80; blood pressure 160/78; respirations 20.

## NEUROLOGICAL EXAMINATION (TAKEN SOON AFTER ADMISSION TO THE EMERGENCY DEPARTMENT)

### Mental Status

Progressive obtundation was noted in the emergency department. At first Mr. C. V. could be aroused, was able to give his name, and knew he was in the hospital, although he was confused. Within an hour the patient was snoring and could be aroused only with a sternal rub (stupor).

### Cranial Nerves

OLFACTION: Not noted.

VISION: Visual fields were full.

OCULOMOTION: There was paralysis of upward gaze on volition, but the eyes tracked vertically during the doll's-eye maneuver.

TRIGEMINAL: Pinprick was perceived from all three divisions bilaterally; masseter muscles were strong.

FACIAL: Grimace was symmetrical. Salivation and lacrimation were present.

AUDITION: Not tested.

VAGOGLOSSOPHARYNGEAL: The gag reflex was present; the voice was not hoarse.

ACCESSORY: Not noted.

HYPOGLOSSAL: The tongue protruded in the midline.

### Station and Gait

Standing, walking, and hopping not tested due to mental status.

### Motor Systems

STRENGTH: Strength seemed normal but could not be quantified because of the patient's inability to cooperate.

TONE: Tone was normal; no spasticity was observed.

BULK: Normal for a sedentary man of his age.

ABNORMAL MOVEMENTS: None observed.

### Sensory Systems

Response to pinprick was symmetrical and seemed within normal limits, given the patient's impaired mental status.

### Reflexes

Bilaterally, the MSRs were (-) from the quadriceps and normal from the brachioradialis, biceps, and triceps. There was no MSR from the gastrocnemius bilaterally.

### Coordination and Control

Not tested.

### Parietal Functions

Not tested.

## ANCILLARY STUDIES

CT was read as normal. Given the history of diabetes mellitus, a hemorrhage (visible by CT) is much more likely than an embolism or thrombosis (not visible by CT), so the normal CT was completely unexpected. The clinical picture of paralysis of upward gaze and alteration of levels of consciousness are classic signs of a lesion in the mesencephalon. Therefore, after considerable deliberation, additional CT images (cut in very thin planes at the mesencephalon) were obtained and the radiologist was asked to read the case again. He immediately amended his previous normal reading because a 1.5-cm intensity in the right side of the quadrigeminal plate was now visible. It was believed to indicate a mesencephalic hematoma in the region of the aqueduct (Fig. 15.10).

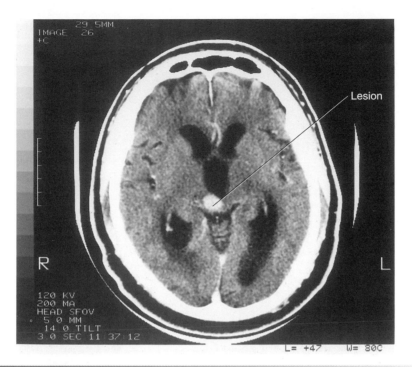

Lesion

**Figure 15.10    Cranial CT from Mr. C. V.**

The abnormality (*L*) in the region of the quadrigeminal plate is small but evident. CT slices on either side of this image do not show the lesion. (CT courtesy of St. Joseph Medical Center, South Bend, IN.)

## SUBSEQUENT COURSE

The patient remained intermittently obtunded, with persistent paralysis of the upward gaze. Each day the patient's wife would express concern over his running nose. This sign seemed trivial, since her husband's survival was in doubt. Mrs. C. V. continued to badger the resident, demanding that he address the issue of the running nose. The resident noted that in fact the patient had considerable nasal discharge. He probed the matter further by sitting down alone face to face with the patient's wife to discuss what he considered the insignificant problem of a running nose. Once seated, the wife told the resident that the nasal symptoms had appeared at about the same time as the neurological symptoms. She asked if there might be a causal association between the two. The resident indulgently replied that it was unlikely. However, she became insistent that a causal relation existed. At this point the resident fixed her gaze and with

exasperation asked why she was so insistent on linking the running nose with the patient's cerebral hemorrhage. Mrs. C. V. replied, "Well, doctor, I just wonder if that cocaine he was taking before he got a runny nose had anything to do with his eyes being buggy and he being so sleepy." This statement finally got the resident's attention. Mr. C. V. eventually made a full recovery. He stopped using cocaine and the other recreational drugs to which he had become accustomed and returned to his ministry. He died a few years later of unrelated causes.

## COMMENTARY

The important clinical signs of supranuclear ophthalmoplegia of vertical gaze combined with the rapid deterioration of consciousness are classic symptoms of a mesencephalic lesion. It is clear that the patient's obtundation was caused by dysfunction of the mesencephalic reticular formation and that his loss of vertical gaze was due to a lesion involving the superior colliculus or pretectal area. These small structures are close together only at the rostral pole of the mesencephalon. Given the rapid onset of symptoms, this lesion is probably due to a stroke.

Two principles of history taking and diagnosis are demonstrated by this case. First, always determine the location of the lesion before seeking ancillary data. If the ancillary data are not congruent with the lesion as you have placed it, determine how the discrepancy occurred. Do not simply take another opinion at face value. In this case, the discrepancy between the clinical picture seen in the emergency department and the opinion of the radiologist arose because the bleed was so small it did not appear on the initial CT. The difference of opinion was resolved by taking subsequent CT images cut at different levels in the mesencephalon, which eventually revealed the lesion. The subsequent CT images had great diagnostic importance in this case because during the early stages of a stroke, CT can reveal only fresh blood, not ischemic infarction. In the absence of a demonstrable lesion by CT, an ischemic event is assumed and anticoagulation with heparin is normally indicated. This course of treatment would have had disastrous results in this case.

Second, the wife's constant badgering had a point. Only after the young doctor took the appropriate amount of time to listen to her carefully and gain her confidence did she confide what she knew all along to be the cause of her husband's illness—cocaine. The cocaine had raised his blood pressure and caused a small hemorrhage in one of his brittle diabetic vessels. Had the patient's use of cocaine been known on the night of admission, hemorrhagic stroke would have been more carefully considered and reevaluation of the CT results would have been easier. This case reveals these important points: listen carefully to the history, believe your patient, and trust your observations.

## FURTHER APPLICATIONS

15.6.  How do you know this lesion is supranuclear ophthalmoplegia rather than nuclear ophthalmoplegia?

15.7.  An ischemic stroke is not revealed by CT during the first 48 hours. The initial read of the CT is consistent with an ischemic stroke. What do you think are the elements in this case that made the emergency department physicians uneasy about the normal CT? How would knowing the history of cocaine use been useful in arriving at a diagnosis?

15.8.  Describe the clinical observations that clearly place this lesion below the tentorium. Particularly discuss the importance of the changing levels of consciousness.

15.9.  Review the risk factors for stroke (see Chapter 7). How are they pertinent in this case?

## SUMMARY

- The cortical columns are collections of cells that form the fundamental computational unit of the cerebral cortex.

The higher-order complex functions of the cerebral cortex are derived from the interactions between the cortical columns. Together the columns create a functional complex more powerful than the individual components. No satisfactory methods for monitoring the properties of ensembles of neurons are yet available.

- The EEG is a crude measure of the electrical events of the cerebral cortex.

The EEG reflects PSP activity in pyramidal cells. For convenience of description this activity can be divided into four frequency bands: the $\beta$-band, 13 to 30 Hz; $\alpha$-band, 8 to 13 Hz; $\theta$-band, 4 to 8 Hz; and $\delta$-band, 0.5 to 4 Hz. The lower frequencies signal synchronization among pyramidal cells; higher frequencies reflect lack of synchronization. High frequencies are associated with states of mental alertness. Despite its limitations, the EEG is a useful clinical tool.

- **The EEG is useful in determining various states of consciousness.**

The most common state of altered consciousness is sleep, a period of intense brain activity that is somehow necessary for normal brain function. Deprived of sleep, the brain becomes dysfunctional, incapable of sustained mental activity during wakefulness. Based on EEG recordings, sleep is divided into five stages, 1 through 4 and REM. During an evening of sleep, a person passes through the stages in sequence in a series of sleep cycles, each culminating with a period of REM. Dreaming occurs only during REM.

- **The various states of brain activity are determined by the brainstem, which drives thalamic nuclei.**

The thalamus in turn sets cortical activity. Lesions to the brainstem, particularly to the PAG, locus ceruleus, and the raphe nuclei, can produce an irreversible cortical state that is similar, if not indistinguishable, from sleep.

- **Sleep disorders are characterized as insomnia, hypersomnia, or parasomnia.**

Most types of insomnia are related to stress and are temporary. Nonobstructive sleep apnea is a disorder in which hypopnea is caused by a depressed central respiratory drive. The resulting hypoxemia wakes the person frequently during the night, disrupting the normal sleep cycle. The most common hypersomnia, obstructive sleep apnea, also produces excessive daytime sleepiness but it does not usually awaken the patient during the night. Narcolepsy, another hypersomnia, is thought to be a REM-like state that intrudes during normally wakeful periods. Disturbances of the normal circadian rhythm can also produce hypersomnia during inappropriate times. Motor disturbances during sleep, such as sleepwalking in children, are considered parasomnia.

- **Brain injury can alter the conscious state.**

In increasing order of severity, the altered states of consciousness are confusion, stupor, coma, and cerebral death. Altered states of consciousness can be caused by a variety of insults, including concussion or contusion, increased intracranial pressure, disruptions in electrochemical balance or pH, hypoxia, hypoglycemia, and drugs or toxins. Supratentorial lesions usually produce altered states of consciousness that progress from confusion to coma in an orderly manner. Infratentorial lesions can produce coma and death immediately, without progressing through less severe stages, if the brainstem centers that control cortical activity and the respiratory centers are affected early in the course of events.

- **Seizures are periods of abnormal, hyperactive, synchronized neuronal activity in the cerebral cortex.**

Seizures may be classified as partial if they initially involve a restricted part of the brain or general if they appear to initially involve the entire cerebral cortex. Partial seizures, which are associated with motor or sensory auras that are appropriate to the locus of the seizure, are considered simple if consciousness is not affected or complex if mental awareness is altered. In the later case, the postaura period is characterized by automatisms. General seizures always affect consciousness. Absence seizures consist of periods of unawareness of one's surroundings. They are brief (seconds) and frequent (several to several hundred times a day). Clonic-tonic general seizures are dramatic events that involve both loss of consciousness and brief periods of altered muscular activity. Febrile seizures are general seizures of infancy associated with a fever of rapid onset. Epilepsy is a condition of repeated seizures that continues throughout life unless successfully treated.

- **The cerebral cortex is not functionally homogeneous.**

Language operations are performed in the left hemisphere in all but 4% of the population. Problems that involve linear, stepwise thinking, such as mathematics, are solved in the left hemisphere. Spatial or pattern problems, such as face recognition and musical skills, that are solved in a parallel, holistic manner are generally performed in the right hemisphere.

- Specific cortical lesions in humans produce functional deficits that are related to the location of the lesion.

Aphasia is produced by lesions (usually) to the left hemisphere in the region of the lateral fissure. Lesions to the posterior area produce receptive aphasia; more-anterior ones involving the frontal operculum produce expressive aphasia. Agnosia results from lesions to the transition areas between the parietal, occipital, and temporal cortical lobes. Asomatognosia is particularly pronounced if the right posterior parietal cortex is lost; visual agnosias are more readily produced by lesions to the inferior occipitotemporal cortex. Lesions to the prefrontal lobes produce perseveration, abulia, release of primitive reflexes, and alterations in personality and strategic planning. Dementia is not related to losses of a specific portion of the cerebral cortex but instead is caused by a general loss of cortical neurons, particularly pyramidal cells. Alzheimer's disease is the most common dementia.

- The technical ability of modern medicine to maintain the viability of major organ systems despite the loss of function of the cerebral cortex and brainstem has raised moral and ethical issues concerning the determination of death.

These issues deal with such questions as the nature of humanity itself and its relation to the brain and brain functions.

## SUGGESTED READINGS

Bellugi U, Poizner H, Klima ES. Language, modality and the brain. Trends Neurosci 1989;12:380–388.

Bernstein L. The Unanswered Question: Six Talks at Harvard. Cambridge, MA: Harvard University, 1976.

Churchland PS, Sejnowski TJ. The Computational Brain. Cambridge, MA: MIT, 1992.

Churchland PS. Neurophilosophy: Toward a Unified Science of the Mind–Brain. Cambridge, MA: MIT, 1986.

Deacon T. The Symbolic Species: The Co-evolution of Language and the Brain. New York: Norton, 1997.

Denny-Brown D. The frontal lobes and their functions. In: Feiling A, ed. Modern Trends in Neurology. New York: Hoeber, 1951.

Edelman GM. Neural Darwinism: The Theory of Neuronal Group Selection. New York: Basic Books, 1987.

Edelman GM. The Remembered Present: A Biological Theory of Consciousness. New York: Basic Books, 1989.

Edelman GM. Bright Air, Brilliant Fire: On the Matter of the Mind. New York: Basic Books, 1992.

Edelman GM, Mountcastle VB. The Mindful Brain. Cambridge, MA: MIT, 1978.

Harlow JM. Recovery from the passage of an iron bar through the head. Mass Med Soc Publ 1868;2:327–346.

Jaynes J. The Origin of Consciousness in the Breakdown of the Bicameral Mind. Boston: Houghton Mifflin, 1976.

Lechtenberg R. Seizure Recognition and Treatment. New York: Churchill Livingstone, 1990.

Llinas R, Churchland P, eds. The Mind–Brain Continuum: Sensory Processes. Cambridge, MA: MIT, 1996.

McCullagh P. Brain Dead, Brain Absent, Brain Donors: Human Subjects or Human Objects. New York: Wiley, 1993.

Plum F, Posner JB. The Diagnosis of Stupor and Coma. 3rd ed. Philadelphia: Davis, 1980.

Scully RE, Mark EJ, McNeely WF, Ebeling SH. A 67-year-old man with three years of dementia. New Engl J Med 1999;340:1269–1277.

Searle J. Minds and brains without programs. In: Blakemore C, Greenfield S, eds. Mindwaves. Oxford: Basil Blackwell, 1987.

Springer SP, Deutsch G. Left Brain, Right Brain: Perspectives on Cognitive Neuroscience. 5th ed. New York: WH Freeman, 1998.

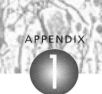

# Neuroembryology

*T. R. Kingsley*

A bit of historical background often goes a long way toward explaining the status quo. In the same way, knowledge of the developmental history of the nervous system, or **neuroembryology**, can clarify the anatomical and functional relations among parts of the nervous system, both anatomical and functional. This introduction to basic embryology is intended to serve these functions. Although recognizable components of the nervous system do not form until the third week of development, a brief review of preneurological embryology is presented first to introduce terms and concepts that set the stage for the discussion that follows.

## EARLY DEVELOPMENT

Human development begins with fertilization, the union of a sperm and egg to form a single-celled **zygote**. The first week following fertilization is marked by rapid cell proliferation via **cleavage**, a type of mitotic division that increases cell number without increasing cytoplasmic mass. After cleavage cells begin to **differentiate**; that is, they become committed to a specific developmental state.

The cells formed as a result of cleavage are **blastomeres** [G. *blastos,* germ, and *meros,* part] (Fig. A1.1). By the fourth day after fertilization, 12 to 16 blastomeres have formed a **morula** [L. *morus,* mulberry], a solid spherical mass. The morula is transformed into a **blastocyst** when it acquires a fluid-filled central

cavity, the **blastocyst cavity.** Two recognizable cell populations are present at this stage, the **trophoblast** [G. *trophe,* nutrition], which forms the surface of the sphere, and the **embryoblast** or **inner cell mass,** a knot of central cells that attaches to the inner surface of the trophoblast. In general, the trophoblast gives rise to the **fetal membranes,** the **amnion, chorion,** fetal components of the **placenta,** and the **primary yolk sac;** the embryoblast gives rise to the embryo itself.

During the second week of development implantation is completed and the formation of the three primary germ layers, or **gastrulation,** begins. The embryoblast is first transformed into the **embryonic disc,** a nearly circular plate of cells. Soon two distinct layers of cells can be discerned within the embryoblast. One layer, which consists of tall columnar cells, is the **epiblast** [G. *epi,* upon]. The other, a layer of cuboidal cells, constitutes the **hypoblast** [G. *hypo,* under]. At this point the embryoblastic tissue may be described as a **bilaminar disc.**

Completion of gastrulation, the formation of a **trilaminar disc,** is signaled by rapid proliferation of cells in the epiblast (Fig. A1.1, *E* and *F*). This proliferation results in the formation of a thick strip of tissue, the **primitive streak,** which extends from the border of the embryonic disc to a point near its midregion. The origin of the primitive streak marks the future caudal end of the embryo, so its location defines the craniocaudal axis. The prim-

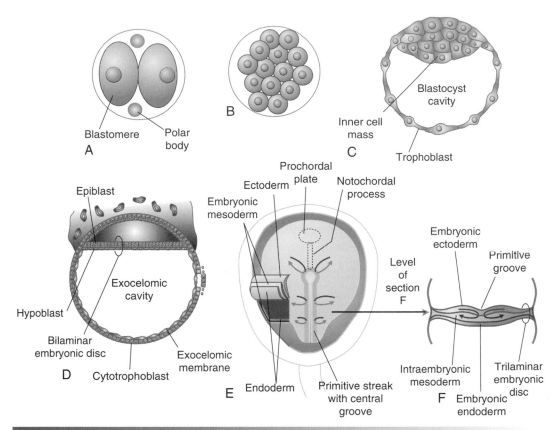

**Figure A1.1    Early embryological development**

**A.** Within 30 hours of fertilization the cell mass subdivides into two blastomeres. **B.** The morula, a solid mass of 12 to 16 blastomeres, forms by the third day. **C.** A fluid-filled blastocyst forms by the fourth day. **D.** During the second week after fertilization, cells of the embryoblast form a bilaminar disc. The upper layer is designated epiblast; the lower, hypoblast. **E.** During the third week cells of the epiblast (ectoderm) proliferate to form a primitive streak. Epiblastic cells migrate down from the region of the primitive streak to form a layer of cells (mesoderm) that intervenes between epiblast and hypoblast. This transforms the embryo into a trilaminar disc (dorsal view). **F.** Transverse section of the trilaminar disc is shown.

itive streak also permits identification of the dorsal and ventral surfaces of the embryo. Epiblastic cells migrate from the deep surface of the primitive streak and form a layer of tissue between the epiblast and the hypoblast. This layer, the **embryonic mesoderm**, progresses to the margins of the embryonic disc. It eventually occupies all areas except for two small axial regions, the **prochordal plate** near the cranial end of the embryo and the **cloacal membrane** near the caudal end of the embryo.

With the formation of embryonic mesoderm the embryonic disc becomes trilaminar.

The layer originally designated as epiblast is now called **ectoderm** [G. *ekdos,* outside, and *derma,* skin]; the layer originally designated as hypoblast is now called **endoderm** [G. *endo,* within]. The three primary germ layers—ectoderm, mesoderm, and endoderm—give rise to all of the more highly differentiated structures of the body. Ectoderm produces the epidermis and nervous system. Endoderm gives rise to the epithelial linings of the respiratory tract and digestive tract and to portions of organs associated with the digestive tract. Mesoderm is the source of the remainder of the organism, including all varieties of connective tissue and muscle, vascular structures, blood cells, bone marrow, and portions of internal organs

After the development of embryonic mesoderm, the primitive streak regresses toward the caudal end of the embryo. Normally it degenerates completely, but occasionally remnants persist, giving rise to a tumor usually in the region of the lower spinal column. Such a tumor is known as a **teratoma** [G. *teras,* monster, and *oma,* tumor]. Since it develops from an embryonic structure that produces a wide variety of tissues and structures, the tumor may exhibit any of a variety of component tissue types.

The first structure to develop within the newly forming embryonic mesoderm is the **notochord** [G. *notos,* back, and *chorde,* string]. This rodlike structure begins to form at the cranial terminus of the primitive streak and extends cranially as far as the prochordal plate. As the primitive streak regresses caudally, the notochord follows. The lengthened notochord now defines the craniocaudal axis of the embryo and lends some rigidity to the embryonic structure. It also has other important functions that are particularly interesting to students of neuroscience. First, the notochord induces the differentiation of a portion of overlying ectoderm to form the primordium of the nervous system. Second, it is the center around which the developing vertebrae form. While the notochord eventually degenerates in the regions where the vertebral bone develops, it persists in the intervertebral spaces, forming the **nucleus pulposus** [L. *pulpa,* flesh] of the **intervertebral disc.**

## DEVELOPMENT OF THE NERVOUS SYSTEM

The term **neurulation** describes the sequence of events that characterizes the formation of the neural plate and neural folds and their conversion into a hollow neural tube (Fig. A1.2). As the notochord begins to develop (approximately day 16 of gestation), it induces the ectoderm dorsal to it to proliferate, forming the **neural plate.**

By day 18 an invagination, the **neural groove,** develops along the midline of the neural plate. At the lateral edges of the groove

are the **neural folds.** By day 21 the neural folds have begun to approach each other in the midline. They eventually meet and form a closed **neural tube.** As they do so, a portion of the tissue found in the area of the neural fold fails to become incorporated into the neural tube. This tissue, the **neural crest,** loses its connection with the overlying surface ectoderm and comes to occupy a midline position between the neural tube and the surface ectoderm. The neural crest rapidly divides into left and right portions that migrate to positions dorsolateral to the neural tube.

Neural crest cells are important to the formation of the peripheral nervous system, since they give rise to all of the sensory cells of peripheral ganglia. They are also the source of Schwann cells and cells of the chromaffin system, including paraganglia, the adrenal medulla, and cells within the carotid and aortic bodies. Neural crest cells can migrate throughout the embryo and may give rise to nonneuronal cell populations as diverse as the melanocytes in the skin, the stria vascularis of the inner ear, and enteroendocrine cells.

## EARLY DEVELOPMENT OF THE CENTRAL NERVOUS SYSTEM

The central nervous system (CNS), which consists of the brain and spinal cord, is derived from the neural tube.

### Development of the Neural Tube

Conversion of the neural groove to a closed tube occurs over several days early in week 4. Closure begins in the region of the fourth to sixth pairs of somites and proceeds both cranially and caudally. The tube is temporarily open at both ends. The cranial opening, the **rostral neuropore,** closes by about day 25. The caudal opening, the **caudal neuropore,** closes by about day 27. The region of the fourth pair of somites marks a dividing point for the CNS. Rostral to this point the neural tube forms the brain; caudal to it the tube develops into the spinal cord.

The neural tube is initially a thin-walled structure having a large central lumen, or

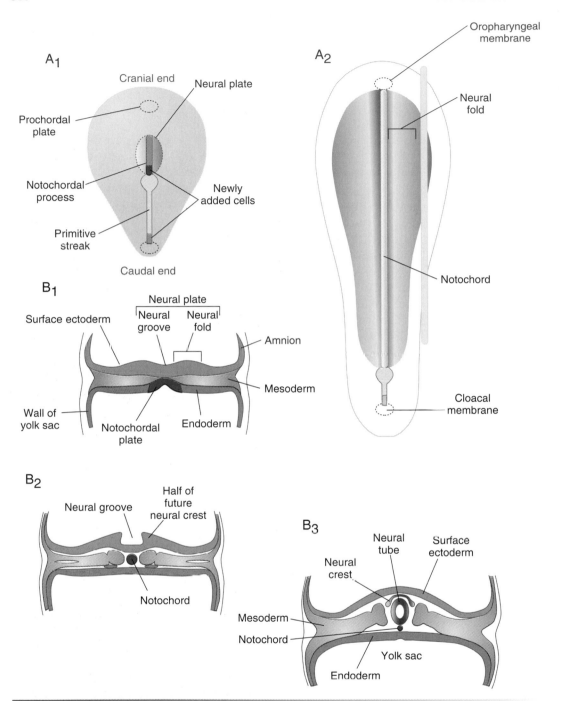

**Figure A1.2    Neurulation**

Development of the notochord induces the overlying ectoderm to transform into neuroectoderm (**A₁** at 17 days, **A₂** at 21 days). This tissue develops as a flat neural plate. A central neural groove with lateral neural folds begins to form by day 18 (**B₁**). The groove deepens (**B₂**), then folds together to form a neural tube by day 21 (**B₃**). Cells from the region of the neural fold separate from the developing tube and from the overlying ectoderm, forming a band of tissue called the neural crest (**B₃**), which later separates into left and right portions dorsolateral to the neural tube.

neural canal. The walls consist of pseudostratified neuroepithelium, each cell of which reaches from the lumen to the margin of the tube (Fig. A1.3, *A* and *B*). Beginning in the fourth week the neuroepithelial cells proliferate rapidly and differentiate into the precursors of categories of cells that will eventually constitute the tissue of the CNS.

As cell replication progresses, the walls of the neural tube thicken. Simultaneously the neural canal diminishes to form a smaller channel that will ultimately form the **ventricular system** of the brain and the **central canal** of the spinal cord. Gradually layers, or zones, of cells become apparent within the tissue of the tube (Fig. A1.3*C*). Remnants of the original neuroepithelial layer remain adjacent to the lumen and form the **ventricular zone**, or **ependymal layer**. This layer will form the epithelial lining of the ventricles and central canal and the epithelium of the choroid plexus. Cells that migrate away from the lumen form the **mantle (intermediate) layer**. All neurons of the CNS and most of the supporting cells, or **macroglia** [G. *makros*, large, and *glia*, glue], are derived

from this layer. A third region, the marginal layer, lies farthest from the lumen. It is composed primarily of axons that grow out from cells of the mantle layer. In the mature nervous system highly cellular regions that are derived from the intermediate zone constitute **gray matter**; regions that are composed primarily of axons constitute **white matter**.

## Origin of Cell Types

Neurons develop from precursor cells that migrate into the intermediate zone. Evidence suggests that primitive neurons, or **neuroblasts**, are assisted in their migration by a population of cells called **radial glial cells**. This cell group differentiates from cells in the parent neuroepithelial cell layer and continues to span the entire width of the neural tube as it thickens. They guide the migration of the newly formed neuroblasts.

Initially the neuroblast has no processes and is therefore called an **apolar neuroblast**. Soon two processes, a primitive axon and a primitive dendrite, develop, after which the cell is termed a **bipolar neuroblast**. The dendritic process de-

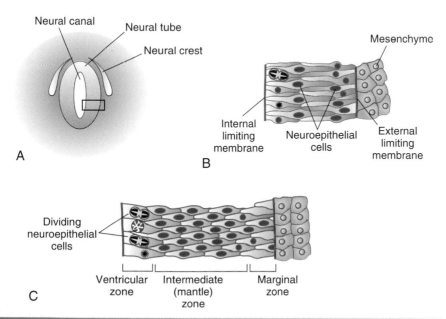

A

B

C

Neural canal

Neural tube

Neural crest

Mesenchyme

Internal limiting membrane

Neuroepithelial cells

External limiting membrane

Dividing neuroepithelial cells

Ventricular zone

Intermediate (mantle) zone

Marginal zone

### Figure A1.3 Development of the cell layers of the primitive CNS

During the fourth week the wall of the neural tube (**A** and **B**) consists of neuroepithelial cells that span the width of the tube from the internal limiting membrane to the external limiting membrane. Continued proliferation of neuroepithelial cells thickens the tube, and three zones gradually emerge (**C**).

generates, leaving a **unipolar neuroblast**, and is replaced with multiple dendrites, transforming the cell into a **multipolar neuroblast**.

After most of the neuroblasts develop, other cells of neuroepithelial origin enter the intermediate zone and differentiate into the macroglia of the CNS. Primitive forms of these cells are called **glioblasts**, or spongioblasts. Some become **astroblasts** [G. *astro*, star], which develop into **astrocytes**. Others become **oligodendroblasts** [G. *oligo*, few, and *dendron*, tree], which mature into **oligodendrocytes**. An additional type of supporting cell found within the CNS, the **microglia**, is not derived from the neuroepithelium; it arises from surrounding primitive mesoderm and migrates into the CNS to become a phagocyte.

### Development of Afferent and Efferent Regions

Continued proliferation of cells along the extent of the neural tube thickens the walls. The pattern of cell proliferation produces a shallow groove along the inner lateral surface of the walls on each side. This groove, the **sulcus limitans** [L. *sulcus*, groove, and *limes*, limit], extends the entire length of the future spinal cord and as far rostral as the future midbrain. It divides the neural tube into a dorsal region, the **alar plate** [L. *ala*, wing] (Fig. A1.4), and a ventral region, the **basal plate**. Structures that develop in the alar plate region mediate **afferent functions** [L. *ad*, to, and *ferre*, carry to] (i.e., information being conveyed into the CNS), and structures found in the basal plate region mediate **efferent functions** [L. *ex*, out] (i.e., information being conveyed from the CNS towards the periphery). Thus, the sulcus limitans forms a handy landmark, neatly dividing the spinal cord and part of the brain into functional regions.

The developing neural tube is surrounded by primitive mesoderm that soon differentiates into connective tissue wrappings called **meninges**. The meninges begin development as a single thick membrane called the **primitive meninx** [G. *meninx*, membrane]. This membrane differentiates secondarily into an outer layer, the **pachymeninx** [G. *pachys*, thick], equivalent to the **dura mater** [L. *dura*, hard, and

*mater*, mother], and a thinner inner zone that forms the **leptomeninges** [G. *lepto*, delicate], which includes the **pia mater** [L. *pius*] and the **arachnoid** [G. *arachne*, spider] layer. The pia mater and arachnoid layer are initially apposed but become separated by the **subarachnoid space**. This space later is filled with **cerebrospinal fluid** (CSF).

### FURTHER DEVELOPMENT OF THE SPINAL CORD

By the sixth week of fetal development the spinal cord begins to assume the morphology that will characterize its adult form. The cell bodies of the mantle layer have produced an area of gray matter that occupies the region near the central canal; their axons in the marginal layer have begun to form a well-defined layer of white matter. **Dorsal root ganglia** cells, which are peripheral ganglia derived from the neural crest, first appear as clumps of cells adjacent to the dorsolateral portion of the spinal cord (Fig. A1.4). Nerve processes from these cells grow into the alar plate region of the developing cord, forming the **dorsal root** of the spinal nerve. **Ventral nerve** rootlets also emerge from the basal plate region. By the fourteenth week of development cells in the central gray matter have organized to form functionally associated groups of cells, or nuclei.

From the time of neural tube formation until the beginning of the third month of fetal development, the spinal cord runs the entire length of the embryo and extends into the developing coccygeal region. Spinal nerves exit through intervertebral foramina at approximately their level of origin (Fig. A1.5A). However, as development progresses, the rate of growth of the vertebral column exceeds that of the spinal cord. This causes the caudal end of the spinal cord to lie at more rostral regions of the vertebral column (Fig. A1.5, B–D). In the adult the spinal cord terminates in the upper lumber region (T12 to L3). Spinal nerves from the lower lumbar, sacral, and coccygeal regions retain their original points of exit between the vertebrae but lengthen as the rate of growth of the vertebral column outstrips that of the spinal cord. As a

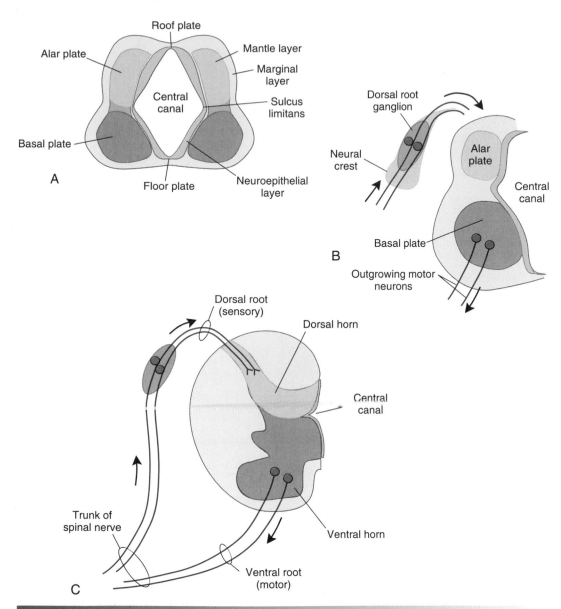

A

B

C

### Figure A1.4 Evolution of the alar and basal plates

The alar and basal plates evolve into sensory and motor regions, respectively. The line that divides the two areas, the sulcus limitans, is an important landmark that extends from the spinal cord through the mesencephalon (**A,** week 6). By the sixth week the sensory ganglion, developing from the neural crest, sends axons into the alar plate region of the CNS. At the same time motor neurons in the basal plate extend axons from the CNS (**B**). The sensory ganglion extends peripheral axons that meet motor axons leaving the CNS. Joined, they form a spinal nerve that contains both afferent (sensory) and efferent (motor) components (**C**).

result, the lower end of the vertebral column is occupied by a sheaf of nerve fibers known as the **cauda equina** [L. *cauda,* tail, and *equinus,* pertaining to a horse]. The dura mater and arachnoid continue to line the entire length of the vertebral column in the adult. The pia mater terminates at the caudal end of the spinal cord, the **conus medullaris** [G. *konos,*

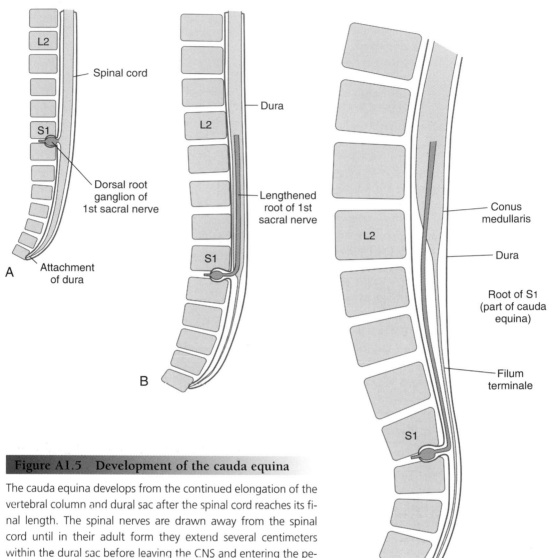

**Figure A1.5  Development of the cauda equina**

The cauda equina develops from the continued elongation of the vertebral column and dural sac after the spinal cord reaches its final length. The spinal nerves are drawn away from the spinal cord until in their adult form they extend several centimeters within the dural sac before leaving the CNS and entering the peripheral space (**A,** third month; **B,** 5 to 6 months; **C,** neonate). The portion of the dural sac between the conus medullaris and its termination at the first coccygeal vertebra forms the lumbar cistern, from which CSF can safely and conveniently be sampled.

cone, and L. *medulla,* marrow]. Only a thin thread of pia mater, the **filum terminale** [L., thread], extends from the conus medullaris to the first coccygeal vertebrae, defining the discrepancy between the initial and final extents of the spinal cord. Because of this anatomical orientation, the subarachnoid space is quite large below the level of the conus medullaris. Consequently, the vertebral column below the level of L3 is a suitable site to insert a needle into the subarachnoid space to obtain a sam-

ple of CSF, a procedure known as a **spinal lumbar puncture.** Inserting a needle in this region carries little risk of damaging the spinal cord.

## CONGENITAL MALFORMATIONS OF THE SPINAL CORD

Failure of the rostral or caudal neuropore to close results in any of a variety of congenital malformations of the brain and spinal cord, respectively. The most common malformation, lack of closure of the caudal neuropore, can produce defects in the spinal cord itself and in structures that lie dorsal to it, including the meninges, vertebral arch, dorsal musculature, and skin. **Spina bifida** [L. *bifidus,* cleft] is a generic term that describes spinal malformations; **crania bifida** describes cranial malformations. Both conditions always include some form of failure of the overlying bone to fuse, but the conditions encompass a hierarchy of severity ranging from asymptomatic to fatal.

**Spina bifida occulta** [L. *occulo,* to cover or hide] (Fig. A1.6*A*) is the minimal degree of defect, in which the halves of the vertebral arch fail to grow together in the medial plane. This produces a dimple often marked by a tuft of hair. The defect is often apparent on the surface and does not involve the underlying meninges or neural tissue. Generally asymptomatic, it is a curiosity found at the L5 or S1 vertebra in approximately 10% of the population.

A more severe malformation, **spina bifida cystica** [G. *kystis,* bladder] is characterized by a saclike protrusion into the cleft between the

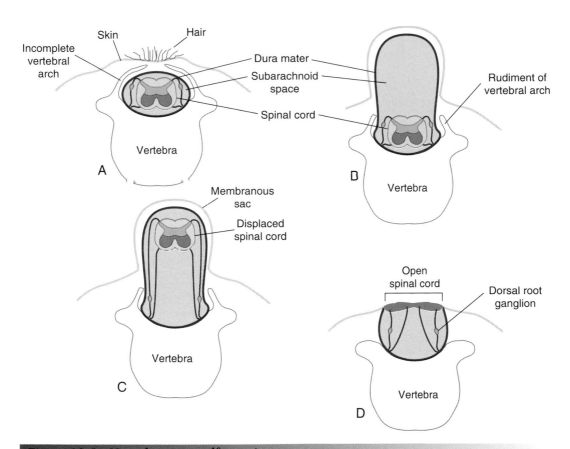

**Figure A1.6  Neural groove malformations**

Common malformations of the spinal cord due to failure of the neural groove to close completely. **A.** Spina bifida occulta. The dural sac and spinal cord are normal. The dorsal aspect of the vertebra is not closed, and a hairy patch over the area is common. **B.** Spina bifida with meningocele. The bony deficit is larger than in spina bifida occulta, resulting in a ballooning dural sac. The neural elements remain in their proper place, and there are usually no neurological deficits. **C.** Spina bifida with meningomyelocele. This condition is similar to spina bifida with meningocele except that the spinal cord and associated spinal nerves are displaced into the expanded dural cavity. This malformation is always associated with neurological deficits. **D.** Spina bifida with myeloschisis. In this case the failure of the neural groove to close is extreme, and the spinal canal does not form. The exposed neural tissue is little more than a malformed neural plate.

unfused halves of the vertebral arch. It has three subtypes. In **spina bifida with meningocele** (Fig. A1.6B), the sac contains only meninges and CSF; in **spina bifida with meningomyelocele** (Fig. A1.6B), the sac also contains tissues of the spinal cord or nerve roots. Both defects can occur at any level of the vertebral column but are most common in the lumbar region. The most severe and rarest form is **spina bifida with myeloschisis** [G. *myelo,* marrow, and *schisis,* cleaving] (Fig. A1.6D). This condition results from a failure of the neural tube to close over an extensive region of the spinal cord, producing an exposed flat mass of neural tissue.

The various forms of spina bifida cystica produce different degrees of neural deficit at levels appropriate to the level of the lesion. Skin sensation is usually lost from regions innervated by nerves at that level; some degree of muscle paralysis is also present. Meningomyeloceles at the lumbosacral level often cause paralysis of bladder or anal sphincters.

Spina bifida cystica can be detected in the developing fetus by measuring the level of **α-fetoprotein** in the amniotic fluid. This protein, normally present in small amounts, is greatly elevated in the presence of spina bifida cystica. The condition may also be seen via ultrasound examination after the 10th week of gestation.

## FURTHER DEVELOPMENT OF THE BRAIN

The region of the neural tube that forms the brain initially resembles the region destined to form the spinal cord. However, beginning in the fourth week of development, the portion of the neural tube rostral to the fourth pair of somites undergoes a series of dilations and foldings that rearrange the tissue into a compact spherical mass and define the functional regions of the adult brain (Fig. A1.7). This process begins when the tube dilates to form three **primary brain vesicles**, the **prosencephalon** [G. *proso,* forward, and *enkephalos,* brain] (or forebrain),

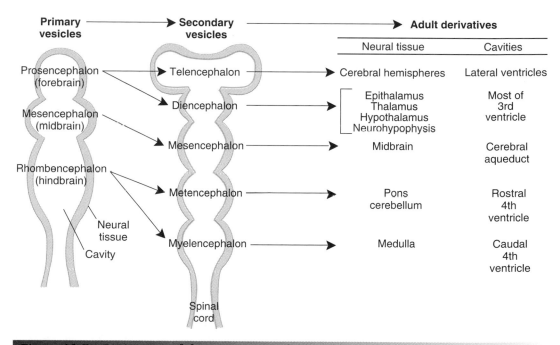

**Figure A1.7   Derivatives of the primary vesicles**

After closure of the rostral neuropore, the neural tube rostral to the level of the fourth somites forms three swellings, the primary vesicles (about day 28). By day 35 the prosencephalon and rhombencephalon divide. This division produces the five secondary brain vesicles from which the definitive brain structures, neural tissue, and cavities develop.

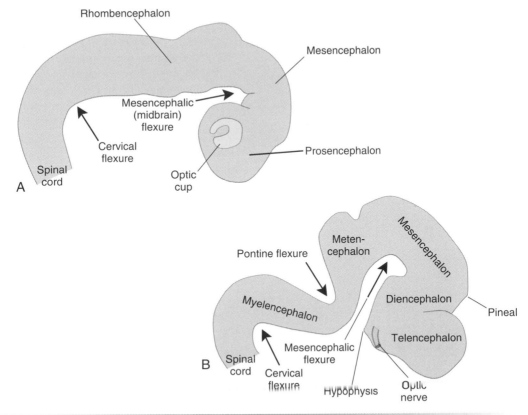

---

#### Figure A1.8    Folding of the rostral neural tube

During the fourth week the rostral neural tube begins to flex at the junction of the spinal cord and rhomben-cephalon, forming the cervical flexure, and at the mesencephalon, forming the mesencephalic flexure (**A**). During the sixth week the pontine flexure develops between the metencephalon and the myelencephalon (**B**). This folding produces a compact mass of tissue that approximates the shape of the adult brain.

---

**mesencephalon** [G. *mesos,* middle] (or mid-brain), and **rhombencephalon** [G. *rhombos,* rhombus] (or hindbrain).

During the fifth week of development the prosencephalon subdivides to form the **telencephalon** [G. *telos,* end] and the **diencephalon** [G. *dia,* through]. The rhombencephalon subdivides to form the **metencephalon** [G. *meta,* after] and the **myelencephalon** [G. *myelo,* marrow]. The mesencephalon does not divide. Each of the resulting five **secondary brain vesicles** consists of a wall of neural tissue bordering a fluid-filled cavity. The cavities persist in the adult as the **ventricular system** of the brain. The sulcus limitans continues rostral from the spinal cord as far as the junction between mesencephalon and the diencephalon,

extending the regional division into alar and basal plates up to that level.

The folding of the brain occurs in two phases (Fig. A1.8). During the fourth week, the prosencephalon bends ventrally, forming a ventrally directed concavity in the mesencephalic region; a similar ventrally directed concavity is formed by a ventral bending at the juncture of the rhombencephalon with the spinal cord. In this manner the **midbrain flexure** and the **cervical flexures** are formed. A third flexure, which has a dorsally directed concavity, forms at the juncture of the metencephalon and myelencephalon during the sixth week. This **pontine flexure** exerts forces that thin the roof of the metencephalon and myelencephalon.

## The Myelencephalon

The tissue of the myelencephalon develops into the **medulla oblongata** of the adult brain. The rostral portion of the myelencephalic cavity becomes part of the **fourth ventricle**, and the caudal portion of the cavity narrows to form the **central canal**, which is continuous with the central canal of the spinal cord. The caudal portion of the myelencephalon retains some of the anatomical characteristics of the adjacent spinal cord (Fig. A1.9A). The lumen remains a small central canal marked by the sulcus limitans, and the division into alar and basal plates persists. However, the arrangement of components of the mantle and marginal layers is different from that of the spinal cord. In the caudal myelencephalon groups of neuroblasts in the mantle layer (gray matter) of the alar plate migrate into the marginal layer (white matter) to become the **inferior olivary nuclei**. At the dorsal border of the myelencephalon, neuroblasts form nuclei on either side of the midline. These nuclei, named from medial to lateral, become the **gracile nucleus**, the **cuneate nucleus**, and the **nucleus of the spinal tract of V.**

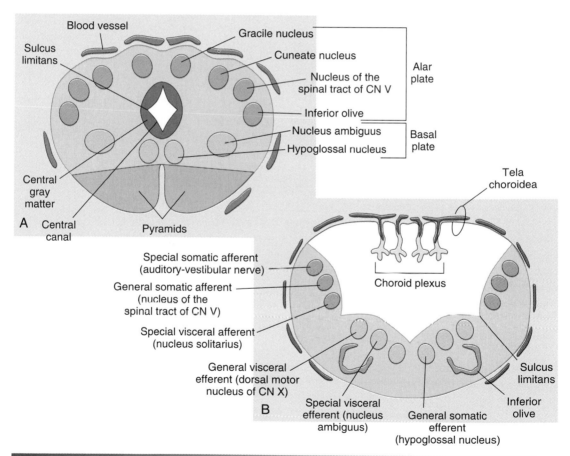

**Figure A1.9   The myelencephalon at 5 weeks**

**A.** Transverse section through the caudal part of the myelencephalon. At this stage it is very similar to the spinal cord: it has a small central canal and a nearly spherical cross-section. The cells of the alar and basal mantle regions begin to migrate and organize into individual nuclei in the marginal layer. **B.** Transverse section through the rostral myelencephalon. The lateral movement of the alar plate has transformed the fourth ventricle into a flat, thin-roofed structure. A series of cell columns is found adjacent to the floor of the ventricle; dorsolateral columns are alar plate derivatives; ventral medial columns are derived from the basal plate.

In the rostral portion of the myelencephalon, the arrangement of components diverges further from the pattern found in the spinal cord (Fig. A1.9*B*). As the result of the development of the pontine flexure, neural tissue originally in the dorsomedial portion of the neural tube is pushed laterally, as if on a hinge at the sulcus limitans. The fluid-filled canal enlarges to form the broad, flat rhomboid-shaped fourth ventricle. The lateral movement of the dorsal neural tissue leaves behind a thin ventricular roof composed only of meninges apposed to ependyma. Along the floor of the fourth ventricle are neuroblasts that form a series of cell columns. Columns that lie dorsolateral to the sulcus limitans are tissue of the alar plate and are associated with sensory function. Those that lie ventral medial to the sulcus limitans are tissue of the basal plate and are associated with motor function. Each column processes neural information of a specific type; that is, its function is associated with a single neural **modality** (at right). The relative positions of cell columns associated with specific modalities remains consistent along the extent of the rostral myelencephalon (Fig. A1.9*B*).

Nerve fibers emerging from the neuroblasts that form these cell columns contribute to structures called **cranial nerves**, which exit from the brainstem and innervate peripheral structures. The 12 pairs, designated CN I to XII, extend from various portions of the brainstem. Some cranial nerves mediate a single modality, such as special somatic sensory information; others mediate a wide assortment of modalities. Cell columns of the myelencephalon develop into nuclei associated with CN XII to IX.

### Metencephalon

The neural tissue of the metencephalon gives rise to the **pons** [L., bridge] and **cerebellum** [L. *cerebellum*, little brain, dim. of *cerebrum*, brain]. Its cavity develops into the rostral portion of the fourth ventricle. Before the eighth week of development the metencephalon resembles the myelencephalon. It has a broad rhomboid-shaped ventricle with a thin roof. Components of the alar plate lie in the dorsolateral region; basal plate components, in the ventral medial region.

## NEURAL MODALITIES

The term *neural modality* describes the nature of the information carried by a given axon. Classical neural terminology defines a number of modalities.

**Afferent** (sensory): transmitted from peripheral sensors, or **receptors**, toward the CNS.

**Efferent** (motor): transmitted from the CNS towards peripheral **effectors**, such as muscle cells or secretory cells that respond to neural stimuli.

Sensory and motor information can be further defined according to the anatomical distribution of the innervation.

**Visceral**: transmitted to or from internal organs (viscera) or regions derived from the branchial arches.

**Somatic**: transmitted to or from the remainder of the body (nonvisceral structures), such as skin and muscles.

A final rather arbitrary distinction is based on the embryological origin of a structure.

**Special**: transmitted to or from a specified subgroup of visceral or somatic structures. **Special visceral** information is transmitted to or from structures derived from the branchial arch region of the embryo. **Special somatic** information qualifies sensory or afferent information transmitted from an organ of special sense, such as the retina, cochlear organ, taste buds, olfactory organ, or vestibular organ.

**General**: transmitted to or from all visceral or somatic structures other than special ones.

A given *axon* is limited to transmitting a single modality; that is, it may be a special somatic or general visceral efferent, for example. *Peripheral nerves* are composed of a mixed population of axons, so a given peripheral nerve may transmit a number of modalities.

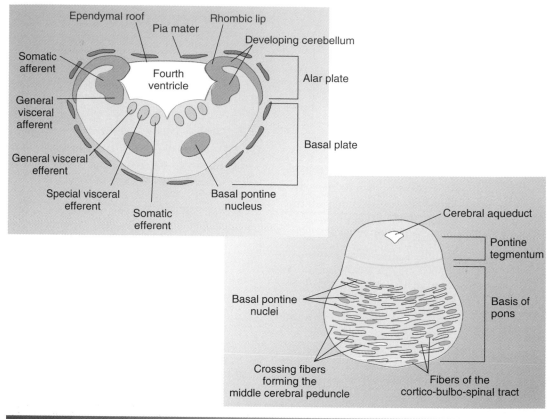

**Figure A1.10   The metencephalon**

**A.** Transverse section through the metencephalon near the end of the fifth week of development. The organization of nuclei across the floor of the fourth ventricle is similar to that in the rostral myelencephalon. In the metencephalon the alar plate further differentiates into the structures associated with the cerebellum. A portion of the alar plate also migrates ventrally to form the basal pontine nuclei. These develop into the principal source of afferent axons to the cerebellar hemispheres. **B.** Transverse section through the adult metencephalon. The greatly expanded basis is formed principally of fibers from the basal pontine nuclei that cross the midline en route to the cerebellum.

## PONS

The pons develops in the region lateral and ventral to the fourth ventricle. The alar plate components form columns of cells in the extreme dorsolateral region of the pons. Some neuroblasts from the alar plate region migrate into the ventral portion of the pontine area, where they join with neuroblasts that migrated from the alar plate region of the myelencephalon to form the **basal pontine nuclei** (Fig. A1.10*A*).

The area that borders the floor of the fourth ventricle constitutes the **tegmentum of the pons** [L. *tegmen*, cover]. This region develops from the basal plate and contains columns of

cells associated with motor function. Ventral to the tegmentum is the **basis of the pons.** This region is initially small and is occupied by the basal pontine nuclei. As development proceeds, large numbers of axons arise from the basal pontine nuclei and cross the midline as they extend toward the contralateral cerebellar hemisphere (Fig. A1.10*B*). These fibers form the **middle cerebellar peduncles,** or **brachium pontis** [G., *brachion*, arm]. The development of this structure greatly enlarges the basis of the pons and is responsible for the predominantly fibrous appearance of the ventral pons in the adult.

The cell columns in the dorsolateral and tegmental portions of the pons give rise to nuclei associated with CN VIII through V, which emerge from the pons.

## CEREBELLUM

The cerebellum begins to develop from the alar plate of the metencephalon. Cells of the alar plate that border the dorsolateral margins of the fourth ventricle form the **rhombic lip** (Fig. A1.10A). Cells at the rostral end of the rhombic lip proliferate, forming a projection into the fourth ventricle. They also grow toward the midline in the area dorsal to the roof of the fourth ventricle. These two projections form the **cerebellar plate**. By the third month the intraventricular projection has regressed, leaving only the plate of tissue covering the roof of the ventricle (Fig. A1.11A). This tissue persists, forming the **vermis** [L. *vermis,* worm] of the cerebellum.

During the fourth month of development the lateral portions of the cerebellar primordium grow and form the **lateral lobes** of the cerebellum (Fig. A1.11B). By the end of the fourth month fissures divide the region (Fig. A1.11C). One fissure segregates tissue of the caudal portion of the cerebellar primordium, defining the caudal **flocculonodular lobe** [L. *flocculus,* small tuft of wool, and *nodulus,* small knot]. The **nodule** forms the medial portion of this lobe, and the **flocculus** forms the lateral portion. Tissue of the lateral lobes lies rostral to the flocculus, and the vermis lies rostral to the nodule. About this time the lateral lobes subdivide into **anterior** and **posterior lobes.**

Within the developing cerebellum, neuroblasts of the mantle layer form the **dentate** and **deep cerebellar nuclei.** Other neuroblasts migrate toward the surface of the developing lobes to form the highly cellular **cerebellar cortex.**

The embryological development of the structure of the cerebellum mirrors its phylogenetic development. The lobes of the cerebellum that are phylogenetically the oldest are concerned with basic, or primitive, function. Thus the **archecerebellum** [G. *archos,* leader,

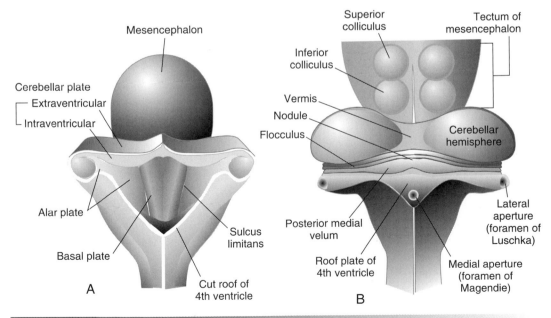

**Figure A1.11   The development of the cerebellum**

**A.** Dorsal view of the metencephalon at 2 months. Its rhombic lip expands medially, merging at the midline and forming the cerebellar plate. **B.** Dorsal view of the metencephalon at 4 months. As development of the cerebellum continues, the three principal divisions of the adult cerebellum become evident: the flocculonodulus, the vermis, and the hemispheres.

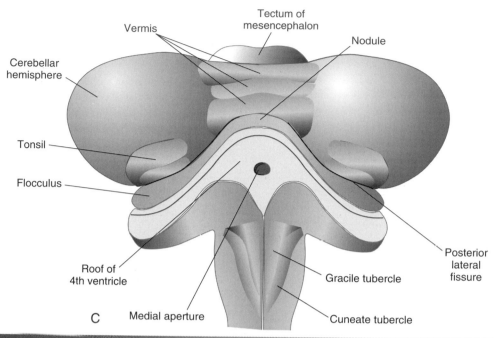

Vermis

Tectum of
mesencephalon

Nodule

Cerebellar
hemisphere

Tonsil

Flocculus

Posterior
lateral
fissure

Roof of
4th ventricle

Gracile tubercle

C          Medial aperture

Cuneate tubercle

**Figure A1.11    The development of the cerebellum—continued**

**C.** Dorsal view of the metencephalon at 5 months. The cerebellum continues to expand dorsally and laterally. The posterior lateral fissure separates the flocculonodular lobe from the remainder of the cerebellum. With further development the puckering on the surface of the vermis leads to the formation of the folia of the adult structure.

chief] is composed of the flocculonodular lobe and is the oldest phylogenetically. It has connections with the vestibular apparatus. The **paleocerebellum** [G. *paleos*, ancient], vermis, and anterior lobes evolved later. The paleocerebellum has reciprocal neurological connections with the spinal cord. The **neocerebellum**, the posterior lobes, is the most recent phylogenetic addition. It has reciprocal neurological connections to the cerebral cortex.

## Mesencephalon

The mesencephalon, or midbrain, undergoes little change during development (Fig. A1.12). The cavity of the mesencephalon is a narrow channel, the **cerebral aqueduct**, that connects the third and fourth ventricles. The dorsal portion of the mesencephalon forms the **tectum** [L. *tectum*, roof]. Neuroblasts of the alar plate proliferate and form paired sets of large nuclei, the **superior colliculi** [L. *colliculus*, dim. of *collis*, hill] (rostral) and the **inferior colliculi** (caudal).

The mesencephalon ventral to the sulcus limitans, which develops primarily from the basal plate, may be divided into a more dorsal tegmentum and a ventral basis. Nuclei associated with CN III and IV, the **red nuclei**, and the nuclei of the reticular formation are found there. The marginal zone at the ventral extreme of the mesencephalon becomes quite prominent as fibers from the developing cerebral cortex pass through the midbrain. These fiber bundles eventually form a prominent landmark, the **cerebral peduncles** [L. *pedunculus*, fr. *pes*, foot]. CN III and IV emerge from the mesencephalic region of the brain.

## The Diencephalon

The diencephalon arises from the thickened walls of the caudal portion of the original prosencephalon. Its cavity forms the **third ventricle**. The sulcus limitans terminates at the junction of the mesencephalon and the diencephalon, and the distinction between alar and basal plates does not extend into the diencephalon and telencephalon. Instead the diencephalon is divided by the **epithalamic sulcus** and the **hypothalamic sulcus**. These sulci separate the tissue of the walls of the diencephalon into three regions that become the **epithalamus, thalamus,** and **hypothalamus** (Fig. A1.13). Major elements within these regions are recognizable by the eighth week of development.

The epithalamus forms from the roof and dorsolateral wall of the diencephalon. This area, which regresses as development proceeds, gives rise to definitive structures including the **pineal gland** [L. *pineus,* pine], a

solid cone of cells that projects into the roof of the third ventricle, and the **habenular nuclei** [L. *habenula,* dim. of *habena,* rein, strap]. Two bands of fibers form transverse commissures, linking the right and left halves of the diencephalon. These are the **habenular** and **posterior commissures.**

The thalamus develops in the midlateral region of the walls of the diencephalon. Neuroblasts proliferate extensively and form groups of **thalamic nuclei** (the anterior, ventral, medial, and lateral groups of thalamic nuclei and the medial and lateral geniculate bodies). These nuclei expand laterally and protrude into the cavity of the third ventricle, reducing

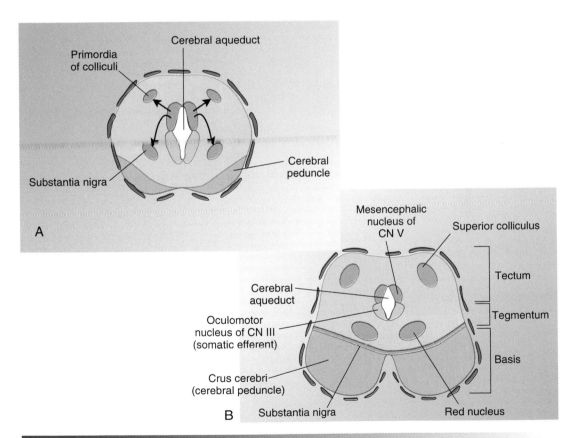

## Figure A1.12   The mesencephalon

**A.** Transverse section through the mesencephalon at 5 weeks. The primordia of the superior and inferior colliculi begin to separate from the alar plate and migrate toward the dorsal margin of the neural tube. Similarly, cells destined to become the substantia nigra, red nucleus, and parts of the reticular formation begin to migrate away from the basal plate. **B.** Transverse section through the mesencephalon at 11 weeks. Fibers originating in the cerebral cortex layer onto the surface of the basis of the mesencephalon, forming the prominent cerebral peduncles. The substantia nigra and red nucleus are recognizable.

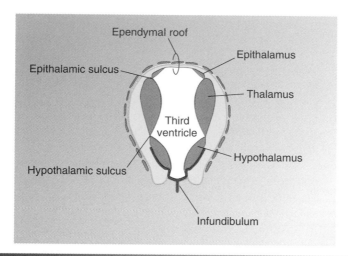

Ependymal roof

Epithalamus

Epithalamic sulcus

Thalamus

Third ventricle

Hypothalamus

Hypothalamic sulcus

Infundibulum

**Figure A1.13    The diencephalon at 8 weeks**

Transverse section showing the division of the region into epithalamus, thalamus, and hypothalamus by the epithalamic and hypothalamic sulci. The sulcus limitans does not exist at this level, and the distinction between alar and basal plates loses its meaning.

it to a narrow slit. The thalamic tissue commonly fuses in the midline, forming the **interthalamic adhesion,** or **massa intermedia.**

The hypothalamus develops from the tissue ventral to the hypothalamic sulcus. In the hypothalamic region neuroblasts of the mantle layer give rise to a number of nuclei that are associated with autonomic or endocrine function. The base of the hypothalamus and a ventral extension of tissue in this region develop into an endocrine gland, the **neurohypophysis.**

### Origin of the Pituitary Gland

Extending from the basis of the hypothalamic region is a glandular structure, the **pituitary gland** or **hypophysis cerebri** [G. *hypo-* and *phyein,* grow, i.e., undergrowth]. Although on gross inspection it appears as a single structure, its embryological development and adult function reveal that the pituitary gland is actually composed of two autonomous glands linked anatomically. During the fourth week the pituitary gland begins to develop from two separate origins, neuroectoderm and oral ectoderm (Fig. A1.14*A*). The neuroectodermal component begins as a down-growth from the ventral surface of the diencephalon, the **infundibulum.** The oral ectodermal component

originates as a diverticulum (**Rathke's pouch**) that projects dorsally from the primitive mouth cavity (stomodeum). Rathke's pouch continues to grow dorsally toward the infundibulum; by the eighth week it reaches a position adjacent to it and loses its connection with the stomodeum.

As development proceeds, the infundibulum expands to form the neural portion of the hypophysis cerebri, or **neurohypophysis** (Fig. A1.14, *B* and *C*). Components of the neurohypophysis include the part of the base of the hypothalamus known as the **median eminence,** a thin stalk (the original infundibulum), and a distended tip, the **pars nervosa,** from which hormones are secreted.

The parts of the hypophysis cerebri that are derived from Rathke's pouch (oral ectoderm) jointly constitute the **adenohypophysis** (Fig. A1.14, *B* and *C*). A small component, the **pars tuberalis,** lies adjacent to the infundibular stalk and wraps around it. The distal portion of the sac expands to form the **pars distalis,** the source of a number of hormones. The posterior wall of the original pouch that lies adjacent to the pars nervosa does not develop extensively in humans. It persists as a small population of cells that make up the **pars in-**

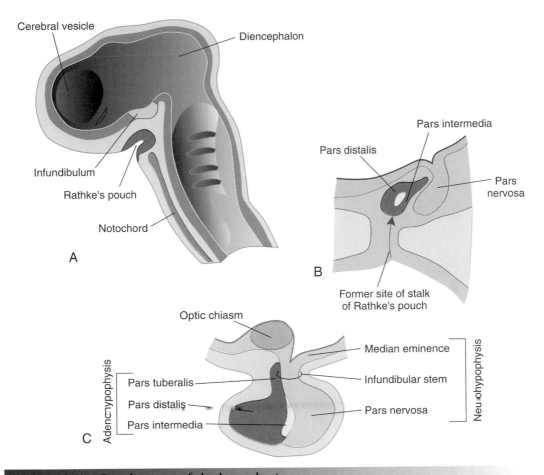

**Figure A1.14   Development of the hypophysis**

**A.** Sagittal section of the cranial end of a 6-week embryo. Tissue of the infundibulum forms on the ventral surface of the diencephalon. Rathke's pouch can be seen extending dorsally from the roof of the stomodeum. **B.** Sagittal section through the region of the developing hypophysis cerebri at approximately 10 weeks. Rathke's pouch has reached a position adjacent to the developing infundibulum, having lost contact with the oral cavity. The anterior surface of the pouch proliferates, forming the pars distalis of the hypophysis. **C.** The definitive structure.

termedia. During development the lumen of Rathke's pouch is commonly obliterated. However, it may persist in the adult gland as a narrow cleft, sometimes occupied by colloidal cysts.

### Origin of the Optic Tract and Retina

During the fourth week of development an **optic vesicle** develops as an evagination from the lateral aspect of each side of the prosencephalon prior to its division into the telencephalon and diencephalon. These vesicles are the primordia of the **optic tract** and **retina**. After the subdivision of the prosencephalon, the fibers that make up the optic tract (axons of the retinal ganglion cells) retain their connection to the diencephalic portion.

### Telencephalon

The telencephalon forms the rostral end of the original neural tube. Its rostral wall is the **lamina terminalis** [L. *lamina*, plate, and *terminus*, boundary]. Large lateral evaginations of the telencephalon form dorsal and rostral to the optic vesicles during the seventh week of development. These **cerebral vesicles** are the primordia of the cerebral hemispheres. Each has a cavity, a **lateral ventricle** that is an extension of the central cavity and is continuous with the third ventricle via the **intraventricular foramen** (Fig. A1.15, *A* and *B*). The cerebral vesicles grow rapidly upward, forward, and backward, overgrowing the diencephalon, mesencephalon, and hindbrain. Above and in front of the diencephalon the medial surfaces of the two vesicles come into contact, forming the flattened medial surfaces of the cerebral hemispheres.

The inferior portion of the cerebral vesicles grows less rapidly and develops into a thick layer of tissue that will become the **corpus striatum** [L. *corpus*, body, and *striatus*, furrowed] (Fig. A1.15, *A* and *B*). Later, nerve fibers leaving the developing cerebral cortex en route to the brainstem and spinal cord form a wide fiber tract, the **internal capsule**, which divides the corpus striatum into the **caudate nucleus** (superior), **putamen** [L., shell] (inferolateral), and **globus pallidus** [L. *pallidum*, pale] (inferomedial). The internal capsule and the caudate nucleus elongate, conforming to the contour of the lateral ventricle as it expands in the rostrocaudal plane.

The nonstriatal portion of the wall of the vesicle, the **pallium** [L., cloak, mantle], remains thin and is the primordium of the cerebral cor-

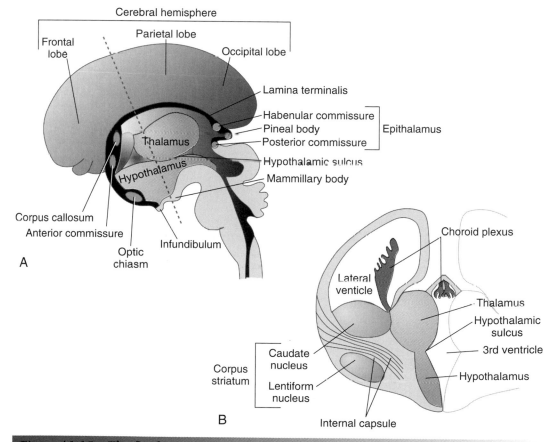

**Figure A1.15   The forebrain at 10 weeks**

**A.** Sagittal section through the developing cerebral hemispheres showing the association with the diencephalon. The various commissures in the region of the lamina terminalis are apparent. **B.** Transverse section through the plane shown in **A.** As the internal capsule develops, it divides the corpus striatum into a superior caudate nucleus and an inferior lentiform nucleus that later become the putamen and globus pallidus.

tex (Fig. A1.15B). The medial pallial wall remains quite thin and invaginates into the lateral ventricle, forming the **tela choroidea** [L. *tela*, web, and *chorioeides*, membranelike]. The line of invagination, which is apparent on the medial surfaces of the hemispheres, is the **choroidal fissure**.

The pallial walls initially have the same layers (ventricular, mantle, and marginal) as the rest of the developing neural tube. Later, cells of the marginal zone migrate outward, forming a highly cellular surface. The surface of the cerebral cortex is therefore composed of gray matter, and the nerve fibers that extend from these cells extend centrally, forming a large mass of white matter.

The area of the lamina terminalis, the original rostral extent of the neural tube, develops into a site in which fiber tracts form and connect corresponding areas of the cerebral hemispheres with one another (Fig. A1.15A). These fiber tracts are called **commissures** [L. *commissura*, join]. The **anterior commissure** is a small fiber bundle that develops early. The largest commissure is the **corpus callosum**, which initially occupies the dorsal region of the lamina terminalis but eventually becomes so large that it extends over the roof of the diencephalon. In the ventral portion of the lamina terminalis half of the fibers from the retina form the **optic chiasm** [G. *chiasma*, crossing of two lines], crossing the midline to join the optic tract of the opposite side.

### The Choroid Plexus

Several regions of the ventricular system of the brain have areas in which little neural tissue intervenes between the ependyma that lines the ventricle and the overlying meninges. As a result, the highly vascular pia mater lies adjacent to the ependyma. At points within these regions the pia mater undergoes extensive proliferation, forming projections into the ventricles that resemble clusters of grapes. These projections retain their ependymal covering. The modified pia mater (vascular connective tissue), together with its ependymal covering, form the **chorioid plexus**. The pia mater component is the tela choroidea; the ependymal component is the **lamina epithelialis** [G. *epi*, upon, and *thele*, nipple; term originally applied to the skin covering the nipple]. The choroid plexus is a secretory tissue responsible for the production of CSF. Areas of choroid plexus lie in the roof of the fourth and third ventricles and in the medial walls of the lateral ventricles (Fig. A1.15B).

## CONGENITAL MALFORMATIONS OF THE BRAIN

Congenital abnormalities of the brain are relatively common. They can result from errors in development of the neural tissue itself or of associated structures (e.g., mesodermal derivatives). Causes include a wide range of genetic and environmental factors. The brain is particularly susceptible to environmental **teratogens** (agents that increase the incidence of congenital malformations) during the first 16 weeks of development.

### Anencephaly

**Anencephaly** [G. *an-* negative prefix], or mero-anencephaly, results from failure of the rostral neuropore to close. The forebrain primordia and the overlying skull do not develop normally and the brain is exposed, a condition known as **exencephaly** [G. *ex-*, out of, away from]. Because components of the brainstem (midbrain, pons, medulla) are usually present, the term **meroanencephaly** [G. *meros*, part] is technically more accurate, but it is not in common use. Anencephaly is a common defect, occurring approximately in 1/1000 births, and it inevitably precludes extrauterine life. The causes are not well understood, but genetic factors undoubtedly play a role, since familial incidence has been well established. Teratogenic agents may also be involved, as suggested by experimental evidence in rats. Anencephaly can be detected by ultrasonography, fetoscopy, and radiography as early as 14 weeks, and like spina bifida, it is usually associated with an elevated level of α-fetoprotein in the amniotic fluid.

### Microcephaly

**Microcephaly** [G. *mikros*, small] is a condition in which the calvaria and brain are abnormally small. The etiology is believed to entail failure of the brain to develop, since pressure from the developing brain normally is responsible for enlargement of the calvaria. The cause of this abnormality is unclear; it may involve genetic or environmental agents. This disorder causes severe mental retardation.

## Hydrocephalus

Hydrocephalus [G. *hydro,* water, and *kephale,* head] describes any abnormality involving expansion of the ventricular system of the brain. It usually results from blockage of CSF circulation that causes an excessive production of CSF relative to its reabsorption. The concomitant increase in intracranial pressure raises the volume of the ventricles. In infants the sutures of the calvaria have not yet fused. Consequently, the increased pressure results in expansion and thinning of the brain and enlargement of the calvaria. This also leads to atrophy of the cerebral cortex and white matter and compression of the basal ganglia and diencephalon. The most common cause of this phenomenon is fetal viral infection by cytomegalovirus or *Toxoplasma gondii.*

## THE PERIPHERAL NERVOUS SYSTEM

The peripheral nervous system consists of a network of **ganglia,** groups of functionally associated neuron cell bodies, and **nerves,** groups of functionally associated axons. Ganglia are composed of neurons that develop from neural crest tissue. They begin to form during the first week of development, and further neuronal proliferation and differentiation continue throughout the course of fetal development and into early childhood.

The axons that constitute peripheral nerves originate from neurons lying in peripheral ganglia, within the brainstem (efferent fibers of cranial nerves), or in the spinal cord (motor neurons in the ventral horn or lateral horn). Their development begins during the fourth week and continues throughout fetal life and early childhood.

Supporting cells of the peripheral system (**Schwann cells**) are also derived from neural

crest tissue. Within ganglia Schwann cells border the cell bodies of the neurons, forming a capsulelike structure. The capsule continues into a **neurilemmal sheath** [G. *neuron,* nerve, and *eilema,* covering] also formed by Schwann cells, that invests the axon.

## Elements of the Peripheral Nervous System

Various types of ganglia and nerves organize to form functional units within the peripheral nervous system.

### PERIPHERAL SENSORY GANGLIA

**Peripheral sensory ganglia** include the 31 pairs of dorsal root, or spinal, ganglia that lie adjacent to each segment of the spinal cord and the peripheral sensory ganglia of CN V, the **trigeminal nerve;** CN VII, the **facial nerve;** CN VIII, the **vestibulocochlear nerve;** CN IX, the **glossopharyngeal nerve,** and CN X, the **vagus nerve.** These ganglia, except CN VIII, are composed of **pseudounipolar neurons,** cells in which the embryonic bipolar status has been modified to form a single process. This process splits in the vicinity of the neuron, forming a peripheral branch that terminates in a sensory ending and a central branch that enters the dorsal horn of the spinal cord. The neurons of the spinal ganglion of the cochlea and the vestibular ganglia of the CN VIII are an exception, remaining bipolar.

### AUTONOMIC GANGLIA

**Autonomic ganglia** are clusters of small multipolar neurons. They include the **sympathetic paravertebral ganglia,** which lie adjacent to the vertebral bodies in the thoracolumbar region of the spinal column, and the **sympathetic collateral ganglia** (e.g., the cardiac, celiac, and mesenteric plexus) in the thorax and abdomen. They also include the **parasympathetic ganglia,** such as the submucosal and myenteric plexus, and other plexus within the tissue of viscera.

### SPINAL NERVES

**Mixed spinal nerves** contain motor elements derived from neuroblasts in the basal plate of the developing spinal cord and **sensory fibers** that develop from neuroblasts in the dorsal root ganglia. Late in the fourth week of development axons grow out from neuroblasts in the basal plate of the spinal cord. Axons emerging at a given level form a group of fibers called a **ventral nerve rootlet** (Fig. A1.4B). A series of rootlets emerge along the length of the spinal cord.

Neuroblasts in the dorsal root ganglion transform from bipolar to pseudounipolar (Fig. A1.4B). The central branch of their process grows toward the alar plate region of the spinal cord. Groups of these fibers from a given dorsal root ganglion form a dorsal root. The distal branch of the process grows toward the periphery, eventually meeting and joining with the axons of the ventral rootlet to form a mixed spinal nerve (Fig. A1.4C).

Each spinal nerve divides immediately into **dorsal** and **ventral primary rami** [L. *ramus,* branch, pl. *rami*]. The dorsal primary ramus innervates the dorsal axial musculature, the vertebrae, the posterior intervertebral joints, and part of the skin of the back. The larger ventral primary ramus innervates the limbs and the ventral lateral parts of the body wall and forms the major nerve plexus. As the limbs develop from **limb buds**, the ventral rami of the corresponding segments grow into the bud and segmentally innervate the muscles and skin of the developing limb. The segmental distribution of the spinal nerves is reflected in the pattern of **dermatomes** that can be mapped on the body surface. Each dermatome corresponds to the region innervated by the dorsal root ganglion associated with one specific level of the spinal cord (see Chapter 5).

## CRANIAL NERVES

The cranial nerves are groups of axons that originate in the brain. With the exception of **CN I, the olfactory nerve,** and **CN II, the optic nerve,** the function of the cranial nerves is associated with nuclei that form from cell columns in the alar and basal plates of the mesencephalon and rhombencephalon. The 12 pairs of cranial nerves are generally divided into three groups according to their embryological origin (see box on pg. 569). The so-

matic efferent cranial nerves include CN IV, the **trochlear nerve,** CN VI, the **abducens nerve,** CN XII, the **hypoglossal nerve,** and most of CN III, the **oculomotor nerve.** The cells of origin of these nerves are in the basal plate region of the brainstem, the region that mediates somatic efferent function. Their axons are distributed to muscles of somite origin.

The **nerves of the branchial arches** include CN V, VII, IX, and X. They serve structures that are derived from embryonic branchial arches. Motor fibers of these nerves originate in the basal plate region, in the cell columns that regulate general and special visceral efferent function. Their sensory fibers terminate in the alar plate region in cell columns that regulate general and special visceral afferent and somatic afferent function.

The **nerves of the special senses** include CN I, the **optic nerve;** CN II, the **olfactory nerve;** and **CN VIII.** CN VIII is a highly specialized somatic afferent nerve whose cells terminate in the alar plate of the brainstem. CN I develops as an evagination of the wall of the brain; consequently it actually is a fiber tract of the brain.

## Subsystems Within the Peripheral Nervous System

The elements of the peripheral nervous system can be functionally grouped into two systems, one that innervates visceral structures, the **autonomic nervous system,** and one that innervates the remainder of the body (e.g., skin and muscles), the **somatic nervous system.**

## THE AUTONOMIC NERVOUS SYSTEM

The autonomic nervous system can be further subdivided into the **sympathetic nervous system** and the **parasympathetic nervous system.** The sympathetic nervous system includes the sympathetic trunks (paravertebral ganglia) and the collateral ganglia. **Preganglionic fibers** arise from neurons in the CNS and synapse within the peripheral sympathetic ganglia; **postganglionic fibers** emerge from the ganglion cells and continue to the target organ. Postganglionic fibers emerging from the sympathetic trunk travel with spinal nerves and mixed peripheral nerves; those emerging from collateral ganglia form purely autonomic **splanchnic nerves.**

The ganglia of the parasympathetic nervous system are small clusters of cells in or near the organ they innervate. Preganglionic fibers arise from neurons in nuclei of the brainstem (associated with CN III, VII, IX, and X) and in the sacral region of the spinal cord. Because of the location of the parasympathetic ganglia, preganglionic fibers are long, while postganglionic fibers have only a short distance to travel before reaching their target cells.

## THE SOMATIC NERVOUS SYSTEM

The somatic nervous system has motor components and a well-developed sensory component. The sensory portion includes peripheral sensory receptors (specialized or simple nerve endings) that form a unit with afferent nerve fibers. Most of these fibers are processes of neurons in the dorsal root ganglia; others are afferent components of cranial nerves. Motor components of the somatic system consist of fibers that emerge from the ventral horn of the spinal cord or fibers that constitute the efferent components of cranial nerves.

## SUGGESTED READINGS

Hamilton WJ, Mossman HW. Human Embryology. 4th ed. Cambridge, UK: Heffer, 1972.

Jacobson M. Developmental Neurobiology. 3rd ed. New York: Plenum, 1991.

Moore KL. The Developing Human: Clinically Oriented Embryology. 6th ed. Philadelphia: Saunders, 1998.

Rowland LP. Merritt's Textbook of Neurology. 9th ed. Baltimore: Williams & Wilkins, 1995.

Sadler TW. Langman's Medical Embryology. 7th ed. Baltimore: Williams & Wilkins, 1995.

Shepherd GM. Neurobiology. 3rd ed. New York: Oxford University, 1994.

# The Neurological Examination

*Robert E. Kingsley and Steven R. Gable*

The neurological examination allows a rapid and accurate assessment of the function of the nervous system. It is elegant in its simplicity. It does not rely on complex or technologically advanced instruments; its power arises from the knowledge and observational skills of the examiner. This is a brief description of the neurological examination appropriate for use in the primary care setting. This standard examination is quite simple, and it is an essential skill for every physician. More detailed explanations of the examination can be found in the Suggested Readings list.

## DESCRIPTION OF THE NEUROLOGICAL EXAMINATION

For purposes of explanation, the neurological examination may be divided into seven categories. However, the examination is never performed in this way. Rather, the elements are combined in a way that is efficient for the physician and that disturbs the patient as little as possible. Therefore, in this appendix, the examination is first described in detail, followed by an outline of the examination as it is practiced. Finally, the format in which the results of an examination (history and physical, including the neurological examination) are presented to other physicians in a stereotyped, formal way that conveys all the relevant information in a concise, efficient manner. The format for this presentation concludes this appendix.

## History of Present Illness

The history of the present illness (HPI) is the most important part of the neurological examination. The patient narrates her difficulties, and the physician thoughtfully interprets the history. Since the history is taken early in the physician's encounter with the patient, it is the best time to establish trust. It is essential to *listen* to the patient. Only by carefully listening with an open mind can one be objective and not impose one's preconceived evaluation of the patient on the history. Although the patient must not be coached or prompted, discreet questions are sometimes necessary to draw out important clinical points that may not seem important to the patient. Almost invariably patients spontaneously describe their condition in a way that leads the knowledgeable physician toward the correct diagnosis. To this end, the physician must be sure to make note of the **chief complaint**, the **time course** of the patient's difficulties, and the **distribution of symptoms**.

Important aspects of the history that may need gentle prompting include family history and possibly embarrassing conditions. For example, the patient may not realize the significance of illnesses of other family members, and most patients are reluctant to describe sexual dysfunction, incontinence, seizures, or drug use (alcohol, tobacco, and prescribed and recreational drugs).

## Mental Status

Evaluation of the patient's mental status is essential. The patient may have a psychiatric disorder or an organic disease process that interferes with the ability to communicate. The physician assesses the patient's mental status while taking the history.

Differentiating psychiatric from organic disorders sometimes is difficult. In general, *the more specific the patient's complaints, the more likely that the disease is organic.* For example, organic neurological illness is suggested if the patient says something like "6 months ago I could lift the salt bags to fill my water softener, but now I can't" rather than, "I feel weak and tired all the time. Some days I just can't seem to get out of bed."

The mental status is frequently described in terms of **levels of consciousness** and **state of memory.** Is the patient awake or comatose? If awake, is he alert, confused, or stuporous? Is the patient oriented to person, place, and time? Ask the patient where she is, what time it is, and what day of the week it is. Finally, give the patient three words to remember—a number, an object or place, and an abstract concept, such as "freedom." Make it clear that he will be asked to recall them later in the examination. After naming these three items, immediately ask the patient to repeat them to ascertain that he heard correctly and understood them.

## Cranial Nerves

During the neurological examination, each component of the cranial nerves is tested.

### OLFACTORY NERVE[1]

Unilateral anosmia is an important clinical sign that may be the only early objective sign of a frontal lobe abscess or tumor (see Chapter 14). The test odor should be chosen with care. Having the patient smell coffee or smelling salts is a poor method of testing olfaction. In the case of coffee, the patient knows by visual association what odor is being presented, and therefore the physician has no independent means of assessing the reliability of the patient's report. Also, some patients may confuse the

warmth of the vapors for the olfactory sensation the physician is testing. Smelling salts are irritating and stimulate the pain receptors of the nasal membranes. The best olfactory stimuli are **methyl salicylate** and **oil of cloves.** Both are colorless aromatic liquids that have a nonirritating, pleasant odor. The patient has no clue to the nature of the odor being presented yet invariably reports in some unambiguous way, describing methyl salicylate as spearmint, Ben-Gay, or another minty odor. To perform the examination, place a vial containing cotton saturated with methyl salicylate or oil of cloves under one nostril while occluding the other with a finger. Ask the patient to sniff and report the odor. Repeat for the other nostril.

### OPTIC NERVE

There are many aspects of the sense of vision, including acuity, color, and scotopic (day) versus photopic (night) vision. The neurologist is not interested in ophthalmological problems, so tests of refraction, glaucoma, and color blindness are not a normal part of the neurological examination. The neurologist is most concerned with signs of **papilledema** and **patterns of visual field losses** (see Chapter 12).

Papilledema can be detected only by a funduscopic examination with an ophthalmoscope. This examination is an essential part of every neurological examination. Visual field disturbances can be crudely determined by standing in front of the patient while the patient fixes the gaze on the examiner's nose. While the patient covers one eye with a hand, the examiner places his two hands in various quadrants of the visual fields and extends some of the fingers. Asking the patient to report how many fingers are extended in each hand can determine whether the patient can see each corresponding quadrant. Avoid moving or twitching the fingers, since motion can be detected in the absence of true visual perception. Each of the four quadrants in both eyes is tested.

### NERVES OF OCULAR MOTION

The three pairs of nerves that innervate the extraocular eye muscles—the oculomotor, the trochlear, and the abducens—can be tested in-

---

[1] The common habit of not testing the olfactory nerve because it is "unimportant" is to be strongly discouraged.

dependently by having the patient gaze approximately 25 to 30° to one side (see Chapter 10). With the eyes in this position, the superior rectus muscle in the abducted eye and the inferior oblique muscle in the adducted eye elevate the gaze. Depression is controlled by the inferior rectus muscle in the abducted eye and the superior oblique muscle in the adducted eye.

The action of the medial and lateral rectus muscles (abduction and adduction of the eye) are tested simply by asking the patient to maintain lateral gaze while testing the other muscles. While testing the eye movements, any nystagmus is noted (discussed later in the appendix).

The parasympathetic component of the oculomotor nerve is tested (see Chapter 10) by shining a light into one eye while observing the two pupils. They should simultaneously constrict (consensual light reflex). This test is not valid if the patient is in a brightly lit room, as the pupils may already be constricted from the ambient light. The size of the pupils before and after constriction should be reported in millimeters.

Because it is not easy to observe both pupils simultaneously, it is suggested that each eye be tested twice in the following manner. The light from the ophthalmoscope is aimed at the forehead and then drawn down to shine the light on the eye while the patient gazes at the wall behind the examiner, not at the light. After a momentary pause during which the examiner watches the pupil of the stimulated eye, the light is raised to the forehead. The process is repeated while observing the contralateral pupil. The same test is performed on the other eye. Note that the light is moved vertically, not horizontally, from eye to eye. This vertical motion gives the pupils time to dilate between stimuli. If the consensual light reflex is weak or absent from one eye, shining the light directly from eye to eye causes the nonreactive pupil (constricted because of the consensual light reflex) to dilate paradoxically. This sign is called the **Marcus Gunn pupil**.

Pupillary constriction also occurs during accommodation and convergence. To test, the patient fixes the gaze on a distant object such as the examiner's finger. As the finger is brought close to the patient, the eyes converge and both pupils should constrict.

## TRIGEMINAL NERVE

The sensory portion of the trigeminal nerve is tested by touching the skin of the face with a wisp of cotton and the cold surface of the tuning fork. The separate dermatomes for all three divisions are tested (see Chapter 10). Because of the discomfort to the patient pinprick testing of the face is usually deferred unless there is a particular reason to do so. The cold tuning fork is an adequate stimulus for the protopathic pathways.

The corneal reflex is always tested. This reflex involves two nerves: the trigeminal, which carries the afferent signal to the brain, and the facial, which carries the efferent component. It is evoked by touching the cornea with the cotton wisp. Since most people blink if they see an object coming directly at their eye, the cotton is brought to the cornea from the side while the patient is looking straight ahead.

The motor component of the trigeminal nerve can be tested by having the patient isometrically bite. Paralysis of a masseter muscle can usually be seen, and flaccidity can be palpated. As an additional test, the jaw deviates to the paralyzed side on opening the mouth due to the paralysis of the external pterygoid muscle.

## FACIAL NERVE

The motor component of the facial nerve innervates the mimetic muscles of the face and the orbicularis oculi (the latter is tested as part of the corneal reflex). The critical observation with respect to the function of the facial nerve is the pattern of paresis or paralysis of the mimetic muscles (see Chapter 10). Paralysis of these muscles is usually quite apparent as facial asymmetry when the patient is asked to grimace. Flattening of the nasolabial fold on the affected side also signifies mimetic weakness. Especially note whether or not the muscles that raise the eyebrows are involved.

The parasympathetic components of the facial nerve affect salivation and lacrimation. Although these functions are not specifically tested during the neurological examination, they can sometimes be inferred from the history if the patient complains of a dry mouth or eye. Corneal ulceration may be secondary to poor lacrimation.

## AUDITORY—VESTIBULAR NERVE

The principal goals in testing the auditory division of CN VIII are first to determine whether hearing is grossly normal and if not, to differentiate between conductive and sensorineural hearing losses. Rubbing the fingers together over the external auditory meatus is commonly used to determine if hearing is grossly present. **Rinne's test** accurately distinguishes between conductive and sensorineural hearing losses but cannot determine the relative sensitivity of hearing. **Weber's test** provides a comparison of hearing efficiency between the two ears but can only be interpreted in light of the results of Rinne's test (see Chapter 11). If these tests indicate conductive hearing loss, the external auditory meatus should be examined with an otoscope for excessive cerumen or other simple obstruction. Central hearing losses can be determined only by special audiological methods, not by routine neurological examination.

The vestibular system is usually not specifically tested. Spontaneous nystagmus, however, may be a sign of vestibular end-organ or nerve disease, particularly if it is accompanied by vertigo, nausea, and unsteadiness with a tendency to fall (see Chapter 10). Nystagmus can also be caused by a cerebellar or brainstem lesion. Therefore, if nystagmus is present, these structures must be carefully examined for corroborative evidence. When vestibular end-organ or nerve dysfunction is suspected, an electronystagmogram (caloric testing) is indicated.

## GLOSSOPHARYNGEAL—VAGUS NERVE COMPLEX

The sensory components of the glossopharyngeal and vagus nerves supply the inside of the pharynx. They can be tested by evoking the gag reflex, which is simply done with a tongue depressor placed at the back of the pharynx. Each side is tested independently. The entire oral cavity can be explored with the tongue depressor to check general sensations if warranted. While eliciting the gag reflex, observe the uvula and pharynx for asymmetries (see Chapter 10). The quality of the voice should be noted for any signs of stridor or hoarseness.

## ACCESSORY NERVE

This nerve is tested by checking the general strength of the sternocleidomastoid and trapezius muscles (see Chapter 10). The sternocleidomastoid muscle is tested by having the patient rotate the head while the examiner offers resistance against the chin. The muscle being tested is contralateral to the direction of head rotation. In addition to checking the strength of the trapezius muscles, the symmetry of the two muscles is noted.

## HYPOGLOSSAL NERVE

The hypoglossal nerve, which innervates the intrinsic muscles of the tongue, is tested by observing the tongue for signs of atrophy or fasciculations and having the patient stick out the tongue in the midline. Deviation from the midline position indicates weakness on the side of the deviation (see Chapter 10).

## Motor Systems

Testing the motor systems is possibly the most illuminating portion of the neurological examination, since few diseases fail to affect motor functions in some characteristic way. Motor system testing can be divided into four categories: observing **gait**, testing **strength** and **tone**, observing **abnormal movements**, and checking for **ataxia**.

### GAIT

To observe the gait, ask the patient to walk several paces away, turn around in place, and return. Normal gait is smooth, on a narrow base, with both arms gently swinging. Weakness may be revealed by circumduction of the leg during the return swing or by a limp. A shuffling gait with the arms held stiffly in one place without swinging suggests parkinsonism. A wide-based, staggering, ataxic gait suggests cerebellar disease. The patient who cannot follow a straight line but meanders back and forth in an almost dancelike manner may have basal ganglion disease.

Next ask the patient to do a deep knee bend, hop on each foot in turn, and walk on the heels and then the toes. These activities test for strength, balance, and coordination. Finally, as a further test of coordination, have the patient walk along a straight line, placing the heel of one foot directly against the toe of the other (**tandem walking**).

## STRENGTH AND TONE

A sensitive test of upper extremity strength is to have the patient stand with the arms held straight ahead and supinated, palms flat and horizontal, with the fingers held together (**drift test**). Any downward or lateral drift, pronation, or separation of the fingers indicates weakness in that extremity.

All major muscle groups should be directly tested for strength by having the patient perform an isometric contraction against resistance offered by the examiner. Strength should be quantified as follows:

0 No movement
1 Any movement less than full range of motion (FROM) that requires support from gravity
2 FROM requiring support from gravity
3 FROM against gravity alone but no other resistance
4 FROM unsustainable against resistance supplied by the physician
5 FROM sustainable against resistance (normal)

Since strength varies considerably from person to person, absolute strength is not measured. The resistance the physician supplies should be appropriate to the age and physique of the patient. Whatever their absolute strength, all normal people can sustain a contraction against resistance. While performing this direct strength testing, the various muscle groups are observed for atrophy and fasciculations (see Chapter 6), spasticity (see Chapter 7), and rigidity (see Chapter 8).

Spasticity and rigidity are directly ascertained by passive joint movement. The examiner slowly lengthens various muscle groups in each extremity separately while the patient is relaxed, for example, by pronating and supinating the arm. Rigidity is steady resistance to passive movement and is usually de-

scribed as feeling like bending a lead pipe. Cogwheel rigidity feels like a series of small catches superimposed on the lead pipe rigidity during passive movement. During the slow, passive motion, the examiner inserts a rapid motion, such as supination or pronation of the arm. Spasticity is revealed as a rapidly developing resistance, or catch, during this rapid passive movement. The catch is caused by the muscle stretch reflex (MSR) elicited by the rapid change in muscle length.

## ABNORMAL MOVEMENTS

Abnormal involuntary movements suggest basal ganglion disease (see Chapter 8). A resting tremor that relents during voluntary movement is a classic sign of parkinsonism. Unusual fidgeting may be an early sign of chorea. Athetosis, dystonia, and tics are usually self-evident.

## ATAXIA

Cerebellar disease is usually quite evident on observation of gait and tandem walk for ataxia To explore the possibility of suspected cerebellar disease, the patient is asked to touch her nose with a finger and then to touch the examiner's finger, which is held in front as a target (dysmetria; see Chapter 9). This movement should be direct, smooth, and coordinated. To challenge the patient the examiner moves her finger as the patient is reaching for it to see if there is a smooth redirection of the intended movement. The lower extremity is tested by having the patient run the heel along the shin of the opposite leg. Finally, have the patient slap his thighs alternately with the palms and the backs of the hands (dysdiadochokinesia).

## Reflexes

The reflexes provide important objective signs of neurological status. Test the five basic MSRs—biceps, triceps, brachioradialis, quadriceps and gastrocnemius—on each side (see Chapters 6 and 7). Also, always check the plantar signs (Babinski) and if there is any doubt, reinforce this with the Bing sign. The other flexion reflex afferent (FRA) reflexes, the cremasteric and abdominal, are occasionally useful. Finally, the atavistic reflexes (rooting, snout, glabellar, palmomental, and grasp) are useful in evaluating the cerebral cortex (see Chapter 15).

## Sensory Systems

Testing the sensory systems can be difficult because it requires the cooperation and understanding of the patient. The examiner cannot directly know the patient's sensations, and the patient's experience of those sensations are inescapably colored by his emotional state. Sensory experiences cannot be objectively reported to the physician. However, many of the sensory tests, such as the methyl salicylate test mentioned earlier, objectively draw out any inconsistencies in the patient's report. Because of the subjective nature of sensory testing, many physicians perform only a cursory examination. This is unfortunate, for the sensory examination is usually the best indicator of the level of a discrete spinal cord or peripheral lesion. Furthermore, learning that the patient is unable to provide a consistent report of sensory perceptions or is malingering is valuable.

The **Romberg test** (see Chapter 5) is an objective sensory test, performed by having the patient stand on a narrow base with eyes open. If the patient is stable, she is asked to close the eyes. A slight increase in instability is normal, but gross instability or falling suggests that proprioceptive sensations from the lower extremities are defective. Instability with the eyes open points to cerebellar disease.

Proprioception can be further tested by shielding the patient's vision from a finger or toe, holding its tip with one hand, and asking the patient to report whether the digit has been moved up or down. Normal patients can detect the slightest movement.

The **epicritic system** (see Chapter 5) is further tested with a wisp of cotton applied very lightly to the skin or to a single hair and asking the patient if it can be felt. The dermatome, peripheral nerve, or stocking-and-glove patterns are checked as appropriate by asking whether the patient can detect a *substantial difference between consecutive touches*, strategically placed on opposite sides of suspected boundaries or in analogous places on opposite extremities.

Finally, the epicritic system is tested with the 128-Hz tuning fork. The stem of the vi-

brating fork is placed on a distal bony prominence of an extremity. When the patient can no longer feel the vibration, the stem is immediately placed on another more proximal prominence. The vibrations should not be felt. Peripheral neuropathy may be present if vibrations are perceived at the more proximal point after distal extinction.

The **protopathic system** (see Chapter 5) is tested by pinprick. A new, clean pin is used for every patient to avoid transmitting blood-borne diseases. As with the epicritic system, draw out any patterns of sensory loss.

## Higher Cortical Functions

Most higher cortical functions (as opposed to primary sensory or motor functions) are tested during the history taking. The various tests are designed to reveal functional differences as they relate to the various lobes and where appropriate, to the left-right differences between the lobes (see Chapter 15). These tests should not be confused with tests for general dementia, which more or less affects the entire cerebral cortex.

Lesions primarily involving the frontal lobes are marked by general deterioration in the personality. The patient may be more belligerent or less respectful than usual. This change is best determined by interviewing a close relative or spouse to determine any deterioration over time. **Perseveration** (see Chapter 15) is an important frontal lobe sign that can be specifically tested during the neurological examination by presenting a series of objects to the patient for identification. If the frontal eye fields are involved, there may be **enhanced fixation** of gaze (see Chapter 10).

**Aphasia**, either expressive or receptive, is usually apparent. **Left-sided neglect** syndrome, associated with right parietal lobe lesions, can be specifically tested by asking the patient to copy drawings provided by the examiner (see Chapter 15). Drawing a clock, a square, and petals on a daisy are all excellent choices. The ability to concentrate is traditionally tested by having the patient subtract 7 serially, beginning with 100 or spelling **world** backwards. More subtle parietal lobe lesions can be determined by evoking the optokinetic reflex (see Chapter 10).

## PRACTICAL APPLICATION OF THE NEUROLOGICAL EXAMINATION

The following outline is a suggested method for performing the neurological examination efficiently. While physicians must develop their own method, it is important that the examination be performed exactly the same way every time. This consistency ensures that nothing will be overlooked. Obtaining data in the same order at every presentation also helps the examiner organize the information systematically.

I. Instruments (Fig. A2.1)
   A. Reflex hammer for reflexes, MSRs
   B. Clean, unused safety pins (use a new pin for each patient) for pain
   C. Wisp of cotton for light touch
   D. Oto-ophthalmoscope for retina, external auditory meatus, light reflex
   E. Methyl salicylate and/or oil of cloves for olfaction
   F. Tuning forks: 128 and 512 Hz for vibration, hearing
   G. Tongue depressors for gag reflex, plantar signs
   H. Optokinetic tape for parietal function, optokinetic nystagmus
   I. Pad and pencil for note taking and patient's drawings

II. Patient seated or in bed in hospital
   A. History. Emphasize chief complaint, time course, and distribution of symptoms. Do not lead the patient; avoid imposing preconceived notions on the patient's narrative. Let the story flow naturally.
   B. Mental status. Evaluate patient's mental status while taking history. Is the patient awake, alert, and oriented to person, place, and time? Give the patient three words to remember.
   C. Note any abnormal movements such as tics, tremor, or fidgeting. Do these movements cease with volition?

III. Patient walking
   A. Evaluate the gait. Ask the patient to do deep knee bends, tandem walk, and hop on each foot.
   B. Feel the head to check for old and new trauma. Use methyl salicylate or oil of cloves to check olfaction and cotton to test corneal reflex and light touch over the face. If warranted, use the tuning fork to test perception of cold over the face.
   C. Facing the patient, combine the Romberg, drift, and finger-to-nose tests.
   D. Use the ophthalmoscope to inspect the fundus and test the light reflex.
   E. Test eye movements and visual fields.
   F. Have the patient grimace, phonate, and protrude the tongue in the midline. While the mouth is open, elicit the gag reflex with the tongue depressor. Observe the muscle tone of the pharynx. Palpate the masseter muscles while the patient is biting.

IV. Patient lying down
   A. Ask the patient to run a heel along the shin of the opposite leg.
   B. Use the safety pin and cotton wisp to test sensations over the arms, legs, and (if warranted) body. Either establish or rule out dermatome, peripheral nerve, and stocking-and-glove patterns to any abnormalities.
   C. If warranted, check the abdominal and cremasteric reflexes.

V. Patient sitting up
   A. Use the 128-Hz tuning fork to test temperature and vibratory sensations.

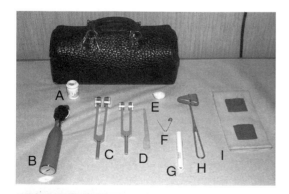

**Figure A2.1   Basic instruments**

A, vial of methyl salicylate; B, oto-ophthalmoscope; C, tuning forks; D, broken tongue depressor; E, cotton; F, pin; G, light; H, reflex hammer; I, OKN tape.

B. Use the 512-Hz tuning fork for Rinne's and Weber's tests. If a conductive hearing loss is found, use the otoscope to examine the external auditory meatus for cerumen and check the tympanic membrane.

C. Test general strength.

D. Check proprioception by testing movement perception of the fingers and toes.

E. Test reflexes and signs.
   1. MSRs. Use the reflex hammer to test the following: biceps, C5, C6; triceps, C6, C7; brachioradialis, C5, C6; quadriceps, L3 to L5; gastrocnemius, S1.
   2. FRAs. Use the tongue depressor to check for the Babinski sign and the safety pin to check the Bing sign.
   3. Atavistic. Good choices for routine examinations are glabellar, grasp, and palmomental.

F. Test higher cortical functions.
   1. Use the optokinetic tape to elicit optokinetic nystagmus.
   2. If indicated, ask the patient make appropriate drawings.
   3. Ask the patient to recall the three memory test items.
   4. Ask the patient to do serial 7 subtractions or spell **world** backwards.
   5. Hold up simple objects for identification to determine whether the patient can correctly identify the objects and has any tendency to perseverate.

VI. Things to Note

A. All of the cranial nerves are tested, and for most of them all components are tested.

B. Important systems (e.g., motor, protopathic, and epicritic) are tested in more than one way.

C. Only simple instruments are needed. Everything is easily carried in a small physician's bag.

D. With the exception of sensory tests, all results are independent of the patient's conscious understanding: the results are signs, not symptoms.

E. The patient is disturbed as little as possible. There are only two major changes in the patient's position.

F. With practice this examination takes very little time, usually no more than 5 minutes.

## PRESENTATION OF A PATIENT

When presenting a patient to another physician, it is useful to use a standard format. A stereotyped presentation helps ensure that no relevant information is omitted or extraneous information included. Over the years the following format, with minor variations, has become nearly universal among physicians. It should be memorized. This format has been used throughout the text, with some parts deleted to conserve space.

I. Chief Complaint

A. State *name, age, sex,* and *race* of patient followed by the *principal reason* the patient sought medical assistance. Use the patient's own words if possible, stating *one (i.e., chief) complaint, distribution, and time course* into a single sentence.

B. Example. "Mr. X, a 45-year-old white man, has been feeling numbness and tingling in his right hand for several weeks."

II. General Mental Status and Informant

A. Indicate the general mental status (orientation) of the patient with respect to *person, place, and time.*

B. Name the *informant,* and if not the patient, identify the relationship of the informant to the patient.

C. Examples. "Mr. X is oriented as to person, place, and time and fully cooperated with the interview and examination." Or, "Mr. X knew who he was but did not know where he was and thought the year was 1983. He believes Ronald Reagan is president. His wife supplied most of the details of the history."

III. History of Present Illness

A. Name each symptom separately, giving *time course, distribution, exacer-*

bating and alleviating conditions, and pertinent positive and negative factors. Symptoms are problems the patient expresses; signs are observations the physician makes. The history contains only symptoms; do not express your observations at this time.

B. Example. "Mr. X has trouble swallowing liquids [first symptom], a problem that began suddenly 2 months ago. This has been getting steadily worse [time course]. The difficulty is worse at the evening meal than at breakfast [exacerbating factor]. He has no difficulty with solids [pertinent negative]. He also complains of a hoarse voice [second symptom], which also began suddenly about 2 months ago and has remained about the same since it began [time course]. The hoarseness is fairly constant [no exacerbating or alleviating factors] and began at the same time as the swallowing difficulty [pertinent positive factor]."

C. Pertinent positive and negative findings require more background knowledge than most first-year students have. These findings are primarily used to narrow the differential diagnosis.

IV. List all medications the patient is taking, along with dosages.

V. Allergies

A. List all allergies, paying particular attention to allergies associated with medications. Elicit the specific allergic reaction (e.g., hives, rash, vomiting). A patient may describe as "allergic" reactions that are not medical allergies. These should be noted anyway.

B. Example. "Mr. X says he is allergic to penicillin, which gives him hives, and to carrots, which make him vomit."

VI. Past medical history. List all psychiatric, medical, and surgical illnesses with dates and resolution of each illness.

VII. Social history. Determine use of *social drugs* (alcohol, tobacco, and caffeine), *il-*

*licit drugs, home environment* (marriage status, children), *occupation,* and *occupational status* (employed, unemployed, retired).

VIII. Family history. Ascertain major diseases and causes of death of first-degree relatives (parents, siblings, and children).

IX. Review of all systems. This review is beyond the knowledge of most first-year students.

X. Physical examination. List only signs (what you have observed). [Only the neurological examination is outlined in this appendix.]

A. Mental status

B. Cranial nerves. Review all components of each nerve in order beginning with olfaction.

1. Olfaction: CN I

a. Test each side separately and report how the patient identified the test substance.

b. Example. "The patient identified the odor of Ben Gay from each nostril independently."

2. Vision: CN II

a. Fundi. Directly examine the retina, paying special attention to the optic discs. Note presence or absence of papilledema.

b. Fields. Report results of confrontation test, noting central and peripheral vision.

c. Example. "The retina appeared grossly normal, without papilledema. The patient correctly reported finger count from all four quadrants. Central vision was grossly intact."

3. Oculomotion: CN III, IV, and VI

a. Pupils. Report direct and consensual light reflex in millimeters. Note constriction on accommodation.

b. Note presence or absence of ptosis.

c. Eye movements. Test all muscles and note presence or absence of palsy, spontaneous movements (nystagmus), and results of smooth pursuit and saccade tests.

   d. Example. "Pupils were equal and constricted from 4 mm to 2 mm to both direct and consensual stimulation. Eye movements were full in all directions. Smooth pursuit and saccade maneuvers were performed normally. There was no ptosis or nystagmus."

4. Trigeminal: CN V
   a. Sensory. Report light touch and cold stimulation (pinprick only if abnormalities are likely) over all three divisions.
   b. Cornea. Report corneal reflex.
   c. Motor. Report masseter and pterygoid strength.
   d. Example. "Light touch and cold were perceived equally and appropriately from all three divisions of the trigeminal nerve. Corneal reflex was bilaterally present and brisk. Masseters were equally strong, and lateral jaw movements were full and symmetrical."

5. Facial: CN VII
   a. Motor. Report facial symmetry at rest, nasolabial fold, and results of facial maneuvers.
   b. Example. "The patient's face was symmetrical, with deep nasolabial folds. Grimace was symmetrical, eyebrows arched together, and I was unable to pry open the eyelids on forced closure."

6. Audition: CN VIII
   a. Auditory. Report finger rub, Rinne's, and Weber's tests.
   b. Vestibular. Cannot be tested in routine examination. Spontaneous nystagmus is reported under ocular motion.
   c. Example. "Air conduction was more sensitive than bone conduction by 10 seconds bilater-

ally. Patient localized Weber's test to the middle of his head and had no difficulty detecting light finger rubs."

7. Vagal—glossopharyngeal: CN IX–X
   a. Report symmetry of pharyngeal arches, position of the uvula, gag reflex, and quality of voice.
   b. Example. "The pharyngeal arches lifted symmetrically, and the uvula was in the midline. Gag reflex was present bilaterally. Voice was normal."

8. Accessory: CN XI
   a. Report strength of sternocleidomastoid and trapezius muscles.
   b. Example. "The sternocleidomastoid and trapezius muscle strength was 15 bilaterally."

9. Hypoglossal: CN XII
   a. Report appearance of tongue and position on extension.
   b. Example. "The tongue extended in the midline. There were no fasciculations."

C. Station and Gait
   1. Report posture, gait, arm swing, and heel, toe, and tandem walk.
   2. Example. "The patient stood erect with a normal posture. Stride was narrow-based and relaxed, with appropriate arm swing. Heel, toe, and tandem walk and deep knee bends were performed without difficulty."

D. Motor Systems
   1. Drift. Report the results of the drift test.
   2. Tone. Passively move the shoulder, elbow, wrist, fingers, knee, and ankle joints and note the following:
   a. Spasticity: increased tone and resistance to rapid passive movement
   b. Rigidity: lead pipe or cogwheel; increased resistance to

slow passive movement. (The terms *spasticity* and *rigidity* convey specific meanings. Do not use these terms casually or interchangeably.)

3. Bulk. Measure two sides if atrophy is noted.
4. Strength. Directly examine and quantify strength at the shoulder, elbow, wrist, fingers, knee, and ankle using the scale described on page 585.
5. Abnormal movements. Describe if present or note if absent.
6. Example. "The patient exhibited no drift for 30 seconds. Muscle tone and bulk were symmetrical and appropriate in all extremities. There was no spasticity or rigidity. Strength was +5 from all muscle groups. No abnormal movements were present."

E. Sensory systems. Note pattern (dermatome, peripheral nerve, stocking-and-glove) of any abnormalities.
1. Report pinprick and temperature results together (protopathic system).
2. Report light touch, proprioception, vibration, and Romberg's test results together (epicritic system).
3. Example. "The patient perceived pinprick and temperature equally and in the same quality in all extremities over all dermatomes. Light touch and proprioception were also perceived normally. The sense of vibration extinguished equally at the distal and proximal test points. Patient was stable on a narrow base with eyes open and closed." (Avoid "Romberg was negative.")

F. Reflexes. Test the following:
1. MSRs from these muscles: triceps, biceps, brachioradialis, quadriceps, and gastrocnemius. Quantify as: clonus, ++, +, normal, −, −−, absent.

2. Babinski and Bing signs
3. Cremasteric, abdominal, and anal wink if indicated; otherwise these reflexes are optional.
4. Example 1. "MSRs were symmetrical and normal; sign of Babinski was absent."
5. Example 2. "MSRs from the right triceps, biceps, and brachioradialis were ++; from the right quadriceps and gastrocnemius, +; all others were normal. Signs of Babinski and Bing were present on the right, absent on the left."

G. Coordination and Control
1. Cerebellum
   a. Dysmetria: finger-to-nose; heel-to-shin
   b. Dysdiadochokinesia: rapid alternating movements
2. CBST: Fine finger-to-thumb
3. Example. "There was no dysmetria or dysdiadochokinesia, and fine finger movements were well coordinated."

H. Parietal functions. Test the following:
1. Memory: three-item test
2. Concentration: serial 7 subtractions or "world"
3. Optokinetic reflex (OKN): if abnormal, state direction
4. Neglect: describe if present; report results of extinction tests
5. Atavistic signs, perseveration
6. As indicated, perform and report the following tests:
   a. Language: note type of any aphasia
   b. Note ability to follow written commands
   c. Note ability to follow spoken commands
   d. Check for graphesthesia
   e. Check for stereognosis
   f. Check for constructional apraxia
7. Example 1. "Mr. X remembered the items three, red, truth; performed serial 7 subtractions to

65; and exhibited OKN in both directions. There was no extinction, atavistic signs, or perseveration."

8. Example 2. "Ms. Y remembered only the word red and could not perform serial 7 subtractions below 93. The OKN could not be elicited toward the right but was present toward the left. The patient did not perceive coincident palm touches on the left. There were no atavistic signs, and she did not perseverate."

## FURTHER APPLICATIONS

A2.1. Make a list of the cranial nerves and their components. Identify where each cranial nerve is tested in the neurological examination. Are any missed? Which?

A2.2. Identify which parts of the neurological examination test the cerebellum, the basal ganglia, the upper motor neuron system, the lower motor neuron system, and the protopathic (anterior lateral [ALS] system) and epicritic (dorsal column system) sensory systems.

A2.3. Practice this examination on a friend until you have it memorized. It is important that you do it exactly the same way every time. Leave nothing out. Get into the habit of taking notes (use the pad and pencil) while performing the examination.

## SUGGESTED READINGS

Adams RD, Victor M. Principles of Neurology. New York: McGraw-Hill, 1993.

Bickerstaff ER, Spillane JA. Neurological Examination in Clinical Practice. Boston: Oxford, 1989.

Bradley WG, Dardoff RB, Fenichel GM, Marsden CD. Neurology in Clinical Practice. Boston: Butterworth-Heinemann, 1996.

DeMeyer W. Technique of the Neurologic Examination. New York: McGraw-Hill, 1980.

Geraint F. Neurological Examination Made Easy. New York: Churchill Livingstone, 1993.

Goldberg S. The Four-Minute Neurological Examination. Miami: MedMaster, 1992.

Joynt RJ. Clinical Neurology. Philadelphia: Lippincott, 1993.

Rowland LP. Merritt's Textbook of Neurology. Philadelphia: Lea & Febiger, 1989.

# Atlas of Magnetic Resonance Images

*Susan Stoddard*

## TRANSVERSE SECTIONS

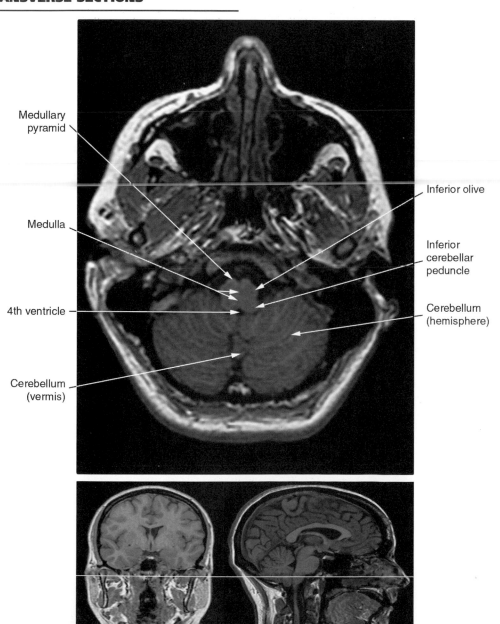

Medullary pyramid

Inferior olive

Medulla

Inferior cerebellar peduncle

4th ventricle

Cerebellum (hemisphere)

Cerebellum (vermis)

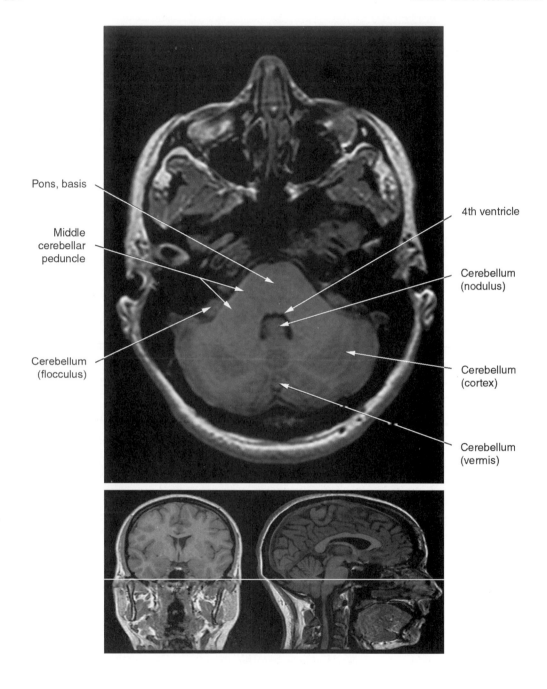

Pons, basis

Middle cerebellar peduncle

Cerebellum (flocculus)

4th ventricle

Cerebellum (nodulus)

Cerebellum (cortex)

Cerebellum (vermis)

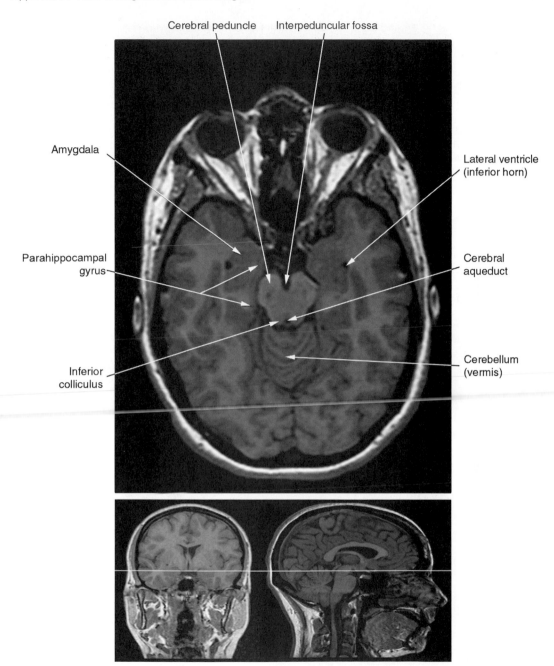

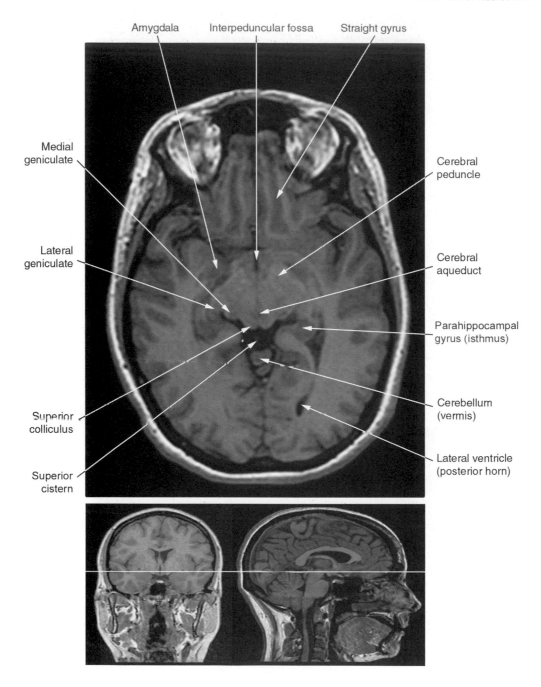

Amygdala   Interpeduncular fossa   Straight gyrus

Medial geniculate

Lateral geniculate

Superior colliculus

Superior cistern

Cerebral peduncle

Cerebral aqueduct

Parahippocampal gyrus (isthmus)

Cerebellum (vermis)

Lateral ventricle (posterior horn)

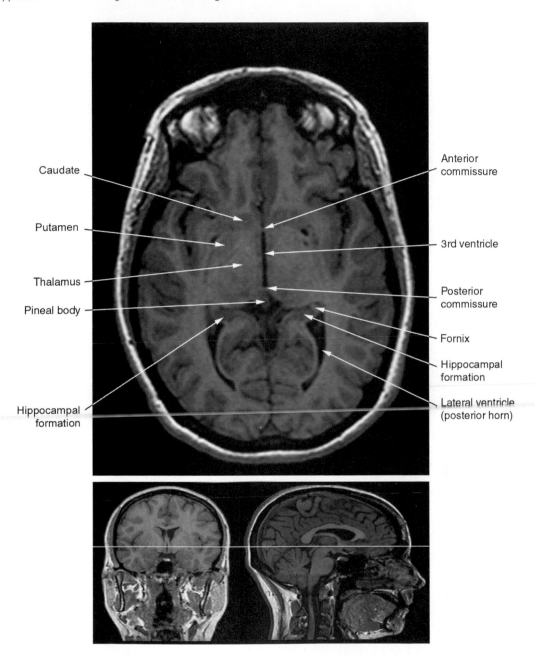

Caudate

Putamen

Thalamus

Pineal body

Hippocampal
formation

Anterior
commissure

3rd ventricle

Posterior
commissure

Fornix

Hippocampal
formation

Lateral ventricle
(posterior horn)

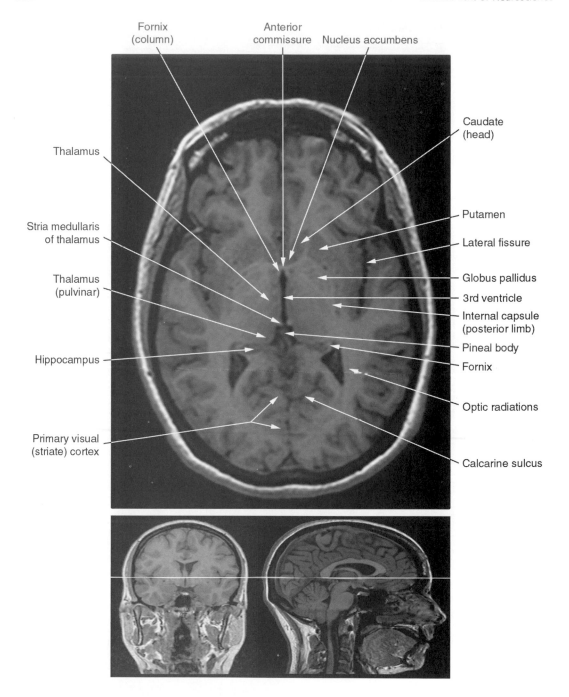

Fornix
(column)

Anterior
commissure     Nucleus accumbens

Thalamus

Stria medullaris
of thalamus

Thalamus
(pulvinar)

Hippocampus

Primary visual
(striate) cortex

Caudate
(head)

Putamen

Lateral fissure

Globus pallidus

3rd ventricle

Internal capsule
(posterior limb)

Pineal body

Fornix

Optic radiations

Calcarine sulcus

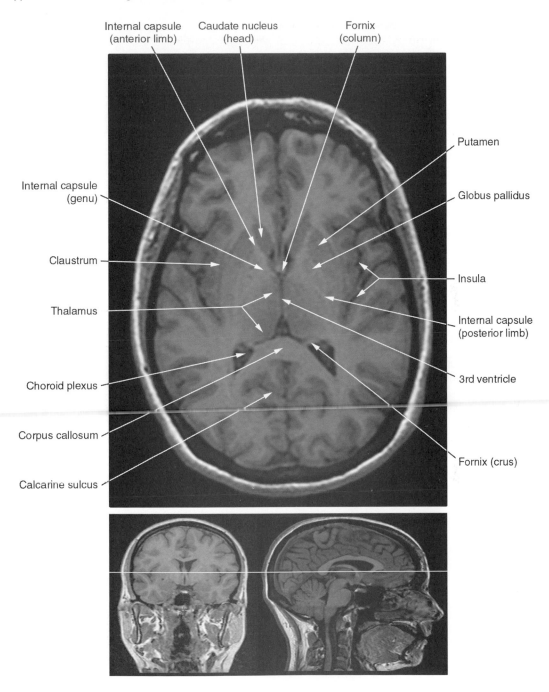

Internal capsule (anterior limb)

Caudate nucleus (head)

Fornix (column)

Putamen

Globus pallidus

Internal capsule (genu)

Claustrum

Insula

Thalamus

Internal capsule (posterior limb)

3rd ventricle

Choroid plexus

Corpus callosum

Fornix (crus)

Calcarine sulcus

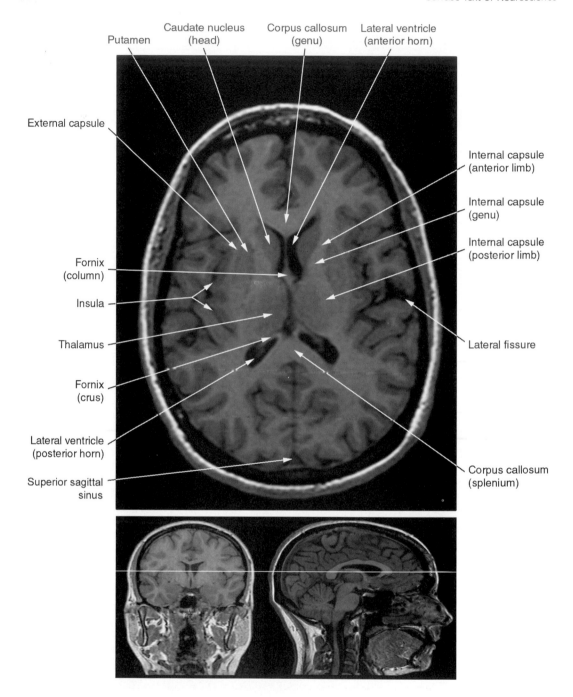

Putamen

Caudate nucleus
(head)

Corpus callosum
(genu)

Lateral ventricle
(anterior horn)

External capsule

Internal capsule
(anterior limb)

Internal capsule
(genu)

Internal capsule
(posterior limb)

Fornix
(column)

Insula

Thalamus

Lateral fissure

Fornix
(crus)

Lateral ventricle
(posterior horn)

Superior sagittal
sinus

Corpus callosum
(splenium)

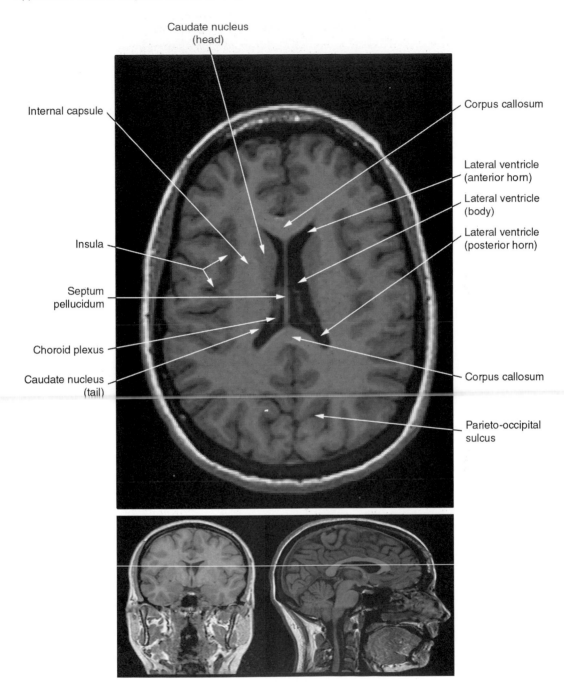

Caudate nucleus
(head)

Internal capsule

Corpus callosum

Lateral ventricle
(anterior horn)

Lateral ventricle
(body)

Lateral ventricle
(posterior horn)

Insula

Septum
pellucidum

Choroid plexus

Caudate nucleus
(tail)

Corpus callosum

Parieto-occipital
sulcus

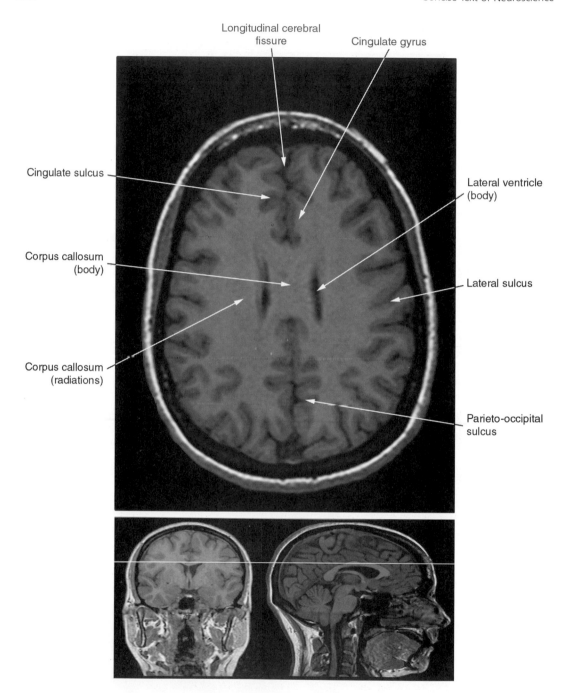

# CORONAL SECTIONS

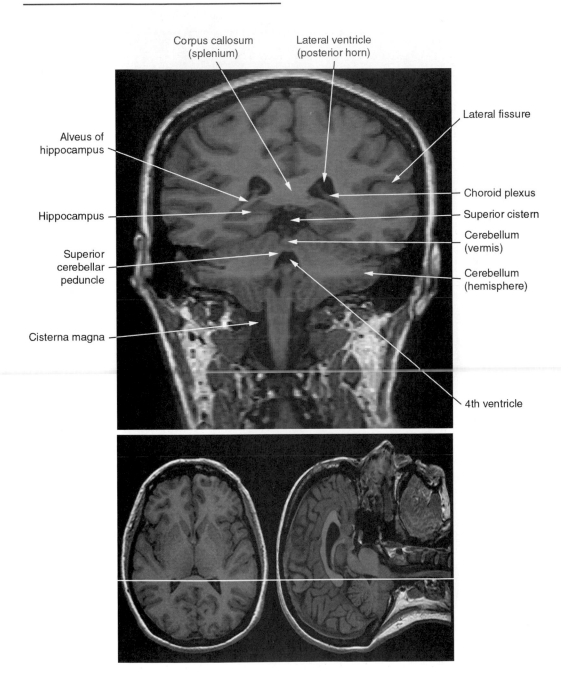

Corpus callosum
(splenium)

Lateral ventricle
(posterior horn)

Lateral fissure

Alveus of
hippocampus

Choroid plexus

Hippocampus

Superior cistern

Cerebellum
(vermis)

Superior
cerebellar
peduncle

Cerebellum
(hemisphere)

Cisterna magna

4th ventricle

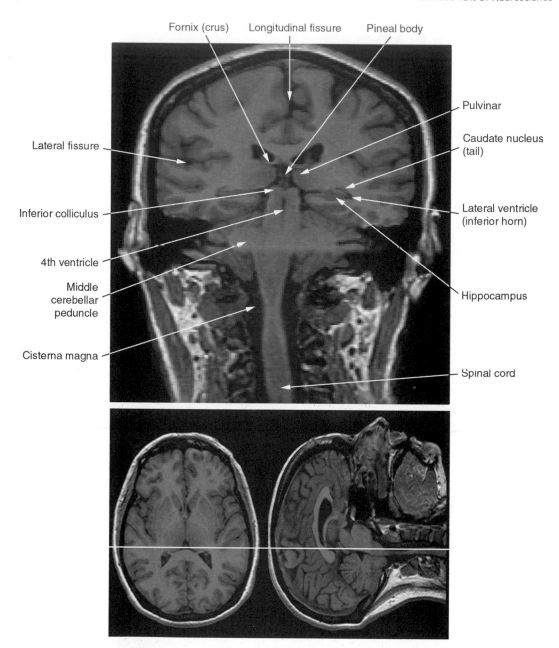

Fornix (crus)    Longitudinal fissure    Pineal body

Pulvinar

Caudate nucleus
(tail)

Lateral fissure

Lateral ventricle
(inferior horn)

Inferior colliculus

4th ventricle

Middle
cerebellar
peduncle

Hippocampus

Cisterna magna

Spinal cord

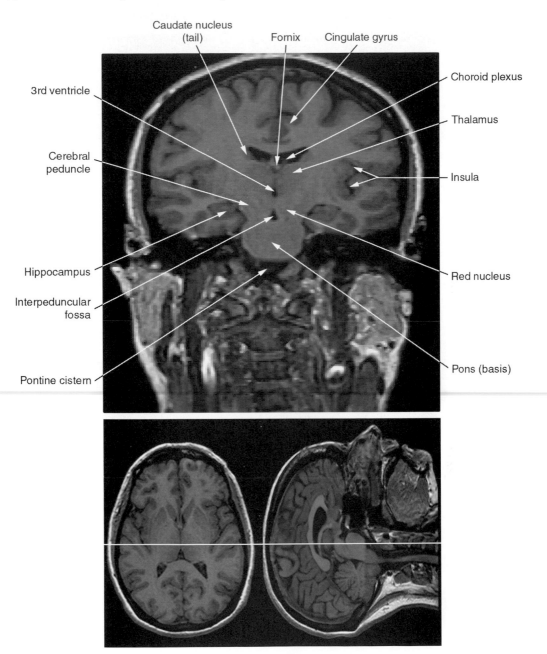

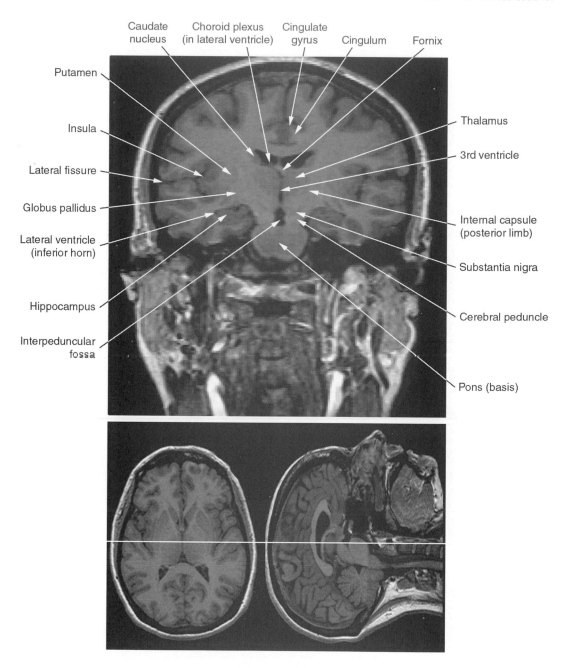

Caudate nucleus

Choroid plexus (in lateral ventricle)

Cingulate gyrus

Cingulum

Fornix

Putamen

Insula

Lateral fissure

Globus pallidus

Lateral ventricle (inferior horn)

Hippocampus

Interpeduncular fossa

Thalamus

3rd ventricle

Internal capsule (posterior limb)

Substantia nigra

Cerebral peduncle

Pons (basis)

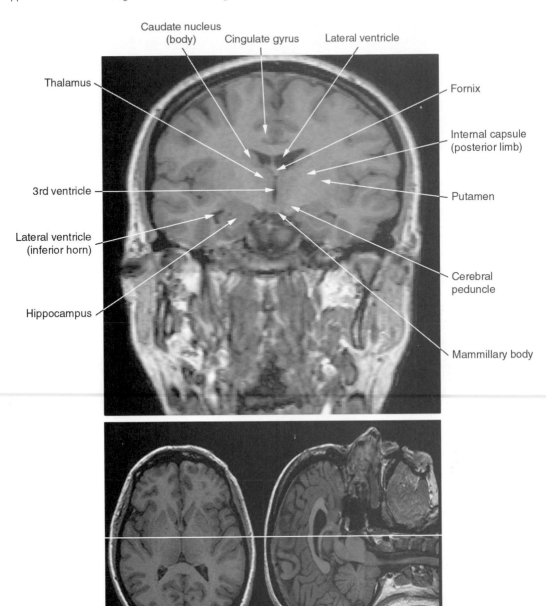

Caudate nucleus (body)

Cingulate gyrus

Lateral ventricle

Thalamus

Fornix

Internal capsule (posterior limb)

3rd ventricle

Putamen

Lateral ventricle (inferior horn)

Cerebral peduncle

Hippocampus

Mammillary body

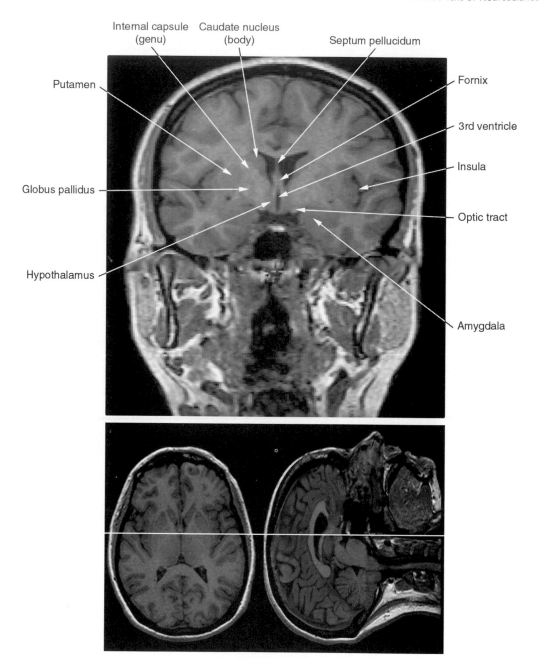

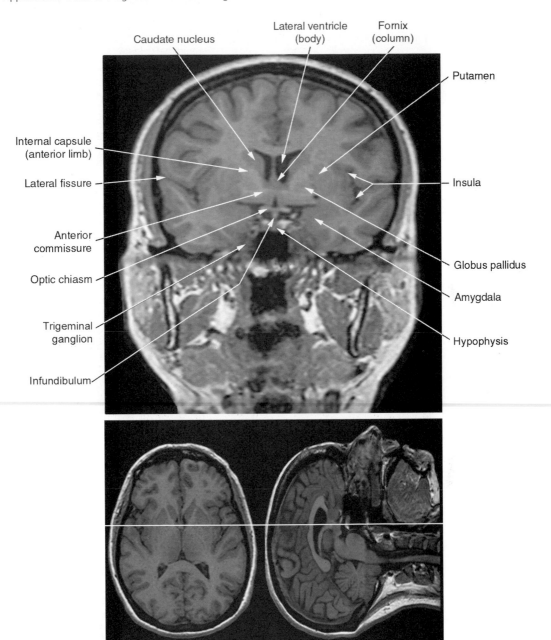

Caudate nucleus

Lateral ventricle (body)

Fornix (column)

Putamen

Internal capsule (anterior limb)

Lateral fissure

Insula

Anterior commissure

Optic chiasm

Globus pallidus

Trigeminal ganglion

Amygdala

Hypophysis

Infundibulum

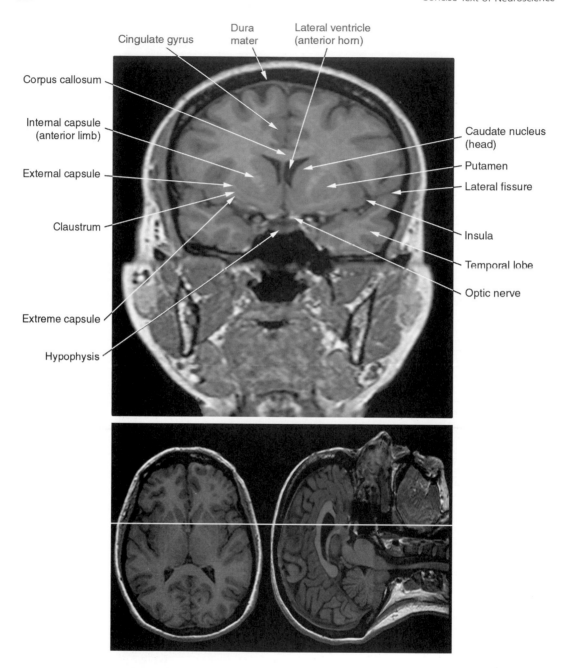

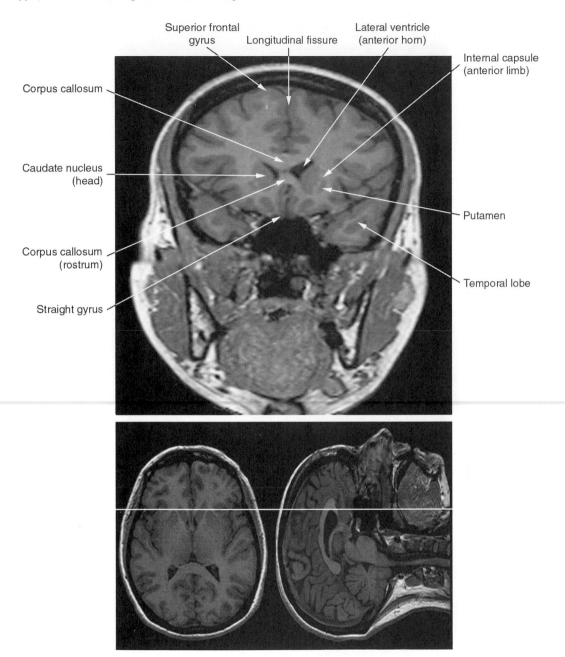

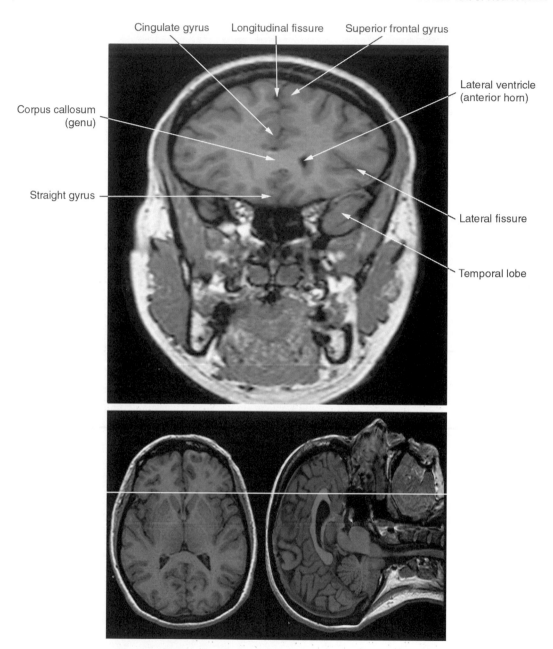

Cingulate gyrus   Longitudinal fissure   Superior frontal gyrus

Lateral ventricle
(anterior horn)

Corpus callosum
(genu)

Straight gyrus

Lateral fissure

Temporal lobe

## SAGITTAL SECTIONS

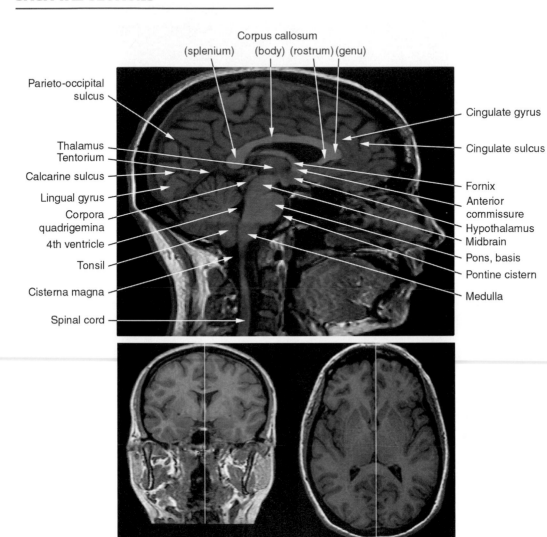

Corpus callosum
(splenium) (body) (rostrum) (genu)

Parieto-occipital sulcus

Cingulate gyrus

Thalamus
Tentorium

Cingulate sulcus

Calcarine sulcus

Lingual gyrus

Fornix

Corpora quadrigemina

Anterior commissure

4th ventricle

Hypothalamus

Tonsil

Midbrain

Pons, basis

Cisterna magna

Pontine cistern

Spinal cord

Medulla

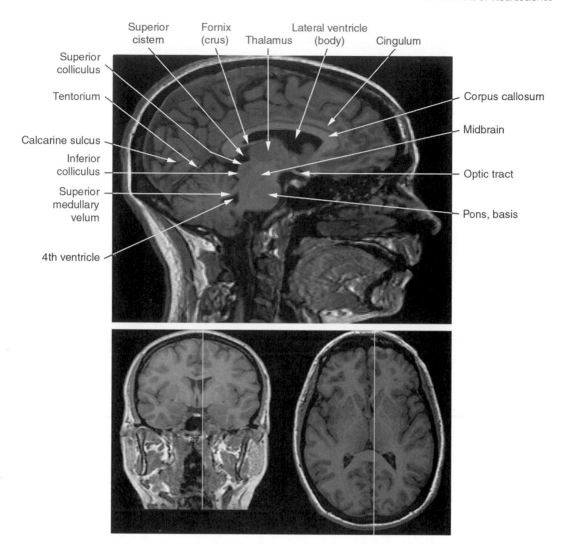

Superior cistern
Fornix (crus)
Thalamus
Lateral ventricle (body)
Cingulum
Superior colliculus
Tentorium
Calcarine sulcus
Inferior colliculus
Superior medullary velum
4th ventricle
Corpus callosum
Midbrain
Optic tract
Pons, basis

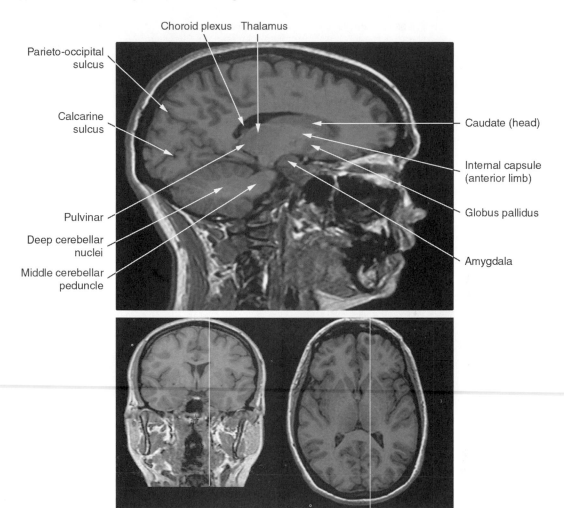

Choroid plexus    Thalamus

Parieto-occipital sulcus

Calcarine sulcus

Pulvinar

Deep cerebellar nuclei

Middle cerebellar peduncle

Caudate (head)

Internal capsule (anterior limb)

Globus pallidus

Amygdala

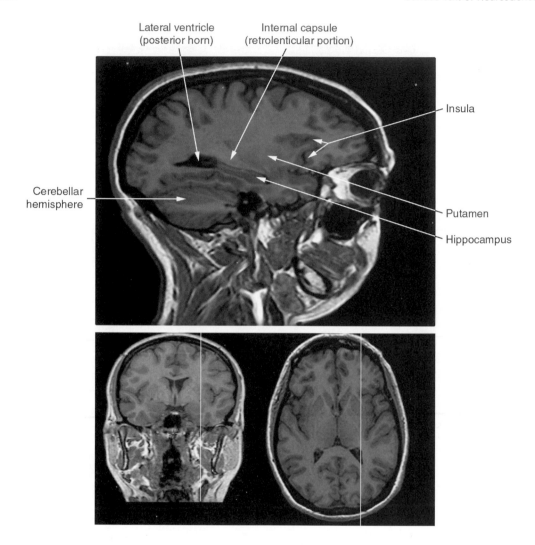

Lateral ventricle
(posterior horn)

Internal capsule
(retrolenticular portion)

Insula

Cerebellar
hemisphere

Putamen

Hippocampus

# Neuroimaging Techniques

## Robert E. Kingsley and Victor F. Jones, II

Although the patient's history and neurological examination remain the bedrock of neurologic diagnosis, modern imaging techniques have revolutionized the practice of medicine, especially neurology and neurosurgery. Images can be formed by the use of several techniques. The mainstay of medical imaging is the radiograph. Newer imaging techniques are based on the magnetic properties of nuclei and the emission of positrons and γ-rays from isotopes injected into the body.

## RADIOGRAPHIC IMAGING

The discovery of x-rays in 1895 by Wilhelm Röntgen revolutionized the practice of medicine almost immediately. For the first time it was possible to look at internal parts of the body without surgery.

X-rays are generated in a vacuum tube. They leave the tube from a single point and fan out as a three-dimensional cone. They pass through the body, losing some of their energy, before finally passing through a sheet of photographic film. The x-rays interact with the silver salts in the film, which when developed, registers an image of the subject.

An image can be formed only when one part of the subject absorbs more of the x-ray energy than adjacent parts. This differential absorption of x-ray photons provides *contrast* to the image. In most images of biological material differential absorption of x-rays is provided by only four materials; *air, water, fat, and mineral* (Fig. A4.1). Because bone contains a

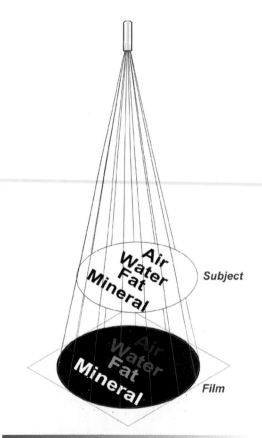

**Figure A4.1 Four contrast densities for radiographs**

X-ray tube at the top sends x-rays through a subject onto photographic film. Air, water, fat, and minerals absorb the energy of the x-rays with increasing efficiency. Because the image on the film is a negative, the image of air is rendered darkest and mineral is lightest.

lot of calcium, which has relatively high atomic mass, bone absorbs more of the electromagnetic energy of the x-ray than the surrounding tissue, which is mostly water. Since

the brain is mostly water, it does not differentially absorb enough of the x-rays passing through it to be registered on film. The little contrast that is available is obscured by the necessity to represent the three-dimensional structure of the brain on a two-dimensional sheet of film. The brain itself cannot be imaged by ordinary x-ray techniques; it is invisible (Fig. A4.2).

## The Pneumoencephalogram

The first successful attempt to image intracranial structures was based on the contrast properties of air. A **pneumoencephalogram**, also called a **ventriculogram**, is made by replacing some of the cerebrospinal fluid (CSF) with air. This can be done by inserting a needle directly into the lateral ventricle and replacing some of the CSF with air. Or CSF can be removed from the lumbar cistern and air allowed to bubble up the spinal dural sac into the fourth ventricle. From there, depending on how the head is tilted, air can be directed into the third ventricle, all horns of the lateral ventricles, and the subarachnoid space (Fig. A4.3). This traumatic procedure is associated with high rates of morbidity and mortality. In addition, the in-

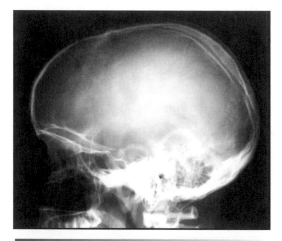

**Figure A4.2    Plain skull radiograph**

This is a lateral radiographic view of the skull. Various densities of mineral, including the teeth, are imaged, but the brain structures are not visible. (Courtesy of Dr. John Harding and the St. Joseph Medical Center, South Bend, IN.)

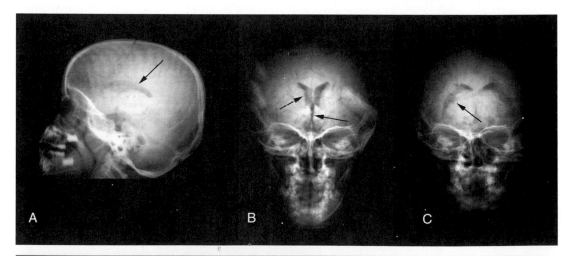

**Figure A4.3    Pneumoencephalogram**

A portion of the CSF has been replaced with air, which shows up darker than the brain. **A.** Lateral view showing the body of the lateral ventricle (*arrow*). The patient is erect, so the air rises to the superior surface of the ventricles. **B.** Anterior posterior view of a supine patient. The air rises to fill the anterior horns of the lateral ventricles (*top arrow*) and the third ventricle (*bottom arrow*). **C.** Anterior posterior view of a prone patient. The air fills the posterior horns of the lateral ventricles (*arrow*). (Courtesy of Dr. John Harding and the St. Joseph Medical Center, South Bend, IN.)

formation provided is limited because only the ventricles and subarachnoid spaces can be visualized. Hence, only expanding masses that distort the ventricular space can be inferred. This procedure has been replaced by computed tomography (CT).

## Angiography

The second method of neuroimaging became possible with the development of iodinated contrast media that could be injected into the vascular system with relative safety. The medium remains in the arteries and veins, and the atomic mass of the iodine is sufficient to provide contrast such that the vessels appear white against the dark background of the brain tissue. This technique, called **angiography** [G. *angeion,* a vessel or cavity of the body, and *graph,* write], allows imaging of the vascular system in great detail.

To image the cerebral vasculature, one introduces a cannula into the femoral artery and threads it to the aortic arch. From there the two carotid and two vertebral arteries can be individually cannulated and injected with the contrast fluid. As the contrast fluid enters the vasculature of the brain, a series of radiographic images of the head are made. By taking the images in temporal sequence, the various branches of the vascular system can be seen at different stages of filling and emptying (Fig. A4.4). Angiograms of the head are taken in two or more planes simultaneously, which facilitates three-dimensional visualization.

Like pneumoencephalography, angiography does not image the brain but only the arteries and veins. Mass lesions can be inferred from angiograms only if the vessels are displaced from their normal position (Fig. A4.5). Angiography is unsurpassed, however, in detecting vascular malformations, aneurysms, and other small vascular lesions (see Fig. 1.37).

## Computed Tomography

The use of x-rays was revolutionized in 1971 when **computed tomography** [G. *tomos,* cutting (section), and *gramma,* writing] (CT) was introduced. CT differs from ordinary x-ray imaging in two important ways. First, CT images are not made on photographic film. Instead,

the x-rays are detected by a photomultiplier tube (PMT) that converts the x-ray energy into an electrical signal. PMTs are more sensitive than film and record a greater range of x-ray energy. Second, the x-rays are not generated by a single source but are produced as an array of very narrow (about 1 mm in diameter), highly collimated beams that do not disperse in a cone shape as ordinary x-rays do. Each beam is aligned with a single PMT. This arrangement ensures that each PMT measures the x-ray absorption of only a small column of tissue (Fig. A4.6).

To generate an image, the x-ray tubes emit a series of beams of x-rays. After passing through the subject, the x-ray energy is recorded by the PMTs and saved in computer memory. The x-ray tube and the associated PMTs are then rotated slightly around the long axis of the body and the process is repeated. This process continues in a 360° arc around the head. The resulting data constitute a set of overlapping vectors of a matrix (Fig. A4.7). The vector data are used to compute the solution for the matrix. Each cell of the matrix (a **pixel**) represents the x-ray absorption of the corresponding volume of tissue (a **voxel**) *as if it were an isolated radiograph.* The entire matrix, when displayed on film or a video screen, becomes an image of the subject as if it had been sliced like a melon, revealing the internal structures (Fig. A4.8). The thickness of each slice is a function of the width of the *x-ray* beam. The table on which the patient rests is moved farther into the gantry holding the *x-ray* tube and PMT array and another image taken. In this manner a series of images are obtained as if the brain had been sliced like a loaf of bread.

CT was the first technique that allowed the direct imaging of the living brain, and it provides good resolution and contrast for the depiction of anatomical features. Before CT, the presence of tumors could only be inferred by the displacement of the ventricles or arteries. With CT, tumors and other focal lesions can be imaged directly (Fig. A4.9).

CT has a number of advantages over other forms of imaging. The images can be obtained rapidly and economically. Brain infarcts, intracranial masses, ventricular size, and ex-

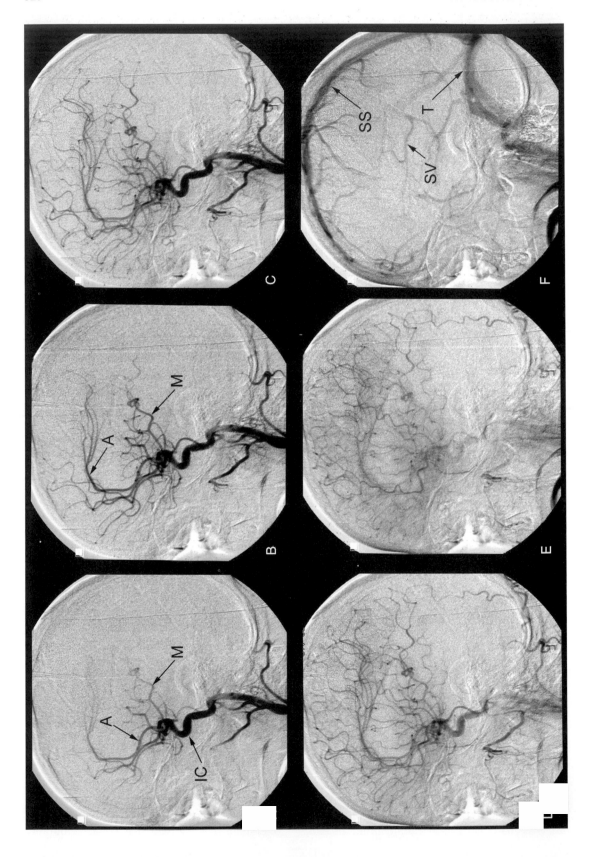

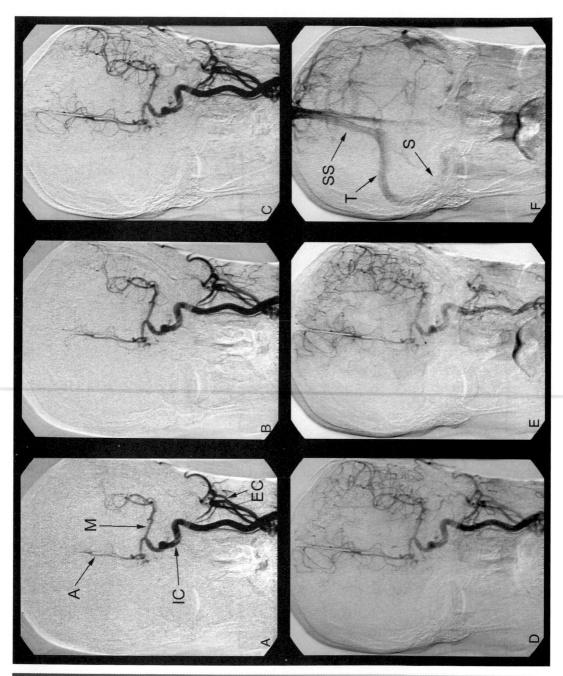

## Figure A4.4   Temporal series of arteriograms

Arteriograms taken in sequence following the injection of contrast fluid into the left common carotid artery. **Left panel.** Lateral views (anterior to the left). **Right panel.** Anterior posterior views. Each pair of images, **A–F,** were taken at the same time. **A–E.** Arteries. **F.** Superficial veins and the sinuses. **D** and **E** of the anterior posterior series clearly show the terminal fields of both anterior cerebral arteries (*A*) because the contralateral anterior cerebral artery is filled through the anterior communicating artery. *A*, anterior cerebral artery; *IC*, internal carotid artery; *EC*, external carotid artery; *M*, middle cerebral artery; *S*, sigmoid sinus; **SS**, superior sagittal sinus; *SV*, superficial vein; *T*, transverse sinus. (Courtesy of Dr. John Harding and the St. Joseph Medical Center, South Bend, IN.)

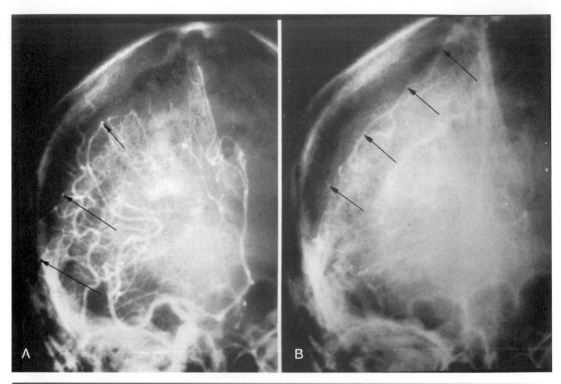

## Figure A4.5    Subdural hematoma

Space-occupying lesions can only be inferred from arteriograms. A subdural hematoma is inferred from the fact that the arteries (**A**) and veins (**B**) do not reach the skull but are displaced from the surface by a hematoma that remains invisible. *Arrows* show limit of perfusion. (Courtesy of Dr. Victor F. Jones, II, St. Joseph Medical Center, South Bend, IN.)

travascular blood are clearly revealed. And because the equipment does not interfere with monitoring or visual observation of the patient, CT is ideal in the emergency department.

CT brain imaging is limited by distortions of the image in areas close to dense bone. Therefore, the view of the brainstem is limited by artifacts. Also, as a practical matter, CT images can be obtained in only one plane, which makes assessing the extent of a lesion in three-dimensional space difficult. Despite these limitations, CT is the imaging study of choice when speed and the ability to monitor the patient are paramount issues.

## NUCLEAR MAGNETIC RESONANCE

**Magnetic resonance imaging** (MRI) *does not depend on the absorption of x-ray energy by tissue.* Instead it forms images according to the mag-netic properties of atomic nuclei. It is important to understand that MRI is based on physical principles that are entirely different from the principles that allow the creation of x-ray images. Therefore, while the images are superficially similar (after all, they depict the same anatomy), the information content of the images is quite different. These differences must be understood if one is to interpret the images.

The nucleons (protons and neutrons) in the nuclei of atoms behave as if they are spinning. When a nucleus has more than one nucleon, they are grouped in pairs. The two members of the pair spin in opposite directions. Because the opposite spins cancel, only atoms with an odd number of nucleons exhibit detectable spin properties.

One of the properties of spin is gyroscopic force. Consider a child's toy gyroscope. When it spins, it balances on its axis. The gyroscope

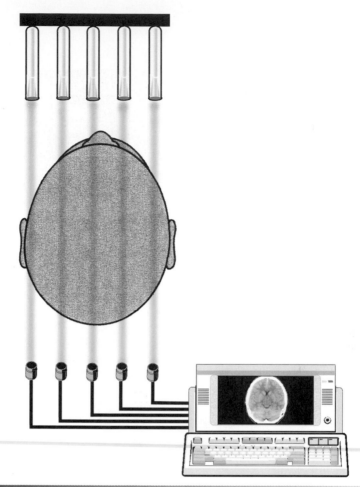

**Figure A4.6  The mechanics of CT**

X-ray tubes (*top*) are aligned with the PMTs (*bottom*) so that each PMT measures the radiographic density of only a small column of tissue. The radiographic density is stored in a computer for subsequent analysis.

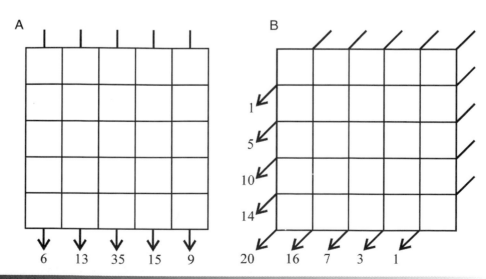

**Figure A4.7  Mathematics of CT**

This schematic illustrates how the radiographic density data for CT are collected and organized. **A.** Each x-ray tube–PMT pair measures the radiographic density of a single column of tissue. These data represent the vectors of a matrix. **B.** The x-ray tube–PMT array is rotated and a new set of data vectors is collected.

C

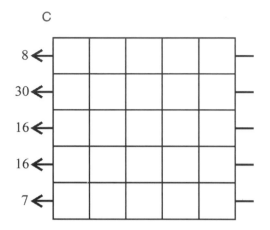

D

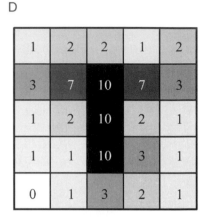

**Figure A4.7    Mathematics of CT—*continued***

**B** and **C.** The x-ray tube–PMT array is rotated and a new set of data vectors is collected. **D.** When the matrix is solved, the radiographic density of a small volume that corresponds with the intersection of all the vectors is revealed as if that volume had been imaged in isolation.

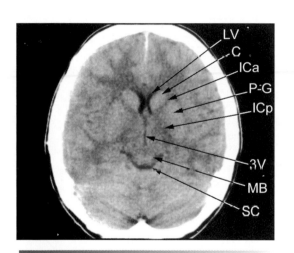

**Figure A4.8    Normal CT**

*LV,* lateral ventricle; *C,* caudate nucleus; *ICa,* anterior limb of the internal capsule; *P-G,* putamen–globus pallidus; *ICp,* posterior limb of the internal capsule; *3V,* third ventricle; *MB,* midbrain; *SC,* superior cistern. (Courtesy of Dr. Victor F. Jones, II, and St. Joseph Medical Center, South Bend, IN.)

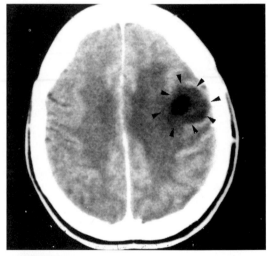

**Figure A4.9    Glioma revealed by CT**

The presence of a glioma (*arrowheads*), a malignant brain tumor, revealed by CT. (Courtesy of Dr. Victor F. Jones, II, and St. Joseph Medical Center, South Bend, IN.)

is not perfectly stationary, however; it wobbles on one of its axes, slowly scribing an imaginary circle in the air. This wobble is called **precession.** The time the gyroscope takes to precess 360°, the **resonance frequency,** is partly a function of the object's mass. Because of the

gyroscopic force, all spinning masses precess on their axes; atomic nuclei precess too.

Another property of spin is magnetism. Spinning nuclei act as small magnets and consequently are affected by the electromagnetic force. For MRI, a strong external magnetic field is used to align the nuclei. In the absence of a strong magnetic field, nuclei are oriented randomly. When placed in the strong magnetic field of the MRI scanner (the magnet used for most MRI imaging is 1.5 tesla (T), which is 30,000 times the magnetic field of the earth), nuclei with an odd number of nucleons align themselves along the axis of the field (the z-axis), just as a compass needle aligns itself with the magnetic field of the earth.

Any magnet that moves through a magnetic field disturbs the electromagnetic force and generates electrical energy. For this reason, *a magnetic nucleus precessing within a magnetic field emits a weak electrical signal at the resonance frequency.* This electrical signal is used to make the MRI.

To create a detectable signal, the nuclei must be precessing coherently; that is, their axes must point in the same direction. Ordinarily the nuclei precess at random; their poles point at random sites around the precession circle. To make the axes all point in the same direction, a brief burst of radio frequency energy is transmitted through an an-

tenna placed close to the subject (**TR pulse**). This burst of energy tilts all the spinning nuclei so that they are aligned 90° to the z-axis. After a brief interval a second burst of energy flips the nuclei 180° and forces them to precess coherently. At a certain time after the 180° pulse (**TE time**), the MR signal is measured. Because the signal is weak, the pulse sequence is repeated several times so that the signals can be averaged, which improves the signal-to-noise ratio.

When the transmission pulse stops, two things happen. First, the nuclei start to realign with the magnetic field. The time it takes them to realign with the magnetic field is called the **T1 relaxation time** (Fig. A4.10). Second, the nuclei start to *dephase* instead of precessing coherently, and the precessions start to become random. The time it takes for coherency to be lost is called the **T2 relaxation time** (Fig. A4.10).

At present all MRI is based on the hydrogen proton bound in water. The T1 and T2 relaxation curves for the hydrogen proton differ according to the hydration of the tissue and the microscopic magnetic environment. There-

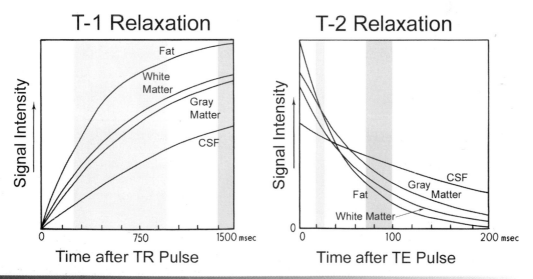

**Figure A4.10   MRI relaxation curves**

The T1 relaxation curves show the time it takes for the nuclei of various tissues to realign with the external magnetic field (z-axis) after being rotated 90° by the TR pulse. The T2 relaxation curves show the rate of loss of coherent precession of various tissues following the TE pulse. *Light gray,* "short" TR and TE periods. *Dark gray,* "long" periods (see Table A4.1). Note how the relative intensity of the CSF signal reverses on the T2 relaxation curve between the light and dark gray areas.

fore, the strength of the MR signal from a particular tissue depends largely on its water content and when during the relaxation period the signal is sampled (Fig. A4.10). Because image contrast in MRI depends on the differences in signal intensity available from different tissues *when the signal is sampled,* the timing of the TR and TE pulses affects the appearance of the image (Fig. A4.11).

Three pulse sequences are commonly used for brain imaging. The *T1-weighted image uses relatively short TR and TE times* (Table A4.1) in which CSF, bone, air, and flowing blood emit almost no signal and are therefore rendered black. Fat and bone marrow emit a very strong signal and are rendered white. Brain tissue emits a signal of intermediate strength, with gray matter slightly darker than white matter. The *T2-weighted images use long TR and TE times.* Bone, air, and flowing blood are again rendered black, but CSF emits a strong signal and is rendered white. Gray matter is rendered lighter than white matter. The *proton density image results from the use of a long TR and short*

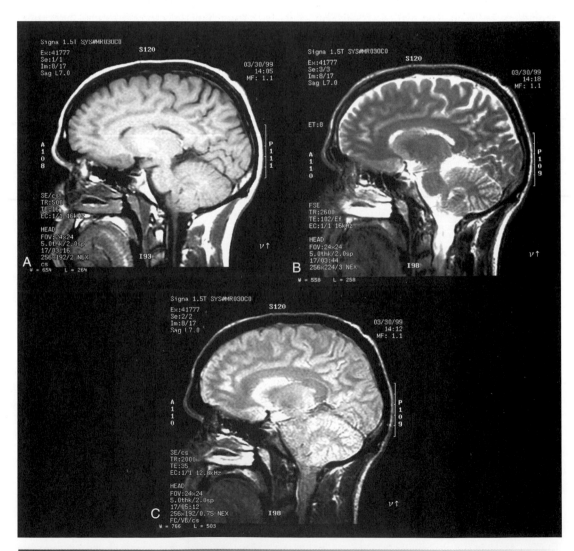

**Figure A4.11. Normal MRIs**

**A.** T1-weighted MRI (TR-500/TE-16, T-1.5). **B.** T2-weighted MRI (TR-2600/TE-102, T-1.5). **C.** Proton density–weighted MRI (TR-2000/TE-35, T-1.5). (Courtesy The Magnetic Resonance Center, South Bend, IN.)

**Table A4.1   Appearance of Various Tissues in MRI with Various Pulse Sequences**

| Common Name | Pulse | Pulse Timing | CNS Structure | Appearance |
|---|---|---|---|---|
| T1-weighted | TR | 200–1000 msec | CSF | Black |
| | TE | 20–25 msec | White matter | Bright |
| | | | Gray matter | Gray |
| T2-weighted | TR | >2000 msec | CSF | Bright |
| | TE | >75 msec | White matter | Dark |
| | | | Gray matter | Gray |
| Proton density | TR | >2000 | CSF | Dark |
| | TE | 20–25 | White matter | Dark gray |
| | | | Gray matter | Light gray |

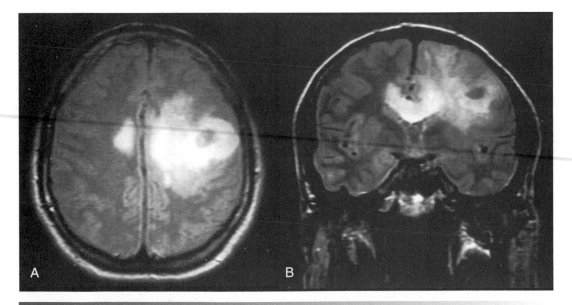

**Figure A4.12   Glioma revealed by MRI**

The glioma (*area of high signal*) revealed in this proton density–weighted MRI is from the patient in Figure A4.9. **A.** Approximately the same plane as the CT in Figure A4.9. Much more of the tumor is revealed by MRI. **B.** The value of the multiplanar imaging capability of MRI is demonstrated. The image clearly shows that the tumor has penetrated the contralateral hemisphere by growing through the corpus callosum rather than by metastasizing, as might be inferred by looking only at **A.** (Courtesy of Dr. Victor F. Jones, II and the Magnetic Resonance Center, South Bend, IN.)

*TE time.* Fat emits a strong signal and is therefore white; CSF is dark but not black. Gray matter appears lighter than white matter. Air, bone, and flowing blood are black.

MRI has a distinct advantage over CT because it demonstrates brain anatomy and lesions in greater detail and with better contrast.

Also, because of the manner in which the MRI data are obtained, images can be produced in any plane. Finally, because MRI is more sensitive to changes in tissue water content, it can expose subtle pathological changes that escape detection with CT (Fig. A4.12). MRI can be enhanced by the use of gadolinium, a lan-

Figure A4.13    Gadolinium
enhancement

The **left** panel of each pair of images is the
unenhanced MRI. Images on the **right** were
made following injection of gadolinium.
**Upper left.** T1-weighted (TR-10002/TE-
137). **Lower left.** Proton density-weighted
(TR-2000/TE-20). **Right.** Both T1-weighted
(**top,** TR-650/TE-30; **bottom** TR-500/TE-
16). This patient has a large meningioma,
(*long arrow*) a nonmalignant tumor originating from the meninges that is enhanced
by the injection of gadolinium. Multiple
small lesions, which do not enhance (*short
arrows*), are also visible. These small lesions
are thought to be infarcts caused by cerebrovascular disease. (Courtesy of The Magnetic Resonance Center, South Bend, IN.)

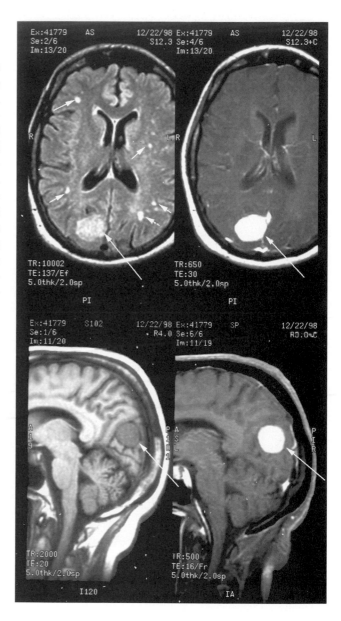

thanide element (atomic number 64) with
paramagnetic properties. Gadolinium com-
pounds used in MRI do not normally cross the
blood-brain barrier; therefore, any lesion that
disrupts the blood-brain barrier displays an increased signal intensity following gadolinium
injection on T1-weighted images (Fig. A4.13).

MRI is becoming useful in angiography. **MR
angiography** (MRA) is used to detect vascular
malformations and aneurysms of the larger intracerebral vessels. Although its resolution of
medium-size arteries and veins cannot match

the resolution obtained with standard *radiographic* angiography, MRA is sometimes preferred over *radiographic* techniques because it
is noninvasive and therefore safer.

**Diffusion MRI** is a new technique that detects areas of acute infarction. Its promise lies
in its ability to facilitate the diagnosis of an ischemic stroke (thrombotic or embolic) in its
earliest stages. Current acute treatment for ischemic stroke requires the administration of
specific clot-dissolving agents within 4 hours
of the onset of symptoms. Since neither CT

nor ordinary MRI can reliably detect infarction at this early stage, the diagnosis of stroke is sometimes difficult. Because the clot-dissolving agents pose definite risks, they are usually not given without a certain diagnosis. Diffusion MRI can provide useful data to support the early diagnosis of ischemic stroke.

Although MRI is considered noninvasive, it does have its limitations. The orifice of the magnet is relatively small and long. Many people become claustrophobic when placed in it, and a few cannot tolerate the confinement. Also, severely obese people do not fit into the magnet. People who are on life support or have cardiac pacemakers cannot be imaged because the magnet interferes with equipment that has ferrous metal parts. Finally, people with ferrous metal implants such as aneurysm clips or metal debris in the eye (common among certain industrial workers) cannot be placed in the magnet because the metal moves in the magnetic field. The effect of strong magnetic fields on the fetus has not been determined; therefore pregnant women are usually excluded from MRI. These limitations are few, however, and MRI has proven to be perhaps the most important adjunct to neurological diagnosis.

# Further Applications Answers

**3.1.** Pyridostigmine blocks the action of acetylcholinesterase, prolonging the action of acetylcholine at the myoneural junction.

**3.2.** No. Anticholinesterase drugs treat symptoms only. Plasmapheresis attacks the cause of the disease in a limited way. Myasthenia gravis is caused by an unknown process that stimulates the production of acetylcholine receptor (AChR) antibodies. Plasmapheresis does remove the antibodies from the bloodstream but does nothing to stop the production of AChR antibodies.

**3.3.** Since antibodies are found in 85 to 90% of patients with myasthenia gravis, measuring antibody titers is a useful adjunct to the edrophonium test. However, antibody titers cannot be used to develop a prognosis or to direct therapy.

**3.4.** Plasmapheresis removes antibodies from the blood, reducing the attack on the myoneural junction. Corticosteroids are anti-inflammatory and therefore help to alleviate the effects of the immune attack on the myoneural junction. Thymectomy is often effective, especially in young patients. The role of the thymus in myasthenia gravis is not known, but almost all people who have myasthenia gravis have pathological findings in the thymus, either hyperplasia or a true thymoma. One hypothesis centers on the "myoid" cells in the thymus, which have histological characteristics of muscle. These cells may trigger an autoimmune response in the thymus.

**4.1.** Important points of peripheral nerve injury are the ulnar groove, carpal tunnel, brachial plexus (Saturday night syndrome), and common peroneal nerve at the head of the fibula.

**4.2.** The muscles governing the movements of the wrist and fingers that were tested are all supplied by the radial nerve. Since the axillary is a branch of the radial nerve, the physician is trying to determine whether the axillary nerve was injured in isolation or the radial nerve central to the axillary branch was injured directly. Normal movement and strength in the fingers and wrist indicate that the main trunk of the radial nerve is intact.

**4.3.** Review the distribution of the radial nerve in any gross anatomy text. Also, see the dermatome map in Chapter 5.

**4.4.** Axoplasmic flow and blood circulation to the nerve itself can be compromised by nerve compression alone. Long-term nerve compression denies to distal targets (e.g., muscles and myoneural junction) transported proteins needed for normal function.

**4.5.** The narrow flexor retinaculum in the wrist contains tendons and nerves in a confined, nondistensible space. Therefore, compression cannot be relieved.

**4.6.** Repetitive movement of the tendons in the retinaculum can cause irritation that leads to edema and swelling. Since there is no room for expansion, the swelling can press on the nerves and lead to a nerve compression syndrome.

4.7. Review the distribution of median and ulnar nerves in any gross anatomy text.

## CHAPTER 5

5.1. Ask your instructor to evaluate your sketch.

5.2. Fine tactile sensations are carried in the dorsal columns in the spinal cord. The preservation of the epicritic senses means that the dorsal columns are spared.

5.3. Romberg's test evaluates how effectively the proprioceptive sense from the lower extremities, especially the ankles, is integrated into the subconscious motor control of balance. The ability to maintain balance in the absence of visual clues is further evidence that the dorsal columns are functional and intact.

5.4. The burn on her shoulder indicates long-standing loss of pain referable to a lesion in the cervical region of the spinal cord.

5.5. Yes. The diagnosis can be made without MRI because the pattern of the sensory and motor losses is so characteristic that the lesion can be delineated quite precisely. Most ancillary procedures should be ordered to verify and quantify results obtained from the history and examination. Ancillary tests are not "fishing expeditions" ordered in the face of ignorance. The MRI was important not only to verify the diagnosis but to evaluate the patient for surgery (which was determined to be useless in this case).

5.6. Intractable pain associated with syringomyelia and syringobulbia can be explained by central sensitization—the development of spontaneous activity in protopathic pathways in the thalamus—that results from deafferentation (secondary fibers cut in the central white commissure in spinal cord).

5.7. The nerve roots have been avulsed from the spinal cord. Removing the arm, and hence its nerves, could not further diminish neural input to the spinal cord. The amputation was performed for cosmetic and practical considerations, not to relieve pain.

5.8. The dorsal columns contain primary afferent axons that were disconnected from their cell bodies (dorsal root ganglion) by the avul-

sion, hence they have already degenerated. Stimulating the dorsal columns can no longer affect the spinal cord neurons that their collateral branches once innervated. Similarly, TENS would not be effective in this case, since the peripheral axons have been separated from the central connections (and the arm was amputated).

5.9. Coagulation of the dorsal horn destroys the soma of the neurons projecting to the thalamus; tractotomy leaves the soma intact. In the latter case, the remaining neuron soma and its amputated axons can sprout and form new, inappropriate synapses in the spinal cord. These new synapses may lead to abnormal activity in other intact neurons that project to the thalamus. Also, coagulation of the dorsal horn destroys all of the interneurons and the inappropriately reorganized interconnections and activity associated with spinal central sensitization. However, both coagulation and tractotomy deafferent the thalamus, so in the long run, coagulation may be no better than tractotomy. Further studies are needed, but this case does make the point that at least some intractable pain originates in the spine.

5.10. Major complications of this surgery are the risk of damage to dorsal columns and lateral white columns (corticobulbospinal tract; see Chapter 7).

5.11. Neurosurgery produces edema in the structures surrounding damaged neural tissue. Edema can press on the dorsal columns (causing ipsilateral paraesthesias) and the lateral white columns that carry the principal descending motor tracts (leading to some loss of motor function). Because the edema dissipates with time, these side effects are short-lasting. Of course, permanent loss of function results if the needle electrode is inappropriately placed during surgery.

## CHAPTER 6

6.1. When evaluating a neurological case, focus your attention on the areas of the nervous system most likely to be involved: brain, brainstem, cerebellum, basal ganglia, spinal cord, peripheral nervous system (PNS), and so on. In this case the bilateral stockinglike pattern of sensory loss virtually eliminates all parts of the nervous system except the spinal cord and PNS. Decreased muscle stretch reflexes (MSRs) can only be caused by lesions to the PNS or the parts of the spinal cord that contribute to the lower motor neuron.

6.2. The loss of position sense from the toes indicates that the large-diameter fibers are compromised, since this sense is carried by large A$\alpha$ and A$\beta$ fibers. The $I_A$ fiber (essential for the MSR) is also large and therefore likely to be affected. The preservation of position sense from the upper extremity is consistent with the preservation of MSRs from the same region. This information helps to limit the locus of the lesion and provides objective information about progression or lack thereof on future examinations.

6.3. The patient's ataxia could be caused by loss of proprioception or a cerebellar lesion (see Chapter 9). In this case the Romberg test demonstrates that the ataxia is due to a sensory loss, because Mr. E. A. became unstable only when he closed his eyes. A patient with a cerebellar lesion would be unstable with the eyes open.

6.4. Fasciculations and atrophy are signs of muscle denervation. In this case the axons are intact and are nourishing the muscle, so there can be no atrophy or fasciculations. The axons are just not conducting normally. Therefore, the other sensory and motor signs associated with the LMN are present.

6.5. Most peripheral neuropathies are caused by toxins. Toxins might first be expected to affect the neurons with the longest and largest diameter axons because they have the largest volume and surface area (remember, most of the neuron cytoplasm is in the axon). Axons with a large volume have the greatest metabolic needs and therefore may be particularly susceptible to metabolic toxins. Also, their large surface area means that they are likely to absorb circulating toxins. The long axons also have a large vascular supply that can be affected by the disease process of diabetes mellitus.

6.6. The S1 spinal nerves leave the sacral spinal cord at approximately the level of the L1 vertebra. It descends to the vertebral S1-S2 interspace and must therefore pass the L5-S1 intervertebral disk. At this point the S1 nerve is more medial than the L5 nerve. Either or both nerves can be pressured by the L5-S1 disk, but the more medial nerve is the most common target. This is true for all the lumbar intervertebral disks.

6.7. The most likely disk is the L4-L5 disk. Symptoms are the dermatome pattern for L5 (see Fig. 5.22) and weakness in the extensor hallucis and to a much lesser degree in the gastrocnemius muscle; MSRs from the gastrocnemius would be diminished somewhat but not as much as with a S1 disk.

6.8. Because of the anatomy of the cauda equina, a medially displaced ruptured disk at the lumbar level causes bilateral symptoms associated with the spinal nerves S1 to S5. These symptoms include bowel, bladder, and sexual dysfunctions (see Chapter 13), problems rarely associated with single nerve entrapments. Because these problems are caused by damage to small, unmyelinated axons that regenerate poorly, quick action is required to avoid permanent loss of function.

6.9. There is no cauda equina in the cervical region; therefore, cervical disk symptoms are associated with the spinal nerve at the same level as the disk, in this case C7. In addition to the C7 dermatome, one would expect to see weakness in the triceps muscle, which receives its primary innervation from this spinal nerve. Cervical disks can also compress the spinal cord, hence cause symptoms in the lower extremity (see Chapter 7).

## CHAPTER 7

7.1. The weakness would involve the left leg more than the arm. The face probably would be spared. There would probably be no aphasia.

7.2. Cerebral hemorrhages usually take place during the day rather than at night. They are typically sudden events (seconds to minutes). Mr. R. B. probably would have had a severe headache, been confused, and possibly had some alteration of consciousness. The CT would show blood in the cranium.

7.3. If Mr. R. B. had had an embolism, it probably would have dislodged during activity. The event would have been sudden (seconds to minutes), but the symptoms (assuming the embolus lodged in the same place as the plaque formed) would be about the same. If the source of the embolism continued to throw debris into the vascular system, one would expect to see succeeding neurological events as more emboli entered the brain.

7.4. The lesion is above the brainstem on the right, perhaps in the internal capsule (pure motor). This location assumes that the signs of incoordination are due to weakness and not signs of cerebellar dysfunction.

7.5. Amyotrophic lateral sclerosis is a purely motor disease. Any alteration in sensory function rules it out in the differential diagnosis. MS is a CNS myelin disease and therefore can cause any findings referable to the CNS.

7.6. Loss of the descending voluntary motor systems is masked by the loss of the motor neurons. With no motor neurons to affect, the UMN signs cannot be present. Loss of motor neurons produces denervation of the muscles, hence flaccid paralysis.

7.7. The difficulties that amyotrophic lateral sclerosis patients face raise a number of ethical, moral, and legal questions for both the patient and the physician. None of these questions have absolute answers. Discuss these issues on a continuing basis with your fellow students, your professors, and other counselors with whom you have rapport.

8.1. The original diagnosis of stroke is not defensible. The patient's initial complaint is tremor that progressed inexorably over several months. The time course for the onset of stroke is minutes to hours. Furthermore, examination of the patient does not reveal UMN signs such as hemiparesis, dysesthesia, paraesthesia, spasticity, sign of Babinski, or other deficits that can be attributed to an infarct within the territory of a single artery.

8.2. Primary parkinsonism is idiopathic. Therefore, identifying any cause of parkinsonism excludes primary parkinsonism from the diagnosis. Correct diagnosis is important because many nonidiopathic forms of the disease respond poorly to L-dopa and have a poorer prognosis. The possibility of carbon monoxide poisoning should always be entertained because it is fairly common, resulting from poor furnace venting. Manganese and carbon disulfide poisoning may be associated with the work environment. The major antipsychotic drug classes, such as the phenothiazines (prochlorperazine [Compazine]), dibenzoxazepines (loxapine [Loxitane]), and butyrophenones (haloperidol [Haldol]) can produce **tardive dyskinesia**, the iatrogenic form of parkinsonism, as a side effect. Tardive dyskinesia is sometimes reversible if the offending drug is discontinued. If drug treatment is not discontinued, tardive dyskinesia can persist indefinitely after drug withdrawal.

8.3. One possible mechanism of failure of L-dopa therapy is that with the continuing loss of the SNc cells, L-dopa can no longer be converted to dopamine, since the conversion (at least in the affected part of the brain) occurs primarily in the SNc cells. In addition, with the loss of the SNc cells, the synapses on the target cells in the striatum degenerate. Without this synaptic contact, the striatal cells may no longer be driven to produce dopamine receptors. With fewer receptors, any dopamine that is present will be less effective. If failure of L-dopa therapy is due to the inability to convert L-dopa to dopamine, MAO inhibitors and dopa agonists can be effective. On the other hand, if the receptors fail, MAO inhibitors and agonists cannot be effective.

8.4. The coadministration of carbidopa with L-dopa reduces the required oral dose of L-dopa by about 75%, since the peripheral metabolism of L-dopa to dopamine is substantially reduced. The peripheral effects of excessive dopamine (nausea, cardiac dysrhythmias, orthostatic hypotension, anorexia, vomiting, and dizziness) are greatly reduced by the coadministration of carbidopa.

8.5. Primary parkinsonism is an adult-onset disease. When it is suspected in a child, a long list of differential diagnoses should be pursued, including exposure to drugs (prescribed, recreational, or accidental) and toxins; head injury; brain tumor; hydrocephalus; and metabolic disease, among others. Dystonia, on the other hand, usually first appears in children. While tremor is a dramatic symptom, parkinsonism has four major characteristics: tremor, bradykinesia, lead pipe or cogwheel rigidity, and postural disturbances. Its diagnosis depends on the presence of two or more of these symptoms. Finally, the rigidity of parkinsonism is lead pipe or cogwheel. The extremity is not locked into a fixed position by sustained muscle contractions, as is the case with dystonia. Tremor has a long list of differential diagnoses; the interested student is referred to standard neurological texts. In the case of Ms. T. L., the diagnosis of juvenile parkinsonism based on tremor alone is not appropriate.

8.6. Yes, it was fortunate that the family physician recognized the relation between metoclopramide and dystonia. His alertness and gentle counseling persuaded Ms. T. L. to seek further (and finally competent) medical attention. Given his alertness to the meaning of the drug's obvious side effects on his patient, it is perhaps surprising that he did not diagnose dystonia sooner. Perhaps, as a primary care physician, he was reluctant to challenge the neurologists' (inaccurate) diagnoses. The lesson is to trust your own observations and draw your own conclusions. If your conclusion conflicts with another person's opinion, resolve the conflict. Don't ignore it.

8.7. PET studies show that dopamine receptors are present in the striatum of dopa-responsive dystonia patients. Therefore, the defect must be caused by the lack of availability of dopamine. Perhaps the nigral cells are producing defective dopamine or competent dopamine in inadequate amounts. A less likely possibility is that normal amounts of competent dopamine are being released but that it is being scavenged by overactive reuptake or catabolic mechanisms.

9.1. Lesions to the cerebral cortex or the internal capsule produce symptoms that are limited to the contralateral side of the body. In this case, because the symptoms are bilateral, a cortical or capsular lesion is unlikely. Lesions to the basal ganglion usually produce hyperkinesia or hypokinesia, which are absent in this case. Thalamic lesions usually produce thalamic pain syndrome or hypesthesia in the contralateral half of the body. This patient has no thalamic pain syndrome, and the hypesthesia is limited to the right half of the face. The brainstem signs exclude the spinal cord and peripheral nervous system. The ataxia, dysmetria, dysdiadochokinesia, dysarthria, and scanning speech all point to the cerebellum or its peduncles; the oculomotor, trigeminal, and facial disturbances all suggest a brainstem lesion.

9.2. Neither CT nor ordinary MRI can reveal the early stages of a neural tissue infarct (however, see diffusion MRI in Appendix 4). Intracranial blood can be imaged by both techniques, hence the initial CT. Infarcts can be imaged about 48 hours after the insult. Ordinarily it is not necessary to image the brain after hemorrhage has been ruled out, but in this case it was necessary to rule out a basilar aneurysm. Therefore, the MRA (magnetic resonance angiography; see Appendix 4) was ordered to study the basilar artery, and MRI was a part of that procedure.

9.3. Emboli that develop in the systemic circulation are filtered by the pulmonary circulation before they reach the brain. Although pulmonary emboli are a serious medical problem, they do not have neurological implications. In this case, however, the patent foramen ovale allows blood to bypass the pulmonary circulation, allowing emboli originating as deep vein thrombi to reach the systemic arterial circulation.

9.4. In the midbrain, the medial lemniscus and the decussation of the superior cerebellar peduncle are side by side. At this level the most medial portion of the medial lemniscus carries the epicritic sensations from the face. Therefore, a small lesion may involve the lateral part of the superior cerebellar peduncle and the medial portion of the medial lemniscus.

9.5. Look up these drugs in the *Physicians' Desk Reference.*

9.6. The use of cocaine is medically significant because it dramatically increases blood pressure. Therefore, patients using cocaine have a higher risk of hemorrhagic stroke. The consumption of the hallucinogenic mushrooms probably has no medical significance.

9.7. Multiple sclerosis is characterized by multiple CNS lesions disseminated in time and space. The exacerbations usually develop over hours to days. In this case multiple sclerosis is unlikely because the symptoms developed too quickly and there is no history of repeated attacks over an extended period.

## CHAPTER 10

10.1. The following structures lie within the territory of the posterior inferior cerebellar artery, with neurological signs in parentheses: nucleus and spinal tract of V (ipsilateral loss of protopathic functions from the ipsilateral face); anterior lateral system (contralateral loss of protopathic functions from the body); dorsal longitudinal fasciculus (ipsilateral Horner's syndrome); inferior cerebellar peduncle (ipsilateral ataxia); nucleus ambiguus and CN IX and X (hoarseness, dysphagia, diminished gag reflex); vestibular nuclei (nystagmus, vertigo, nausea, and vomiting); solitary nucleus and tract (loss of taste on the ipsilateral side).

10.2. The following structures lie within the territory of the lower medulla (the neurological signs associated with the anterior spinal artery are in parentheses): medullary pyramid (contralateral spastic hemiparesis); medial lemniscus (contralateral loss of epicritic functions except for the face); hypoglossal nerve and nucleus (ipsilateral paresis and subsequent atrophy of the intrinsic muscles of the tongue).

10.3. Neurological signs associated with occlusion of the vertebral artery are varied for two reasons. First, the branching pattern of the arteries arising from the vertebral artery is variable. Second, depending on its size, a thrombus or embolus may occlude one or more of these branches. Third, if the occlusion is proximal to the first branch, the circulation to the lower medulla and cervical spinal cord can be provided by the intact vertebral artery. If a vertebral occlusion spares the posterior inferior cerebellar artery and the anterior spinal artery, the structures affected are usually lim-

ited to the nucleus and spinal tract of V (loss of protopathic sensations from the ipsilateral face); anterior lateral system (loss of protopathic sensations from the contralateral body); fasciculus cuneatus and the internal arcuate fibers (loss of protopathic sensations from the ipsilateral body, sparing the face).

10.4. Mesencephalic structures (and the neurological signs associated with the paramedian branches of the basilar or posterior communicating artery) are the oculomotor nerve and nucleus (ipsilateral third nerve palsy, anisocoria, and loss of light reflex); medial half of the cerebral peduncle (contralateral spastic hemiparesis); decussation of the superior cerebellar peduncle (ataxia).

10.5. Pineal tumors can press on the superior colliculus and neighboring structures, especially the pretectal nuclei. Disruption of these structures can produce supranuclear ophthalmoplegia of vertical eye movements. Also, the cerebral aqueduct can be occluded, which produces signs of increased intracranial pressure (see Chapter 15). Although this patient does not exhibit any signs of increased intracranial pressure, he does have signs of basal ganglion disease. These signs cannot be attributed to the superior colliculus or its immediate neighbors.

10.6. The pineal body is immediately superior to the mesencephalon and cerebral aqueduct. Therefore, an increase in its size may occlude the aqueduct.

10.7. Aneurysms of the carotid artery commonly present as sixth nerve palsy.

10.8. Given the high incidence of positive findings associated with third nerve palsy, a CT study revealing no lesion should not be considered definitive. The CT can rule out many intracranial masses and hemorrhage, but not aneurysms.

## CHAPTER 11

11.1. The most common sequence of symptoms in patients with acoustic neuroma is (a) unilateral hearing loss affecting especially the high frequencies; (b) chronic vertigo (as opposed to intermittent vertigo seen in Ménière's disease); (c) ipsilateral facial palsy; and (d) ipsilateral facial numbness.

11.2. Cranial nerve involvement usually follows the same order as the symptoms: cochlear, vestibular, facial, and trigeminal. The vagal and glossopharyngeal nerves may also become involved in advanced cases (about 2%).

11.3. Had Mr. R. W. been right-handed, there might have been both noise-induced and tumor-induced hearing loss in the left ear, a finding that could have confounded the diagnosis. With a reasonable explanation for the unilateral hearing loss (noise-induced trauma due to firearms), the MRI might have been delayed.

11.4. The most common causes of unilateral hearing loss are conductive. Most causes of sensorineural hearing loss affect both cochleas; notable exceptions are Ménière's disease, sudden deafness syndrome, neuromas, and exposure to the noise from the use of long guns. Because of the extensive bilateral divergence of the central acoustic pathways, unilateral central hearing loss is nearly impossible. Unilateral hearing loss must always be vigorously investigated.

11.5. Following an abnormal audiogram and BAER, MRI is the most appropriate next step.

12.1. The first symptom, vertigo, is probably caused by a lesion to the vestibular nuclei or the flocculus or fastigial nucleus of the cerebellum (nystagmogram indicated a CNS lesion). The second episode includes trouble with balance, which could be an exacerbation of the vestibular-cerebellar lesion. However, the poor coordination and dysarthria are new symptoms. Neither symptom is referable to the suspected vestibular-cerebellar lesion but can be localized to a small lesion of the corticobulbospinal tract, which innervates the cervical spinal cord and brainstem (UMN to the right $\alpha$-motor neurons and the hypoglossal nucleus). The third episode is papillitis of the right eye, which is referable to the right optic nerve.

12.2. Papillitis is an inflammation of the optic nerve (optic neuritis) with swelling of the papilla. It is caused by an immunological attack on the myelin of the optic nerve axons. Because the optic tract, optic nerve, and retina are embryological outgrowths of the primitive diencephalon, they are CNS structures, and their axons are myelinated by oligodendrocytes, not Schwann cells.

12.3. For practical purposes brain images based on the MRI properties of nuclei are formed by the signals received from hydrogen protons. Most hydrogen in the brain is found in water molecules, so MRI reveals the distribution of water in the brain. Myelin is formed from lipids, which are highly hydrophobic. The inflammation process disturbs the structure of myelin, allowing water to penetrate, making edematous myelin appear quite different from normal myelin on MRI. CT is based on the electron density of molecules. There is not enough difference in electron density between edematous and normal myelin to be detected by CT.

12.4. There is no definitive test on which to base the diagnosis of MS; it is a clinical diagnosis. The diagnosis is based on documentation of CNS lesions disseminated in space and time. Because MS cannot be definitively diagnosed without the demonstration of multiple lesions, many physicians consider it inappropriate to burden a patient with the anxiety even a tentative diagnosis of MS creates. Two recent advances are altering that attitude. First, MRI often reveals multiple white matter lesions that are consistent with MS in patients who have had only a single clinical manifestation of a CNS lesion. Second, interferon-$\beta_1$ reduces the frequency of relapses and the progression of disability in many people with MS. Therefore, with effective therapy available for the first time and a useful but not definitive ancillary study (MRI), many physicians no longer consider it appropriate to withhold the diagnosis of MS until it is clinically obvious.

14.1. The patient's diabetes insipidus was probably initially caused by an interruption of the axons from the supraoptic and/or paraventricular nuclei to the neurohypophysis. The unstable body temperature can be related to invasion of the anterior hypothalamus by the tumor. Anterior hypothalamic lesions can be expected to increase body temperature. The decreased endocrine functions can all be correlated with the destruction of the median eminence. The hyperphagia and rage in this case correlate well with animal studies in which destruction of the medial region of the ventral hypothalamus produces similar effects. Lateral lesions in animals produce aphagia.

14.2. The disruption of the patient's emotional continence may be related to connections of the septal nuclei with the basal nucleus and substantia innominata. These latter structures project to the frontal lobes and also have connections with the caudate and putamen, which may affect nonmotor cortical functions.

14.3. Pneumoencephalograms have been entirely replaced by CT and MRI. Had these newer techniques been available in 1962, their use would probably have precluded the craniotomies performed in this case.

14.4. Amplitude of the action potential in the bouton modulates the influx of calcium ions, which in turn modulates the amount of neurotransmitter released. The amplitude of the action potential is a function of the external sodium ion concentration. Therefore, a decrease in extracellular sodium concentration may decrease transmitter release, globally diminishing the effectiveness of neurotransmission.

14.5. In addition to the hypothalamic structures that regulate autonomic functions, the subfornical organ (sensor of plasma antidiuretic hormone [ADH]) and the organum vasculosum (sensor of plasma osmolarity) play an important role as well. Also, arteriole oxygen tension affects vasopressin release.

14.6. The bitemporal hemianopia is caused by disruption of the crossing fibers in the optic chiasm at the anterior portion of the hypothalamus. The anterior region of the hypothalamus helps to regulate body temperature (see next question).

14.7. Involvement of the anterior hypothalamus can disrupt the temperature regulation control system. If thermal signals cannot be processed, the thermoregulatory system may interpret the body temperature to be below

the set point and initiate compensatory physiological and behavioral mechanisms to raise body temperature, such as shivering and seeking blankets. From a clinical standpoint, elevated body temperature usually indicates infection, so that possibility must be investigated.

14.8. Discuss this question in a small group.

## CHAPTER 15

15.1. The key observations are ascending paraplegia, decreased muscle tone, and downgoing toes (no Babinski). Although decreased tone and the absence of the Babinski sign are LMN signs, they are consistent with acute spinal trauma due to spinal shock. The rapid time course, pattern of paralysis (paraplegia), and ascending progression of weakness all point to strangulation of the spinal cord. Cerebral trauma (in the absence of spinal shock) produces spastic hemiplegia, increased muscle tone, and up-going toes.

15.2. An epidural hematoma is caused by arterial bleeding, so the neurological signs develop rapidly (within minutes to hours). If the hematoma is caused by a blow to the head, there may be a history of initial unconsciousness due to the blow, followed by a period of lucidity. The lucid period is succeeded by confusion, stupor, and coma *in that order.* The delayed changes in consciousness are due to the rapidly expanding mass of the hematoma causing an equally rapid increase in intracranial pressure and displacement of the intracranial structures. Hemotympanum (blood in the middle ear) following head trauma strongly suggests a basal skull fracture and possibly laceration of the middle meningeal artery. A subarachnoid hematoma can bring about the same progression of neurological signs, but slowly (days to months), in which case hemotympanum is unlikely.

15.3. With intracranial bleeding, any resulting paralysis is directed to the contralateral side, with increased muscle tone, hyperactive MSRs, and up-going toes (Babinski's sign). Severe headache and alteration of consciousness are also commonly associated with intracranial bleeding.

**15.4.** As with paralysis, intracranial lesions produce contralateral hemihypoesthesia. In the present case sensory losses were bilateral and affected the lower extremities before the upper extremities (i.e., ascending).

**15.5.** Intracranial lesions do not always produce findings related to the cranial nerves because the brainstem is well protected. Most often the cerebral cortex is traumatized, sparing the brainstem. However, expanding masses, such as hematoma, if large enough, can press on the upper brainstem. Such pressure is most commonly manifested in signs associated with the third nerve (dilated pupil, third nerve palsy). For that reason, anisocoria (one pupil larger than the other) is an important sign that should never be ignored.

**15.6.** The doll's eye sign indicates that the nuclei of ocular motion and their connections with the vestibular system (via the medial longitudinal fasciculus) are intact.

**15.7.** This was a close call. However, given the patient's history of diabetes mellitus and rapidly deteriorating mental status, a hemorrhagic stroke is more likely. An ischemic stroke was not out of the question, and given the CT findings, the emergency department physician prepared a syringe of anticoagulant to be given to the patient. Only after further reflection and consultation with a colleague did he order additional CT. Had the history of cocaine use been known at the time, the decision to investigate the possibility of hemorrhage further would have been much easier to justify, because snorting cocaine greatly increases blood pressure.

**15.8.** The supranuclear ophthalmoplegia is the most critical observation. This sign is almost always associated with tectal or quadrigeminal lesions. This diagnosis is reinforced by the sudden alteration of consciousness. Stupor was one of the first neurological signs to appear. Had the lesion been supratentorial, one would have expected to observe an extended period of confusion before the stupor. Therefore, the pontine reticular formation or its ascending tracts must also be involved in the lesion.

**15.9.** The principal risk factors for stroke are hypertension, hyperlipidemia, diabetes mellitus, heart disease, and cigarette smoking. In this case, diabetes mellitus and hypertension are present, the latter being exacerbated by the use of cocaine.

# Glossary

*Virginia Hellenga and Robert E. Kingsley*

The selection of terms in this glossary is necessarily arbitrary. We have skewed the selection toward medical terms that may be unfamiliar or that have a specific medical connotation different from the general use of the term. We have not included anatomical terms except for common synonyms for the usual term. Almost all of the items in this glossary appear in boldface type in the text. We recommend the resources listed at the end for those whose interest in medical terminology extends beyond the scope of this glossary.

**aboulia** [G. *a-*, without, and *boule*, will] Lack of will power. A condition associated with frontal lobe lesions in which the affected person is apathetic and slow in speech and other motor actions. The profoundly affected may lie motionless for weeks.

**absence seizure** Loss of conscious awareness without loss of muscle tone. Absence seizures have a frequency of several to several hundred a day. There are no obvious motor signs. Formerly known as *petit mal* seizures.

**accommodation** In ophthalmology, the ability of the lens to change its shape to bring a near object into focus.

**achromatopsia** [G. *a-*, without; *chroma*, color; and *opsis*, vision] The inability to tell one color from another. Also called achromatopsy.

**ACTH** See adrenocorticotropin.

**action potential** The rapid reversal of a neuron's membrane potential and its recovery. The action potential is a signal that conveys information within the nervous system.

**action tremor** Unsteadiness in target-directed movements, also called intention tremor. The amplitude of the tremor increases as the movement progresses. See resting tremor, postural tremor.

**adequate stimulus** The notion that a stimulus of a unique energy form is required to activate a specific receptor designed especially to receive that form of energy. In fact, receptors can be activated by any of a number of energy forms, but their lowest threshold is usually reserved for only one type of energy.

**ADH** See antidiuretic hormone.

**adrenocorticotropin (ACTH)** The pituitary hormone that affects the adrenal cortex by stimulating steroid synthesis.

**Aesculapius** The Roman version of Asclepius, the Greek god of medicine. The staff of Aesculapius, a stick with a single snake coiled around it, is the symbol of the medical profession. See caduceus.

**afferent** [L. *afferens*, bringing to] Approaching the central nervous system. Afferent fibers are axons that carry afferent signals to the central nervous system from elsewhere in the body. See efferent.

**agnosia** [G. *a-*, without, and *gnosis*, knowledge, knowing] Inability to recognize or attach meaning to various sensory stimuli.

**alar plate** Region of the embryonic nervous system dorsal to the sulcus limitans from which sensory neurons intrinsic to the central nervous system develop. See basal plate.

**AM** See amplitude modulated.

**aminoglycoside antibiotics** A class of antibiotics that interfere with protein synthesis in prokaryotic cells.

**amplitude modulated (AM)** A type of information coding. Amplitude-modulated signals convey information by coding the intensity of the carrier signal in proportion to the information signal. See frequency modulated, analogue, digital.

**analogue** [G. *analogos*, according to ratio, proportionate] Of signals, varying in proportion to the energy content of the stimulus. See digital, amplitude modulated, frequency modulated.

**anastomosis** [G. *anastomo*, furnish with a mouth or outlet] Connection between two vessels or channels forming a connecting cross-branch uniting two tubular structures.

**aneurysm** [G. *aneurysma*, wide] Weakness in the arterial wall that widens the artery. In a dissecting aneurysm the layers of the artery separate. A berry aneurysm is a small balloonlike dilation in the artery that communicates with the main branch by means of a narrow passage, making the aneurysm look like a berry on angiography.

**anisocoria** [G. *an*, not; *iso*, equal; and *kore*, pupil] Inequality in the size of the two pupils.

**anterograde** [L. *antero*, in front, and *gradior*, go] Forward; to the front. See orthograde, retrograde.

**antidiuretic hormone** A circulating hormone that increases the permeability of the collecting duct cell membranes in the kidney. This increase in permeability allows water and electrolytes to be reabsorbed into the circulation.

**aphasia** Inability to communicate by reading, writing, speaking, listening, or signing because of loss of cerebral function independent of motor or sensory losses.

**aponeurosis** [G. *aponeurosis*, end of a tendon, fr. *apo*, from, and *neuron*, sinew] A flat white fibrous membrane functioning as the sheath of a muscle, sometimes forming the connection between muscle and tendon.

**arteriovenous malformation (AVM)** An inappropriate anastomosis between an artery and vein without an intervening capillary bed.

**aspartate** A climbing fiber neurotransmitter that opens calcium ion channels in the soma of Purkinje cells, producing excitatory postsynaptic potentials.

**atavism** [L. *atavus*, remote ancestor] Literally, disease that can be attributed to a remote ancestor. In neurology it refers to reflexes that are present in infancy but not thereafter unless function of the cerebral cortex deteriorates.

**ataxia** [G. *a*, without, and *taxis*, order] In neurology, lack of coordination because of diminution or loss of cerebellar function. Most commonly seen in inebriated persons.

**atherothrombotic infarction** Infarct caused by arterial thrombosis. See infarct, thrombosis.

**athetosis** [G. *athetos*, without position or place] A type of involuntary movement characterized by continuous, slow, writhing motor activity in one or more parts of the body.

**atrophy** [G. *a*, without, and *trophe*, nourishment] In neurology, wasting away of muscle mass. Atrophy of disuse follows immobilization and is relatively minor. Denervation atrophy is profound and is an important clinical sign of lower motor neuron disease (see).

**AVM** See arteriovenous malformation.

**BAER** See brainstem auditory evoked response.

**basal plate** Portion of the embryonic nervous system, ventral to the sulcus limitans from which efferent neurons develop. See alar plate.

**Beevor's sign** Rostral movement of the umbilicus during contraction of the rectus abdominis muscles when there is paresis or paralysis of the caudal portions of this muscle. In normal persons there is no movement of the umbilicus.

**bilaminar disc** The embryoblast during the early phase of gastrulation, when it consists of two layers, the epiblast and the hypoblast.

**brachium conjunctivum** Synonym for the superior cerebellar peduncle.

**brachium pontis** Synonym for the middle cerebellar peduncle.

**brainstem auditory evoked response (BAER)** A sensory evoked potential elicited by auditory stimuli. The response provides information about the integrity of the auditory brainstem nuclei.

**brainstem coma** Coma induced by a lesion in the brainstem that deprives the cerebral cortex of essential activation by subcortical structures.

**Brown-Séquard syndrome** The characteristic set of signs and symptoms produced by hemisection of the spinal cord.

**caduceus** [L. *caduceus,* staff of Mercury] Staff with two snakes coiled around it and with two wings at the top. It is the symbol of the U.S. Army Medical Corps. See Aesculapius.

**canal of Schlemm** A large cavity with a meshwork of collagen fibers encircling the anterior chamber of the eye through which the aqueous humor is returned to the vascular system.

**carpal tunnel syndrome** Paresthesias in the hand, particularly within the distribution of the median nerve, caused by compression of that nerve by the flexor retinaculum.

**CBS tract** See corticobulbospinal tract.

**central hearing loss** Hearing loss from damage to retrocochlear structures. See conductive hearing loss, sensorineural hearing loss.

**central nervous system (CNS)** The part of the nervous system whose axons are myelinated by the oligodendrocyte. See peripheral nervous system.

**cerebral death** Usually, death of the cerebral cortex while lower areas of the central nervous system, particularly brainstem structures, remain viable.

**cerebral embolism** The passage of a blood clot from a remote structure, such as the heart, into the vasculature of the brain, causing infarction (see).

**cerebral hemorrhage** Arterial bleeding into cerebral tissue or the subarachnoid space. Not to be confused with a contusion or bleeding into the epidural space.

**chorea** [G. *choros,* dance] Involuntary movement that appears to be a fragment of purposeful movement.

**chromaffin cell** [G. *chroma,* color, and L. *affinis,* affinity, closeness] Cell in adrenal medulla and paraganglia of the sympathetic nervous system that stains with chromic salts, giving a brownish-yellow reaction.

**chromatolysis** [G. *chroma,* color, and *lysis,* dissolution] Dispersion of the Nissl substance (rough endoplasmic reticulum) after the separation of the axon from the soma.

**circumventricular organs (CVO)** Small areas within the brain containing modified capillaries that allow blood-borne signals (hormones) to reach and affect neurons. They lie near the midline and at the ventricular surface, giving them their generic name.

**Clarke's column** Synonym for nucleus dorsalis of the spinal cord.

**clasp knife reflex** Reflex evoked by stimulating the Golgi tendon organs, which in turn inhibit the homonymous motor neuron pools.

**clonus** [G. *klonos,* a tumult] The rapid (5 to 10 Hz) beating of an extremity such as a hand or foot when one of the muscles controlling it is placed under rapid and sustained tension. Clonus occurs only after injury to the corticobulbospinal tract innervating the motor neuron pool controlling the muscle. See spasticity.

**CNS** See central nervous system.

**cogwheel rigidity** Rigidity to passive movement that is released in small steps, giving the impression of a cogged wheel being turned. It primarily affects patients with certain basal ganglion diseases, particularly parkinsonism. See lead pipe rigidity, spasticity.

**coma** State of unconsciousness from which the patient cannot be aroused by sensory stimuli although cerebral cortical activity remains.

**concussion** [L. *concussio,* to shake violently] State of brief cerebral cortical dysfunction resulting from a violent blow to the head.

**conductive hearing loss** Hearing loss caused by the inability of sound pressure waves to reach the cochlea. See central hearing loss, sensorineural hearing loss.

**confusion** In medicine, the state of decreased cerebral cortical function in which the patient is conscious and aware but not entirely oriented to time and place.

**contusion** [L. *contusio,* a bruising] A bruise of the brain tissue resulting from a severe blow to the head but that does not cause cerebral hemorrhage.

**corona radiata** Portion of the cerebral white matter that lies superior to the internal capsule and radiates like a crown into the cerebral cortex.

**corticobulbospinal tract (CBS)** Motor tract that originates in the cerebral cortex and terminates on the brainstem and the spinal interneurons and motoneurons that produce voluntary movement.

**CVO** See circumventricular organs.

**decomposition of movement** [L. *de,* down from, less than, and *compono,* put together] Poor timing of motor acts that accompanies cerebellar lesions.

**decussation** [L. *decusso,* make an X] Any paired bundle of axons that crosses the midline.

**déjà vu** Literally, already seen. In neurology an epileptic aura characterized by a sensation that one's surroundings are unusually familiar or have been seen previously, even if one knows objectively that the familiarity is false.

**dementia** The loss of cognitive capabilities without objective loss of sensory or motor functions.

**digital** Pertaining to signals that code the stimulus in the time domain, their energy content remains constant. See analogue, frequency modulation.

**doll's-eye sign** Tendency of the eyes to maintain their orientation while the head is moved. While the unconscious patient is lying supine, the head is rotated. Normally the eyes rotate in the opposite direction, giving the impression that gaze is fixed straight ahead, much like the weighted glass eyes in a doll.

**dorsal spinocerebellar tract (DSCT)** A principal fiber tract carrying sensory information from the proprioceptors in the lower half of the body to the spinocerebellum. See proprioception.

**DSCT** See dorsal spinocerebellar tract.

**dysarthria** The inability to speak because of lack of coordination, spasticity, or weakness of the muscles of speech.

**dysdiadochocinesia** [G. *dys,* difficult; *diadochos,* working in turn; and *kinesis,* movement] (also spelled dysdiadokokinesia) The inability to perform smooth, rapidly alternating movements requiring the coordination of antagonistic muscle groups.

**dyskinesia** [G. *dys,* bad, and G. *kinesis,* movement] General term describing any difficulty in performing voluntary motor activity.

**dysmetria** [G. *dys,* bad, defective, and *metron,* measure] Inability to fix the range of movement in muscular activity, a form of incoordination and timing derangement related to cerebellar dysfunction. Performance deteriorates as the motor act progresses. Dysmetria resembles a tremor that is expressed only during a voluntary act. See intention tremor.

**dystonia** [G. *dys,* bad, and *tonos,* tension] Condition in which a set of antagonistic muscles is involuntarily kept in prolonged isometric contraction.

**Eaton-Lambert syndrome** Autoimmune disease affecting the voltage-gaited calcium ion channels, characterized by motor weakness and an incrementing electromyographic response to repetitive stimulation.

**efferent** [L. *efferens,* bringing out] Leaving, or *evading,* the central nervous system. Efferent fibers are axons that convey efferent signals away from the central nervous system. See afferent.

**embolus** [G. *embolos,* a wedge or stopper] A blood clot or other foreign object that is detached from its site of formation and has occluded a distant vessel.

**emmetropia** [G. *emmetros,* according to measure, and *opia,* vision] Refraction of a normal spherical eye, in which distant objects are brought into focus when the ciliary muscles are relaxed.

**endogenous opioids** Neuroactive peptides produced by the body that bind to the receptors in the brain that bind morphine.

**envelope of sound stimulus** Timing, intensity, and spectral variation of animal vocalizations. Dynamic variations of the sound envelope are essential to one's overall perception and discrimination of sound.

**epilepsy** Chronic disorder of the central nervous system characterized by seizures that repeat periodically.

**EPSP** See excitatory postsynaptic potential.

**excitatory postsynaptic potential (EPSP)** A hypopolarizing postsynaptic potential. See postsynaptic potential.

**fasciculation** [L. *fascis,* bundle] Involuntary twitching of a motor unit, frequently but not always the result of muscle denervation.

**feedback control system** A control system in which the error signal is computed from the deviation of the controlled variable from the desired steady-state value. The control signal modifies the action of the control system after an action takes place.

**feed-forward control system** A control system in which the error signal is computed without direct reference to the controlled variable but from other variables. The control signal modifies the action of the control system before an action takes place.

**flexion reflex afferent (FRA)** Receptor that elicits a polysynaptic reflex facilitating flexor motor neuron pools.

**flocculus** [L. *flocculus,* dim. of *floccus,* tuft (of wool or hair)] Lobe on the undersurface of the cerebrum behind the middle peduncle.

**FM** See frequency modulated.

**folia** [L. *folium,* pl. *folia,* leaf; thin, broad leaflike structure] Folds on the surface of the cerebral cortex or cerebellar cortex that increase the surface area. Deep folds separate the cerebrum and cerebellum into lobes.

**Fourier analysis** Mathematical analysis of an arbitrarily complex waveform from which a series of pure sinusoidal waveforms are extracted, the sum of which reconstruct the original.

**FRA** See flexion reflex afferent.

**frequency modulated (FM)** A type of information coding. Frequency-modulated signals convey information varying the timing of elements of the carrier signal in proportion to the information signal. See amplitude modulated, analogue, digital.

**general seizure** Seizure affecting the entire brain from the onset. See partial seizure.

**Gilles de la Tourette's syndrome** A neurological disorder characterized by involuntary tics and repetitive compulsive behavior, often including involuntary cursing (coprolalia). Thought to be carried by an autosomal dominant gene with variable penetrance, it is associated with abnormally low levels of dynorphin and defective dopamine uptake mechanisms.

**glabrous skin** [L. *glaber,* smooth] Smooth, hairless skin.

**glaucoma** Disease of the eye in which intraocular pressure is elevated because the rate of production of intraocular fluid exceeds the rate of removal.

**glomerulus** [L. *glomerulus,* little ball or cluster] In neuroscience, a complex cerebellar synaptic structure within a glial capsule.

**glutamate** [L. *gluten,* glue or paste] Granule cell neurotransmitter.

**Golgi cell** Multipolar nerve cell in the cerebral cortex and posterior horns of the spinal cord.

**grand mal seizure** See tonic-clonic seizure.

**Guillain-Barré syndrome** Autoimmune disease directed against peripheral myelin. Also known as Landry-Guillain-Barré syndrome, acute inflammatory polyneuropathy, acute autoimmune neuropathy, postinfectious polyneuritis. See multiple sclerosis.

**habenula perforata** [L. *habenula,* a small strip of hide, strap or thong, and *perforatus,* pp. of *perforare,* pierce] Small perforations in the temporal bone through which distal axons of auditory neurons enter the scala media.

**hemiparesis** Weakness of half of the body divided along the midsagittal plane. See paresis.

**hemiplegia** Paralysis of half of the body divided along the midsagittal plane. See plegia.

**Hertz (Hz)** The unit of frequency of sound, that is, the number of compression and rarefaction events per second, measured in cycles per second.

**homonymous hemianopia** [G. *homos,* same, and *nomos,* law; *hemi,* half; *an,* not; and *opia,* vision] The loss of vision in half of the visual field divided by the vertical meridian. The same hemifield is affected in both eyes.

**Horner's syndrome** The unilateral constellation of three symptoms—miosis, ptosis, and anhidrosis—resulting from sympathectomy. Enophthalmos is also present but is subtle and often overlooked.

**hypercapnia** Increased arterial carbon dioxide tension.

**hyperopia** [G. *hyper,* over, beyond, and *ops,* eye] Farsightedness, in which only objects far from the eye can be brought to focus. The image falls behind the retina because the eyeball is flattened.

**hypesthesia** or **hypoesthesia** [G. *hypo,* under, less than normal, and *esthesia,* feeling, sensation] Diminishment or partial loss of sensitivity to stimulation.

**hypotonia** Decrease in resting muscle tone.

**hypoxia** Decrease in arterial oxygen saturation.

**hysteresis** [G., *hysteresis,* coming later] Delay in effect of the application of a force.

**ictal** [L. *ictus,* a blow or a stroke] Relating to a seizure.

**idiopathic** [G. *idios,* individual, and *pathos,* suffering] Without known cause.

**infarct** [L. *infarcio,* stuff into] Death of tissue due to loss of vascular perfusion.

**infarction** Formation of an infarct. See atherothrombotic infarction.

**inhibitory postsynaptic potential (IPSP)** Alteration in the membrane permeability that buffers the membrane potential of neurons against hypopolarization. Generally but not always a hyperpolarizing postsynaptic potential.

**intention tremor** See action tremor.

**intraocular pressure** Pressure of fluid within the eye, determined by the regulation of the ratio of production to reabsorption of aqueous humor.

**IPSP** See inhibitory postsynaptic potential.

**isometric** In physiology, the contraction of a muscle held at constant length.

**isotonic** In physiology, the contraction of a muscle under constant tension.

**jamais vu** Literally, never seen before. In neurology, an epileptic aura characterized by a sensation that one's surroundings are unfamiliar or have never been seen previously, even if one objectively understands that the sensation is false.

**keratoconus** [G. *keras,* horn, and *konos,* cone] Deformation of the normally spherical cornea into a cone shape because of thinning of the cornea at the margin.

**Korsakoff's amnesic state** Anterograde amnesia characterized by inability to consolidate short-term memory into long-term memory. Correlated with specific damage to the CA regions of the hippocampus.

**lateral corticospinal tract** A subset of the corticobulbospinal tract in the lateral white columns of the spinal cord.

**lateral geniculate nucleus (LGN)** Nucleus of the thalamus, a laminated structure having six layers of cells, that receives bilateral visceral input.

**lead pipe rigidity** Rigidity to passive movement that gives slowly to constant pressure, giving the impression of bending a lead pipe. Patients with certain basal ganglion diseases, particularly parkinsonism, display lead pipe rigidity. See cogwheel rigidity, spasticity.

**leukodystrophy** Generic term describing any degeneration of the white matter of the brain.

**LGN** See lateral geniculate nucleus.

**Lhermitte's sign** A sensation of electric shocks descending the spine upon flexion of the neck. A sign of meningeal irritation.

**ligand-gated ion channel** Membrane protein that adjusts its permeability to one or more ions when a specific ligand is bound to a specific receptor on the protein.

**line of Gennari** An unusually prominent band of white matter in layer IV of the primary visual cortex (Brodmann area 17) that is visible to the naked eye and gives this area its name, the striate cortex.

**Lissauer's tract** Synonym for dorsolateral tract.

**LMN** See lower motor neuron.

**lower motor neuron (LMN)** Not a single structure but all of the structures in which lesions decrease the muscle stretch reflex. See upper motor neuron.

**Marcus Gunn pupil** In neurology, a pupil that paradoxically dilates when light is shone into the eye.

**meatus** [L. *meo,* flow, run] A small tubular passage or channel.

**Ménière's disease** A neurological disorder characterized by extreme vertigo because of inappropriate unilateral stimulation of the labyrinth.

**metabolic coma** Coma of chemical as opposed to structural origin; common causes are hypoxia, hypnotic drugs, and hypoglycemia.

**miosis** [G. *meiosis,* lessening] Constriction or contraction of the pupil.

**monoplegia** [G. *monos,* single, and *plege,* stroke] Paralysis of a single extremity.

**monosynaptic reflex** Synonym for muscle stretch reflex.

**mossy fibers** The most numerous type of axon entering the cerebellum. Mossy fibers excite granule cells that in turn excite Purkinje cells via parallel fibers. A single mossy fiber innervates approximately 600 granule cells.

**motor learning** See motor plasticity.

**motor plasticity** The ability of the nervous system to use experience to modify the way motor acts are coordinated. Conscious regulation of motor acts becomes directed more to strategy and less to tactics. This capacity is particularly well developed in the cerebellum.

**MSR** See muscle stretch reflex.

**multiple sclerosis (MS)** An autoimmune disease directed against central myelin. See Guillain-Barré syndrome.

**muscle stretch reflex (MSR)** A reflex initiated by the rapid stretch of a muscle that stimulates the primary receptors of the muscle spindle apparatus and facilitates the motor neuron pools serving the homonymous muscle.

**myasthenia gravis** [G. *mys*, muscle, and *astheneia*, weakness; L. *gravis*, heavy] Autoimmune disease directed against the acetylcholine receptors in the motor end plate of striated muscle. Weakness increases with activity in this disorder of neuromuscular transmission.

**myelogram** A radiographic procedure in which the cerebrospinal fluid in the lumbar cistern is replaced with a radiopaque fluid. Subsequent spinal radiographs reveal the outline of the dural sac.

**myopia** [G. *myo*, to half close, and *ops*, eye] Nearsightedness. A condition in which only objects close to the eye can be brought to focus because of nonuniform growth of the eye. The eyeball is elongated, and the focal plane is in front of the retina.

**narcolepsy** [G. *narkoo*, benumb, deaden, and *lepsis*, seizure] A form of hypersomnia characterized by uncontrollable napping during the day, cataplexy, hallucinations while falling asleep, and sleep paralysis.

**neurofibrillary bodies** Collections of tubules found within neurons of patients with Alzheimer's disease. These tubules are slightly different from the microtubules normally found in neurons and other cells.

**neurohypophysis** [G. *neuron*, nerve; *hypo*, under; and *physis*, growth] An extension of the central nervous system composed of the infundibulum and the posterior division of the pituitary gland.

**Nissl substance** Historical name for the rough endoplasmic reticulum of neurons.

**nociceptor** [L. *noceo*, injure, and *capio*, take, seize] Receptor that is most sensitive to noxious stimuli, including tissue-killing stimuli such as heat and the byproducts of tissue destruction. Such receptors should not be called pain receptors because pain is a perception, not a stimulus.

**nodulus** [L. *nodulus*, dim. of *nodus*, knot] Small knotlike protuberance on the anterior portion of the vermis cerebelli.

**nystagmus** [G. *nystagmos*, nod] Rhythmic oscillation of the eyes, the oscillation being fast in one direction and slow in the other. The nystagmus is named right or left according to the direction of the fast phase.

**OKN** See optokinetic nystagmus.

**operculum** [L. *operculum*, cover or lid] The part of the cerebral cortex that covers the insula, obscuring and forming a cover over it.

**optokinetic nystagmus (OKN)** Nystagmus produced by a series of images passing before the eyes.

**orthograde** [G. *orthos*, correct, straight, and L. *gradior*, walk] Moving in the normal direction. In neuroscience, moving along an axon beginning at the soma, as in orthograde conduction. See anterograde, retrograde.

**orthograde axonal degeneration** Disintegration of an axon once it has been separated from the soma. Because the distal portion is removed from its source of metabolic nourishment, the axon soon dies and then disintegrates. Also called Wallerian degeneration.

**otosclerosis** Disease characterized by pathological growth of bone at the margin of the oval window. Initially this growth only impedes the movement of the stapes, but eventually the stapes becomes fixed in place.

**ototoxic** Toxic to the hair cells of the vestibular apparatus or cochlea.

**oxytocin** [G. *oxys,* sharp, keen; *tokos,* birth; and *-in,* suffix denoting an activator] Circulating hormone that initiates milk letdown from the mammary glands and causes contraction of the uterine muscles during parturition.

**papilledema** [L. *papilla,* nipple, and G. *oidema,* swelling] Protrusion of the papilla (the point of entry of the optic nerve) into the eye, caused by an increase in intracranial pressure. Not to be confused with papillitis.

**papillitis** Inflammation of the head of the optic nerve where it enters the eye, usually caused by exacerbation of multiple sclerosis. Not to be confused with papilledema.

**paraparesis** Weakness of the two lower extremities.

**paraplegia** [G. *para,* beside, and *plege,* stroke] Paralysis of the two lower extremities.

**paresis** [G. *paritemi,* let go, slacken] Weakness or partial paralysis.

**Parkinson's disease** Progressive neurological disorder characterized by bradykinesia, a 4- to 7-Hz tremor of rest and lead pipe or cogwheel rigidity. Described by James Parkinson. See primary parkinsonism.

**paroxysm** [G. *paroxyno,* to sharpen, to irritate] Sharp or sudden onset and recurrence of the manifestations of disease.

**partial seizure** Seizure that is at least initially confined to a small part of the cerebral cortex. It may expand and become a general seizure (see).

**peduncle** [ML. *pedunculus,* a little foot, stalk, or stem] Protuberance caused by a fiber tract (collection of axons) connecting parts of the brain.

**Pelizaeus-Merzbacher disease** Neurological disease characterized by lack of development of central nervous system myelin with normal peripheral myelin because of a genetic error that prevents the correct assembly of proteolipid protein.

**peripheral nervous system** The part of the nervous system whose axons are myelinated by the Schwann cells. See central nervous system.

**peritrichal receptor** [G. *peri,* around, and *thrix,* hair] Sensory receptor at the base of a hair shaft that is sensitive to movement of the hair.

**perseveration** [L. *persevero,* to persist] In neurology, repeated and inappropriate naming of each object in a series by the name given to the first object, even though they are all different.

**petit mal seizure** See absence seizure.

**phase locking** Firing characteristic of auditory neurons. Timing between groups of action potentials at various frequencies as determined by the frequency of the stimulus.

**piebaldness** Patchy loss of pigment in the hair. An autosomal dominant trait. See vitiligo, Waardenburg's syndrome.

**plegia** [ Gr. *plege,* stroke] Profound weakness or paralysis.

**pluripotential** [L. *plus, pluris,* several, more, and *potentia,* power, ability] Flexible regarding potential development; capable of differentiating into various types of tissue elements. Applies to embryonic tissue.

**PNS** See peripheral nervous system.

**poikilothermal** [G. *poikilos,* varied, and *therme,* heat] Thermal variance in accordance with the environment.

**poliomyelitis** [G. *polios,* gray; *myelos,* marrow; and *itis,* inflammation] Literally, inflammation of the gray matter of the spinal cord. A viral disease that among other things, kills α-motor neurons, particularly those of the lumbosacral spinal cord.

**postictal** [L. *post,* after, and *ictus,* blow or stroke] Following a seizure.

**postsynaptic potential (PSP)** Alteration in membrane potential produced by electrochemical events originating at synapses terminating on that neuron.

**postural tremor** Tremor that occurs while an extremity is actively held in certain static positions. See resting tremor, action tremor.

**presynaptic inhibition** Electrochemical alteration in the bouton membrane that reduces the efficiency of transmitter release from that bouton, reducing its effect on the postsynaptic neuron.

**presbyacusis** [G. *presby,* old, and *akouo,* to hear] Decrease in sensitivity to high-frequency sound that occurs with advancing age.

**presbyopia** [G. *presbys,* old, and *ops,* eye] Decreased elasticity of the optic lens that results in inability to bring near objects into focus; a process of advancing age.

**primary parkinsonism** A generic term for diseases of the basal ganglia with the common features of resting tremor, bradykinesia, and rigidity; includes Parkinson's disease and a number of other significantly different illnesses, such as supraoptic ophthalmoplegia.

**primitive reflexes** See atavism.

**primordium** [L. *primus,* first, and *ordior,* begin] In an embryo, the gathering of cells in a group, indicating the first trace of an organ or structure.

**proprioception** [L. *proprius,* self, and *capio,* take] The perception of position, length, and tension and changes of position, length, and tension in muscles and joints without the use of sight; the ability to sense the position of the body.

**prosopagnosia** [G. *prozapine,* countenance, face, and *gnosis,* knowledge, knowing] Inability to recognize familiar faces.

**PSP** See postsynaptic potential.

**ptosis** [G., a falling] Drooping of the eyelid.

**Purkinje cells** Cells in the cortex of the brain having a large, goblet-shaped body and an immense, fan-shaped dendritic tree that extends toward the cerebellar surface into the molecular layer.

**pyramidal tract** *Obsolete.* Corticobulbospinal tract (see).

**pyramidal tract syndrome** *Obsolete.* Upper motor neuron syndrome (see).

**quadriplegia** [L. *quadri-,* four, and G. *plege,* stroke] Paralysis of all four extremities.

**radicula** [L. dim. of *radix,* root] Spinal root; hence *radicular pain,* pain following the distribution of the axons of a spinal root.

**Raynaud's syndrome** Paroxysms of pain and cyanosis in the distal portions of the extremities, brought on by emotion or cold. Commonly associated with sympathectomy of the extremities, as in peripheral neuropathy or peripheral nerve compression.

**restiform body** See inferior cerebellar peduncle.

**resting tremor** A tremor that occurs while the extremity is relaxed and subsides during voluntary motor activity. See action tremor, postural tremor.

**retrograde** [L. *retro,* behind, and L. *gradior,* go] Proceeding backward. See anterograde, orthograde.

**Rinne's test** Comparison of hearing by bone conduction and by air conduction. A vibrating tuning fork is first placed on the mastoid process to stimulate the cochlea by bone conduction, then held near the ear to stimulate the ear by air conduction. See Weber's test.

**satellite cells** Supporting cells that surround the neuron soma in ganglia. Now usually called Schwann cells.

**Schwann cells** The only type of supporting cells in the peripheral nervous system. Schwann cells wrap around the axons of peripheral nerve fibers and form the myelin sheath. They effectively isolate the neuron from the general extracellular environment.

**scotoma** [G. *skotos,* darkness] A blind area of the visual field that may be natural, as the blind spot, or due to disease.

**seizure** [O. Fr. *seisir,* grasp] Literally, a sudden attack. In neurology, the transient appearance of inappropriate, synchronous, repetitive activity of a large number of neurons in the cerebral cortex.

**sensorineural hearing loss** Hearing loss from damage to cochlear structures or the auditory nerve. See conductive hearing loss, central hearing loss.

**serous otitis media** The accumulation of fluid in the middle ear, often seen in children. It is neither infectious nor painful, but the accumulation of fluid does cause hearing impairment.

**sign** In medicine, an abnormality observed by the physician and independent of the report of the patient. See symptom.

**sign of Bing** Flexion of the foot in response to stabbing a pin into the dorsum of the foot. A sign of upper motor neuron disease. The normal response is to extend the foot away from the pin.

**sign of Babinski** Extension and flaring of the toes in response to scraping the lateral margin of the sole of the foot. A sign of upper motor neuron disease. The normal response is to flex the toes.

**sound pressure level (SPL)** Sound pressure of 0.0002 dynes/cm$^2$ used to establish a 0-decibel reference for audiological testing.

**spasticity** Increase in muscle tone resulting from increased sensitivity of the muscle stretch reflex; cardinal sign of an upper motor neuron lesion. See cogwheel rigidity, lead pipe rigidity.

**spina bifida** [L. *bifidus,* cleft] The generic term for any of a set of developmental disorders in which the structures dorsal to or derived from the neural tube do not close during development.

**spinal disk syndrome** The constellation of signs of unilateral (rarely bilateral) radicular pain and weakness of muscles innervated by the same spinal root, caused by compression of the spinal nerve by a prolapsed spinal disk.

**SPL** See sound pressure level.

**stereocilia** Tubelike evaginations of the membranes of hair cells of the receptors in the inner ear. Stereocilia are bathed in endolymph and filled with extensively crosslinked actin, which stiffens them. Stereocilia are connected to one another and move as a unit.

**strabismus** [G. *strabismos,* a squint] Lack of parallel tracking of the two eyes resulting in diplopia.

**stroke** Rapid loss of neural function that can be explained by infarction of a portion of the brain within the territory of a single artery and that does not resolve within 24 hours.

**stupor** A state of unconsciousness from which the patient can be aroused but not brought to full awareness.

**subiculum** [ L. *subex,* layer] An area of transitional cerebral cortex between the hippocampus proper and the entorhinal cortex.

**symptom** In medicine, an abnormality felt by the patient and reported to the physician. Symptoms are necessarily subjective. See sign.

**TENS** See transcutaneous electrical neural stimulation.

**thrombotic stroke** Occlusion of a cerebral artery by formation of a thrombus within that artery as opposed to an occlusion by an embolism.

**thrombus** [G. *thrombosis,* a curdling or clotting] A clot in a vessel that may or may not occlude the vessel but that remains in place. See embolus.

**TIA** See transient ischemic attack.

**tic** Involuntary rapid and repeated contraction of a small group of muscles that results in spasmodic movement.

**tic douloureux** [F. *tic,* spasmodic movement, and *douloureux,* painful] See trigeminal neuralgia.

**tinnitus** [L. *tinnio,* pp. *tinnitus,* jingle, clink, ring] The nonhallucinatory perception of sound where none exists, caused by damage to the cochlea.

**tonic-clonic seizure** A type of general seizure characterized by an initial tonic contraction of the skeletal muscles and loss of consciousness, followed by a prolonged rhythmic contraction and relaxation of the skeletal muscles that gradually subsides, followed by a period of stupor, confusion, and eventual recovery. Formerly called grand mal seizure.

**tonotopic mapping** Organization and mapping of core pathways in central connections of the auditory system according to the characteristic frequency of the neurons. These core pathways are the fastest and most direct in the auditory system.

**Tourette's syndrome** See Gilles de la Tourette's syndrome.

**transcutaneous electrical neural stimulation (TENS)** Stimulation of a nerve by passing electrical current noninvasively through the skin.

**transient ischemic attack (TIA)** Rapid loss of neural function attributable to dysfunction of a portion of the brain located within the territory of a single artery that resolves within 24 hours.

**trigeminal neuralgia** Paroxysms of severe pain in the territory of the trigeminal nerve, usually the ophthalmic or mandibular division. The pain is intense, often described as burning, tearing, cutting, or stabbing. It lasts for several seconds and occurs frequently. Synonym for tic douloureux.

**UMN** see upper motor neuron.

**uncinate fasciculus** [L. *uncinatus,* hooked, and *fasciculus,* dim. of *fascis,* bundle] Arch of fibers connecting the frontal and temporal lobes of the cerebellum.

**upper motor neuron** All of the structures in which lesions increase the muscle stretch reflex. See lower motor neuron.

**vasopressin** See antidiuretic hormone.

**ventral spinocerebellar tract (VSCT)** Principal fiber tract carrying proprioceptive information from the muscles and lower half of the body surface to the spinocerebellum.

**vestibulocerebellum** Lobe composed of the flocculus and the nodulus that receives most of its afferent fibers from the vestibular nuclei. These fibers terminate as mossy fibers.

**vestibulo-ocular reflex (VOR)** The reflex movement of the eyes in the opposite direction of the movement of the head. See doll's-eye sign.

**vermis cerebelli** [L. *vermis,* worm] A wormlike process continuous with the two hemispheres of the cerebellum at the midline.

**vitiligo** [L. *vitium,* blemish, vice] Depigmented patches on the skin due to the loss of epidermal melanocytes by an autoimmune attack. Hair in the affected area may or may not be affected. See piebaldness, Waardenburg's syndrome.

**VOR** See vestibulo-ocular reflex.

**VSCT** See ventral spinocerebellar tract.

**Waardenburg's syndrome** The association of several of the following characteristics: widely spaced eyes, wide root of the nose, sensorineural hearing loss, and pigment anomalies, such as heterochromic irides, white forelock, vitiligo, piebaldness, and retinitis pigmentosa.

**Wallerian degeneration** See orthograde axonal degeneration.

**Weber's test** A method of comparing the auditory sensitivity of the two ears. A necessary adjunct to Rinne's test (see).

## ADDITIONAL RESOURCES

Stedman's Medical Dictionary, 26th ed. Baltimore: Williams & Wilkins, 1995.

Taber's Cyclopedic Medical Dictionary, 18th ed. Philadelphia: Davis, 1997.

Dorland's Illustrated Medical Dictionary, 28th ed. Philadelphia: Saunders, 1994.

Lockhard I. Desk Reference for Neuroscience. New York: Springer-Verlag, 1992.

# Index